Circulation of the Blood

MEN AND IDEAS

Circulation of the Blood

MEN AND IDEAS

*Edited by Alfred P. Fishman
and Dickinson W. Richards*

NEW YORK
Oxford University Press
MCMLXIV

Copyright © 1964 by Oxford University Press, Inc.

Library of Congress Catalogue Card Number: 64-12605

PRINTED IN THE UNITED STATES OF AMERICA

TO THE MEMORY OF HOMER WILLIAM SMITH
(1895 - 1962)

Contributors

RICHARD J. BING, *Professor of Medicine,*
Wayne State University College of Medicine, Detroit, Michigan

STANLEY E. BRADLEY, *Bard Professor of Medicine,*
Columbia University College of Physicians and Surgeons, New York, New York

ANDRÉ COURNAND, *Director, Cardiopulmonary Laboratory,*
Columbia University Division, Bellevue Hospital, New York, New York

GEOFFREY S. DAWES, *Director of the Nuffield Institute for Medical Research,*
University of Oxford, Oxford, England

ALFRED P. FISHMAN, *Director of the Cardiorespiratory Laboratory,*
Columbia University College of Physicians and Surgeons, New York, New York

BJÖRN FOLKOW, *Professor of Physiology,*
University of Göteborg, Göteborg, Sweden

WILLIAM F. HAMILTON, *Professor of Physiology Emeritus,*
Medical College of Georgia, Augusta, Georgia

HERMAN K. HELLERSTEIN, *Assistant Professor of Medicine,*
Western Reserve University School of Medicine, Cleveland, Ohio

CORNEILLE J. F. HEYMANS, *Professor of Pharmacology Emeritus,*
University of Ghent, Ghent, Belgium

LOUIS N. KATZ, *Director, Cardiovascular Institute,*
Michael Reese Hospital and Medical Center, Chicago, Illinois

SEYMOUR S. KETY, *Chief, Laboratory of Clinical Science,*
National Institute of Mental Health, Bethesda, Maryland

EUGENE M. LANDIS, *George Higginson Professor of Physiology,*
Harvard Medical School, Boston, Massachusetts

WILFRIED F. H. M. MOMMAERTS, *Professor of Medicine and Physiology,*
The University of California, Los Angeles, California

SIR GEORGE PICKERING, *Regius Professor of Medicine,*
University of Oxford, Oxford, England

DICKINSON W. RICHARDS, *Lambert Professor of Medicine Emeritus,*
Columbia University College of Physicians and Surgeons, New York, New York

HOMER W. SMITH, *Late Professor of Physiology and Biophysics Emeritus,*
New York University School of Medicine, New York, New York

Foreword

'Science like life feeds on its own decay. New facts burn old rules; then newly developed concepts bind old and new together into a reconciling law.'

WILLIAM JAMES

THIS book presents twelve chapters in the history of cardiovascular physiology. The primary objective in its design has been to provide a study of the origins, discovery, and progress of certain of the great ideas of this branch of science, and to bring to life, insofar as possible, the great men who made these discoveries and achieved this progress.

The authors of the twelve chapters are all distinguished in cardiovascular physiology. Each brings to his essay a lifetime of study in his field of special interest as well as a personal achievement in its more recent advances.

The treatment of the subject matter, chapter by chapter, is quite varied, each author having been free to choose not only the manner of his presentation, but also the span of history which he would review. Some accounts close with work done thirty years ago; others continue on to the present day.

Dr. Cournand, writing on Air and Blood, starts almost at the dawn of classical philosophy, with pneuma, the breath or spirit. The origins of Dr. Bradley's chapter go back even further, since, in certain curious beginnings of our particular form of civilization in the West, the liver was of primary importance as an organ of divination. Dr. Kety goes back to the Egyptians for early records of the anatomy of the brain.

Other chapters begin much later: Dr. Landis and Dr. Smith with early observations with the microscope; Dr. Hamilton and Dr. Richards with Wm. Harvey's discovery of the circulation. Dr. Katz and Dr. Hellerstein give a brief survey of the early history of electricity, then start their definitive account of electrophysiology with the experiments of Galvani and Volta. Sir George Pickering begins with Stephen Hales and the famous mare tied down on a gate. Dr. Bing surveys the early knowledge of the anatomy of the heart as a prelude to consideration of the discovery of the coronary circulation by the great pathologists and clinicians of the seventeenth and eighteenth centuries. Drs. Mommaerts, Dawes, Heymans, and Folkow are concerned chiefly with the modern era.

The authors have made these chapters much more than a historical record. Each is a critical review in depth of the whole physiology of the subject, based on the developments of the past, considering the knowledge and theory of the present, and in some instances even looking toward the future. They are written for the physiologist as much as for the historian.

In a series of essays such as these, it is inevitable that some great historical figures will appear many times; the more important the man, the more frequently will he be mentioned. Since each author has stressed a different aspect of the man's work there has been little duplication.

With the amount of careful study, scholarship, and critique that has gone into the preparation of these chapters, one would expect a number of new historical disclosures and original interpretations, and such is indeed the case. These the reader can discover for himself.

In the composition of this book, both the authors and the editors have devoted a large amount of time and effort to the illustrations. The portraits we have used are authentic, with three exceptions: Hippocrates, Galen, and Richard Lower. The recently discovered "Hippocrates of Ostia," though a first century A.D. Roman copy, seems to be at least what antiquity believed to be a portrait of the Father of Medicine. There is only one ancient representation of Galen, in a sixth century A.D. manuscript, but there is no evidence of its authenticity. We have chosen instead a typical medieval picture of the Prince of Physicians. The only available engraving supposedly representing Richard Lower is probably that of someone else.

Where more than one portrait, bust, or photograph are available, we have chosen one taken during the man's active years; where possible, we have used a picture of him at work.

In selecting illustrations from published books or papers, we have gone back to the originals in all instances. We are especially grateful to the Meriden Press for their skilful, and indeed beautiful, reproductions of illustrations from ancient books.

We are profoundly indebted to the many who have helped us in this venture. First, to the authors of the chapters of the book, not only for their excellent contributions, but also for their patience with the slow progress of the editors in completing their editorial task. Also, and particularly, to the United States Public Health Service, the New York Heart Association, and the Commonwealth Fund, for financial aid in getting the project under way. Very specially to our colleagues in the Oxford University Press, for their unfailing consideration, generosity, and assistance. Finally, to the many libraries and librarians, and the host of correspondents and friends who have helped us with the location, loan, or reproduction of books, references, portraits, photographs, medals, and the like, that form so important a part of this volume. We have acknowledged these individually, to the best of our ability, in a special section at the end of the book.

Table of Contents

Part One THE HEART

I *Air and Blood* — 3
ANDRÉ COURNAND

II *The Output of the Heart* — 71
WILLIAM F. HAMILTON AND DICKINSON W. RICHARDS

III *Heart Muscle* — 127
WILFRIED F. H. M. MOMMAERTS

IV *Coronary Circulation and Cardiac Metabolism* — 199
RICHARD J. BING

V *Electrocardiography* — 265
LOUIS N. KATZ AND HERMAN K. HELLERSTEIN

Part Two BLOOD VESSELS

VI *The Capillary Circulation* — 355
EUGENE M. LANDIS

VII *Vasomotor Control and the Regulation of Blood Pressure* — 407
CORNEILLE J. F. HEYMANS AND BJÖRN FOLKOW

VIII *Systemic Arterial Hypertension* — 487
GEORGE PICKERING

CONTENTS

PART THREE   SPECIAL CIRCULATIONS

IX   *Renal Physiology*   545
HOMER W. SMITH

X   *The Splanchnic Circulation*   607
STANLEY E. BRADLEY

XI   *The Cerebral Circulation*   703
SEYMOUR S. KETY

XII *Physiological Changes in the Circulation after Birth*   743
GEOFFREY S. DAWES

Notes and Acknowledgments, 817

List of Illustrations and Sources, 821

Name Index, 835

Subject Index, 851

Part One

THE HEART

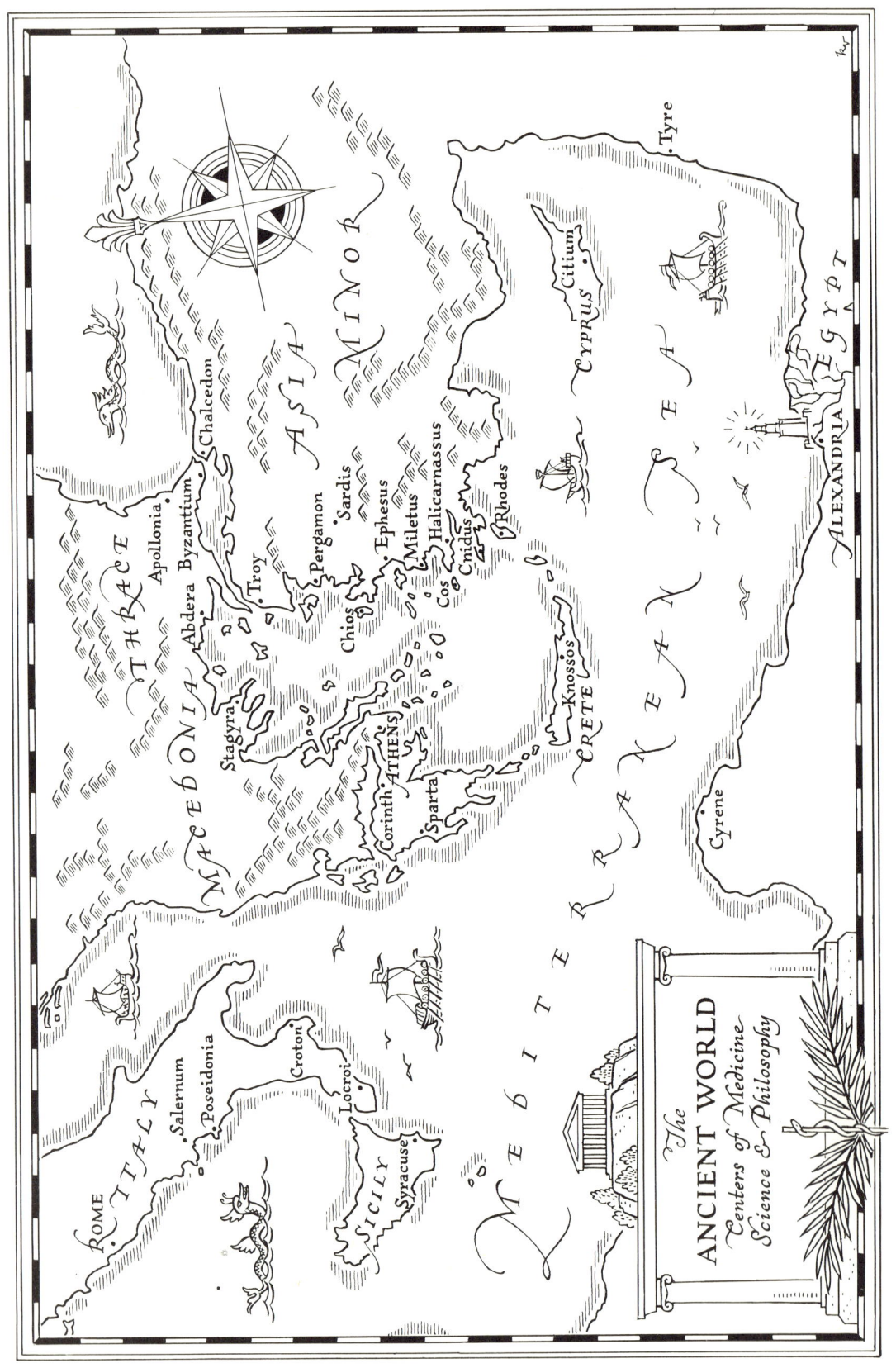

I

Air and Blood

THE idea that air and blood meet within the lungs and that from this conjunction blood gains a vital essence for distribution throughout the body is an old one. Indeed, it can be traced back to Ionia, the cradle of Greek science. Nonetheless, despite the antiquity of the idea, our present knowledge of this subject is still incomplete and in the process of development. Accordingly, it is reasonable to ask if it may not be a needless distraction for modern scientists to look back to the state of knowledge of ancient or even recent times.

The danger in such a negative attitude, which presupposes a dogmatic concept of science and implies the image of a final state of knowledge, has been crisply stated by J. B. Thornton (*119*): "The more we treat the theories of our predecessors as myths, the more inclined we shall be to treat our own theories as dogmas." It is my conviction that no limit should be set on the intellectual content of scientific research. In our quest for meanings we should look for a unifying tradition, for a continuity of ideas evolved by great men, for their grasp of and their addition to what their predecessors knew, and also for the large schemes that are sometimes elaborated. In such an endeavor, we must be familiar with and apply a method that is scientific in its spirit of inquiry based on checking, confronting, even doubting what appears certain to others, and historical in the sense that predominant periods and large syntheses must be identified, and that creative men must not be separated from their surroundings, or from the prevailing ideas and events of their time.

With this in mind, I have recognized several stages in the history of the conjunction of air and blood in the lungs, corresponding more or less to well-defined historical periods, and animated by men searching for an elusive truth.

THE HEART

Identification of Pneuma, Blood, and Blood Vessels

In the ancient Greek world, metaphysically elaborated philosophical systems defined the nature of reality, the subject matter of science. Therefore, direct observations of phenomena were on the whole of secondary importance.

As early as the sixth century B.C., Ionian philosophers living in the prosperous city and harbor of Miletos (Asia Minor) had raised the fundamental question of the nature of a First Principle. For Anaximenes (*115, 116*) it was Pneuma, or Air. Tangible and yet intangible, compressible and yet indefinitely expansible, it permeated everything, and in the body it submitted to the rhythmic phases of breathing, comparable to the great rhythm of the Cosmos. Soon thereafter, according to an early Hippocratic treatise—*On breath*—Diogenes of Apollonia (*116, 130*) conceived of pneuma as possessing properties essential to man and animals, in that they could not live without it. The semantic progression from air to breath, from breath to life, and from life to spirit was already in the minds of thinking men.

Empedocles of Agrigente (*115, 116*), the creator of the doctrine of the four elements: Air, Fire, Water, and Earth, "the roots of things," demonstrated the corporeality of pneuma by observing the appearance of bubbles on the surface of water into which a vessel with holes at opposite ends had been immersed. He also contributed the idea of rhythmic motion and interrelation of pneuma, source of health in the body, with blood, carrier of innate heat, issuing from the heart and returning to it, moving backward and forward by tides and pulsations.

The notion of blood transport by vessels originating in the heart was, however, not original with Empedocles. Alcmeon of Croton (*115, 116, 130*), the first Greek known to have practiced dissection, distinguished two types of vessels (phlebos) carrying blood, as early as the sixth century B.C. This member of the Pythagorean sect, primarily interested in the relationship between the brain and the sense organs, taught that, during sleep, blood retreated from one set of vessels. Having observed the vacuity of some vessels after death, he assumed that in similar fashion the same vessels became bloodless during sleep.

The separation of vessels into two types is found early in the Hippocratic Corpus (fifth century B.C.). At first the term "artery" was used to

AIR AND BLOOD

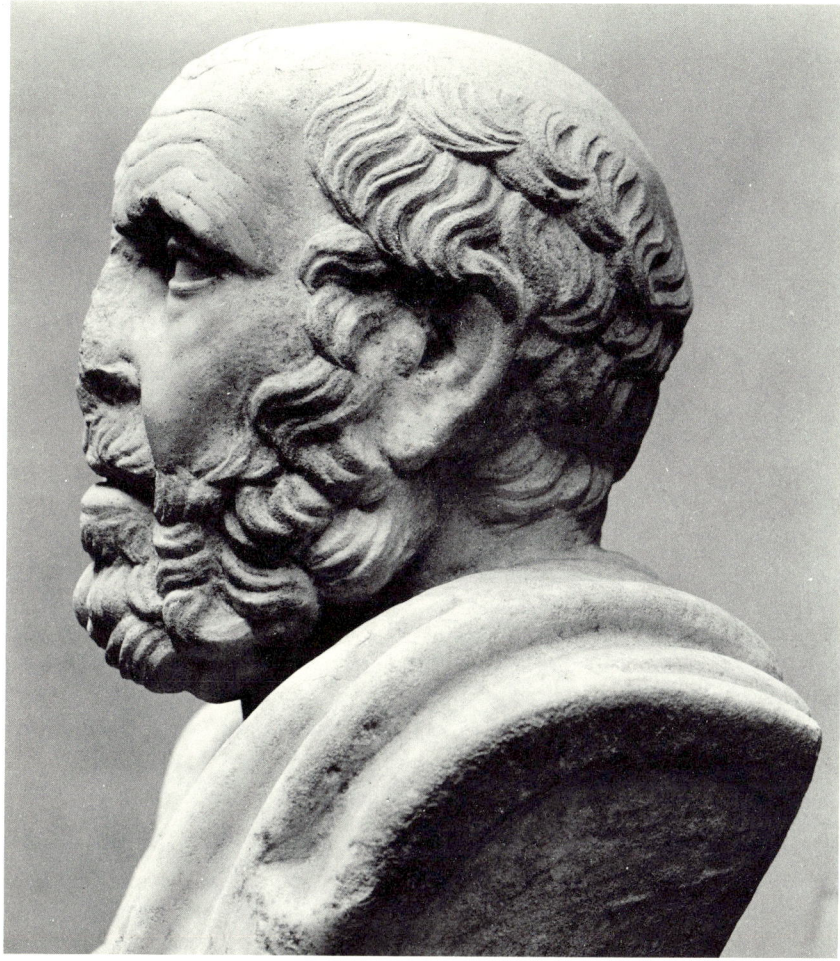

Figure 2. The "Hippocrates of Ostia." This remarkable head was discovered in 1940, in excavations near Ostia, the ancient seaport of Rome. It was found in the family tomb of a Greco-Roman physician of the first century, A.D. For the several items of evidence identifying the bust with Hippocrates, see section on notes and acknowledgments at the end of the book.

designate the trachea and bronchi, which transported pneuma to the heart. Since some of the vessels originating from the heart cavity were found more or less empty of blood after death, they too were soon called arteries; but they were also said to transport blood and to be connected with the veins. Indeed, in the treatise *On the localities of man*

[5]

(130), one finds the first mention of these connections, as well as a suggestion that blood circulates.

THE HEART

"The vessels communicate with one another and the blood flows from one to another. I do not know where the commencement is to be found, for in a circle you can find neither commencement nor end, but from the heart the arteries take their origin and through the vessel, the blood is distributed to all the body, to which it gives warmth and life; they are the sources of human nature and are like rivers that purl through the body and supply the human body with life; the heart and the vessels are perpetually moving, and we may compare the movement of the blood with courses of rivers returning to their sources after a passage through numerous channels."

An extraordinary Hippocratic document—On the heart—has been attributed to Philistion of Locroi, a disciple of Empedocles of the fourth century B.C. *(115, 116)*. It contains the first complete description of the heart and of its valves. The authorship of this document is considered by some historians of science, particularly Littré, to be apocryphal. Leboucq *(85)*, a French Hellenist, claims that the text genuinely belongs to the Hippocratic Corpus and believes that it represents student notes taken at a lecture given by Philistion. *On the heart* is divided into twelve paragraphs that contain several statements of amazing accuracy as to the anatomy and the physiology of the heart and of the large vessels. This may be judged by the following quotations:

"The heart is a powerful muscle . . . [with] two distinct ventricles quite dissimilar; the right lies in front . . . is spacious and less firm than the left; it does not reach the apex. The left ventricle is located beneath, exactly behind the left nipple where its beat can be felt; it has a thick wall. The lungs envelop the ventricle . . . [and] thus moderate the excess heat, since [they] are cold and refreshed by respiration.

". . . soft and hollow structures surround the ventricle . . . called auricles . . . thanks to them the heart regulates respiration; . . . [after the ventricles cease to contract] they may continue to be inflated and deflated isolatedly.

". . . after resection [of the apex of the ventricles and the upper part of the auricles] two apertures appear in each ventricle.

"It remains to speak about hidden membranes and of fibers stretched in the ventricles like spider webs completely surrounding the apertures. At the origin

of the two arteries [which originate from the ventricles] are placed very ingeniously on the right and on the left side three rounded membranes, with their free edge disposed in semicircle; when these come together, it is admirable to observe how they obstruct the lumen of the arteries. If someone . . . after extracting the heart from a human cadaver, first separates and then brings together the leaflets, neither the injection of water nor of air will force these in the heart; this is particularly true of the left side where the leaflets are built with great precision.

"With regard to the vessel originating from the right ventricle, it also presents the commissure of the leaflets, but they do not obliterate the orifice completely because they are too weak. This vessel opens up also toward the lung to supply it with blood which serves as its nourishment, whereas it is closed toward the heart, not hermetically sealed, but enough, however, to let some air pass through in small quantity" (85).

Thus, if Leboucq is correct, Philistion, writing five centuries before Galen, knew of the heart's exact location in the chest, its relation to the lungs, the structure of its cavities, muscular walls, and valves, and had observed the long survival of its auricular contractions after the ventricles ceased to beat. Since the authenticity of this document has been doubted, and since it is so much in advance of its time and breaks the continuity of the development of ideas, it seems more likely that it was a much later addition to the Hippocratic Corpus (*106*). It is nonetheless an ancient writing and of great interest, regardless of its precise date and origin.

Be that as it may, Philistion was probably visited in Syracuse by Plato, who gathered from him some information about the lungs and heart, which can be found in the *Timaeus* (*116, 85*):

". . . and the heart is the junction of the veins and the source of the blood that has been carried around vigorously down all the limbs. . . . As a means of relief from the leaping heart when the passion is excited . . . from the action of fire they [the engendered sons of God] contrived and implanted the form of the lung—soft and bloodless . . . it contains within perforated cavities like those of a sponge so that when it receives the breath and the drink it might have a cooling effect. . . . To this end they drew the channels of the round pipe to the lungs and placed the lungs as a kind of padding around the heart . . . ."

THE HEART

Aristotle, the other great Athenian philosopher of this period, discovered nothing new about breathing, described the heart inaccurately by ignoring the interauricular septum, and asserted that the heart was the center of the intelligence and that the brain secreted phlegms in order to cool it. He emphasized, however, that the heart was the source of motion of blood in the vessels and that blood was the distributor in the body of transformed food. To explain his lack of curiosity about human anatomy, the suggestion has been made that, like many other sons of physicians, the founder of Biology had a strong dislike of medicine and a great enthusiasm for other physical sciences (*116*).

Nonetheless the philosophy of Aristotle and his scientific method immediately influenced the course of medicine. His contemporary, Diocles of Caryostos (*116, 74*), a famous Athenian physician, reorganized the traditional Hippocratic and Cnido-Sicilian knowledge in a systematic and logical order. His disciple Praxagoras, in the second half of the third century B.C. (*115, 116, 130*), became the renovator of the teaching of the school of Cos. He made the unequivocal distinction between arteries and veins and introduced a scheme of the cardiovascular system according to which the left ventricle and the arteries carried only air, while the right ventricle and the veins transported blood. He studied systematically the pulsations of the arteries and wrote a treatise on the pulse.

The relations of the pulse to the heart beat, almost entirely neglected by the Hippocratic school, were known in Egypt in the seventeenth and sixteenth centuries B.C., according to the Smith Papyrus. Praxagoras deserves lasting credit for rescuing this important source of information from oblivion. During his lifetime he witnessed the early stages of the prodigious renaissance of Hellenic medicine, as its center shifted from Cos to Alexandria, and one of his disciples became the chief author of this rebirth.

Concept of a Dual System for Transport of Blood and Air

Endless internecine wars among the Greek city states made possible their subjugation by Philip, king of the Macedonian barbarians. His son, Alexander, who had been educated by Aristotle, conquered a large part of the known world, spread Hellenism into Asia, and orientalized eastern Europe. After the death of Alexander (June 327 B.C.), one of his generals proclaimed himself king of Egypt, as Ptolemy I Soter. In Alexandria, Ptolemy built the Museum, which was completed under his son, and the Library, which became a unique center of documentation. Both kings attracted the greatest scientists and physicians of their time to the Museum. In this institute, scientific research became independent of philosophy and pursued its proper object: in particular, the explanation of natural mechanisms. Anatomical investigations were pursued with continuity and method and with almost unrestricted facilities, and dissection was openly practiced with the help of assistants and in the presence of students. In this period of exceptional freedom from religious prejudices and with the patronage of the rulers, a complete survey of the human body, which was probably preserved according to the ancient art of embalming, was soon on its way. These unique opportunities were exploited by two great physicians, Herophylos of Chalcedon and Erasistratos of Chios, both of whom we know only through Galen.

AIR AND BLOOD

Herophylos (*115, 118, 9*), born on the shore of the Bosphorus in the fourth century B.C., had studied in Cos with Praxagoras, then went to Alexandria, where he spent the rest of his life. Above all an observer who maintained complete independence of traditional observations, he was careful in his inquiries as to the causes of phenomena and extended his skepticism toward theoretical concepts and ideas. His anatomical studies ranged from the cranium and the brain, to which he restored the seat of intelligence, to the sensory nerves, the meninges, the eye, the digestive tract, and the genital organs. The observations on the cardiovascular system, some of them of a physiological nature, are remarkable for their accuracy. Herophylos demonstrated that arteries, thicker than veins (six times or more!) contained blood during life and that after death they were flat and empty of blood. He identified the pulmonary artery as the *arterial vein* and the pulmonary vein as the *venal artery*. Furthermore, he taught that the heart transmits its blood and its pulsations to the arteries and he studied in detail the rhythm and force of the arterial pulse with the clepsydra. He also described the pulmonary function according to a four-phase rhythm: absorption of fresh air, distribution of air in the body, collection of air returning from the body, evacuation of vitiated air to the exterior. This is an insight of genius into the combined mechanism of breathing and respiratory gas transport.

His former assistant and younger rival at the Museum, Erasistratos (*118, 9*), was responsible for the concept of two separate systems for the transport of blood and air. Born on one of the Cyclades in the fourth century B.C., he studied in Athens, where he was under the influence of the Aristotelians, and at the school of Cnidus, where the atomistic doctrine was then taught. He settled at the Museum in Alexandria, and probably died in that city in the middle of the third century B.C. Galen, who may have misrepresented some of his ideas, was well acquainted with Erasistratos' experimental method, which included some attempts at quantitative measurements. Galen gave him credit for his anatomical descriptions and terminology, which extended those of Herophylos, and for his studies of comparative and pathological anatomy. In his anatomical studies of the human heart, Erasistratos gave an excellent description of the tricuspid valve and of the sigmoid valves located at the origin of the "artery-like vein" and of the aorta.

His most ambitious attempt was to give a synthetic explanation of vital processes: blood, *the source of matter*, nourished all constituents of the body with the natural spirit that it carried; and *pneuma*, in its two

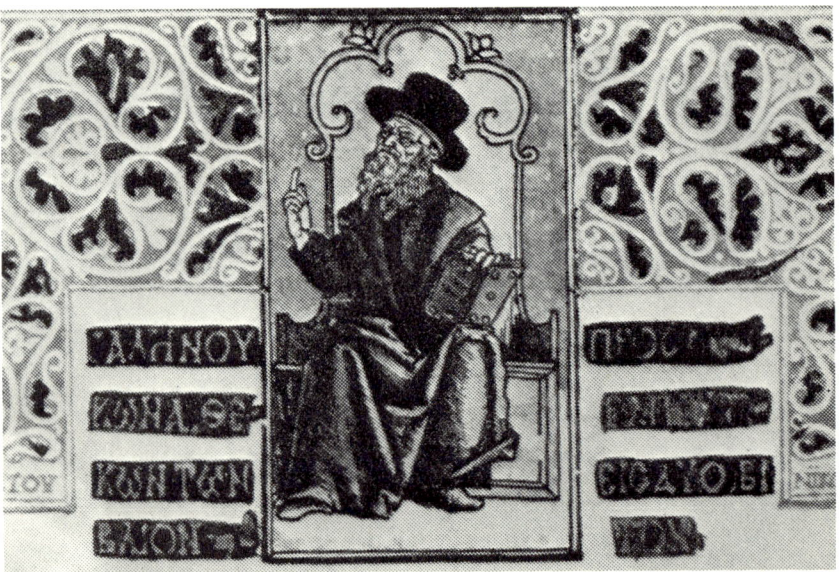

Figure 3. Galen of Pergamon, as he was depicted in medieval times. From Galen's Therapeutica, published in Venice in 1500. No authentic ancient representation of Galen exists.

forms—vital spirit and animal spirit—was *the source of energy* animating matter. He conceived of two separate systems to transport these fundamental elements: (1) blood manufactured in the liver moved through the veins toward all organs; a small fraction of it that reached the right ventricle, unable to return to the vena cava because of the tricuspid valve, was directed through the "artery-like vein" toward the lungs for their nourishment, (2) pneuma inspired into the lungs flowed through the vein-like artery to the cavity of the left ventricle, where it became vital spirit, and was then distributed to the body through the aorta and the arteries; the part of the vital spirit that reached the brain was transformed into animal spirit, accumulated in the cerebral ventricles, and was transported through the hollow nerves to the entire body. In this schema, motion of blood to the lungs and of pneuma in the left cavity was assured by the diastolic activity of the heart, and the reflux from or to the ventricles of both blood and pneuma was prevented by the valves. The unidirectional motion of blood to the lungs and of air to the left ventricle was, for the first time, explicitly recognized. In his system, Erasistratos also emphasized that veins, arteries, and nerves were juxtaposed in all parts of the body and that the finest divisions of the veins and arteries intercommunicated.

Four centuries later, the anatomical and physiological discoveries of the two Alexandrian physicians were utilized and improved upon by one of the great men of antiquity, Galen of Pergamon.

The Galenic System of Motion of Blood and Air

Pergamon, located in Asia Minor opposite the Isle of Lesbos, had become during the second century B.C. the rival of Alexandria, and during the first century B.C. the ally of Rome, which was then on its way to conquering the Greek and the Hellenistic world. The Roman conquest was mainly political, economic, and administrative; international law, peace, and order prevailed. But Greek was still used as the language of philosophers and scientists, and the existing schools and institutes remained prosperous.

Galen (*115, 118, 9, 117*), "the Serene," was an intellectual giant. He inherited, discussed, and synthesized all philosophical, scientific, historical, philological, and medical knowledge accumulated during eight centuries of Greek and Hellenistic civilization. His greatest achievement in cardiovascular physiology was his concept of the unidirectional movement of blood and air through the lungs, which endured until Harvey.

He was educated in the foremost philosophical systems of his time, Academic, Lycean, Epicurean, and Stoic, and also in mathematics and logic. Galen's education was strongly influenced by his father, a learned man of the highest personal qualities, and by his city of birth, Pergamon, in which the famous temple to Asklepios was located. At seventeen years of age, apparently prompted by his father's vivid dreams, he added the study of medicine to his study of philosophy. After several years of medical study, which included the dissection of animals, he left Pergamon to travel throughout Greece and Asia Minor, exploring the medical customs of each of the areas that he visited. Included in his itinerary was Alexandria, where he encountered the scientific tradition established by Herophylos and Erasistratos, and where he found human dissection used in anatomical teaching. After twelve years of study abroad, he returned to Pergamon to become physician to the gladiators, a position which provided ample experience in traumatic surgery and medicine. Four years later he moved to Rome, then at the zenith of its power. There he soon achieved great renown for his skills in medical practice and in dissection, and became the physician and friend of the Emperor, Marcus Aurelius. Although his medical colleagues were well aware of his scientific talents and accomplishments, they found his arrogance and ostentation insufferable. His scientific legacy consisted of many papers and books, but no disciples.

His views on the movement of blood reflect his eclecticism, his capacity for assimilating observations, whatever their origin, for testing them experimentally, and for presenting them with order and logic. They culminated in a large synthesis of knowledge.

His physiological scheme was obviously inspired by Erasistratos. The venous, the arterial, and the nervous systems, with the liver, the heart, and the brain as their respective centers, were still considered to be separate, and the function of each was to distribute through the body one of the three spirits: respectively, the natural, the vital, and the animal. In one fundamental aspect, however, Galen disagreed with his Alexandrian precursor: he affirmed that blood was carried both within the venous system and the arterial system. His description of the venous system will be discussed in a later chapter. He had almost complete knowledge of the anatomy of the heart, save that he considered the auricles as dilatations of large veins. He knew that the direction of blood flow was governed by the one-way valves situated at the four openings of the heart's ventricular cavities: "Nature ... provided the cardiac openings of the vessels with membranous attachments to prevent their content from being carried backwards" (De nat. fac. 3, XII) (37). One pair of valves "expels matter from the heart so that it cannot get back again ... and the other pair admits matter in such a way that it cannot get out again by the same channel" (De usu partium 6, XI) (49). Galen believed that the heart was not a muscle, for unlike a real muscle it could not be moved at will, but its dilatation, caused by the "pulsific" activity possessed by its tissues, drew some blood from the vena cava into the cavity of the right ventricle; only an insignificant portion of this blood returned to the vena cava whence it came. Most of the blood, but not all, as we shall see presently, leaving the right ventricle moved into the *arterial vein* [pulmonary artery] and thence forward into the *vein-like arteries* [pulmonary veins], by means of fine "openings." He explained the mechanism of the motion of the blood in the following manner:

"*If the great orifice of the arterial vein [pulmonary artery] were always open, and if Nature had not invented a means for alternately closing and opening it at appropriate times, the blood would not penetrate into the pulmonary arteries [pulmonary veins] on contraction of the thorax. When the thorax contracts, the pulmonary arteries with their veinlike structure, crowded and pushed from all sides with great force, instantly expel the Pneuma which they contain and in return are filled through these narrow channels with particles of blood ... as it is, the blood, finding its passage cut off through the great orifice ... [of] ... the arterial vein on the side of the heart ... penetrates in the form of minute drops into the arteries ....*" [De usu partium 6, x].

The concept of one-way traffic in the lungs and the structures that prevent reflux are thus well defined: "*Otherwise, the blood would always be coming and going, to no purpose and without end like tides in a strait.*" (italics added). In a remarkably well-documented analysis of what Galen wrote and meant, Fleming (37) has recently shown that the actual metaphor of ebb and flow, misconstrued by many historians of science, is used by Galen to illustrate the kind of absurdity that Nature would *not* fall into.

Galen did not clearly state whether the blood, once it passed into the pulmonary veins, was transmitted to the left ventricle, although the statement cited above regarding the role of the two pairs of valves in admitting matter could be interpreted in this sense. Be that as it may, Galen held that inspired air in some form or other, or some quality derived from air, was transferred from the lung through the venous artery into the left cavity of the heart by means of the diastolic active dilatation of the ventricle, and that there was a movement of waste products in the opposite direction, from left ventricle to the lung through which they were expired. "The venous artery [pulmonary vein] has no advantage of being closed since it has rather the mission of letting pass from the heart into the lungs the sooty residues which the natural heat necessarily produces in that organ [the heart] and which have no shorter means of exit. This discharge is made possible by the comparative weakness of the mitral valve" (*49*).

Compounding this unfortunate assumption with another that has been a blot on his fame, Galen stated that some blood passed directly from the right ventricle into the left through invisible pores located in the interventricular septum.

Once in the cavity of the left ventricle, and only there, were blood and pneuma elaborated into the *vital spirit*. Through their own pulsific properties, the aorta and the arteries drew the spiritous blood from the left ventricle and distributed it throughout the body.

Galen's scheme was a decisive step toward the understanding of the movement of blood through the lungs. To be sure, it introduced the paradox of two-way traffic in the pulmonary vein, and of the selective permeability of the mitral valve for sooty wastes but not spiritous blood, both of which led William Harvey to reconsider the Galenic system. But was not this paradox the first attempt to explain the two simultaneous functions served by the movement of blood through the lungs: the acquisition of a useful substance, and the elimination of a wasteful one? One wonders why Galen, a keen observer, should have assumed the existence of pores between the ventricles too small to be visible. Prendergast (*113*) has suggested that this assumption was based on a sound anatomical observation and mechanical explanation: The orifice of the pulmonary artery being smaller than that of the tricuspid, and the mitral orifice being smaller than that of the aortic, parity between the quantity of blood in both ventricles was re-established by a trickle of blood through pores; therefore, the pits visible on the wall of the ventricular cavities corresponded to pores and were not fortuitous but developed according to a design and to serve a purpose.

The Spread of Galen's System

An enthusiastic and outstanding investigator during his youth, Galen later became dogmatic and prone to invoke unverifiable forces and teleological concepts in order to explain natural phenomena, and ended by praising Divine Providence for the marvels of its creation. Hence, his authoritative pronouncements in all fields of medicine were readily acceptable to theologians, whether Moslems, Jews, or Christians.

The spread of Galen's system has been traced back to Oribasios of Pergamon, the physician of Julian the Apostate; it was carried later by the Aryans and Nestorians, refugees from Christian persecution. These scholars brought back Greek and Hellenistic science to the Near East, first to Edessa, where Galen's works were translated into Syriac, and from there to Baghdad (*118*).

In the eleventh century, Ibn Sina (Avicenna), who had integrated all Greek and Moslem knowledge in his famous Canon, still adhered strictly to the description of the heart and lungs given by Galen. This was considered sound doctrine until the middle of the thirteenth century, when Ibn Nafis, an Arab physician born in Damascus in 1210, who

لو خلط بالـدم . . . . وهذا التجويف هو التجويف
الأيمن من تجويفى القلب و إذا لطف الدم فى هذا التجويف فلا بد من نفوذه إلى التجويف الأيسر
حيث تتولد الروح ولـكن ليس بينهما منفذ فان جرم القلب هناك مصمت ليس فيه منفذ ظاهر
كما ظنه جماعة ولامنفذ غير ظاهر يصلح لنفوذ هذا الدم كما ظنه جالينوس فان مسام القلب هناك
مستخصفة وجرمه غليظ فلا بد وأن يكون هذا الدم إذا لطف نفـذ فى الوريد الشريانى إلى
الرئة لينبث فى جرمها ويخالط الهـواء ويتصفى الطف مافيه وينفـذ إلى الشريان الوريـدى
ليوصله إلى التجويف الأيسر من تجويفى القلب . . . . . . : : . . . . . . :

Figure 4. Pulmonary circulation. A page from the manuscript of Ibn Nafis.
"The blood (of the right ventricle) passes through the vena arteriosa (= pulmonary artery) to the lung, spreads through its substance, mixes with the air and becomes completely purified; then it passes through the arteria venosa (= pulmonary vein) to reach the left chamber of the heart."

was also a philologist and a theologian, presented some divergent points of view in his *Commentary on the Anatomy of Avicenna's Canon* and rejected Galen's assumption of interventricular pores.

This document remained unknown to the Western world until 1922, when it was discovered in the Prussian State Library by an Egyptian medical student, Muhyi el din At Tatawi. In 1924 he published the relevant part of the *Commentary* in his thesis for the degree of Bachelor of Medicine of the University of Freiburg in Breisgau (*120*). This rather confused text, the first complete translation of which was made in German (*102*), reveals that Ibn Nafis rejected Galen's description of interventricular pores, and also remarked, somewhat cryptically, that the aeration of blood takes place in the lungs. The following significant passage is quoted from the thesis of E. Bittar, a graduate of Yale Medical School, who has recently translated the entire *Commentary* (*13*) from Arabic into English:

"What we say (and God knows better) is that whereas one of the functions of the heart is the generation of the spirit, which consists of highly rarefied blood, extremely mixable with an airy substance, it is essential that such highly rarefied blood and air meet in the heart to facilitate the evolution of the spirit from the compound formed of their mixture. This meeting takes place in the left cavity of the two cavities of the heart, where the animal spirit is generated.

"It is also essential that there be in the heart of man, and other animals possessing lungs, another cavity in which the blood is rarefied to be fit for mixing with air. For if air were mixed with blood when thick, a homogeneous compound could not result. This cavity is the right cavity of the two cavities of the heart.

"After the blood has been rarefied in this cavity, it must of necessity pass to the left cavity, where the animal spirit is generated. But there is no opening, as some thought there was between these two cavities, for the septum of the heart there is watertight without any apparent fenestrations in it [emphasis added]. *Nor, as held by Galen, would an invisible opening be suitable for the passage of this blood, for the pores of the heart there are not patent and its septum is thick. The blood, therefore, after thinning, passes via the vena-arterialis* [pulmonary artery] *to the lung for circulation and mixes with air in the pulmonary parenchyma. The aerated blood gets refined and*

passes through the arteria-venalis [pulmonary vein] to reach the left cavity of the two cavities of the heart, after having mixed with the air and become suitable for the evolution of the animal spirit.

"The residuum of less rarefied blood is used up by the lungs for its nourishment. Accordingly, the vena-arterialis was made strongly impermeable with two layers, so that what seeps through its interstices be then highly rarefied, while the arteria-venalis was made thin, with a single layer, to facilitate the absorption of whatsoever filtrated into this vein. For this reason obvious openings between the two vessels were established."

Besides this passage, the whole text is redundant with repetition of the same statements in different forms. They add nothing but confusion to the main thesis—namely, that (a) blood is rarefied in the right ventricle so that it may be fit to mix with the air in its passage through the lung; (b) blood and air are transported to the left cavity where the animal spirit is generated; (c) pores, through which blood might trickle from the right to left ventricular cavities, do not exist, and (d) the lungs are nourished by a special fraction of blood, issued from the right ventricle.

On the basis of this document, some Arab scholars have made extravagant claims about the extent of the Arabic challenge to Galenic doctrine (*31, 102-105, 52, 134*). One of these claims, which deserves serious consideration, purports to establish a probable connection between the teaching of Ibn Nafis and the origin of the anti-Galenic trend in Padua early in the sixteenth century (*14*). It points out that Andreas Alpagos and Paulus Alpagos, his nephew, after having spent thirty years in the Arab world and having acquired a good knowledge of the Arabic language, had translated into Latin most of Ibn Nafis's *Commentary on Avicenna's Canon*, and returned to Padua around 1520. The thesis seems plausible, but unfortunately the relevant part of the translation, i.e. the section on anatomy, has not been recovered; the whole matter is still based largely on circumstantial evidence.

With the fall of the Roman Empire practically all of Greek science was lost to the West, although much of it survived in the Byzantine Empire. Recovery was slow: it came first from the Arab world by way of reconquered Spain, along with the significant contributions of Arab medicine. Arabic translations of Galen and Hippocrates and the Canon of Avicenna were translated in turn into Latin by Gerard of Cremona. Another source was the School of Salerno in southern Italy, a way station for the Crusaders, and the place where the Arab scholar Constantine of Africa established himself in the eleventh century. More accurate knowledge came later, when Italian scholars had direct access to Greek texts. In the thirteenth century the entire Aristotelian corpus was translated and published by Albertus Magnus. He added extended observations of his own in plant and animal biology (*129*). The search for a unifying physical theory of Nature was then renewed by men of learning, who strove to reconcile the facts of natural experience with the perfect and unchallengeable systems of knowledge inherent in Christian theology.

Galen's System in Question

By the sixteenth century the Humanists were investigating the original texts of the Scriptures and beginning frankly to question the truthfulness of Christian dogma. One of them, Michael Servetus, in a book inspired by his search for true religion, described the passage of the blood through the lungs and its change of color in the process, in no ambiguous terms. He was the first in Western Christendom to question parts of Galen's scheme (*13, 39, 26, 73, 125, 5, 6, 46*).

But this account does not give the full measure of Michael Servetus. What transcends is the man himself, his urge to investigate texts as well as facts, his intellectual capacity, his spirit of revolt against dogma.

Michael Servetus as a theologian (*6*) could not accept blindly the official interpretation of Biblical texts and could not find support for the doctrine of the Trinity in the Greek and Hebraic Bibles. As a philosopher, he believed that all forms of human knowledge—theology, psychology, anatomy, physiology, mathematics, geography, astronomy, and astrology, with each of which he was familiar—were ultimately to be unified in one single coherent system of the universe, not only penetrated by Reason, as the Stoics held, but by a creative dynamic energy, the very Being of the Creator Who infuses all with His Spirit. He was a Christian, with reverence and love for the Supreme Harmonious Being, who fought for the return to a simple faith, that of the early Christian era. A man of indomitable courage and absolute intellectual integrity, he was forthright in the expression of his views.

Up to his final agony at the stake he spoke his innermost, uncompromising belief, even though to have said "Jesus, the Eternal son of God," instead of "Jesus, son of the Eternal God," might have saved him.

His life was almost a continuous flight. He was born in 1511, in Tuleda in the province of Navarre in Spain, and was reared in Villanueva; he went to Toulouse to study law. As the protégé of a Franciscan scholar, Servetus traveled to Bologna, where he was depressed by the outrageous pomp of the coronation of Charles V of Spain by Pope Boniface VI. From there he went to Basel, where he studied Aryanism,

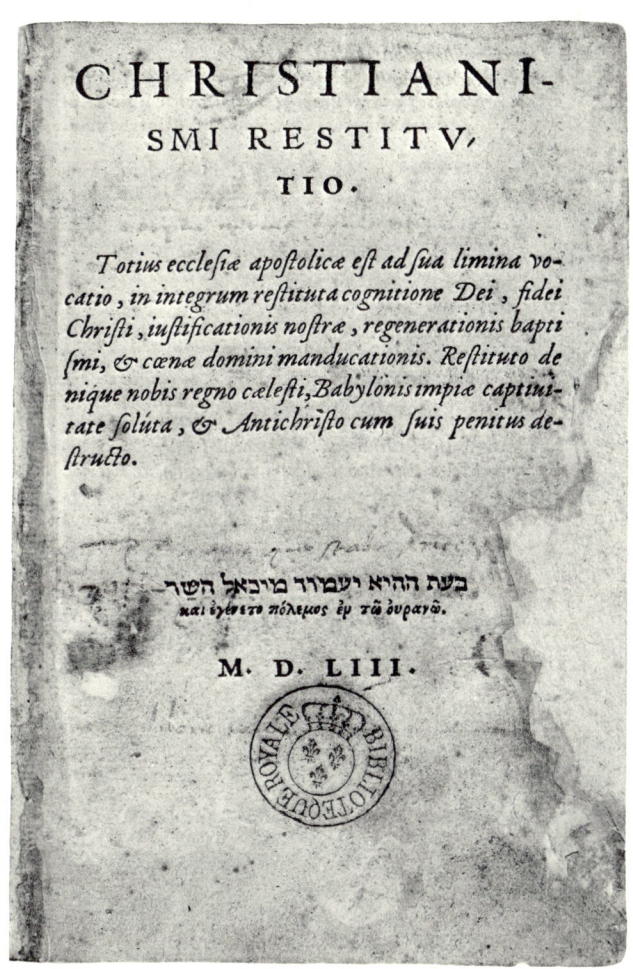

Figure 5. Title page of Christianismi Restitutio of Michael Servetus. 1533.

to Strasbourg, where in 1531 at the age of twenty he published his treatise *Errors of the Trinity*, and from there to Basel again, where he assumed the name of Villanovanus in order to hide from the Inquisition. In 1532 he paid his first visit to Paris, where he taught mathematics, and where in 1536 he had his first encounter with Calvin, who attempted to modify some of his theological views. He went then to Lyons, where he re-edited the *Geography of the Ptolemees*. Later he returned to the University of Paris, and in 1537 he began to study medicine under Dubois (also known as Sylvius), Jean Fernel, and Guinther of Andernach. It was under the last that he learned anatomy by dissection. Here he met Vesalius, whom he succeeded as prosector. In the preface of a new edition of his *Institutiones Anatomicae* (1539), Guinther praised Servetus's general culture, his skill in dissection, and his profound knowledge of Galen (6). During his medical studies Servetus wrote on syrups, disputing Fuchs, and on astrology, bringing upon himself the wrath of the Dean of the Medical Faculty. A lonely man, never secure, Servetus, after living three years in Charlieu, finally settled as a physician near Lyons in the town of Vienne in 1541. Claims that around that time he went to the University of Montpellier (*13*), or even to Padua (*106*), are unsupported. He practiced medicine in Vienne for twelve years, pursuing his theological investigations in private. Outwardly content with his medical practice and editorial work, he spent considerable time in research and in writing his theological beliefs. He communicated his ideas to Calvin, who summarily rejected them. In early 1553 he published anonymously his *Christianismi Restitutio*. This led to his arrest by the Inquisition, upon denunciation by a friend of Calvin. Thus both the Calvinists and the Roman Inquisition charged Servetus with heresy. Escaping from prison, Servetus took flight to Geneva, where, while attending church on a Sunday morning, he was recognized, expeditiously judged, and burned at Champel (on the outskirts of Geneva) on October 27, 1553, with a copy of the book that caused his doom attached to his arm. Of one thousand books printed in 1553, only three authentic copies remain and only two are complete, all others presumably having been seized and destroyed. The copy preserved at the Bibliothèque Nationale in Paris was probably once in the hands of Colladon, Calvin's friend, who was the chief witness against Servetus throughout his trial.

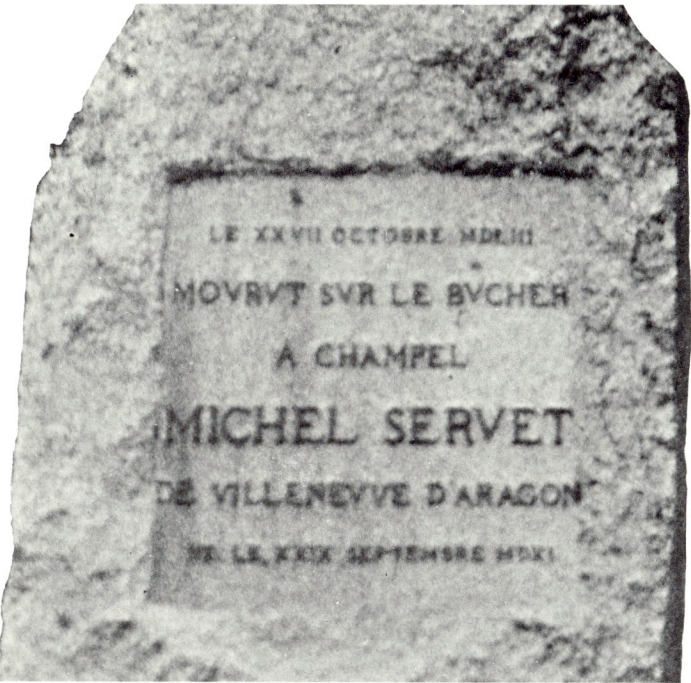

Figure 6. Stone tablet in Geneva, marking the place where Servetus was burned at the stake.

In Chapter v, from page 169 to 171, one reads the description of the transit of blood through the lungs in a few luminous and concise sentences:

"... *It is not said that the divine spirit is principally in the walls of the heart, or in the body of the brain or of the liver, but in the blood, as is taught by God Himself in Gen. 9, Levit. 8, Deut. 12.*

"*In this matter there must first be understood the substantial generation of the vital spirit which is composed of a very subtle blood nourished by the inspired air. The vital spirit had its origin in the left ventricle of the heart, and the lungs assist greatly in its generation. It is a rarefied spirit, elaborated by the force of heat, reddish-yellow* (flavo) *and of fiery potency, so that it is a kind of clear vapor from very pure blood, containing in itself the substance of water, air, and fire. It is generated in the lungs from a mixture of inspired air with elaborated, subtle blood which the right ventricle of the heart communicates to the left. However, this communication is made not through the middle*

THE HEART

wall of the heart, as is commonly believed, but by a very ingenious arrangement the subtle blood is urged forward by a long course through the lungs; it is elaborated by the lungs, becomes reddish-yellow and is poured from the pulmonary artery into the pulmonary vein. Then in the pulmonary vein it is mixed with inspired air and through expiration it is cleaned of its sooty vapors. Thus finally the whole mixture, suitably prepared for the production of the vital spirit, is drawn onward to the left ventricle of the heart by diastole.

"*That the communication and elaboration are accomplished in this way through the lungs we are taught by the different conjunctions and the communication of the pulmonary artery with the pulmonary vein in the lungs. The notable size of the pulmonary artery confirms this; that is, it was not made of such sort or of such size, nor does it emit so great a force of pure blood from the heart itself into the lungs merely for their nourishment; nor would the heart be of such service to the lungs, since at an earlier stage, in the embryo, the lungs, as Galen teaches, are nourished from elsewhere because those little membranes or valvules of the heart are not opened until the time of birth. Therefore that the blood is poured from the heart into the lungs at the very time of birth, and so copiously, is for another purpose. Likewise, not merely air, but air mixed with blood, is sent from the lungs to the heart through the pulmonary vein; therefore the mixture occurs in the lungs. That reddish-yellow color is given to the spiritous blood by the lungs; it is not from the heart.*

"*In the left ventricle of the heart there is no place large enough for so great and copious a mixture, nor for that elaboration imbuing the reddish-yellow color. Finally, that middle wall, since it is lacking in vessels and mechanisms, is not suitable for that communication and elaboration, although something may possibly sweat through. By the same arrangement by which a transfusion of blood from the portal vein to the vena cava occurs in the liver, so a transfusion of the spirit from the pulmonary artery to the pulmonary vein occurs in the lung. If anyone compares these things with those which Galen wrote in Books* VI *and* VII, De usu partium, *he will thoroughly understand a truth which was unknown to Galen*" (119).

For over a century the existence of this important text remained undisclosed. Then in 1694, Wotton (*132*), an English antiquarian, obtained a transcription from an English surgeon who had received it from an unnamed friend. Wotton later had access to the manuscript now at the Bibliothèque Nationale in Paris.

In the light of this text, the most important physiological contributions of Michael Servetus are these: first, the passage of blood through the lungs, its mixing there with air, and its change in color; second, his emphasis on the size of the pulmonary artery, from which he deduced that it must serve some purpose other than transporting blood for the nourishment of the lungs; and third, his twice-repeated statement that there is no communication allowing blood to move through the interventricular septum.

Because of the context in which this description is given, many commentators (*13, 39*) have belittled its importance. This attitude attests a lack of objectivity, since we must admit that the center of gravity of a man's thought may be different from ours. Bainton (*6*) has dealt at great length with the question why Servetus's description appeared in a book devoted to the return to true Christianity. This is not the place to review his theological argument, except to cite its conclusion: "He who really understands what is involved in the breathing of man has already sensed the breath of God and thereby saved his soul."

I have mentioned previously that some Arab writers contend that Michael Servetus knew of Ibn Nafis's writings. One even went so far as to state, "He who reads the work of Servetus cannot help noticing that it is almost a literal translation of [a passage in] Ibn Nafis's [*Epistle on the Perfect Man*]" (*52*). However, a translation of this *Epistle* (*13*) reveals not a single word relative to the pulmonary circuit. Moreover, Meyerhof (*105*) and Temkin (*121*), who denied any link between Ibn Nafis and Servetus, have been vindicated recently by Bittar, who translated the *Epistle* (*13*) and found no evidence of a connection between the writings of Ibn Nafis and the anti-Galenic teachings of the medical school of Padua (*14*).

The school of Padua was the most celebrated in Europe. There, in the sixteenth century, two anatomists, Vesalius and Realdus Columbus, contributed further to the elaboration of the concept of the passage of blood through the lungs.

Of Andreas Vesalius there is little to say in this chapter, but that he expressed discreet skepticism about the pores in the interventricular septum. In the first edition of his great treatise *De humanis corporis fabrica* (1543) he wrote: "the septum of the ventricles, as I said, formed from the thickest substance of the heart, abounds in pits impressed into

[23]

both sides of it. None of [them] penetrates from the right ventricle, so we are compelled to wonder at the industry of the Creator of all things by which the blood sweats from the right ventricle into the left through invisible passages." In the second edition (1555) the skepticism is more overt: "I have not found even the most hidden passages" and again, "not long ago I would not have dared to turn aside even a nail's breadth from the opinion of Galen, the prince of physicians.... But the septum of the heart is as thick, dense, and compact as the rest of the heart" (*132*).

His assistant, Realdus Columbus (1516-80), succeeded him as professor of anatomy, and was considered by Harvey to be "a most skilful and learned anatomist.' In his *De re anatomica* (1559) he presented his views on the pulmonary passage and supported his observations with well-designed experiments. He confirmed the fundamental observation made by Jean Fernel in 1542 that cardiac systole and diastole coincide respectively with expansion and contraction of the arteries, and he demonstrated also that the mitral valve was completely closed during systole and that the transmission of pulsations back to the pulmonary vein was thus checked. After opening these veins, he found not fumes but spiritous blood:

> "Between these ventricles there is placed the septum through which almost all authors think there is a way open from the right to the left ventricle.... But these make a great mistake: for the blood is carried by the artery-like vein to the lungs, and being made thin is brought back thence together with air by the vein-like artery to the left ventricle of the heart. This fact no one has hitherto observed or recorded in writing; yet it may most readily be observed by anyone" (*29*).

The question of priority between Realdus Columbus and Michael Servetus regarding the true passage of blood through the lungs and the change in color which takes place there has been discussed at great length. On this subject Bainton (*6*) has wisely written: "Here, as so often in the history of Science, independent investigators came upon the same truth almost coincidentally. There can be no rivalry between Servetus and Columbus, the other contestant, for it has been established that neither knew the discovery of the other. Insofar as the announcement, there is no problem at all." Indeed, Servetus's text dates back to

1553, whereas Columbus's *De re anatomica* was published six years later. Furthermore, with regard to the time of the observation, Bainton in a short and searching paper (*4*) has given convincing proof that a manuscript of Servetus in the Bibliothèque Nationale in Paris containing a statement on the pulmonary passage of blood is probably a faithful copy of an earlier draft sent, in 1546, to Calvin, who never returned it.

Two other anatomists, Juan Valverde and Andreas Caesalpinus (1519-1603), have also been linked with the discovery of the pulmonary circulation. The Spaniard, Valverde, was a pupil of Columbus. Since Columbus's manuscript was many years in preparation, Valverde must have had knowledge of its content. However, instead of waiting for its publication, which took place after Columbus's death, Valverde incorporated in his own book what he had learned. Not only did he present the concept of his teacher as his own, but he also boasted that "nobody before me has said this," namely, that there is no communication through the interventricular septum (*4*). Caesalpinus, in his description of the passage of blood in the heart and in the lungs (*Quaestionum Medicarum*, book 2, question 7) added very little to that given by Columbus, except that he emphasized the pumping character of the ventricular action and the important role of the valves, which he had already mentioned twenty-two years previously in his *Quaestionum Peripateticarum* (1571) (*23*).

The Pulmonary Passage in Harvey's Scheme

For fourteen centuries the Galenic concept of the vascular system had prevailed. Owing to the resumption of human dissection, and also to greater freedom from dogma, new details had been introduced in the description of the unidirectional passage of blood through the lungs. But the validity of the scheme itself had not been questioned.

The concept of blood circulation, its significance, and something of its discoverer's life and philosophy will be discussed in other chapters of this book. My comments will therefore be limited to the importance of the pulmonary circulation in Harvey's discovery (*25, 134, 60*), a subject which has been excellently analyzed by Fleming (*38*).

Although, in the Introduction of *De motu cordis* (*60*), William Harvey (1578-1657) ridiculed Galen for his account of the motion of air in one direction and of waste in the other during their transit through the venous artery, he praised Galen for having provided clear evidence of the pulmonary passage of blood: "From Galen, that great Prince of Physicians, it seems clear that the blood passes through the lungs from the arterial vein into the minute branches of the venous artery, urged to this both by the beatings of the heart and by the movements of the lungs and thorax." But Harvey defined the precise mechanism of the heart beat and of the effects of lung motion.

"When the right ventricle is contracting and expelling during systole its content of blood, the artery-like vein is pulsating and being dilated synchronously with the other arteries of the body ... by this inthrust [of the right ventricle] the vessels and porosities of the lungs must be distended. Moreover, in breathing the lungs rise and fall, movement that necessitates the opening and closing respectively of the porosities and vessels...."

Harvey also paid tribute to Columbus, who was "convinced of the truth ... of the passage of blood through the lungs ... from the size and the structure of the lungs, from the fact that the vein-like artery and likewise the [left] ventricle are always full of blood, which must have come to them through the veins and by no other path than an intrapulmonary one."

From the consideration of a unidirectional and continuous movement of blood from the artery-like vein to the vein-like artery, Harvey reached an important conclusion:

"... and I finally saw that the blood was forced out of the heart and driven by the beating of the left ventricle through the arteries into the body at large and into its several parts, **in the same way** *as it is sent by the beating of the right ventricle through the arterial vein [pulmonary artery] into the lungs, and that it returns through the veins into the vena cava and so to the right ventricle in the same way as it returns from the lungs through the venous artery [pulmonary vein] to the left ventricle"* [emphasis added].

Thus, the passage of blood from the arterial vein into the venous artery was illuminating to him, since by analogy he could explain the passage of blood at the periphery from artery to veins.

But what the nature of the communication was he did not then know. Much later, in fact only a few years before his death, he wrote to his friend Slegel in Hamburg (58), describing perfusion experiments on the heart and lungs, in which he demonstrated conclusively the passage of blood from the pulmonary artery to the left ventricle. This will be discussed more fully in the next chapter.

At this point it is very important to emphasize that pulmonary circulation was not essential to Harvey's conception of the general circulation. In his dissection of eighty species of animals he had found some without lungs which had no right ventricle, and yet had demonstrated that the blood moved from the vena cava to the aorta. The presence of lungs, therefore, implied the concomitant existence of a right ventricle:

> *"However, when nature wished the blood to be filtered through the lungs, she was forced to make the extra provision of a right ventricle so that its pulsation would drive the blood through these very lungs from the vena cava to the region of the left ventricle. Thus one has to regard the right ventricle as having been made for the sake of the lungs and the transfer of blood . . . and not merely for nutrition."*

The role of the pulmonary circulation in his scheme puzzled him greatly. Why should the same amount of blood be sent to the lungs at each systole that is sent to the rest of the body? Obviously, this amount was not needed for the nutrition of the lungs, as he repeatedly asserted: "It is altogether incongruous to suppose that the lungs need for their nourishment so large a supply of food, so pulsatorily delivered." He therefore had recourse to the traditional Galenic explanation when he stated that "the hot blood is carried to and through the lungs, to be tempered by the inspired air and to be freed from bubbling to excess."

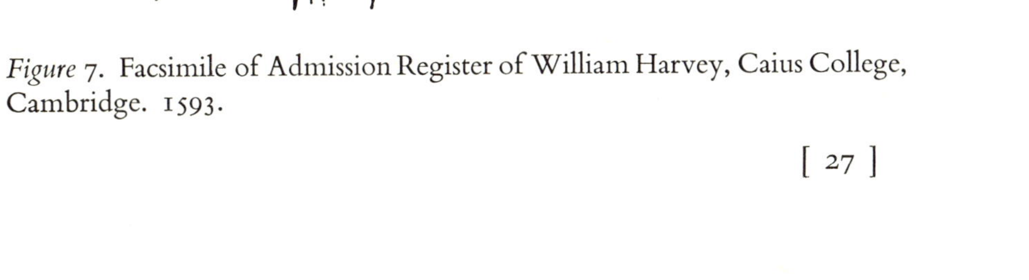

Figure 7. Facsimile of Admission Register of William Harvey, Caius College, Cambridge. 1593.

Throughout his life the problem of the relation of the respiration to the pulmonary circulation was on his mind. One can read in *Praelectiones* that "life and respiration are convertible terms, for there is no life without breathing, and no breathing without life . . ." and on a marginal note of the same work, "why and how air is needed by animals which breathe . . . ," and also, "air is necessary to a candle and to a fire" (*59*). However, he was not able to give a reasonable interpretation at the time *De motu cordis* was published in 1628: "But to settle these points and to give a full explanation is merely to explore the purpose of the lung's fabrication. It is here that by very numerous observations I have discovered much about these organs and their function and movement, about ventilation as a whole, the need for and function of the air . . . . I will leave these matters for more suitable exposition later in a special treatise." He never did write a treatise on this subject, although shortly before his death he modified the antique and traditional views somewhat: "[those who] consider more closely the nature of air will, I think, readily grant that air is given to animals neither for cooling nor as a nutriment. Thus much merely by the way, on the subject of respiration. Perhaps I shall treat of it more fully in its proper place" (*Exercitationes de generatione animalium*, 1651).

Whatever his queries and doubts, they could not be dispelled in his own lifetime for lack of proper knowledge of chemistry. Although in his time the microscope was already in use, Harvey did not live to learn that Malpighi, who was born the year his first great book was published, would discover the capillaries of the lungs and observe the movement of blood through them.

Discovery of the Pulmonary Alveoli and Capillaries

While holding the chair of Theoretical Medicine at Pisa, Marcello Malpighi (1628-94) addressed two memorable letters, *De pulmonibus* (*96*), to his close friend Borelli, a mathematician who was interested in physiology as a branch of physics. These letters, translated into English by James Young (*133*), contain, among other things, observations on the pulmonary alveoli and capillaries seen with the help of a compound microscope. With humility Malpighi announced "a few little observations that might increase the things found out about the lungs." These little observations were no less than the first description of the air sacs in the lungs of a dog, and of the pulmonary capillaries of the tortoise and frogs, "the whole race" of the latter, he claimed jokingly to "have almost destroyed." We may well admire the technical ability and the ingenuity which he displayed in observing the movement of blood in the capillary network of the lungs of a living frog while the heart was beating, and in examining, after ligature of the pulmonary veins, its lungs, turgid with blood and dried in that state:

"It is clear to sense that the blood flows away through the tortuous vessels, that it is not poured into spaces but always works through tubules and is dispersed by the multiple winding of the vessels."

We may also admire his suggestion that "the lungs are created by nature as if for a storehouse of blood, so that it may constantly in turn give forth blood to the heart . . . ." As to the function of the lungs, he was as much in the dark as Harvey and his predecessors, although he made an original suggestion:

"Concerning the use of the lungs, I know that many views are held from the ancients onwards, and about them there is very much dispute—especially about the cooling which is taken to be the principal purpose when it strives with the imagined excessive heat of the heart, which may require eventation; wherefore these things have made me diligently inquisitive in the investigation of another purpose, and from these things which I subjoin I can believe that the lungs are made by nature for mixing the mass of blood."

All the structures contributing to the passage of blood into the lungs had now been described, but it took more than 150 years to understand exactly the nature of the exchange which took place within the lungs between air and circulating blood. The question had been begging for solution since Empedocles. The correct answer had to wait for progress in physics and chemistry, and for successive and often combined inquiries, experiments, and discoveries. This was the achievement of the English scientists, Boyle, Hooke, Lower, and later, Priestley, and of Lavoisier, the founder of respiratory physiology.

Aeration of Blood in the Lungs

Chemistry has been developed through the centuries by empirical methods but was plagued by mystico-spiritualist explanations. At the end of the sixteenth century, the traditional concept of the four elements, and of their four associated principles, still prevailed; from their combinations were derived spirits, and from these all known forms of matter. The search for a unifying chemical entity was on: it led first to the unfortunate assumption of a universal agent, phlogiston, intervening in all chemical reactions, and released into the ambient air in the course of combustion.

A fundamental distinction was made by van Helmont (1577-1644) between air, an uncoercible element, and *gas* (*Geist* in German, meaning spirit). This "*gas sylvestre*," that emanated from matter of which water was the ultimate constituent, was unique, yet possessed of many different qualities, depending on its preparation (distillation, fermentation, action of acid on carbonates, decomposition by heat). Air could be charged with the particles of gas, and hence acquire various qualities of the gas, but after the destruction of those qualities by burning, air resumed its initial state. Therefore, this Belgian physician assumed that air itself did not play any part in combustion or respiration.

Among chemical substances, *nitre*, potassium nitrate, was long known for its fertilizing and explosive properties, which were applied in agriculture and in pyrotechnics. Since snow and rain, lightning and thunder also possessed these same properties, some sort of nitre was assumed to exist in the ambient air. By decomposing nitre, the Dutch physicist, Cornelius Drebbel (1572-1633), prepared a gas capable of maintaining life. However, the fundamental demonstration that a gas already in the air participated in respiration, as well as in combustion, was not forthcoming until Robert Boyle (1627-91) investigated the properties of air (*33, 44*).

This genius, son of an Irish nobleman, educated in England, France, Switzerland, and Italy, decided early in life to devote himself to science. He settled in Oxford in 1654. Stimulated by von Guericke's description of the air pump, and with the aid of his brilliant young assistant Robert Hooke, Boyle built a pneumatic air pump with which he investigated "the spring of air and its effects." This great work, continued over many years, had far-reaching consequences. It was published in two communications (*17, 18*), the first in 1660, "New Experiments Physico-Mechanical, touching the Spring of the Air and its Effects," and the second in 1682, "A Continuation of New Experiments, Physico-Mechanical,

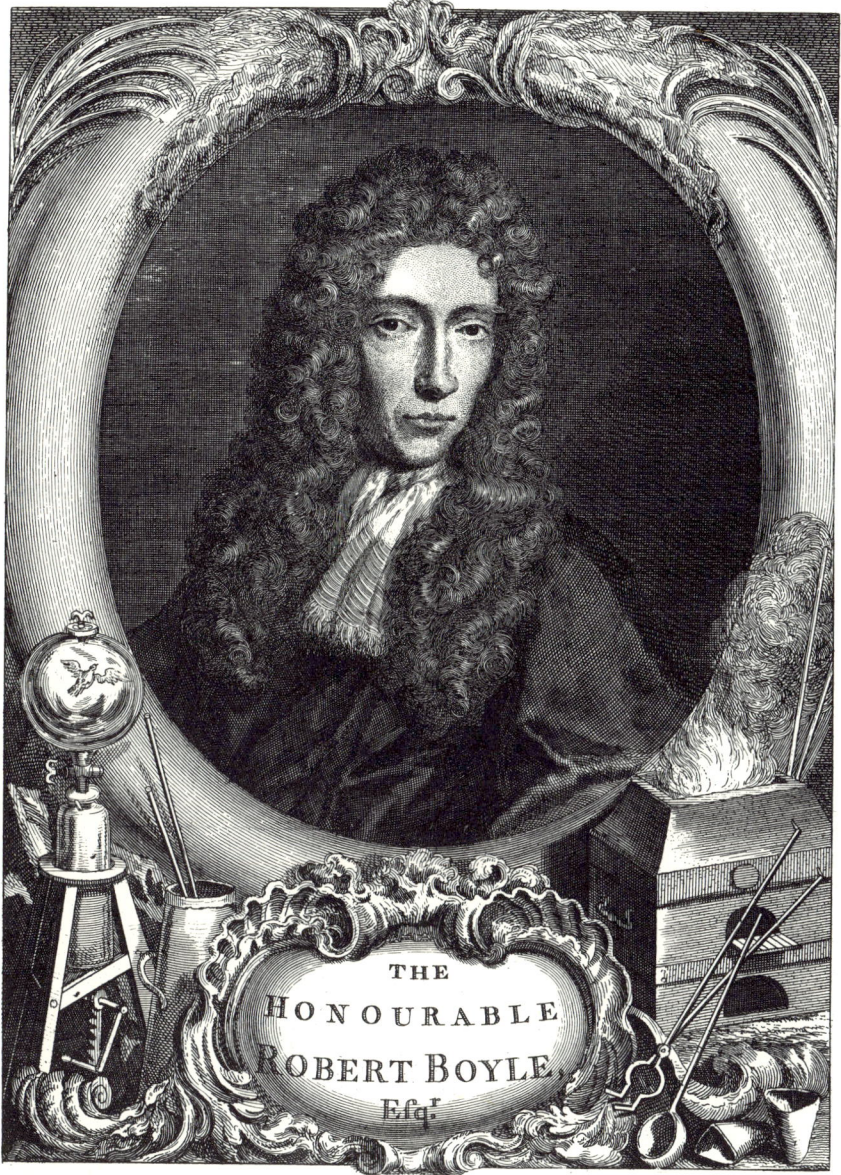

Figure 8. Robert Boyle (1627–91). Of a multitude of portraits of Boyle, this engraving, from an original painting by Johann Kerseboom, hangs in the Royal Society, London.

THE HEART

touching the Spring and Weight of the Air, and their Effects." In these studies he explored not only the physical properties of air, but also its fundamental role in combustion and respiration, through the use of physiological experiments.

Boyle found that, besides being cooled by air ventilated through the lungs, the blood during its "passage ... is disburdened of those excrementitious steams proceeding for the most part from the superfluous serosities of the blood." He commented on the statement of Paracelsus, that "the lungs consume part of the air and proscribe the rest so that ... we may suppose that there is in the air a little [of that] vital quintessence." He added also that "since most of the air is unserviceable, it need not seem strange that an animal stands in need of almost incessantly drawing on fresh air. But though this opinion is not ... absurd ... it should not be barely asserted but explicated and proved." To this end, he supplied the convincing evidence that an animal placed in the evacuated pump could not survive. As a logical step, the analogy between life and combustion was strengthened by the demonstration that sulfur, a highly combustible substance, was no longer inflammable in the vacuum; a lighted substance was also soon extinguished in it. As a further observation, he pointed out that "Air lurks in water ... and of it fishes may make some use by separating it when they strain the water through their gills."

Boyle became, at Oxford, the teacher and the adviser of Richard Lower, a young man who was destined to make the next important advance in the physiology of air and blood. Hooke, likewise, was Lower's friend and fellow student at Christ Church. These associations undoubtedly helped Lower in his fundamental and inspiring work, which demonstrated the influence of the gas "Spiritus Aeris Nitrosus" on the color of the blood.

Richard Lower (1631-91) was born of an affluent family at Tremeer, near Bodmin, in Cornwall, and at the age of seventeen was elected to studentship at Christ Church in Oxford (*45, 93, 109*). Soon thereafter he became research assistant to Thomas Willis, a position he held for ten years, to his and his teacher's great benefit. Indeed, Willis praised him in the introduction of his *Cerebri Anatome* (1664) as "a doctor of outstanding learning and an anatomist of supreme skill. The sharpness of his scalpel and of his intellect ... enabled me to investigate better both the structures and the functions of bodies, whose secrets were previously concealed" (*131*).

The first evidence of Lower's interest in the problem of the effect of air on blood appears in a letter (*109*) written to Boyle on June 24, 1664, in which he proposed to investigate "the reason for the different color of the blood of the veins and arteries: the one being florid and purple red, the other dark and black." In 1665, the year Lower became bachelor and doctor of physics, he published *Diatribae de febribus* (*91*), a tract written to vindicate Willis after a book of his had been attacked by an Irish physician. On that occasion Lower erroneously stated that pulmonary venous blood and pulmonary arterial blood were the same dark color, and that the florid tinge of the peripheral arterial blood therefore required passage through the left ventricle. This misconception was later corrected in *De corde* (*92*), his treatise published in London early in 1669, three years after he had moved there.

In the third chapter of *De corde*, Lower proved beyond any doubt that the function of the pulmonary circulation is the arterialization of

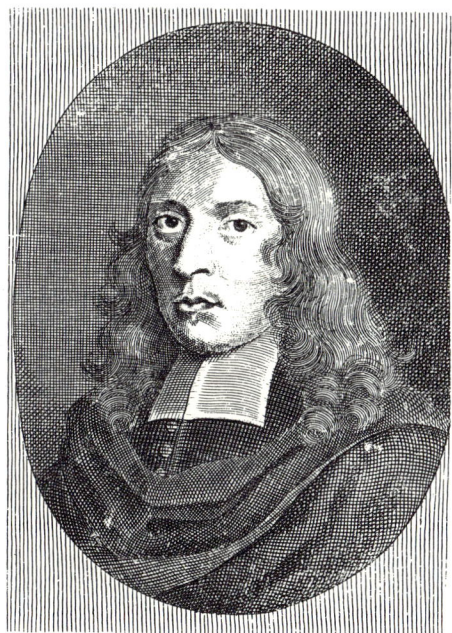

Figure 9. Richard Lower (1631–91). This, the only available portrait supposed to be that of Lower, is probably spurious.

THE HEART

the venous blood. This text, one of the most important in the history of physiology, by the nature of the observations, the rigor of the experimental design and demonstrations, the simple and convincing form of the presentation, the honesty with which his previous error is admitted, and the candid expression of indebtedness to a fellow investigator, deserves to be read in its entirety. Following is a selection from the English translation by K. J. Franklin (93).

"I have spoken elsewhere of the different returns of the two kinds of blood, and of the sources from which they are derived. I have also in the same place discussed their colour-variation, and the cause of this very noticeable difference between them. But as I relied more in this matter on the authority and preconceived opinion of the learned Dr. Willis than on my own experience, and confused too far the torch of life with its torchbearer; as, too, the lapse of time has now taught me differently, I shall not be loth to exchange my former view for a better one. It is not my intention to attack the beliefs and opinions of others, or to bring scorn on myself by changing my own, but what is suggested by reason and confirmed by experience carries more weight with me and will always have my allegiance.

"It is certain then, that the difference in colour, which is found between venous and arterial blood, is quite independent of the heating of the blood in the heart (even if some such heating must be conceded there); for, granted that heating does occur chiefly in the heart, then, as the function of both ventricles is the same, and they do not differ in any other respects than, as stated above, in the strength and thickness of their fibres, why should the colour not undergo a similar change in the right ventricle? But it is quite certain that blood withdrawn from the pulmonary artery is similar in all respects to venous blood, and is only reddish on the surface. Indeed, it will be shown by a very convincing experiment that this fresh red colour is not conferred on the blood by the left ventricle either. For, if the trachea is exposed in the neck and divided, a cork inserted, and the trachea ligatured tightly over it to prevent any ingress of air into the lungs, then the blood flowing from a simultaneous cut in the cervical artery (or, at least, such blood as comes out some time after the asphyxiation of the lung) will be seen to be as completely venous and dark in colour, as if it had flown from a wound in the jugular vein. I have tried this fairly often, and the same truth is more evident still from the fact that the blood within the left ventricle of the heart and the trunk of the aorta of an animal, which has been strangled or has

died a natural death, and in which air is prevented from passing into the blood, is found to be entirely akin to venous blood.

"*Finally, to abolish any possible room for doubt, it occurred to me to make an experiment on a strangled dog, after sensation and life had completely deserted it, and to see if the still-fluid blood in the vena cava would all return equally bright in colour through the pulmonary vein, after being driven to the right ventricle and to the lungs. So I drove on the blood, and carried out a simultaneous insufflation of the perforated lungs. The result corresponded very well with my expectation, for the blood was discharged into the dish as bright-red in colour, as if it were being withdrawn from an artery in a living animal.*

"*I have shown that the bright red colour of arterial blood is not acquired through any heating in the heart or anywhere else at any time. In like manner also the dark colour of venous blood is independent of any extinction of its heat within the veins. For, if this were so, why should the arterial blood not take on a like colour after it has left its vessels, since it has now beyond all doubt lost its heat?*

"*This being so, we must next see to what the blood is indebted for this deep red colouration. This must be attributed entirely to the lungs, as I have found that the blood which enters the lungs completely venous and dark in colour, returns from them quite arterial and bright. For, if the anterior part of the chest is cut away and the lungs are continuously insufflated by a pair of bellows inserted into the trachea, and they are also pricked with a needle in various places to allow free passage of air through them, then, on the pulmonary vein being cut near the left auricle, the blood will flow out into a suitably placed receptacle completely bright red in colour. And, as long as the lungs are supplied with fresh air in this way, the blood will rush out scarlet, until the whole perfusate reaches several ounces, nay pounds, just as if it were being received from a cut artery. What I had written earlier about the blood withdrawn from the pulmonary vein being like venous blood was said as a result of experimental work, but at a time when I did not yet know from experiment that one could keep life in an animal by continuous insufflation of pricked lungs; so that all the air had been forced out of the lung before I was able to seize and to lance the pulmonary vein. I acknowledge my indebtedness to the very famous Master Robert Hooke for this experiment—by which the lungs are kept continuously dilated for a long time without meanwhile endangering the animal's life—and the opportunity thereby given me to perform this piece of work.*

"*If anyone, however, argues that this bright colour of the blood is to be*

[35]

attributed to its fragmentation in the lungs rather than to the mixture of air with the blood, he should consider whether the blood can really be broken into fragments better in the lungs than in the muscles of the body, or even as well. For the lungs are kept constantly dilated for the right conduct of this experiment, and I fail therefore to see how the blood can undergo fragmentation save in passing through their pores, as in the rest of the body-framework.

"Further, that this red colour is entirely due to the penetration of particles of air into the blood, is quite clear from the fact that, while the blood becomes red throughout its mass in the lungs (because the air diffuses in them through all the particles of blood, and hence becomes more thoroughly mixed with the blood), when venous blood is received into a vessel, the surface and uppermost part of it takes on this scarlet colour through exposure to the air. If this is removed with a knife, the part lying next below will soon change to the same colour through similar contact with the air.

"Indeed, if the cake of blood is turned over after remaining stationary for a long while, its outer and uppermost layer takes on the red colour in a short space of time, provided the blood is still fresh. It is a matter of common knowledge that venous blood becomes completely red when received into a dish and shaken up for a long time to cause a thorough penetration of air into it. And let no one be surprised at a loss or admixture of air causing such marked colour-changes in the blood, since we see other fluids also acquiring various colorations, according as their pores take up or refract in greater or lesser amounts the rays of light.

"If you ask me for the paths in the lungs, through which the nitrous spirit of the air [spiritus aeris nitrosus] reaches the blood, and colours it more deeply, do you in turn show me the little pores by which that other nitrous spirit, which exists in snow, passes into the drinks of gourmets and cools their summer wines. For, if glass or metal cannot prevent the passage of this spirit, how much more easily will it penetrate the looser vessels of the lungs? Finally, if we do not deny the outward passage of fumes and of serous fluid, why may we not concede an inward passage of this nitrous foodstuff into the blood through the same or similar little pores?

"On this account it is extremely probable that the blood takes in air in its course through the lungs, and owes its bright colour entirely to the admixture of air. Moreover, after the air has in large measure left the blood again within the body and the parenchyma of the viscera, and has transpired through the *pores of the body, it is equally consistent with reason that the venous blood, which has lost its air, should forthwith appear darker and blacker.*

"From this it is easy to imagine the great advantage accruing to the blood from the admixture of air, and the great importance attaching to the air taken in being always healthy and pure; one can see, too, how greatly in error are those, who altogether deny this intercourse of air and blood. Without such intercourse, any one would be able to live in as good health in the stench of a prison as among the most pleasant vegetation. Wherever, in a word, a fire can burn sufficiently well, there we can equally well breathe."

In the other chapters of *De corde* there are many observations which add to Richard Lower's stature as a great physiologist. For instance, in the first chapter he gives a detailed and accurate description of the anatomical disposition of the cardiac muscle fibers which anticipates by 250 years that given by Hall. The relation of these structures to their function during heart contraction is discussed in the second chapter, where Lower also states that

"*. . . for a proper and regular lung circulation more blood must not be poured out by the right ventricle than can be dispatched by the left; and that the left ventricle designed as it was for heavier work and greater effort than the right had necessarily to excel it far in the strength and thickness of its wall.*"

Finally, in the fourth chapter, he gives an account of a blood transfusion from dog to dog, the first demonstration of the potential safety of a method which three centuries later was to revolutionize surgery.

The merits of Boyle, Hooke, and of Lower particularly, have been somewhat overshadowed by the extraordinary praises indiscriminately lavished upon one of their younger contemporaries at Oxford, John Mayow (1640-74) (*33, 45, 93, 109, 110*).

Mayow has been stamped by many modern commentators (*50*) as one of the greatest of scientists, one who had discovered the compound nature of air, the existence of a special gas essential both for life and for combustion and responsible for the change in color of the blood; in short, one who had preceded Scheele and Priestley in their discovery of oxygen and Lavoisier in his correct interpretation of the role of this gas in combustion and respiration. These claims have been cut down to measure and placed in their proper perspective by T. S. Patterson (*109,*

110) and by J. F. Fulton (45). From their searching examination of the scientific atmosphere and of the contemporary setting in Oxford, and from their comparison of the content and dates of his *Tractatus duo* (99) and *Tractatus quinque* (100) with the work published by Boyle, Hooke, and Lower, Mayow emerges as a very brilliant, precocious, and somewhat unprincipled young man, remarkably adept at grasping and absorbing the ideas and observations of others whose experiments he was privileged to witness, eager to make them his own, and more than reticent in acknowledging their true sources. According to Patterson's convincing arguments, Mayow was decidedly not the first to show that a candle enclosed in a flask goes out while there is still an abundance of air; to infer that air is heterogeneous; to suggest the existence in air of a vital substance to be found also in nitre and nitric acid; to call this substance nitro-aerial spirit; to demonstrate that an animal placed in a closed vessel died more quickly if a live candle were also placed in the vessel; to prove that animals exhaust the air of some constituent necessary to life which entered the blood during breathing; and to deduce that this part of the air was the nitro-aerial spirit. It appears also that Mayow was endowed with a considerable imagination. He thought that the nitro-aerial spirit, posited by Lower before him as a gas necessary to maintain life, was some kind of a *deus ex machina* in chemistry and physics, playing a role somewhat similar to that attributed later to the phlogiston by Stahl's followers. There are, however, two undisputed achievements to his credit: he was the first to demonstrate experimentally the reduction of the volume of air contained within a vessel during respiration, and he extended the law derived by Boyle from his experiment on air to two gases which we now call hydrogen and nitric oxide. These are truly fundamental observations and all his own. Mayow's excellent technique of handling gas was later improved by Stephen Hales, who is usually considered to be the founder of quantitative gasometry.

Properties of Air

Stephen Hales, the clergyman of Teddington (1677-1761), who was particularly interested in plant physiology, made significant observations on the exchange between air and blood. Lavoisier later said that he was "the first who examined the problem from the quantitative point of view; he developed several devices, simple and easy to handle, in order to measure exactly the volume of air." In Vol. I of his *Statical Essays* (1731) (55), Hales described the apparatus making it possible to "take an estimate of the quantity of Air absorbed or fixed or generated by the breath of living animals." In Experiment CVII he measured the amount of air absorbed by breathing, and in Experiment CX he defined the site of absorption, marveling at the vast expanse of the alveolo-capillary membrane:

"... *but some of the elasticity of air which is inspired is destroyed and that chiefly among the vesicles . . . whence probably . . . acid spirits . . . are conveyed in the blood which we see by an admirable contrivance spread into a vast expanse commensurate to a large surface of air from which it is parted by very thin partitions; so very thin as thereby probably to admit the blood and air particles . . . within the reach of each other's attraction, whereby a continued succession of fresh air must be absorbed by the blood.*"

Two years later, in Vol. II of *Statical Essays* (56), he reported measurements made by direct observation of the rate of flow in the lung capillaries of frogs, and he stated that the blood must traverse the lungs with "vastly greater rapidity than through other parts of the body."

With improvement in chemical methods, progress in the characterization of gas was fairly rapid. In 1757 the Scottish chemist, Joseph Black, demonstrated that reactions involving magnesia and other carbonates resulted in a loss of weight and volume of these compounds, and concluded that they contained a *fixed gas* (carbon dioxide) different from atmospheric air. Like Boyle and Hales, Black had also observed the effects of respiration upon the atmospheric air, the reduction in its volume, the change in its nature, and the loss, in the process, of its property of maintaining the life of animals. Eight years later, Henry Cavendish differentiated a second gas from air, which he called *inflammable air* (hydrogen) (33). At this time the picturesque figure of Priestley came upon the scene.

Joseph Priestley (*124, 128, 122, 30*) a Presbyterian minister, interested in theology, history, and grammar, had come to London at the age of thirty in order to meet Benjamin Franklin. Priestley was encouraged by the famous diplomat-scientist to write the *History and Present State of Electricity.* This started him on a scientific career. He became interested in gas chemistry because he lived at Leeds near a brewery, the odoriferous product of which he began to investigate. A self-taught chemist, he acquired an extraordinary skill in manipulating gases, which he applied to his chemical researches. His liberal bent of mind, generous character, and impetuous personality, on the other hand, soon involved him in discussions of religious dogma, in the defense of the American colonists, and in the enthusiastic support of the French Revolution. Indeed, he had to flee for his life from Birmingham after he joined with friends in celebration of the second anniversary of Bastille Day. Two years later he joined his sons in Pennsylvania, where he was greeted with enthusiasm and where he became probably the first Unitarian minister.

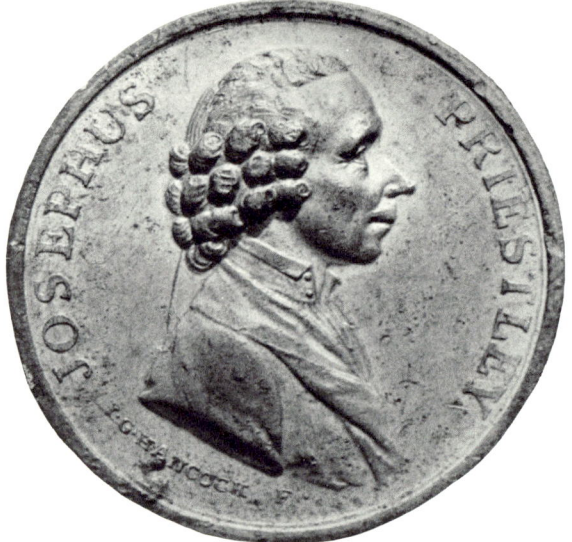

Figure 10. Joseph Priestley (1733–1804) from a silver medal in his honor, cast in 1783.

Although in his religious and political beliefs he was a radical, in his theoretical scientific thinking he was extremely conservative. Because of this conservatism he was never able to interpret his major discovery correctly.

Between 1772 and 1774 he had rediscovered Black's *fixed air* and characterized several nitrous gas compounds (*30*). On August 1, 1774, he isolated, by heating *mercuric red oxide* in a closed container, a gas in which a candle "burned ... with remarkably vigorous flame ... and a piece of red hot wood sparkled in it ... and consumed very fast." In March, 1775, he demonstrated that mice lived longer in the new gas than in an equal volume of atmospheric air. This gas he called *dephlogisticated air* (oxygen), and shortly thereafter he characterized a second gas in the atmospheric air, *phlogisticated air* (nitrogen). Although in the remarkable experiments described in *Experiments and Observations in Different Kinds of Air (30)*, Priestley had shown that *dephlogisticated air* was essential for the maintenance of life, and although he demonstrated that this gas was given off by plants, his contribution to the elucidation of the process of exchange between air and blood in the lungs was not crucial. Intellectually unprepared to break with the traditional theory of the *phlogiston*, the universal chemical entity created by Stahl, Priestley clung to an explanation of the phenomena of respiration and of calcination of metals that was exactly the reverse of what is known now to be true: "the function of the blood is not to receive the phlogiston of the air, or to meet with the phlogisticated air while it circulates, but to communicate phlogiston to air. One should therefore not expect that air is corrected by red blood in the same way that it is vitiated by dark blood" *(114)*. According to this theory, in heating a pure metal, which was then considered to be a complex substance, phlogiston was given off to ambient air and thereby the volume of dephlogisticated air was reduced. The metallic oxide thus formed was considered to be the simple substance and the question of weight change was simply solved by invoking the property of "levity" or negative weight possessed by phlogiston. Similarly, venous blood, in its passage through the lungs, lost its phlogiston, and its arterialization was accompanied by a reduction of the *dephlogisticated air*. A new light was needed to give a "clear and economical explanation instead of a confused one" *(124)*.

Antoine Laurent Lavoisier (1743-94) was born in Paris and spent all his life there. After a brilliant education, humanistic and scientific, he showed himself to be an exceptional man by the breadth of his activities and by his intellectual and practical gifts. A great administrator who served his government, a successful financier, a political economist, a versatile scientist who contributed to mineralogy, agronomy, pure and applied chemistry, and physiology, Lavoisier was able to pursue his several and parallel enterprises not only with order and method but

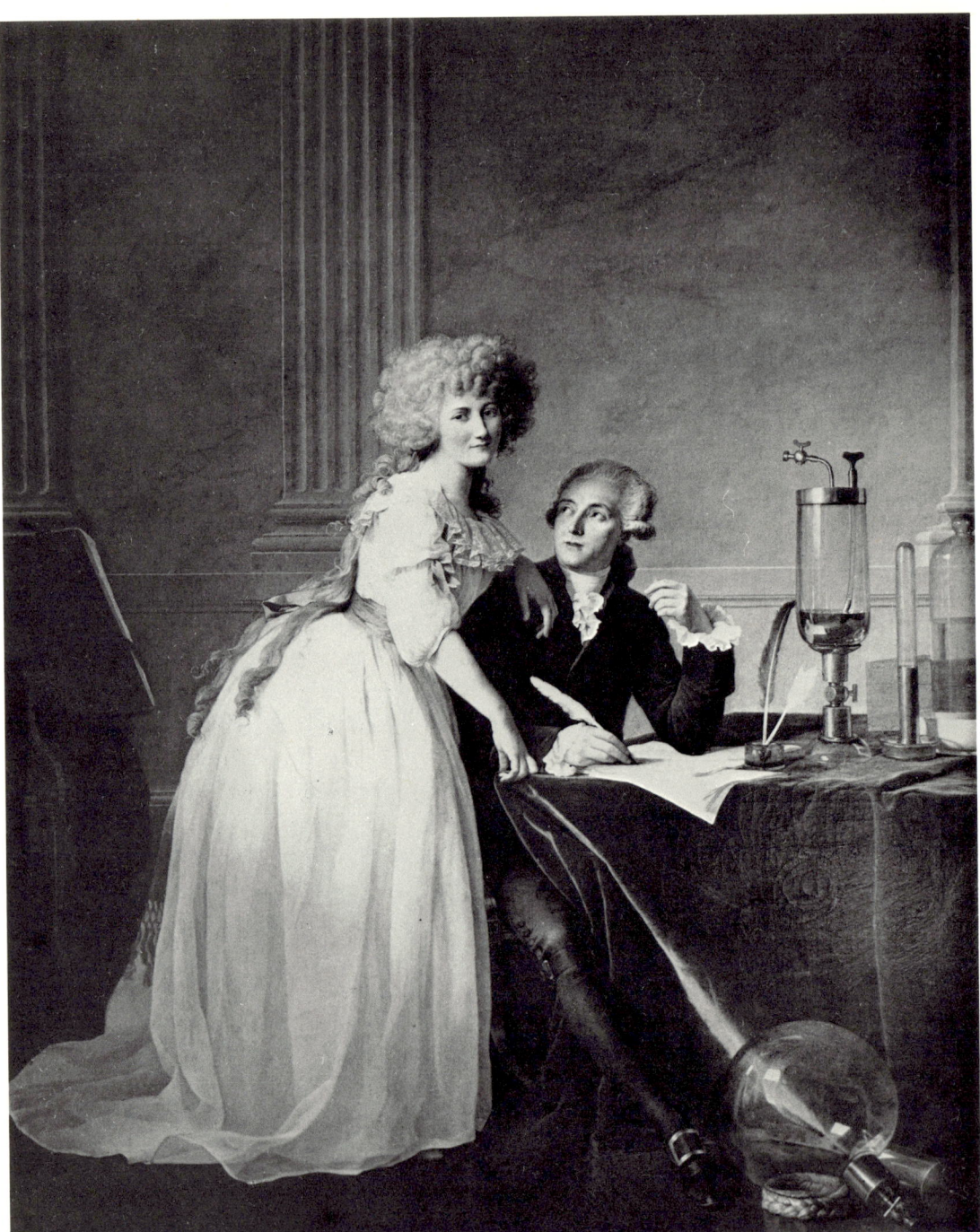

with considerable effectiveness and authority. Happy in all his endeavors, his marriage to a girl of fourteen, Marie Anne Paulze, proved to be a great asset to his career: she took notes of his experiments, translated scientific articles by English chemists, sketched and engraved illustrations for his publications, and also acted as a hostess in their luxurious home, open to French and foreign philosophers, writers, and scientists. Lavoisier maintained close relations with the physiocrats, and became one of the most active representatives of the enlightened and liberal *haute bourgeoisie*, who played an essential role in bringing about reforms to the authoritarian monarchic institutions. At the advent of the Revolution, he collaborated with the governing body of the National Assembly, but when demagogy, violence, and dictatorship prevailed, he became one of the victims of the Terror. Arrested on the denunciation of one of his former subordinates and convicted on a false charge, he was guillotined on May 8, 1794, at the age of fifty. Hearing of this tragic death, the famous mathematician Lagrange exclaimed, "It took only one moment to sever that head, and perhaps a century will not be enough to produce another like it" (*124, 128, 32, 21, 34*).

His research in chemistry, begun at the Académie des Sciences, to which he was elected at the age of twenty-five (1768), proceeded from 1775 in the laboratory he built at the Arsenal (the seat of the state controlled manufacture of gunpowder) of which he was, for practical purposes, the director. This research, which culminated in the discovery that respiration is a combustion, is impressive for its continuity in design, perseverance in effort, and application of precise physical methods. The inflexible law which dominated its progress was:

"... *to simplify as much as possible the mental process of reasoning* ... *which is the only source of error; to test theory continuously against experience: never to retain facts which are not given by Nature; to look for truth in the natural development of experiment and observation in the same manner that mathematicians reach the solution of a problem by arranging the given premises in the most simple way and reducing reasoning to so elementary an operation and so short a judgment that they never lose sight of the evidence which*

Figure 11. Portrait by David of Lavoisier and Madame Lavoisier.

guides them ... never to proceed but from the known to the unknown, never to deduce any consequence that does not derive immediately from experiments or observations" (*77*).

THE HEART His lucid mind and his education in mathematics and the physical sciences were reflected in the clarity of his style and by the choice of the proper term to define his thought. He was well informed and made use of the experimental results obtained by other scientists, benefiting from the improvement in communications among scientific men, which made science more and more a co-operative effort. The conversation that he held in Paris with Priestley, whom he met in the fall of 1774, and the thorough analysis that he made of the translation of the second edition of Priestley's book (*114*) undoubtedly provided precious food to his power of reasoning (*30*). He may also have used some valuable suggestions included in a letter from Scheele (*10*), the extraordinarily talented Swedish pharmacist, who probably anticipated Priestley in isolating and characterizing the "*fire air,*" analogous to the *dephlogisticated air*. Between 1772 and 1786, Lavoisier discovered an impressive number of organic compounds.

Be that as it may, ideas, and not facts alone, were to revolutionize the problems of combustion, calcination, and respiration. By combining "a rigorous technique of analysis [with] an incomparable synthetic mind," Lavoisier was able "to group in a coherent system, separated facts [observed by him or] discovered by his predecessors and his contemporaries" (*128*).

On November 1, 1772, Lavoisier deposited at the Académie des Sciences a sealed note containing his observations on the weight gained by sulfur and phosphorus by burning, which was "due to prodigious quantities of air which [are] fixed" (*78*). He immediately extended this notion to the process of metallic calcination and demonstrated its reversibility: "during the transformation of a calx to metal a considerable quantity of air was liberated." Soon after he met Priestley he started to use mercuric red oxide in his experiments. At the Easter meeting (1775) of the Academy (*79*), he reiterated that "the principle combining with metals during their calcination and augmenting their weight is nothing else than the pure portion of air which surrounds us [and] which we breathe ..." and he established the fundamental distinction that reduction of the metallic calx with coal resulted in the production of *fixed air*, whereas its reduction without coal resulted in the production of the *eminently respirable air*. He concluded therefore "that the principle, called up to now *fixed air*, is the combination of the portion of *eminently respirable air* [liberated by heating the calx] with the carbon." From then on the links of his discovery that respiration is a combustion were forged slowly but solidly.

In his essay, *Experiments on the respiration of animals and on the changes affecting air in its passage through the lungs (80)*, read at the Academy on May 3, ·1777, Lavoisier was not yet ready to make an unequivocal statement on respiration, but his ideas on this subject were near to attaining their final form. By a series of beautiful experiments that

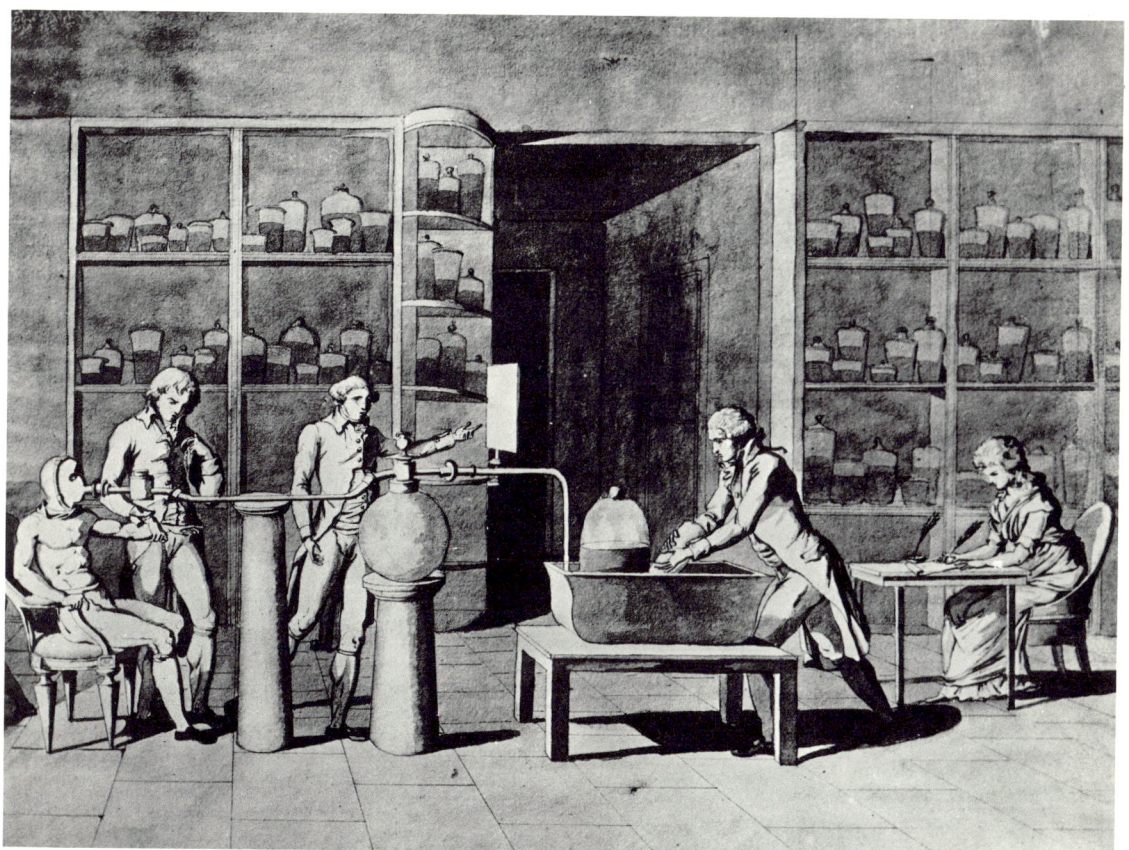

Figure 12. Lavoisier in his laboratory. A drawing by Madame Lavoisier. Séguin is the subject.

display his physiological and chemical mastery, he developed conclusions that still hold true:

"Eminently respirable air that enters the lung, leaves it in the form of chalky aeriform acid [CO_2] *... in almost equal volume....*

"Respiration only acts on the portion of pure air that is eminently respirable ... the excess, that is, its mephitic portion [nitrogen], *is a purely passive medium which enters and leaves the lung ... without change or alteration.*

"The respirable portion of air has the property to combine with blood and its combination results in its red color."

As to the source of chalky aeriform acid he was still in doubt. In the same year, in an essay *On combustion in general (81)*, he supported the hypothesis that the *eminently respirable air* participates in the lung in a reaction similar to that observed in the combustion of carbon; between inspiration and expiration the *chalky aeriform acid* is formed, and *the matter of fire* (which he later called *caloric*) is distributed with the blood in the whole animal economy to maintain body temperature. In the essay *On heat (82)*, published three years later in collaboration with Laplace, in which precise methods of calorimetry are presented, it is specified that maintenance of animal heat is due, at least in great part, to the heat produced by the combination of pure air breathed by animals with the *base of fixed air* supplied by the blood. "Respiration is a combustion, indeed very slow and perfectly similar to that of carbon."

Finally, in his first publication with Séguin, *On the respiration of animals (83)*, there is no longer any equivocation as to the mechanism of the combustion characteristic of respiration:

"Respiration is not limited only to the combustion of carbon but causes a combustion of part of hydrogen contained in blood, and therefore results not only in the formation of the gas carbonic acid but of water, which explains perfectly well the phenomenon observed [in collaboration with Laplace, i.e. a larger release of heat than that expected from the formation of carbon dioxide alone].

"On the basis of what we know, and in limiting ourselves to simple ideas, that anyone can easily understand, we shall generally state that respiration is a slow combustion of carbon analogous to that operating in a lamp or in a lighted

candle, and that *from this point of view animals which breathe are really combustible substances burning and consuming themselves.*

"*In respiration, as in combustion, the atmospheric air supplies the oxygen and the* caloric; *but since, in respiration it is the substance itself of the animal, the blood which supplies the combustible, if the animals were not replacing usually by food what they lose by respiration, the lamp would be short of oil, and the animal perish, just as the lamp goes out when it lacks nourishment.*"

The concluding paragraph of this essay is revealing:

"*No experiment decisively proves that carbonic acid exhaled during expiration is formed in the lung itself or in the circulation by combination of the oxygen of the air with the carbon of the blood. It is possible that carbonic acid is formed by digestion, introduced in the circulation by the lymphatics, finally that* reaching the lung it is released from the blood while oxygen combines with it (the blood) by means of a superior affinity" (emphasis added).

In April, 1790, he reiterated that, in addition to occurring in the lung, combustion of the blood might take place "perhaps in other parts of the body" *(84).*

At the peak of his scientific career Lavoisier summed up the development of his physiological studies:

"*The animal machine is governed by three main regulating systems: respiration, which consumes oxygen and carbon, and supplies the caloric; the transpiration, which increases or diminishes, depending on whether it is necessary to eliminate more or less of the caloric; finally, digestion, which returns to the blood what it loses by respiration and transpiration.*"

New terms mark the development of his ideas: the *eminently respirable* portion of the common air became vital air, which supplied the *principle oxygine*—later called oxygen (etymologically, to engender acid)—together with the *caloric* element. These replaced the phlogiston, discarded because of its vagueness, its explaining too much rather than too little, like "a real Proteus changing its form every minute." But Lavoisier had not overthrown the theory without paying tribute to Stahl for two fundamental observations: that metals are combustible, and that this combustible property is transmissible; these indeed had served him as a beacon.

Lavoisier's theory that a gas was made of a principle (oxygen or nitrogen, etc.) that supplied its physico-chemical characteristics and properties, and of caloric, a fundamental constituent of matter included with light among the elements, was useful, but eventually was also laid aside. What endured was an assimilation of biological processes to chemico-physical reactions and the emphasis on quantitative measurements in physiological research.

Nearly half a century after Lavoisier's death, Gustav Magnus (95) properly placed the site of combustion in the body tissues, by determining and comparing the oxygen and the carbon dioxide content in the veins and in the arteries.

Adaptation of Pulmonary Circulation to Respiratory Gas Exchange

By the middle of the nineteenth century, physiology was on its way to becoming a major science: it had by then defined its method and renounced vitalistic explanations; and it was invigorated by novel developments in experimental design and instrumentation. Progress was particularly impressive in the German universities, where administrative autonomy and largesse in supplying equipment favored the assertion of strong personalities. Through the efforts of the French and German physiologists, the physiologic features of the pulmonary circulation began to be recognized and to be distinguished from those of the systemic circulation. Foremost among the contributions of this period were the blood pressure measurements obtained in Ludwig's laboratory in Leipzig on open chest preparations, and by Chauveau and Marey in Paris in the intact animal. These measurements provided experimental support for the explanation advanced by Harvey for the difference between the wall thickness of the two ventricles:

"[The] wall [of the right ventricle] is three times as thin as that of the left ventricle.... The lungs are spongy, loose in texture and soft, and hence less force is required to extrude blood into them ... the left ventricle needs greater strength and force to have extended its influence upon the blood throughout the whole of the body" (De motu cordis, Chapter 17).

The major contributions to cardiovascular physiology of Carl Ludwig (1816-95) and his school are reserved for another chapter. It is sufficient to note here that in 1852, one of Ludwig's early students, A. Beutner, using Ludwig's manometer, recorded pressures in the pulmonary artery of rabbits, cats, and dogs (*17*). After opening the chest, a cannula was inserted in the left pulmonary artery and all or most branches were tied; under these conditions the mean blood pressure was found to be four to five times lower than that in the aorta, the values varying from 14 to 23 mm. Hg according to the size of the experimental animal.

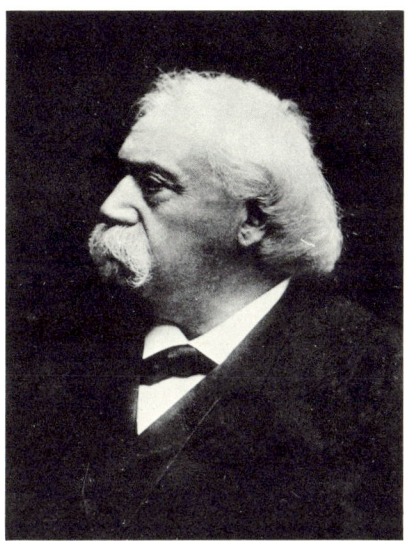 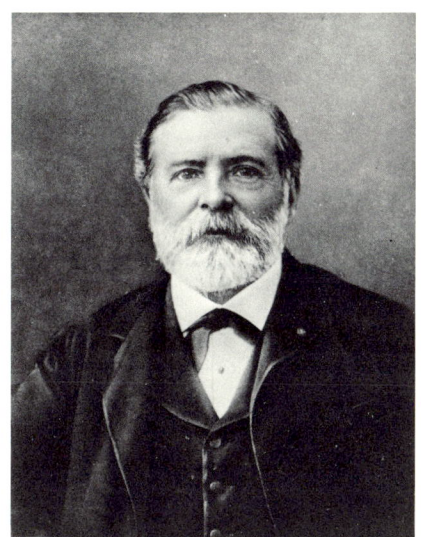

Figure 13. Auguste Chauveau.   *Figure* 14. Étienne Jules Marey.

Auguste Chauveau (1827-1917), a professor of veterinary medicine in Lyons, who had previously performed many experiments on the horse, collaborated in 1861 (*24*) with Jules Marey (1830-1904), a brilliant Parisian physician who, extending the instrumentation created by Ludwig, devised air-filled manometers for the graphic registration of biological phenomena. In order to record pressures in the pulmonary circulation, the French physiologists had the idea of introducing a long catheter with a double lumen through the jugular vein into the right heart cavities of an unanesthetized horse. In some experiments they simultaneously introduced a second, specially designed catheter into the left ventricle through the carotid artery. They then recorded systolic pressures in the right and left ventricles. These averaged 27 and 129 mm. Hg, respectively, whereas the end diastolic pressure in the left ventricle was nearly atmospheric. In two cases they also reported (97) a mean pressure in the pulmonary artery five times lower than in the aorta. There has been much debate about the significance of the contour of the curves obtained by the use of long catheters connected with air-filled manometric systems. It was only in 1912 and in 1914 that Wiggers, using high frequency manometers built according to the specifications of Frank, obtained, in the exposed pulmonary artery, curves worthy of detailed hemodynamic analysis. Nonetheless, the blood pressure levels recorded by Chauveau and Marey were correct and the general form of the curves was not grossly distorted.

Chauveau later performed important research in body energetics. It is not generally known that in 1863 he had prophetically written: "Contagion proceeds always from a special agent, the *virus, organism or organite, which cannot be created spontaneously*" (italics added). Marey (23), on the other hand, continued to create innumerable and ingenious laboratory instruments; he also used photography in order to record and analyze motion in many of its physiological aspects, and was far along in developing moving-picture photography when this process was first described by A. Lumière (23).

In the second half of the nineteenth century a method of measuring pulmonary blood flow also became available. This will be discussed in another chapter.

The question of the effects of respiratory movements upon the pulmonary blood flow and vascular resistance was the next to arouse interest. As a matter of fact, the correct answer to the question had in the main already been given by Albrecht von Haller (1708-77) in the second half of the eighteenth century.

This Swiss naturalist and poet had been the librarian of the city of Bern and president of the Academy of Hanover before he became the first holder of the chair of Medicine at the University of Göttingen. In 1760, he reported some experiments on the perfusion of frog lungs with dye (57). By varying the ventilatory volume of their exposed lungs, he observed that when moderately inflated, the pulmonary blood flow was greater than when the lungs were collapsed or ventilated under pressure. Thus began a controversy which was finally terminated, more than one hundred years later, in 1881, by two Belgian physiologists, Héger (*61, 62*) and Spehl (*62*), who presented rather conclusive evidence that the observations of Haller held true in the closed chest animal. In their well-controlled experiments on rabbits, Héger and Spehl used a procedure employed previously by Claude Bernard, which permitted the simultaneous ligature of pulmonary artery and veins after closure of the chest. They concluded that "the amount of blood inthrusted in the lungs during natural respiration is the greatest; the greatest amount coming from the venous return and the rest from distension of the pulmonary vessels."

Between 1760 and 1881 the effects of respiration upon the circulation had been studied exhaustively in several laboratories; these studies led to important technological and experimental developments, to the collection of valuable data concerning the pulmonary circulation, and to heated arguments among investigators engaged in them.

Early in the nineteenth century, François Magendie (1783-1855), the French physician and physiologist who was the teacher of Claude Bernard, had supported Haller's idea.

". . . the actual cause of the progression from artery to vein is the right ventricular ejection. . . . During inspiratory distension the passage is easy, during expiration when the lungs contain less air it is more difficult. It is also more likely that these vessels are dilated and contracted according to the volume of blood flow, and possibly for other reasons. When the lung expands it attracts air and blood at the same time" (*94*).

Magendie's opinion was not based on new experimental evidence; it was disputed in the year of his death by J. Poiseuille (1799-1869), the French physicist and physician, who, after completing his studies on the law regulating the flow of fluid in small tubes, was engaged in transferring his experimental results from the field of physics to that of physiology. By an a priori reasoning he postulated the elongation of capillaries during inspiration; he did not consider the possibility of simultaneous radial traction. He studied the effects of ventilation upon the herniated frog lung, and observed that blood flow was slower during chest distension (*112*). However, he failed to implicate positive inflation and to contrast its effect with that of natural inspiration. The same lack of discrimination between these opposite effects caused considerable confusion until Lichtheim (*86*) produced experimental evidence that natural inspiration and insufflation under positive pressure had opposite effects upon the blood pressures in the pulmonary artery.

The controversy was nonetheless very fruitful in several respects. First, a method of artificial circulation with defibrinated blood was developed and perfected; its use was extended later to the heart-lung preparation, which was adapted by Fühner and Starling to the study of the pulmonary circulation. With this method it became possible to control and to vary all mechanical factors and to measure pulmonary arterial, left atrial, and systemic pressures under selected conditions and combinations of inflow and outflow (43). Second, the separate and joint effects of thoracic pressures on venous return and of the lung's elasticity on the resistance to flow in the small vessels were assessed; in this respect the work of Jacques Arsène d'Arsonval (1851-1940) was particularly convincing. This physician, Claude Bernard's assistant, had a solid background in physics, of which he made liberal use later in medicine. In 1877, in his inaugural thesis (2), d'Arsonval objectively demonstrated that, in the animal with closed chest and perfused with blood through the vena cava, blood flow through the right heart and through the lungs increased during distension of the chest cage produced by traction on the diaphragm. He remarked significantly, "the largest amount of air in the lungs coincides with the largest amount of blood present." Third, an important observation was made by Cohnheim and Litten (28) when they noted that all small vessels in the lungs are not perfused at the same time and with equivalent volume. As a result, they postulated that in the low pressure pulmonary circulation the least variation of resistance in the lungs would affect local flow, thus anticipating the modern concept of interrelations between alveolar ventilation and capillary perfusion.

In addition to concluding a period during which much had been learned of the pulmonary circulation and of its relation to the mechanics of the thorax and of the lungs, Héger and Spehl (62) also provided the first estimation of the pulmonary blood volume during inspiration and expiration, amounting respectively to one-twelfth and one-seventeenth of the total blood volume. These figures would correspond, in a man of average size, to approximately 350-400 ml. of blood within the pulmonary blood vessels exclusively; they agree with estimates based on precise anatomical measurements.

By 1880 the mechanical factors affecting blood circulation through the lungs were known and had been experimentally analyzed, and the notion of low resistance in the small vessels relative to that in the systemic vessels was established. These characteristics were consistent with the large volume of blood flow and also constituted a necessary condition for the maintenance of respiratory gas exchange between alveolar air and capillary blood. In 1872, Brown-Séquard had described a sympathetic supply to the lung vessels; shortly thereafter, the question of whether it played a role in controlling pulmonary vascular resistance became an important issue.

Badoud (3), in Fick's laboratory, was the first to demonstrate a pressure rise in the pulmonary artery after stimulation of the sympathetic track in the cervical region and along the brain stem up to the pons. However, since the pressure in the aorta rose simultaneously, the significance of the rise was questioned. Indeed, Badoud suggested that the rise in the pulmonary artery was secondary to the pressure rise in the aorta and left ventricle following generalized vasoconstriction of the

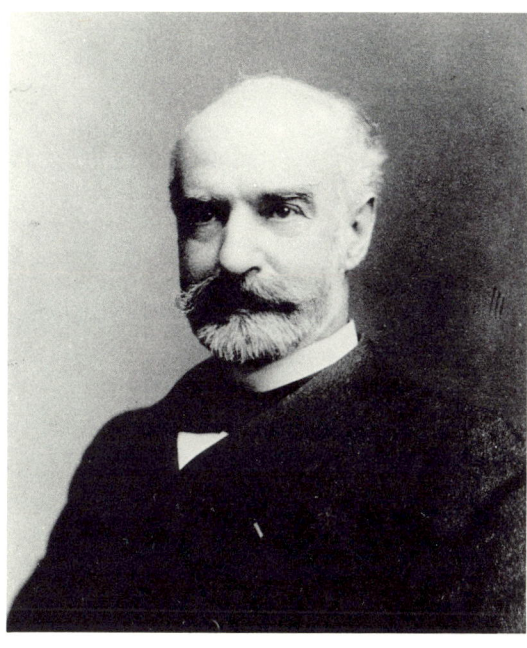

Figure 15. Charles Émile François-Franck (1849–1921).

systemic arterioles. To Charles Émile François-Franck (1849-1921) must be attributed the merit of having been the first to emphasize the difficulties encountered in investigating the pulmonary vasomotor system and the importance of controlling the backward effects of simultaneous change in the systemic circulation.

The results of François-Franck's experiments were first presented at the Société de Biologie in 1880, and recorded in its transactions (*40*); they were discussed in detail by Lalesque in his medical thesis (*76*), published in 1881. Lalesque, who worked in François-Franck's laboratory and reported his opinions and experiments, wrote:

"It is therefore essential to eliminate modifications in the systemic circulation in order to recognize the localized effects on the pulmonary vessels. This can be done by stimulation of the first dorsal ganglia, after section of their connection above and below, or by stimulation of the branches issuing from the ganglia. Under these conditions, if one records simultaneously the pressures in the left atrium and in the right ventricle, it will be observed that during stimulation the pressure drops in the left atrium and the systolic pressure increases in the right ventricle."

In order to magnify the variations of pressure in the left atrium, François-Franck had substituted sodium sulphate for mercury in the U-tube manometer.

In two subsequent papers (*41, 42*), published in 1895, François-Franck called attention to his prior work, added some new information, illustrated his findings abundantly, and finally paid tribute to the conclusiveness of the observations made by Bradford and Dean (*20*) between 1889 and 1894 on the effect of sympathetic stimulation on pulmonary vasomotricity. He also recorded an increase in the pulmonary blood volume by oncography during the period of stimulation. He gave a most provocative interpretation of this finding, which was somewhat unexpected in view of the drop in left atrial pressure; he assumed that the dilated vessels upstream to the constricted small vessels had incarcerated enough blood to more than compensate for the expected downstream reduction in blood volume.

In the introduction to these two papers, François-Franck commented that "there is still some doubt among physiologists as to the exact influence of the sympathetic system upon the vasomotricity of the pulmonary vessels." After his experiments and those of Bradford and Dean, there could be no more doubt that this action could be elicited in experimental preparations. Nonetheless, eighty years later, there is still some question as to whether under normal physiological conditions the autonomic nervous system participates to any significant degree in the control of pulmonary vascular resistance. By and large, this resistance, although influenced by lung elasticity, appears chiefly dependent upon the balance between right and left ventricular inflow and outflow, and their effects upon the vascular walls.

In the course of their investigation, Bradford and Dean had observed that during asphyxia the pulmonary arterial pressure rose, but the experimental conditions did not then permit an exact analysis of a phenomenon which has led recently to one of the most fruitful hypotheses concerning the control of the pulmonary circulation, namely, that respiratory gases themselves affect pulmonary vascular resistance and local blood flow.

In severe asphyxia, as induced by Bradford and Dean, the resulting failure of the left heart had rendered difficult the interpretation of the effects of hypoxia and of hypercapnia upon the pulmonary vascular resistance. Local effects on the lung vessels had to be distinguished from their general effects. It was not until 1942 that the action of hypoxia upon isolated dog lung was studied by Beyne (*12*) in Leon Binet's laboratory in Paris; he attributed the observed pressure rise in the pulmonary artery to the increase in blood flow. Then, in 1946, von Euler and Liljestrand (*36*) started a series of experiments on cats which demonstrated that hypoxia and hypercapnia caused an increase in pulmonary vascular resistance, even after sympathetic denervation. Enlarging the problem, Liljestrand (*88*) formulated the hypothesis that the partial pressure of respiratory gases in the alveoli and in the capillary blood regulated the vascular resistance locally, in such a manner that an optimum relationship was maintained between local alveolar ventilation and blood perfusion. This attractive hypothesis has received experimental support very recently. It is quite fitting that it should have been formulated by Liljestrand, one of the only two now surviving of the great physiologists of the early twentieth century who investigated the factors influencing the transfer of gases between alveolar air and capillary blood.

Physico-chemical Basis of Alveolar-capillary Gas Exchange

The branch of cardiovascular physiology dealing with the precise physico-chemical relation between the respiratory gases in the alveoli and in the capillary blood in the lungs, which was first given substance by Priestley and Lavoisier, had to wait, for further definition, upon new knowledge of the blood itself.

The early period of this development began in the nineteenth century in Germany, as the intense scientific renaissance of that country was gathering momentum. Most of the important discoveries in the beginning were isolated findings, separate and individual strands which only later were woven into the whole fabric.

It has been noted that Gustav Magnus (95), as early as 1837, measured oxygen, nitrogen, and carbon dioxide in blood, finding oxygen higher and CO_2 lower in arterial blood than in venous blood. In 1851, Otto Funke (47, 48) found hemoglobin in the blood of the spleen. Six years later, Lothar Meyer (101), working with Carl Ludwig in Vienna, made measurements of oxygen uptake by hemoglobin; this relation was further developed by Hoppe-Seyler (71, 72) who demonstrated, in 1864, the loose combination of oxygen with the hemoglobin of the red blood cell. The most fundamental fact of all, that the tissues use oxygen and discharge CO_2—lungs and blood being therefore no more than a conveyor system—was realized gradually by a succession of discoveries. Mayer in 1845 showed that animals draw energy from oxidative processes (98); Liebig started his extended studies of the chemical components of tissues and their metabolism at about the same time (87). Final proof of energy exchange in tissues was provided by Pflüger in 1872 (111).

The time was ripe for a first-class investigator to devote himself continuously to the large problem of the physiology of respiratory gas exchange. This task was undertaken by Christian Bohr (1855-1911) (123). In 1883, this young physiologist from Copenhagen came to study with Carl Ludwig in Leipzig, and two years later, on a return visit to the same laboratory, he became interested in the combination of oxygen with hemoglobin. When he was called back to Copenhagen to head the department of physiology in 1885, he decided to institute a methodical inquiry into the relations both of oxygen and carbon

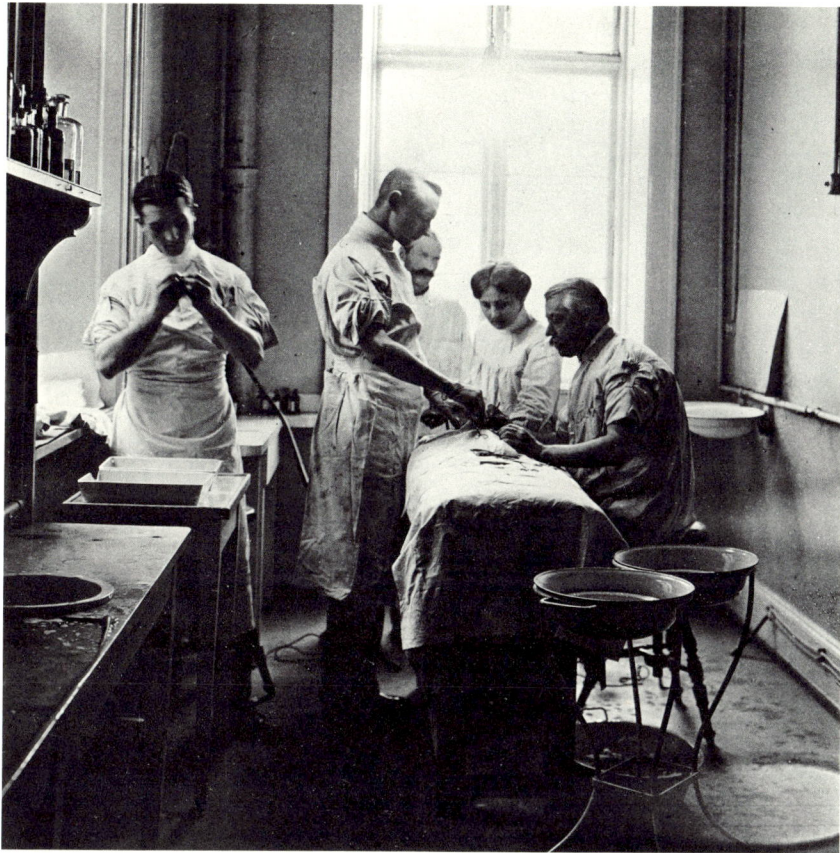

Figure 16. Christian Bohr (seated, right) and his associates, at work in his laboratory. The young man at the left, by the window, is George Fahr.

dioxide in blood and other fluids. This occupied him, in its many aspects, for twenty years. His crowning achievement was the paper published in 1904, with his two brilliant young students, August Krogh and K. A. Hasselbalch (*16*), in which the effects of CO_2 tension on the binding of oxygen by hemoglobin was demonstrated, with a full set of oxygen dissociation curves at varying CO_2 tensions.

Further inquiry led Bohr to the conclusion that alveolar-arterial oxygen differences were inadequate to explain oxygen uptake in the arterial blood, and that therefore there must be active "secretion" of oxygen by the lungs into the blood (*15*).

THE HEART

The commanding figure of August Krogh (1874–1949), leading the way in so many fields of comparative and human physiology, will be met with repeatedly in the succeeding chapters of this book. Here, at the beginning of his career, it is interesting to note how promptly and powerfully he concentrated on one of the central problems. Having first assumed, with his chief, the secretion of oxygen in the lungs, he soon came to doubt this. In the course of the ensuing decade, using his invention of the microtonometer for measurement of gas tensions in blood, and aided by his wife, Marie Krogh (75), he was able to show that oxygen pressure was always higher in alveolar air than in arterial blood, and that diffusion alone therefore was enough to explain pulmonary gas exchange. "In a series of papers," wrote Barcroft, "which are at once a model of certainty of touch and modesty in presentation, [Krogh] has revised the whole field of the relation of oxygen pressures in the blood and the alveolar air, insofar as it can be revised by methods of this kind" (8).

During the early decades of the twentieth century, Krogh and his students, especially J. Lindhard and G. Liljestrand, continued their activities, particularly on the problem of blood as carrier of oxygen and carbon dioxide in exercise, and on the measurement of the output of the heart. This will be reviewed in the next chapter.

The further study of the physical chemistry of the blood in relation to the respiratory gases became a special objective of the British-American school of cardio-circulatory and respiratory physiologists, a group then at the height of their achievements. In its long history, physiology has brought together many interesting men, but it is doubtful whether any such group of individuals has been at once more brilliant, more broadly and philosophically inclined, or more varied in character from one individual to another than the members of this British-American school.

In the particular field before us, the three notable contributors whose work we shall look into are Haldane, Barcroft, and Henderson.

Early in his career, John Scott Haldane (1860–1936) was interested in the problems of coal miners, and the gases to which they were exposed. With Lorrain Smith (54), he studied the question of whether there were "poisonous" gases liberated in the expired air itself. He found that there were not, but he also noted the remarkable sensitivity of respiration to one of the gases in the "vitiated" expired air, namely, carbon dioxide. This led to an extended series of brilliant investigations (53), involving both CO_2 and oxygen, their concentrations in air and blood, and the relations between them; much of it concerned with respiration, but much with respiration and circulation together. An important milestone in this work was the measurement of the CO_2 dissociation curves of blood, which demonstrated that the curve of reduced blood is some seven volumes per cent higher than that of oxygenated blood in the physiological range (27).

Haldane insisted, throughout his life, upon oxygen secretion by the lungs into the blood as a necessary mechanism, especially under conditions of stress, and he very plainly found fault with the techniques of Krogh, Barcroft, and others who doubted this (53).

Joseph Barcroft (1872–1947), was born in Dublin, went to Cambridge as a young man, studied physiology under Michael Foster, and worked

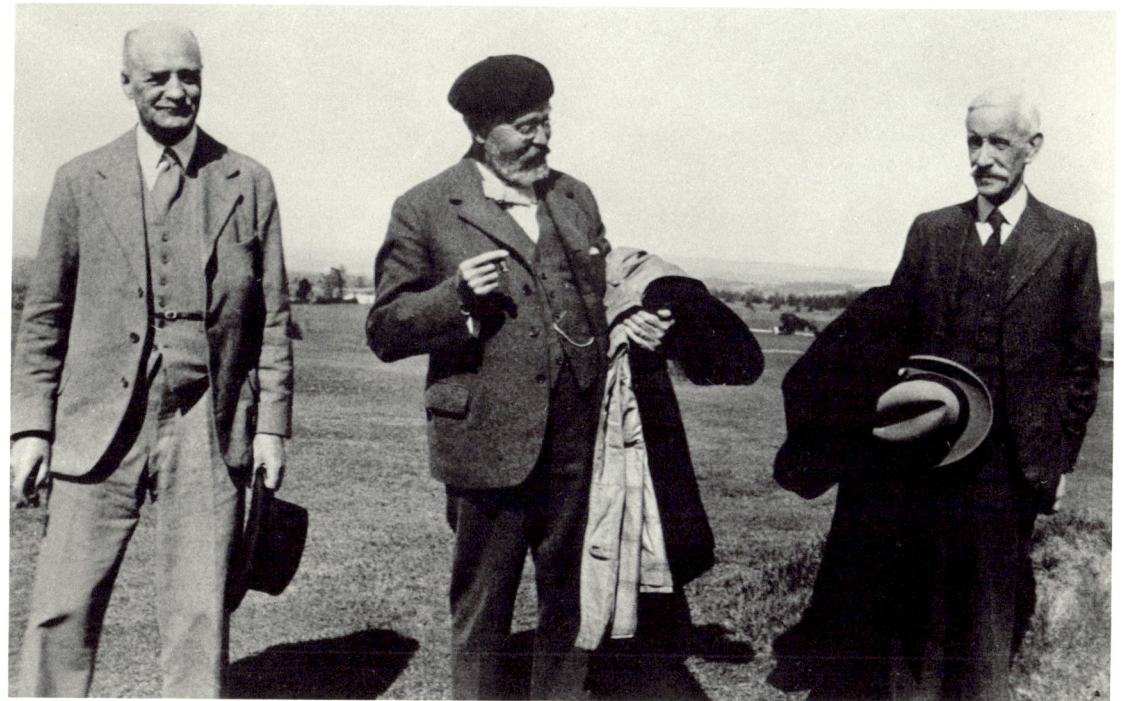

Figure 17. Joseph Barcroft, Lawrence J. Henderson, and F. Gowland Hopkins, in 1936.

at Cambridge the rest of his active life. In his early years he took as his special field (*7*) the "respiratory function of the blood." He measured oxygen dissociation curves and showed the influence of salts and acids upon them. Later he discovered different kinds of hemoglobin, and inquired into the effects of high and low atmospheric pressures upon blood gases and gas exchange. On the subject of diffusion versus oxygen secretion in the lungs, he agreed with Krogh, as we have seen, and disagreed with Bohr and Haldane. At various times in his career he organized expeditions to high altitudes, and he and his colleagues made notable contributions in high altitude physiology (*8*).

His enterprise, his free and prolific imagination, and his experimental skill were joined with an unfailing kindness and a whimsical and gay good humor. Barcroft's charming and lovable character set the tone for this entire group of kindred spirits. Their relations were spirited, friendly, stimulating, and argumentative, and they all enjoyed themselves immensely. Who could forget those meetings of the Physiological Society, when Barcroft's little terriers were scampering around the laboratory, their externalized spleens alternately swelling in contentment, or shrinking with excitement; especially when Barcroft would bring forth a cat at an appropriate moment, just to add zest to their canine emotions?

All the studies thus far mentioned, relating to the physical chemistry of the blood, have been threads of the fabric, but the fabric was not yet one piece. The synthesis, the integration of "blood as a physico-chemical system" had still to be done. This was the achievement of Lawrence J. Henderson (1878–1942) of Harvard. After taking his undergraduate and medical degrees there, he visited the chemist Hofmeister in Germany for a brief period; then returned to Harvard, and began, more or less on his own, an inquiry into the equilibrium between carbon dioxide, carbonic acid, and bicarbonate in water solutions (*63–65*). Great things came from Henderson's contemplation of this apparently simple system. The concept of the acid-base balance in biological systems, hitherto no more than hinted at, took form. It was further developed by many others. Henderson advanced his fundamental idea also into a broader philosophical expression with his essay, *The Fitness of the Environment* (*66*). In a second, *The Order of Nature* (*67*), he pursued the concept of fitness to its logical conclusion and argued for teleology as a positive and necessary tenet in the philosophy of organic mechanism.

The development in physiology itself is summed up in Henderson's classic, *Blood: A Study in General Physiology* (*69*). In this he also described much of the progressive sequence of his thought:

> *"When years ago Barcroft completed his studies which defined the relation between oxygenation of blood, oxygen pressure, and carbon dioxide pressure, and I explained the condition of the acid base equilibrium, each of us not unnaturally supposed that the problems we had studied were solved. We were studying different aspects of the same thing, but we did not recognize the fact, for the nature of the phenomenon escaped us."*

> *"To those who have not themselves experienced that state of bewilderment which is the usual condition of the investigator, it must seem strange that the physiologists who were studying the respiratory function of the blood should not have drawn from the discovery of the variation of oxygen saturation with carbon dioxide pressure, the conclusion that since carbonic acid influences the oxygen equilibrium, oxygen must influence the carbon dioxide equilibrium."*

> *"The discovery by Christiansen, Douglas, and Haldane of the effect of oxygenation of blood upon its carbon dioxide dissociation curves finally led me to the conclusion which should have been drawn a decade earlier, that every one of the variables involved in the respiratory exchanges of blood must be a mathematical function of all the others."*

There were other important facts which Henderson had in mind that had to be brought in, some of them of long standing: Zuntz's demonstration (1868) that the alkali available for the formation of bicarbonate is chiefly contained in the cells, but that the bicarbonate thus formed is not found in the cells but in the plasma (*135*); Limbeck's finding (1894) that cell volume increases with CO_2 pressure (*90*); Gürber's (1895) that chloride, bicarbonate, and water move in and out of red cells, but base does not (*51*). By this time, as Henderson noted, F. G. Donnan had stated his principle of equilibrium with nondiffusible ions.

By 1921, Henderson had worked out the general plan of the system (*68*). The variables whose values in cells and serum required definition were oxygen, carbon dioxide, bicarbonate, H-ion, total base, protein (as anion), chloride, and water. Any two values would fix the rest. But there was much to do: the experimental data, in great part, and their quantitative formulation were still to be obtained. To this end, Henderson and his associates at Harvard joined forces with Donald D. Van Slyke and his associates at the Rockefeller Institute in New York in a broad and intensive program. The achievement of the next three years was remarkable. The equilibrium conditions between cells and plasma of all the variables were experimentally determined, and with the aid of certain simplifying assumptions, Van Slyke, Wu, and McLean (*126*), in an historic monograph, went on to formulate simple equations by which the entire system could be described.

The final synthesis was Henderson's large nomogram upon which all the following were set forth: chloride concentration in plasma and cells, cell volume, per cent water in cells, base bound to protein, cell and plasma bicarbonate, total CO_2, CO_2 tension, plasma pH, cell pH, R.Q., oxygen tension, oxygen saturation, and hemoglobin concentration. As the blood moves from the pulmonary arterial to the pulmonary venous vessels in its passage through the lungs, uptake of oxygen renders hemoglobin more acid, and thus binds more potassium; bicarbonate, chloride, and water leave the cells; loss of CO_2 to the alveoli decreases bicarbonate both of plasma and cells; the plasma sodium can now accept the added chloride and bicarbonate from the cells; thus there is a minimum shift in plasma pH.

The studies thus far had included only normal subjects at rest. During the next several years, Henderson and his associates in the Harvard Fatigue Laboratory worked out nomograms for exercise, and for such pathologic states as anemia, nephritis, diabetic acidosis, and cyanotic congenital heart disease, as well as for the blood of various animal species (*69*).

During the generation since Henderson's publication, further progress has been achieved, in various directions, but this great synthesis that described the physical chemistry of air and blood in the circumstances where these elements meet would seem to be an appropriate place for this account to end.

However, before concluding this chapter, I wish to return briefly to the question raised in its introduction: Is it of benefit to revive the knowledge of the past? In unfolding the common patrimony which unites successive generations of inquiring men, in meeting them as individuals, in attempting to understand the problems they had to face, the intellectual climate in which their investigations were pursued, and the historical and social conditions under which they lived, it is my belief that a sharper consciousness of our own nature is brought forth, and the continuous doubt of the truths which we are building is revealed as our main motivation.

Finally, with a regard to the positivist attitude which does not recognize the value of a return to the sources of scientific knowledge, let me quote the recent judgment of a great modern scientist and natural philosopher, R. A. Oppenheimer (*107*):

"Logical positivism in limiting and restricting its field has reached a definition of truth which it has monopolized . . . criteria of order, harmony, generalization and cohesion are just as much part of science as the accuracies of the observations or the validity of a logical development. . . . [Our goal] is not to reach a certainty; it is to explore a signification."

BIBLIOGRAPHY

1. ANDRADE, E. N. DA C. Robert Hooke. Proc. roy. Soc., A. 201:439, 1950.
2. D'ARSONVAL, J. A. Recherches théoriques et expérimentales sur la rôle de l'élasticité du poumon dans les phénomènes de la circulation. Thèse. Paris, 1877.
3. BADOUD, E. Ueber den Einfluss des Hirns auf den Druck in der Lungenarterie. Arb. Physiol. Lab. Würzburg, 3:237, 1876.
4. BAINTON, R. H. The smaller circulation: Servetus and Colombo. Sudhoffs Arch. Gesch. Med., 24:371, 1931.
5. BAINTON, R. H. Michael Servetus and the pulmonary transit of the blood. Bull. Hist. Med., 25:1, 1951.
6. BAINTON, R. H. Hunted Heretic. The Life and Death of Michael Servetus, 1511–1553. Boston, Beacon Press, 1953.
7. BARCROFT, J. The Respiratory Function of the Blood. Cambridge, University Press, 1914.
8. BARCROFT, J. Features in the Architecture of Physiological Function. Cambridge, Cambridge University Press, 1934.
9. BEAUJEU, J. La science hellénistique et romaine. In Histoire générale des sciences. I. La Science antique et médiévale (des origines à 1450). Paris, Presses Universitaires de France, 1957, pp. 301–305, 386–390, 399–403.
10. BEKLUND, U. A lost letter from Scheele to Lavoisier. Lychnos, p. 39, 1957-1958.

11. BEUTNER, A. Ueber die Strom- und Druckkräfte des Blutes in der Arteria und Vena pulmonalia. Z. rat. Med., N.F. 2:97, 1852.
12. BEYNE, J. Influence de l'anoxémie sur la grande circulation et sur la circulation pulmonaire. C. R. Soc. Biol. (Paris), 136:399, 1942.
13. BITTAR, E. E. Ibn Nafis—A Study with Translations of Two of His Works. Thesis, Yale, 1955.
14. BITTAR, E. E. The influence of Ibn Nafis: a linkage in medical history. Univ. Mich. med. Bull., 22:274, 1956.
15. BOHR, C. Ueber die spezifische Tätigkeit der Lungen bei der respiratorischen Gasaufnahme und ihr Verhalten der durch die Alveolar-Wand stattfindenen Gasdiffusion. Skand. Arch. Physiol., 22:221, 1909.
16. BOHR, C., K. HASSELBALCH, and A. KROGH. Ueber einen in biologischer Beziehung wichtigen Einfluss den die Kohlensäurespannung des Blutes auf dessen Sauerstoffbindung übt. Skand. Arch. Physiol., 16:402, 1904.
17. BOYLE, R. New Experiments Physico-mechanical, Touching the Spring of the Air, and its Effects. Oxford, Hall, 1660.
18. BOYLE, R. A Continuation of New Experiments Physico-mechanical, Touching the Spring and Weight of the Air, and their Effects—The Second Part. London, Flesher, 1682.
19. BOYLE, R. A Disquisition about the Final Causes of Natural Things. London, Taylor, 1688.
20. BRADFORD, J. R., and H. P. DEAN. The pulmonary circulation, J. Physiol. (Lond.), 16:34, 1894.
21. BROGLIE, L. DE. Savants et découvertes. Paris, Michel, 1951.
22. CAESALPINUS, A. Quaestionum peripateticarum libri quinque. Venetiis, Iuntas, 1571.
23. CAULLERY, M. Les Grandes Étapes des sciences biologiques. In M. Daumas, Ed. Histoire de la science des origines au XXe siècle. (Encyclopédie de la Pléiade). Paris, Gallimard, 1957, p. 1224–5, 1232.
24. CHAUVEAU, A., and J. MAREY. Détermination graphique des rapports du choc du coeur avec les mouvements des oreillettes et des ventricules: expérience faite à l'aide d'un appareil enregistreur (sphygmographe). C.R. Acad. Sci. (Paris), 53:622, 1861.
25. CHAUVOIS, L. William Harvey, 1578–1657. Sa vie et son temps—ses découvertes, sa méthode, Paris. Société d'Édition d'Enseignement Supérieur, 1957.
26. CHEREAU, A. Histoire d'un livre, Michel Servet et la circulation pulmonaire. Paris, Masson, 1879.
27. CHRISTIANSEN, J., C. G. DOUGLAS, and J. S. HALDANE. The absorption and dissociation of carbon dioxide by human blood. J. Physiol. (Lond.), 48:244, 1914.

28. COHNHEIM, J., and M. LITTEN. Ueber die Folgen der Embolie der Lungenarterien. Virchows. Arch. path. Anat., 65:99, 1875.
29. COLOMBO, R. (Realdus Columbus), De Re anatomica libri XV. Venetiis, Beuilacquae, 1559.
30. CONANT, J. B. The overthrow of the Phlogiston Theory. In his Harvard Case Histories in Experimental Science. Cambridge, Mass., Harvard University Press, 1957.
31. CROMBIE, A. C. Medieval and Early Modern Science, II. Science in the Later Middle Ages and Early Modern Times, XIII–XVII Centuries. Garden City, N.Y., Doubleday, 1959.
32. DAUMAS, M. Lavoisier, théoricien et expérimentateur, Paris, Presses Universitaires de France, 1955.
33. DAUMAS, M. Les Sciences physiques aux XVIe et XVIIe siecles. In Histoire de la science des origines au XXe Siècle. (Encyclopédie de la Pléiade). Paris, Gallimard, 1957. p. 857.
34. DUJARRIC DE LA RIVIÈRE, R., and M. CHABRIER. La Vie et l'œuvre de Lavoisier d'après ses écrits, Paris. Michel, 1959.
35. ELSBERG, C. A. The Edwin Smith Surgical Papyrus and the diagnosis and treatment of injuries to the skull and spine 5000 years ago. Ann. med. Hist., n.s., 3:271, 1931.
36. EULER, U. S. VON, and G. LILJESTRAND, Observations on the pulmonary arterial blood pressure in the cat. Acta physiol. scand., 12:301, 1946.
37. FLEMING, D. Galen on the motion of the blood in the heart and lungs. Isis, 46:14, 1955.
38. FLEMING, D. William Harvey and the pulmonary circulation. Isis, 46:319, 1955.
39. FLOURENS, J. P. M. Histoire de la découverte de la circulation du sang. Paris, Baillère, 1854.
40. FRANÇOIS-FRANCK, C. É. Sur l'innervation des vaisseaux des poumons et sur les effets produits dans la circulation intracardiaque et aortique par le resserrement de ces vaisseaux. Séances et Mémoires, Soc. Biol. 7e serie, 2:231, 1880.
41. FRANÇOIS-FRANCK, C. É. Nouvelles recherches sur l'action vaso-constrictive pulmonaire du grand sympathique. Arch. physiol. norm. path., ser. 5, 7:744, 1895.
42. FRANÇOIS-FRANCK, C. É. Nouvelles recherches sur l'action vaso-constrictive pulmonaire du grand sympathique. (2e mémoire). Arch. physiol. norm. path., ser. 5, 7:816, 1895.
43. FÜHNER, H., and E. H. STARLING. Experiments on the pulmonary circulation, J. Physiol. (Lond.), 47-286, 1913.
44. FULTON, J. F. A Bibliography of the Honourable Robert Boyle, Oxford, Oxford University Press, 1932.

45. FULTON, J. F. A Bibliography of Two Oxford Physiologists, Richard Lower, 1631–1691, John Mayow, 1643–1679. Oxford, Oxford University Press, 1935.
46. FULTON, J. F. Michael Servetus, Humanist and Martyr, New York, Reichner, 1953.
47. FUNKE, O. Ueber das Milzvenenblut. Z. rat. Med., N.F. 1:172, 1851.
48. FUNKE, O. Neue Beobachtungen über die Krystalle des Milzvenen- und Fisch-Blutes. Z. rat. Med., N.F. 2:198, 1852.
49. GALEN, CLAUDIUS. Opera Omnia. Tr. by C. G. Kühn. Lipsiae, Cnoblochii, 1822. v. 3, pp. 460, 457, 454, 486.
50. GOTCH, F. Two Oxford Physiologists, Richard Lower, 1631 to 1691, John Mayow, 1643 to 1679. Oxford, Clarendon Press, 1908.
51. GÜRBER, A. Ueber den Einfluss der Kohlensäure auf die Vertheilung von Basen und Säuren zwischen Serum und Blutkörperchen. Maly's Jber. 25:164, 1895.
52. HADDAD, S. Who is the discoverer of the lesser circulation? Muktataf J., 89:264, 1936.
53. HALDANE, J. S. Respiration. New Haven, Yale University Press, 1922.
54. HALDANE, J., and J. L. SMITH. The physiological effects of air vitiated by respiration. J. Path. Bact., 1:168. 1893.
55. HALES, S. A specimen of an attempt to analyze the air by a great variety of chymo-statical experiments which were read at several meetings before the Royal Society. In his Statical Essays, vol. I, Vegetable Staticks, 2nd ed., London. Woodward and Peale, London, 1731.
56. HALES, S. Statical Essays, vol. II, Haemastaticks. London, 1733.
57. HALLER, A. VON. Elementa physiologiae corporis humani, v. 3, Lausanne, Bousquet, 1760.
58. HARVEY, W. The Works, Tr. by R. Willis. London, Sydenham Society Publication, v. 10, 1847, p. 597.
59. HARVEY, W. Prelectiones anatomiae universalis. Ed. by Committee of the Royal College of Physicians of London. London, Churchill, 1886.
60. HARVEY, W. Movement of the Heart and Blood in Animals, an Anatomical Essay. Tr. by K. J. Franklin. Oxford, Blackwell Scientific Publications, 1957.
61. HÉGER, P. Recherches sur la circulation du sang dans les poumons. Ann. Université Libre Bruxelles, Fac. med., 1:117, 1880.
62. HÉGER, P., and E. SPEHL. Recherches sur la fistule péricardique chez le lapin. Ligature des vaisseaux de la base du cœur pendant la respiration naturelle: évaluation de la quantité de sang contenue dans les poumons. Arch. Biol., 2:153, 1881.

63. HENDERSON, L. J. Equilibrium in solutions of phosphates. Amer. J. Physiol., 15:257, 1906.
64. HENDERSON, L. J. The theory of neutrality regulation in the animal organism. Amer. J. Physiol., 21:427, 1908.
65. HENDERSON, L. J. Gleichgewicht zwischen Basen und Säuren im tierischen Organismus. Ergebn. Physiol., 8:254, 1909.
66. HENDERSON, L. J. The Fitness of the Environment. New York, Macmillan, 1913.
67. HENDERSON, L. J. The Order of Nature. Cambridge, Harvard University Press, 1917.
68. HENDERSON, L. J. Blood as a physicochemical system. J. biol. Chem., 46:411, 1921.
69. HENDERSON, L. J. Blood: a Study in General Physiology. New Haven, Yale University Press, 1928.
70. HOOKE, R. An account of an experiment made by Mr. Hooke, of preserving animals alive by blowing through their lungs with bellows. Phil. Trans. 11:539, 1667.
71. HOPPE-SEYLER, F. Ueber die chemischen und optischen Eigenschaften des Blutfarbstoffes. Zweite Mittheilung. Virchows Arch. path. Anat., 29:233, 1864.
72. HOPPE-SEYLER, F. Ueber die chemischen und optischen Eigenschaften des Blutfarbstoffes. Dritte Mittheilung. Virchows Arch. path. Anat., 29:597, 1864.
73. IZQUIERDO, J. J. A new and more correct version of the views of Servetus on the circulation of the blood. Bull. Hist. Med., 5:917, 1937.
74. JAEGER, W. W. Diokles von Karystos. Die griechische Medizin und die Schule des Aristoteles. Berlin, De Gruyter, 1938.
75. KROGH, A., and M. KROGH. On the rate of diffusion of carbonic oxide in the lungs of man. Skand. Arch. Physiol., 23:236, 1910.
76. LALESQUE, F. Études critiques et expérimentales sur la circulation pulmonaire, Paris, Thèse, 1881.
77. LAVOISIER, A. L. Oeuvres, Tome I, Traité élémentaire de chimie, Paris, Imprimerie Impériale, 1864.
78. LAVOISIER, A. L. Analyse du mémoire sur l'augmentation du poids des métaux par la calcination. In his Oeuvres, Tome II. Mémoires de chimie et de physique. Paris, Imprimerie Impériale, 1862, p. 97.
79. LAVOISIER, A. L. Mémoire sur la nature du principe qui se combine avec les métaux pendant leur calcination et qui en augmente le poids. In his Oeuvres, Tome II. Mémoires de chimie et de physique. Paris, Imprimerie Impériale, 1862, p. 122.
80. LAVOISIER, A. L. Expériences sur la respiration des animaux et sur les changements qui arrivent à l'air en passant par leur poumon. In

his Oeuvres, Tome II. Mémoires de chimie et de physique. Paris, Imprimerie Impériale, 1862, p. 174.

81. LAVOISIER, A. L. Mémoire sur la combustion en général. In his Oeuvres, Tome II. Mémoires de chimie et de physique. Paris, Imprimerie Impériale, 1862, p. 225.

82. LAVOISIER, A. L., and P. S. DE LAPLACE. Mémoire sur la chaleur. In his Oeuvres, Tome II. Mémoires de chimie et de physique. Paris, Imprimerie Impériale, 1862, p. 283.

83. LAVOISIER, A. L., and A. SÉGUIN. Premier mémoire sur la respiration des animaux. In his Oeuvres, Tome II. Mémoires de chimie et de physique. Paris, Imprimerie Impériale, 1862, p. 688.

84. LAVOISIER, A. L., and A. SÉGUIN. Premier mémoire sur la transpiration des animaux. In his Oeuvres, Tome II. Mémoires de chimie et de physique. Paris, Imprimerie Impériale, 1862, p. 704.

85. LEBOUCQ, G. Une anatomie antique du cœur humain. Philistion de Locroi et le Timée de Platon. Rev. Et. Grecques, 57:7, 1944.

86. LICHTHEIM, L. Die Störungen des Lungenkreislaufs und ihr Einfluss auf den Blutdruck. Breslau, Jungfer, 1876.

87. LIEBIG, J. VON. Familiar Letters on Chemistry. London, Taylor and Walton, 1845.

88. LILJESTRAND, G. Regulation of pulmonary arterial blood pressure. Arch. intern. Med., 81:162, 1948.

89. LILJESTRAND, G. Obituary Notice. August Krogh, 1876–1949. Acta physiol. scand., 20:109, 1950.

90. LIMBECK, R. VON. Ueber den Einfluss des respiratorischen Gaswechsels auf die rothen Blutkörperchen. Arch. exp. Path. Pharmak., 35:309, 1894.

91. LOWER, R. Diatribæ de Febribus. London, Martyn and Allestry, 1665.

92. LOWER, R. Tractatus de Corde. London, Allestry, 1669.

93. LOWER, R. Tractatus de Corde. Tr. by K. J. Franklin. In R. T. Gunther, Early Science in Oxford, vol. IX. Oxford, Clarendon Press, 1932.

94. MAGENDIE, F. Phénomènes physiques de la vie. Leçons professées au Collège de France. Paris, Baillière, 1842.

95. MAGNUS, G. Ueber die im Blute enthaltenen Gase. Sauerstoff, Stickstoff und Kohlensäure. Ann. Phys. Chem., 12:583, 1837.

96. MALPIGHI, M. De Pulmonibus, Observationes Anatomicae, Bologna, 1661.

97. MAREY, É. J. Physiologie médicale de la circulation du sang, basée sur l'étude graphique des mouvements du cœur et du pouls artériel avec application aux maladies de l'appareil circulatoire. Paris, Delahaye, 1863.

98. MAYER, R. Die organische Bewegung in ihrem Zusammenhange mit dem Stoffwechsel. Heilbronn, 1845.
99. MAYOW, J. Tractatus Duo: De Respiratione, De Rachitide. Oxford, Hall, 1668.
100. MAYOW, J. Tractatus Quinque: De Sal Nitro et Spiritu Nitro-Aero, De Respiratione, De Respiratione Foetus in Utero et Ovo, De Motu Muscularis et Spiritibus Animalibus, De Rachitide, Oxford, 1674.
101. MEYER, L. Die Gase des Blutes, Z. rat. Med., 8:256, 1857.
102. MEYERHOF, M. (Review of) El-Tatawi, Mohyi, El-Din, Der Lungenkreislauf nach el Koraschi. Mitt. Gesch. Med. Naturw., 30:55, 1931.
103. MEYERHOF, M. Ibn an-Nafis und seine Theorie des Lungenkreislaufs, Quellen Studien Gesch. Naturwiss. Med., 4:37, 1933.
104. MEYERHOF, M. La découverte de la circulation pulmonaire par Ibn an-Nafis, Médecin Arabe du Caire. (XIII. Siècle). Bull. Inst. Egypte, 16:33, 1934.
105. MEYERHOF, M. Ibn an-Nafis (XIIIth cent.) and his theory of the lesser circulation. Isis, 23:100, 1935.
106. MICHEL, P. H. La Science Hellène. In Histoire générale des sciences. I. La Science antique et médiévale (des origines à 1450). Paris, Presses Universitaires de France, 1957, p. 288.
107. OPPENHEIMER, R. A. Science, culture et expression. Prospective No. 5, p. 79, 1960.
108. PARTINGTON, J. R. The life and work of John Mayow (1641–1679). Isis, 47:217, 1956.
109. PATTERSON, T. S. John Mayow in contemporary setting: A contribution to the history of respiration and combustion. Isis, 13:47, 1931.
110. PATTERSON, T. S. John Mayow in contemporary setting. II. Mayow's views on combustion. Isis, 13:504, 1931.
111. PFLUGER, E. Ueber die Diffusion des Sauerstoffs, den Ort und die Gesetze der Oxydationsprocesse im thierischen Organismus. Pflügers Arch. ges. Physiol., 6:43, 1872.
112. POISEUILLE, J. L. Recherches sur la respiration, C.R. Acad. Sci. (Paris), 41:1072, 1855.
113. PRENDERGAST, J. Galen's view of the vascular system in relation to that of Harvey. Proc. roy. Soc. Med., 21:1839, 1928.
114. PRIESTLEY, J. Expérience et observations sur differentes espèces d'air. Tr. by H. Gibelin. vol. 2. Paris, 1777–80, p. 290.
115. SARTON, G. Introduction to the History of Science, v. 1. From Homer to Omar Khayyam. Baltimore, Williams and Wilkins, 1927.
116. SARTON, G. A History of Science, I. Ancient Science through the Golden Age of Greece, Cambridge, Mass., Harvard University Press, 1952.

117. SARTON, G. Galen of Pergamon. Lawrence, Kans., University of Kansas Press, 1954.
118. SARTON, G. A History of Science, II. Hellenistic Science and Culture in the Last Three Centuries B.C. Cambridge, Mass., Harvard University Press, 1959.
119. SERVETUS, M. A Translation of His Geographical, Medical, and Astrological Writings. Tr. by C. D. O'Malley. Philadelphia, American Philosophical Society Memoirs, v. 34, 1953.
120. TATAWI, M. E. D. Der Lungenkreislauf nach el Koraschi. Dissertation. Freiburg im Breisgau, 1925.
121. TEMKIN, O. Was Servetus influenced by Ibn an-Nafis? Bull. Hist. Med., 8:731, 1940.
122. THORPE, T. E. Joseph Priestley. New York, Dutton, 1906.
123. TIGERSTEDT, R. Christian Bohr. Ein Nachruf. Skand. Arch. Physiol., 25:v, 1911.
124. TOULMIN, S. E. Crucial experiments: Priestley and Lavoisier. J. Hist. Ideas, 18:205, 1957.
125. TRUETA, J. Michael Servetus and the discovery of the lesser circulation. Yale J. Biol. Med., 21:1, 1948.
126. VAN SLYKE, D. D., H. WU, and F. C. MCLEAN. Studies of gas and electrolyte equilibria in the blood. V. Factors controlling the electrolyte and water distribution in the blood. J. biol. Chem., 56:767, 1923.
127. VESALIUS, A. De humani corporis fabrica libri septem. Basileae, Oporini, 1543.
128. VIALLARD, R., and M. DAUMAS. L'Édification de la science classique. In M. Daumas, Ed. Histoire de la science des origines au XXe siècle (Encyclopédie de la Pléiade). Paris, Gallimard, 1957, p. 883.
129. WEISHEIPL, J. A. The Development of Physical Theory in the Middle Ages, London, Sheed and Ward, 1959.
130. WIBERG, J. The medical science of Ancient Greece: The doctrine of the heart. Janus, 41:225, 1937.
131. WILLIS, T. Cerebri Anatome. London, Martyn, 1664.
132. WOTTON, W. Reflections upon Ancient and Modern Learning. London, J. Leake for P. Buck, 1694.
133. YOUNG, J. Malpighi's "De Pulmonibus," Proc. roy. Soc. Med., 23:1, 1929.
134. YOUNG, R. A. The pulmonary circulation—before and after Harvey, The Harveian Oration 1939. Brit. med. J., I:1, 41, 1940.
135. ZUNTZ, N. Beiträge zur Physiologie des Blutes. Dissertation. Bonn, 1868.

II

The Output of the Heart

UNDERSTANDING the mechanisms that control blood flow is the central problem of circulatory physiology. Factors that affect the size of the aortic stream and its distribution determine the environment in which the tissues function. In this complex process, the initial effort is the total output of blood by the ventricles of the heart.

It is logical for the present account to begin at the moment in history when the "motion of blood in a circle" was in the course of its discovery.

Discovery of the Circulation

William Harvey lived and worked in a fortunate country at a fortunate time. Twenty years before his birth, Elizabeth I, declaring that she "wished to open no window into men's consciences," guided her first Parliament through the Religious Settlement in the Acts of Supremacy and Uniformity (51), which, among other things, laid the foundation for England's intellectual freedom. In his most active years, Harvey enjoyed the special favor of James I and was the personal physician to Charles I. Even when the latter's fortunes declined, and he was defeated and deposed, Harvey himself was not persecuted (77), although many of his writings were lost in the course of the Civil War.

Other men were less fortunate. Leonardo da Vinci (1452–1519) lived in a political and social turmoil, constantly changing his patron, his place of living, and the form and direction of his activities (9). His vast compilation of notes and drawings, which he expected to assemble in the last years of his life, were never published. Left to a friend, they were little by little divided and scattered in the generations that followed; they exerted little influence on the advancement of science and were of value to very few except the historians and antiquarians of modern times. Vesalius (1514–64), opposed by his peers and drawn away by a

THE HEART

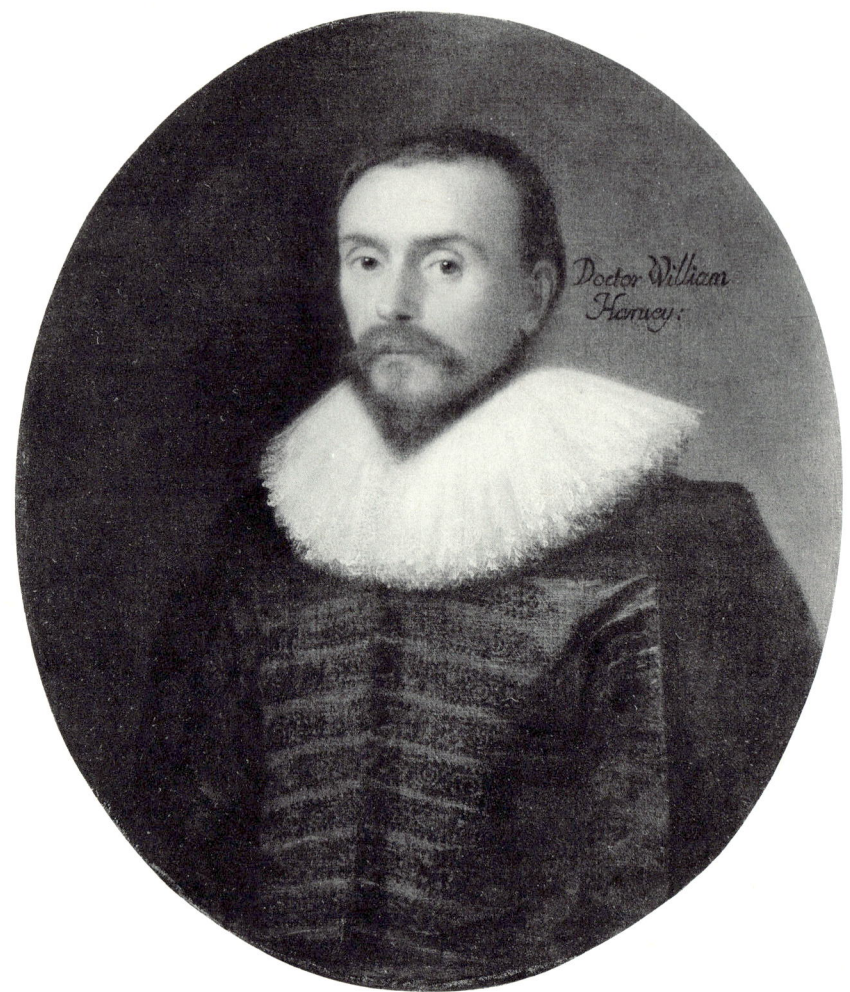

Figure 1. William Harvey (1578–1657). The Rolls Park portrait, painted by an unknown artist in 1626. This was part of a family group, with William's father Thomas in the center, surrounded by portraits of each of his six sons.

mighty patron, abandoned his scientific inquiries at the age of thirty. Servetus and his books were burned. Even Galileo (1564–1642), six years after Harvey had published *De motu cordis*, was forced by the Inquisition at Rome to read, on his knees, the recantation of his "heresy" supporting the theories of Copernicus (*8*).

The historian is fortunate in having enough authentic material about William Harvey so that one can follow his education and reconstruct, at least in part, the progressive development of his ideas about the heart and the flow of blood. He was born in Folkestone, England, on April 1, 1578. When he was ten years old, in the same summer that saw the defeat of the Spanish Armada, Harvey entered King's School in Canterbury (77). He was admitted to Caius College, Cambridge, at sixteen, and was graduated four years later. In 1600 he journeyed to Padua, then the Mecca of science in the civilized world. Here he studied for two years and became the favored pupil of the anatomist Hieronymus Fabricius, who was then completing his great work on the valves of the veins. The young student, as it turned out, made a more profound deduction than his master on the significance of the venous valves. Many years later, as an old man, Harvey told Robert Boyle that the observations of Fabricius first gave him the idea that blood must flow from arteries to veins, and so back to the heart (5).

Returning to London in 1602, Harvey began the arduous climb up the academic and professional ladder. In 1607 he was admitted as Fellow of the College of Physicians, in 1609 he was appointed physician to St. Bartholomew's Hospital, and in 1615 he was named Lumleian lec-

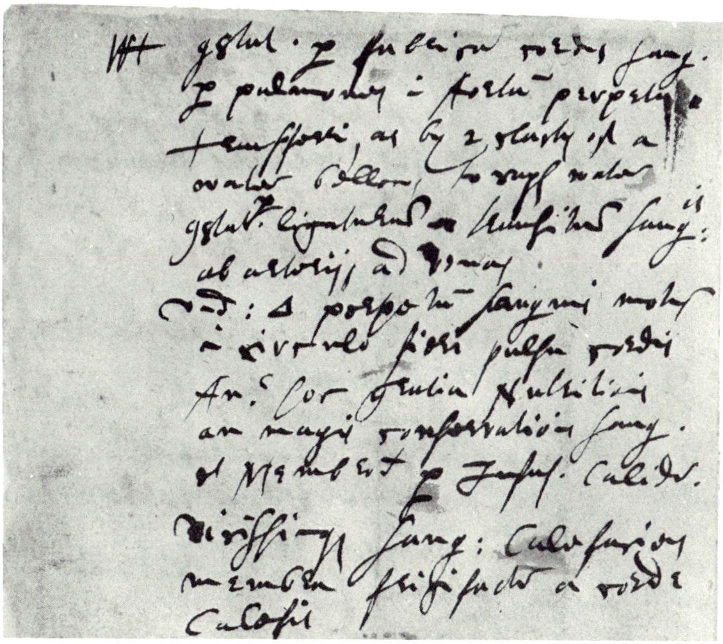

THE OUTPUT
OF THE HEART

Figure 2. William Harvey's notes for his Lumleian Lecture in 1616.

THE HEART

turer of the College. By an extraordinary chance, the notes of his Lumleian lecture of April 17, 1616, found their way into the British Museum, where they were discovered in 1886, some 270 years later. These notes, written originally in a mixture of Latin and English, are worth quoting (*28*):

"*It is plain from the structure of the heart that the blood is passed continuously through the lungs to the aorta as by two clacks of a water bellows to raise water. It is shown by application of a ligature that the passage of blood is from the arteries into the veins. Whence it follows that the movement of the blood is constantly in a circle, and is brought about by the beat of the heart. It is a question, therefore, whether this is for the sake of nourishment or of heat, the blood cooled by warming the limbs, being in turn warmed by the heart.*"

The ligature and the flow of blood in the limbs are not new arguments here, but are more or less an extension of Fabricius; a new and interesting thought, however, is the analogy of the heart to the water pump. This is not mentioned in *De motu cordis*, yet may be important, and the point perhaps justifies a small digression.

Though invented and described as early as the first century A.D., in Alexandria (*84*), the double-valve one-way pump was not familiar to the ancients. Erasistratos and Galen both failed to appreciate the heart as a systolic pump. From the *De re metallica* (1555) of Agricola (*1*) it would appear that this general mechanism was developed in the late fifteenth and early sixteenth centuries as a practical instrument to draw water out of deep mines. The pump, was, of course, employed by Galileo in his experiments, and in Harvey's time was doubtless in common use in ships, mines, and elsewhere. This simple device, the "water bellows," appears to have provided an essential concept in Harvey's eventual discovery.

We come now to the book, *Exercitatio anatomica de motu cordis et sanguinis in animalibus*, Guilielmi Harvei, Angli, Francofurti, sumptibus Guilielmi Fitzeri, anno M.DC.XXVIII (*42*). This great work stands by itself. In the medical sciences there is nothing else in the same class. Its seventeen brief chapters, in seventy-two pages, are an inexhaustible source of enlightenment, stimulus and pleasure, with its revelation of clear premises, cogent and skillful experiment, precise deduction, and incontrovertible conclusions. Its achievement was more than a discovery: it was a revolution.

THE OUTPUT
OF THE HEART

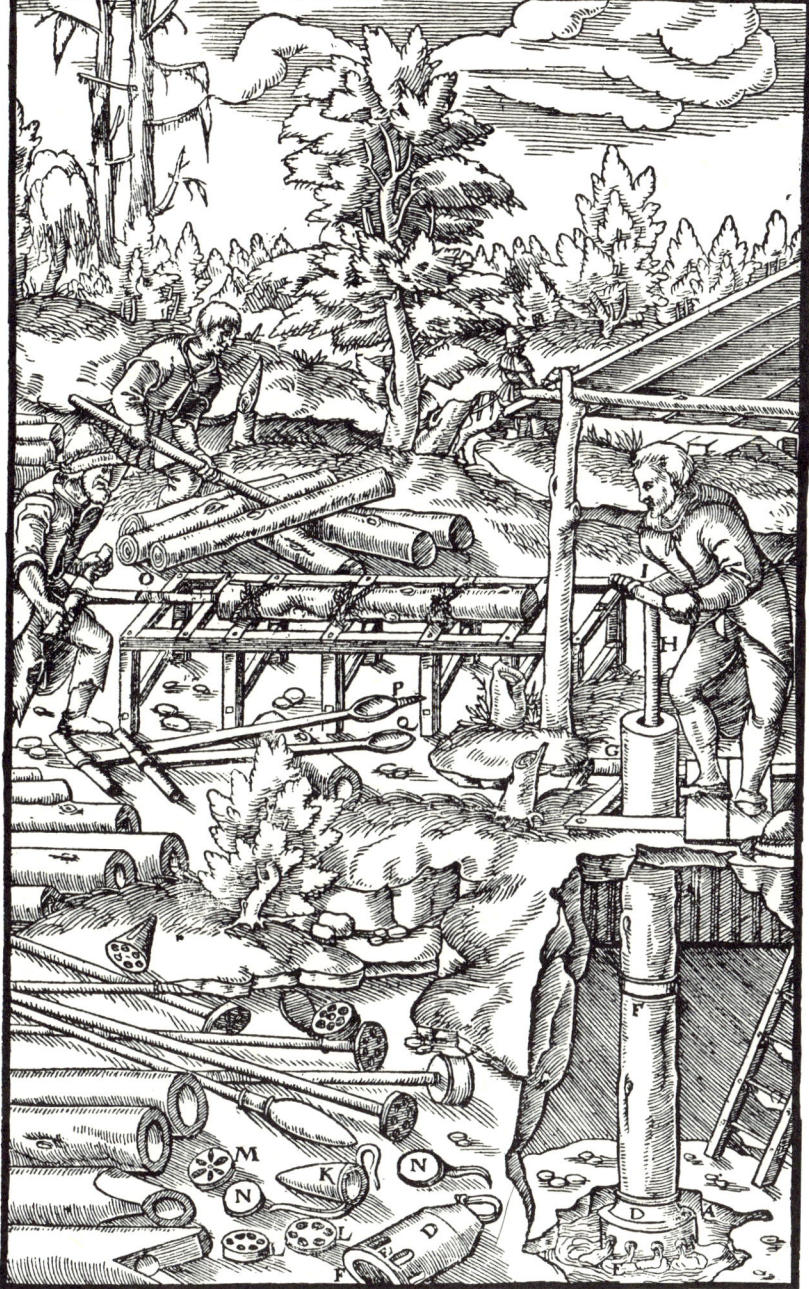

Figure 3. Structure of a one-way-valve water pump. From Georgius Agricola's book, *De re metallica*, first published in 1555.

[75]

THE HEART

Its very style sets it apart. Its manner is swift, trenchant, decisive. The author had brought from Padua much knowledge and a well-trained mind, but not his literary style. There is little here of Fabricius's measured prose (*15*), still less of the gracious dialogue of the *Two New Sciences* (*30*). This style is English, and in a sense Elizabethan: Harvey is terse, vigorous, and outspoken. He always says just what he thinks, whether in agreement or in disagreement, in praise or in derision.

He had worked and lectured on the circulation for twelve years before he ventured to set his argument before the scientific world. The book is put together with immense care; the author was well aware of the intellectual inertia of his contemporaries, both in his own country and abroad. He holds to Galen, the "Prince of Physicians," as much and as long as he can, and in his broader philosophy he remains conservatively and stoutly Aristotelian.

The argument of the book moves with precision. In the Introduction he seeks what aid he can in tradition: he notes that Galen found only blood, not blood and air, in pulmonary veins and aorta; and that Realdus Columbus had observed that the pulmonary artery was unduly large, and inquired the cause thereof. But in general he found traditional theories illogical: if there were both blood and air in the heart, how could blood, and not air, reflux backward through the mitral valves? "What has so far been said is obscure, inconsistent, impossible to the thoughtful student."

The first chapter states simply that, having gained accurate information on the motion of the heart and arteries, he proposes to publish his findings. Chapter 2 notes that the heart contracts in systole, relaxes in diastole, expels blood in systole, receives it in diastole. Chapter 3 adds the observation that when the heart contracts the pulmonary artery and aorta dilate. Then he follows Jean Riolan in observing that the auricles force blood into the ventricles. Here are observations also from Harvey's wide experience in comparative anatomy, on fish, chick embryo, and insect hearts, and on the independent rhythmic contractions of excised bits of heart muscle.

In Chapter 5 the threads of the fabric begin to be drawn together. Both auricles contract, sending blood into ventricles; both ventricles contract, sending blood to arteries. There is no interventricular passage.

How does blood reach the left heart? How does blood get from veins to auricles? "A new path is to be found."

Chapters 6 and 7 are most skillful, and astonishingly sophisticated. In considering the passage of blood from the right side of the heart to the left, why, said Harvey, should one generalize from one animal species alone, that is, from the adult human? There are many more animals without lungs than with them. In many there is but a single ventricle, and the passage occurs right there. In the fetus, with nonfunctioning lungs, there are two passages of transfer; and he described with remarkable accuracy the foramen ovale and the ductus arteriosus, and explained how the blood moves through them, and how they close after birth. Why not conclude, he said, that in adult large animals, the blood—all of it—does pass through the spongy lung tissue through "porosities." Harvey knew of the work of Realdus Columbus, but not that of Michael Servetus. (The three surviving volumes of *Christianismi Restitutio* would not be rediscovered for another seventy years.)

In Chapter 8, the center of his discourse, the argument rises to its tremendous climax: *Coepi egomet mecum cogitare, an motionem quandam quasi in circulo haberet.* ("I began to think within myself whether it might have a sort of motion, as it were, in a circle.") This he afterward found to be true, and he described the course of the blood, out of the ventricles to the arteries, thence onward to the veins, and so back to the heart.

Ordinarily Harvey kept aloof from philosophy, but upon the enunciation of this new principle he was moved to ally his discovery with the cosmic theories of his master Aristotle. "The motion of the blood may be called circular in the way that Aristotle says air and rain follow the circular motion of the stars." As Dr. Leake notes, in his excellent translation of *De motu cordis* (42), Harvey is here somewhat behind the times, neglecting the prime discoveries of the preceding century, of Copernicus, Kepler, and his onetime teacher Galileo. Again, "so the heart is the center of life, the sun of the Microcosm, as the sun itself might be called the heart of the world." One must admit that the further Harvey strayed into cosmic philosophy, the less his genius was displayed.

But in Chapter 9 he returns to the battle, and this time with a new and mighty weapon. Up to this point Harvey had been, as he always

THE OUTPUT
OF THE HEART

professed himself, an anatomist, though a powerfully dynamic one; and in the chapters that follow, his argument again rests upon anatomic grounds. But here in Chapter 9, he steps out of the traditional anatomist's role and makes his one brilliant and purely physical and physiological quantitative hypothesis.

Let us suppose, Harvey said, either in thought or by experiment, that the filled ventricle contains two or three ounces, or even an ounce and a half of blood, and that in systole some quantity is ejected—say, a dram, or two, or half an ounce, or an ounce; then a thousand beats in half an hour will propel from ten to eighty pounds of blood—vastly more than the entire body contains. Ergo, the blood must move around in a circle. It is to be noted that no experimental evidence is adduced, though Harvey commented that he had made "many observations" on the amount of blood ejected at a single beat, and "the factors involved in increasing or diminishing it."

Harvey was quite aware of the importance of this calculation to his argument, for this chapter is entitled, "The circulation of the blood is proved by a prime consideration."

The subsequent chapters of the book deal with further proofs of the direction and force of blood flow in arteries and veins, by the skillful use of tight (arterial) and medium (venous) ligatures, by experiments with various species of animals, and by exploring again the properties of the venous valves of Fabricius. These need not be detailed here.

Harvey's concern over the primary question of all, the basic function of the circulating blood, has been reviewed in the first chapter. He did not forget the one large gap in his experimental proof in *De motu cordis*, the question of flow of blood through "porosities" in lungs and tissues. Undoubtedly he continued his experiments, though it is difficult to determine just what these were and when he did them. An elegant experiment in perfusion of the pulmonary circulation is described, in typically brusque and spicy Harveian style, in a letter written late in his life (1651) to his academic friend, Paul Marquart Slegel of Hamburg (41):

"In a strangled human body, the pulmonary artery and aorta are ligated, the left ventricle opened, and a cannula placed in the vena cava, and water forced in. Quid fit? [*What happens?*] *The right ventricle is vehemently tumefied. Through the opening in the left ventricle, however, not a drop of water or blood escapes.*

> "*So now (the solution having been predicted), the syringe is introduced into the pulmonary artery, with a ligature around it lest water regurgitate into the right ventricle. We force the water in the syringe against the lungs and immediately water with copious amounts of blood leaps out of the cleft in the left ventricle, so that, as much water as is expressed into the lungs, so much flows out of the hiatus mentioned. You can experiment as often as you like, and know for certain that this is so.*
>
> "*By this one experiment, I have easily butchered all the arguments of Riolan on this question.*"

As for the "porosities" in lungs and tissues, it is remarkable that through entirely separate avenues of inquiry, Malpighi (born the same year *De motu cordis* was published) and Leeuwenhoek, four years younger, should have provided, so precisely and so convincingly, and at so timely a moment, a clear demonstration of their structure in solid tissues. This was, in a sense, a sign of the times, a part of the extraordinary outburst of discovery in what Whitehead has called the "Century of Genius" (*90*). It would be difficult to recapture the intensity of interest and excitement that prevailed over Europe at that time, as this new society of natural philosophers, freeing themselves from the restraints of tradition and the bondage of the Church, began to explore the "fabric of Nature" with new methods of experiment. It is noteworthy, as many have observed, that this was in great part a movement outside the universities (*28*). A few of them, such as those of northern Italy, and to some extent those in Holland, supported scientific endeavor, but in most instances neither the stimulus nor the freedom for such inquiries was to be found in the traditional academic atmosphere. It was fostered rather in independent learned societies, which were founded and operated at first more or less secretly, then later in the open. The Secret Academy at Naples (1560) founded by Giovanni della Porta (a botanist who also invented the camera obscura) was followed by the Academy of the Lynxes in Rome (Accademia dei Lincei), in 1603, to which Galileo later belonged, and which continues now as one of the great scientific societies. In 1645 an "Invisible College" was founded in London by Boyle, Wren, and others, which combined later with an Oxford philosophical society to form the Royal Society of London in 1660. The Accademia del Cimento (Experiment) was established by Borelli and Malpighi in 1657, the French Académie des Sciences by Colbert in 1665, and so forth.

Structure and Movement of the Heart

THE HEART

Richard Lower (1631–90) was one of the early members of the Royal Society. His careful studies of the musculature of the heart and the form of its contraction exhibited his extraordinary powers of observation, matching in skill if not in originality his observations on the oxygenation of blood in the lungs. Here Lower has probably received less credit than he has deserved. This may well have been in part because of his irascible personality and barbed pen, and the numerous enemies that he acquired. When he died, among the poetic tributes was the following (63):

"UPON DR. LOWER'S DEATH, BEING A MAN OF A MOROSE DISPOSITION:

> *Had not good nature o'er ye ill prevail'd*
> *Death in attempting Dr. Lower had fail'd*
> *Who might have lived with us many a year*
> *Prepared (in his own pickle) vinegar.*
> *But when ye Alkali had killed ye soure*
> *His blood being sweetened, off went Dr. Lower.*"

Lower's dissections of the heart revealed the inner and outer ventricular muscle layers, disposed obliquely, one extending upward toward the right, the other toward the left; the whorl-like conformation around the apex; and the positions of the papillary muscles, holding out the "sail-like" valvular leaflets. About the lesser size of the left auricle, compared with the right, he said: "Hence the [left auricle's] only requisite is, apparently, that a more forceful movement shall be imparted to the blood as it flows past into the left ventricle, and that its passage shall be somewhat assisted. Thus there is no need of the help of so large an auricle on this side."

In his chapter on the movement of the heart, Lower notes, as Harvey had before him, that heart muscle has independent contractility. He does not find the source of body heat in the heart, but is perplexed by this problem, finally finding an escape in that "the learned Dr. Willis is giving the matter some thought in his book on 'The Spirit, and also the heating of the Blood.'" He describes the contraction of the ventricles, the final movement being one in which the apex "comes nearer" the base.

In the latter part of this chapter, the eminent Dr. Lower ranges far and wide with all sorts of advice, both medical and social, from the reasons why people should sleep with their heads higher than their feet to the pernicious and harmful effects of heavy drinking late at night.

THE OUTPUT OF THE HEART

Quantitative Experiment

The Royal Society was also the intellectual environment that stimulated, guided, and encouraged the next contributor of primary importance to the knowledge of the output of the heart, Stephen Hales (1677–1761).

Hales entered Benet (now Corpus Christi) College, Cambridge, at nineteen, took his master's degree seven years later, and in 1711 became a bachelor of divinity (33). During these years he formed a close friendship with another young man a few years his junior, William Stukeley (the antiquarian who first explored the Druidical mysteries of Stonehenge), and the two young enthusiasts worked together on experiments in anatomy and "chemistry." Hales had the good fortune to receive, as early as 1708, the perpetual curacy of the vicarage of Teddington, a few miles outside London, and he continued his experiments there. For an ordained minister of the church to spend his time in biological experiment was not as strange then as it would be now. This was the eighteenth century, the "Age of Reason based on Faith" (90), and for Stephen Hales at the beginning of the century, just as for Joseph Priestley at its close, the study of Nature was but another way of inquiring into and demonstrating the wisdom of the Almighty; Hales in his writings constantly reminded his readers of this great truth.

He was soon presenting his experiments before the Royal Society, to which he was elected a fellow in 1717. His ingenuity in experiment and his passion for measurement were the mainsprings of his remarkable achievements in the new science of physiology. It would be interesting to know how Hales came by these qualities of mind and character. It may have been in part because he had no formal training in medicine or anatomy, and brought to the problems a fresh and unprejudiced

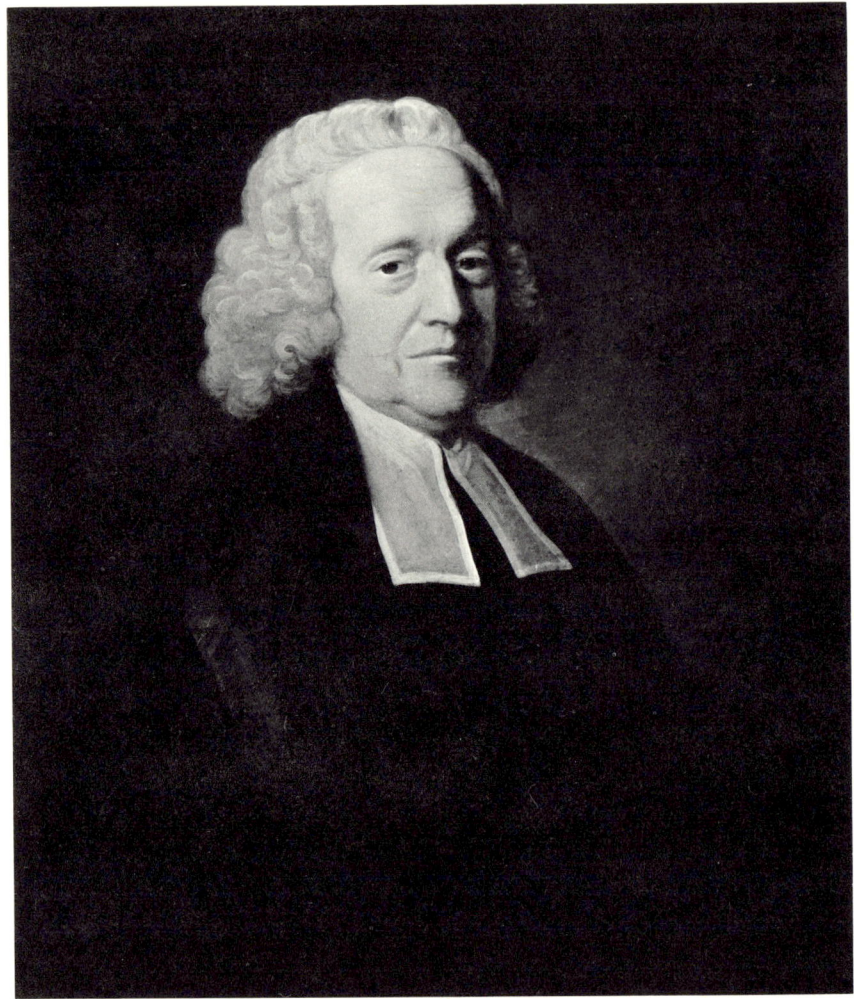

Figure 4. Stephen Hales (1677–1761).

mind. It is probable, also, that he received help from fellow scientists in the Royal Society. Boyle, Hooke, and Lower had passed from the scene, but others had taken their places. The greatest of them all, Isaac Newton, was active during the period of Hales's early studies. It was in the last year of Newton's life, but while he was still president of the Society, and at his direction, that Hales's first volume, *Vegetable Staticks* (*34*), was published.

Hales's mathematics, actually, were simple, but he set up his experiments so that measurements could be made; he made them carefully and verified them by repeated experiment, then used his measurements in physiological calculations and deductions.

His early studies of the physiology of plant life, and his brilliant discoveries in the field of plant and animal respiration, were referred to in part in the previous chapter. The experiments in animal physiology formed a second series, published in 1733, and entitled *Haemastaticks* (35).

The familiar and engaging description—which starts right out as Experiment 1, page 1, in his book—of "the Mare, fourteen hands high," and the measurement of the arterial blood pressure, belongs properly to another chapter. The point to be recorded here is that this same experiment was repeated on "a gelding, thirteen hands high," and again on "a white mare, fourteen hands, three inches high," with the same results; and that at the end of this third experiment, Hales took the next step in his experimentation. The animal having expired, following exsanguination, he filled the left ventricle with melted beeswax and on its solidifying, measured its volume—10 cubic inches, or 160 cc. Assuming complete emptying of the ventricle in systole (we recall that Harvey, a more careful observer, did not make this assumption), and having found the pulse rate of a normal horse at rest to be 36, Hales calculated the cardiac output of the horse at rest to be 360 cubic inches or 6 liters per minute. This is a low figure, caused in part no doubt because the animal had bled to death, and the ventricular cavity was small. Further blood pressure and ventricular volume measurements in other species gave proportionate figures. For man, Hales took Harvey's estimates of two ounces as a likely volume of ventricular ejection, and calculated a cardiac output of about four liters per minute.

He noted that systole occupied only one-third of the cardiac cycle, and concluded that the run-off was therefore accomplished by the elasticity of the large vessels. He calculated the velocity imparted to the aortic column of blood in systole to be 86.7 feet per minute. He was impressed by the variability of blood pressure and heart rate under different circumstances. Hales's further studies of the peripheral circulation, the properties of the "capillary arteries," will be considered in a later chapter.

THE OUTPUT
OF THE HEART

Hæmastatics.

The several Animals.	Quantities of Blood = to the Weight of the Animal in what Time.	How much in a Minute.	Weight of the Blood sustain'd by the left Ventricle contracting.	Number of Pulses in a Minute.	Area of the transverse Section of descending Aorta.	Area of the transf. Section of ascending Aorta.
	Minutes	Pounds	Pounds		Square Inches	Square Inches
Man	36.3 18.15	4.37 8.74	51.5	75		
Horse 3d	60	13.75	113.22	36	0.677	0.369
Ox	88	18.14		38	0.912	0.85 Ri. left
Sheep	20	4.593	35.52	65	0.094 0.383	0.07 0.012 0.246 Ri. left
Dog 1	11.9	434	33.61	97	0.106	0.041 0.034
2	6.48	3.7			0.102	0.031 0.009
3	7.8	2.3	19.8		0.07	0.022 0.009
4	6.2	1.85	11.1		0.061	0.015 0.007
					0.119	0.7 0.031
					0.125	0.062 0.031
7	6.56	4.19			0.109	0.053 0.032

Figure 5. A table from Stephen Hales's *Haemastaticks*, 1733, giving measurements of ventricular volume and estimates of cardiac output.

A broad concept of blood pressure, blood flow, blood velocity, and their relations, and quantitative measurements or calculations of each—these were the great contributions made by Stephen Hales to the knowledge of the output of the heart, a contribution which has oriented all future work.

It is interesting that in this same period the physicist, Daniel Bernouilli (1700–82), in Basel, gave mathematical expression to the laws of hydraulics for ideal fluids. One might speculate to what extent the advancement of hemodynamics would have been accelerated if the concepts of the pioneer mathematical physicists had been applied to the circulation. Such mathematics was far beyond the capacity of Stephen Hales, and had to await Poiseuille a century later.

But in these hundred years there was little advance even from the simple hemodynamics of Hales. The work of the great clinicians of the eighteenth century, so important to the knowledge of pathology and clinical disease, added little to that of the output of the heart, since there were no methods of measurement available. Basic physiological knowledge again had to await the advent of new methods.

THE OUTPUT OF THE HEART

New Instruments and New Methods

The history of graphic recording, prior to and leading up to the epoch-making invention of the kymograph by Carl Ludwig, has been told in a series of fascinating papers by Hoff and Geddes; what follows are brief notes from their work (*48, 49, 50*).

Mechanical devices registering the passage of time can be traced back as far as the clepsydra, or water clock, of the ancients. This was simply a container of water emptying through a narrow orifice. (The old Greek lexicon of Liddell and Scott tells us that it was first used to time speeches in law courts! (*56*)). It was well known in Plato's day. Ctesibios in the third century B.C. is said to have placed a float on the water, with a pointer that recorded against a column—perhaps the first recording timepiece. Through the Middle Ages clock makers were the skilled artisans of all sorts of instruments. With the onset of the era of scientific discovery, the need for recording devices became urgent. There were undoubtedly countless inventions and apparatus developed in many places, most of them never described in publication. There is a letter written by Christopher Wren to his father in 1647, when he was a youth of fifteen, in which he describes the possible use of a revolving cylinder, on which continuous records of weather changes might be inscribed (*98*). More elaborate "weather clocks," recording wind direction and velocity, temperature, etc., were developed in the Royal Society, with Sir Christopher's continued interest, and under the direction of Robert Hooke (1662–72); later models were designed by Leupold of Leipzig in 1726, and Ons-en-Bray in Paris in 1734 (*50*).

New dimensions of speed were required when the science of ballistics began to be applied in practical gunnery. Bullets were fired through paper pasted on the rims of rotating wheels or discs, the use of a smoked drum for recording was described by Duhamel in 1841, and by Wertheim in 1844, electric time signals by Breguet in 1844 and Wheat-

[85]

stone in 1845; in 1845 also the extraordinarily precise ballistic galvanometer of Pouillet was described in publication, both in a French and an English journal (49). These inventions were the immediate precursors of the kymograph.

In 1828, Poiseuille in France invented the mercury manometer for blood pressure recording (15). He connected the manometer to the blood vessel by a rigid tube filled with bicarbonate solution. A different but even more widely important achievement was his analysis, published in 1842, of the flow of viscous fluids in narrow tubes (76): the general relation that resistance is equal to pressure difference divided by flow, and the specific formulation that flow varies as the fourth power of the radius.

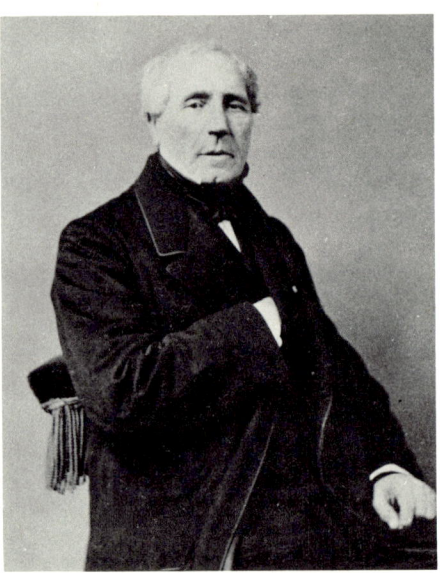

Figure 6. Jean Léonard Marie Poiseuille (1799–1869).

In the years to follow, these diverse methods and observations, and others such as the measurements of blood gases, described in the previous chapter (65), were brought together and applied to the study of the physiology of the circulation.

Dynamics of the Circulation

The prodigious advances in all science, including the biological sciences, during the latter half of the nineteenth century, had their origins in many parts of Europe. So far as the advancement of knowledge of the circulation is concerned, and particularly the action of the heart, Carl Ludwig and his school probably contributed a larger share than any other group.

Born in the small town of Witzenhausen in central Germany, Carl Ludwig received his early education in Hanau, then entered the University of Marburg, and began the study of medicine. He became dissatisfied with the teaching there, and his ardent spirit soon took him instead to the student fencing clubs. This promptly brought him in conflict with the disciplinary authorities of the University, and he was asked to leave. Returning again after an interval, Ludwig was greatly stimulated by the chemist Bunsen, pursued his studies zealously, and eventually received his M.D. degree in 1839, at the age of twenty-three. He became a prosector in anatomy under Ludwig Fick (eldest brother of Adolf Fick). In 1842 he published his remarkable dissertation on renal function, which will be discussed in a later chapter. Still working on his own, Ludwig's next large achievement came five years later when he published the description of his kymograph and recording manometer. Ludwig knew about and mentioned Poiseuille's mercury manometer, but did not mention the recording devices of the French, not even those described in Pouillet's paper, published two years earlier. It is probable that he had read these reports; they certainly were current in Germany. Two other young Germans, soon to be close friends of Ludwig's—Helmholtz and Du Bois-Reymond—knew of them and used them. But regardless of origins, Ludwig's kymograph and recording manometer marked a milestone in biological science; a considerable proportion of the discoveries in physiology and pharmacology in subsequent generations were recorded by their aid (*28*).

In 1849 Ludwig was appointed professor of anatomy and physiology in Zurich, where young Adolf Fick joined him two years later. In 1855 Ludwig went to Vienna, and ten years later to Leipzig, where a new Institute of Physiology was built under his direction and for his use. Holding that physiology arose out of anatomy, and was moving forward along with physics and chemistry, Ludwig had all three disciplines in his institute; one wing of his building for anatomy, one for biological chemistry, and the center for physiology. Contributions from all three branches continued to issue from this institute during the next thirty years.

We wish that it were possible to re-create a living picture of this remarkable man: the kindly, plain, bespectacled face with its great beak of a nose; the spare, brown-coated figure, constantly at work at one or another of the many experiments in progress; the wide sweep of his

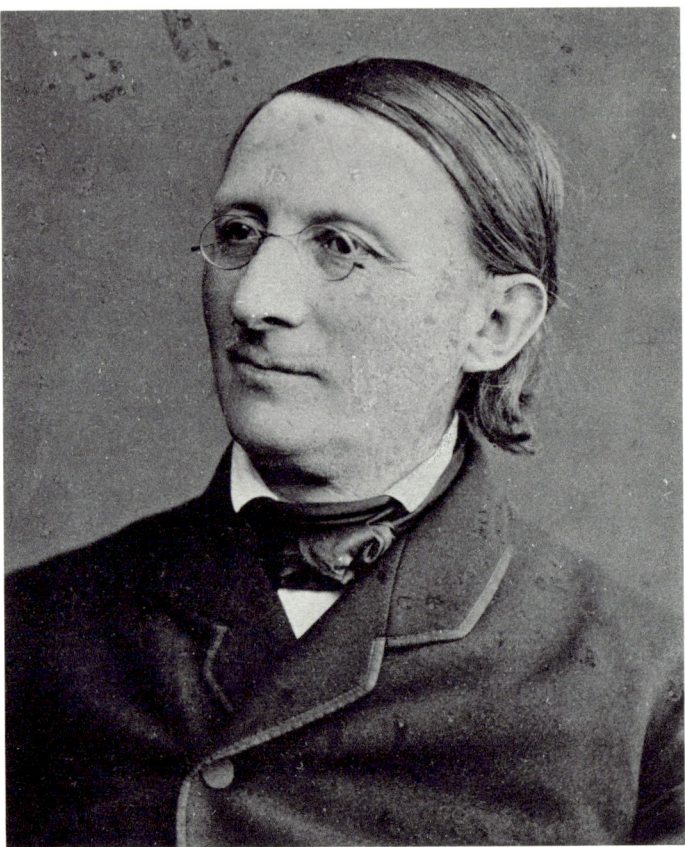

Figure 7. Carl Friedrich Wilhelm Ludwig (1816–95).

interest, the inexhaustible fertility of his experimental imagination; his expert knowledge of anatomy, his attention to detail and insistence on precision; his enthusiasm—the shout of delight with which he would greet some new finding, summoning everyone to come and see (*80*); his charm, his seriousness, and his searching yet kindly humor; his generosity, always giving his students the full credit for the work—

even though he might have done nine-tenths of it himself; his loyalty to all his friends, young and old. It is doubtful whether the science of physiology ever had a more inspiring teacher, or one who filled the academic world in succeeding generations with as many first-class teachers and scientists.

THE OUTPUT OF THE HEART

The contributions of Ludwig and his school to the physiology of the heart and circulation covered an extraordinary range. A long list is always tedious, but it is difficult in this case to give an idea of the activity of Ludwig's laboratory without mentioning at least some of the investigators and their work (*28*). In neurophysiology these included Ludwig's own discovery of ganglion cells in the interatrial septa (1848), von Cyon and Ludwig on the depressor nerve (1866), von

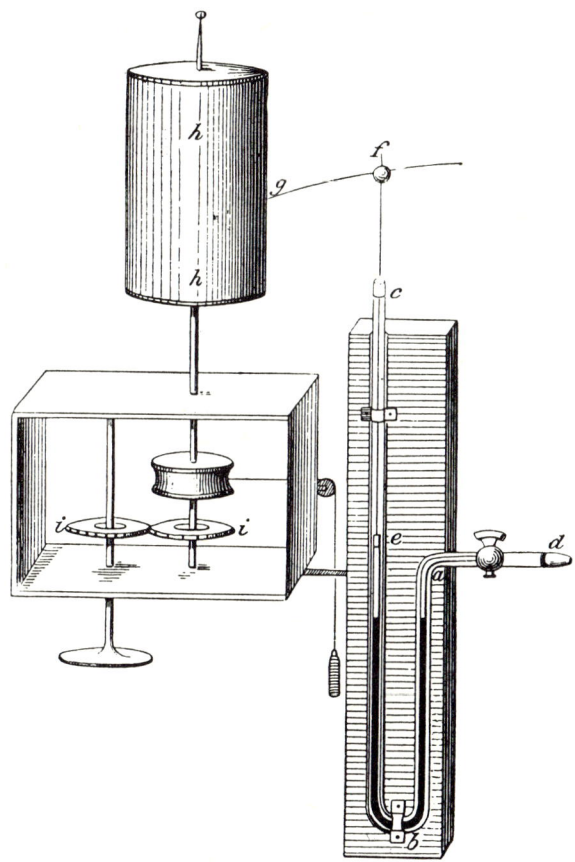

Figure 8. Ludwig's kymograph, described and published in 1847.

Cyon and Gaskell on the sympathetic fibers (1866), and Ludwig and Dittmar on the vasomotor center (1873). More directly in hemodynamics were the invention of the stromuhr, a double vessel on a swivel, for measurement of volume flow, by Ludwig and Dogiel (1867); the discovery by Bowditch of the "all-or-none" activity of cardiac muscle, and of the "staircase" phenomenon (1874); and many studies on skeletal muscle by von Kries, from which Otto Frank derived much help in the next generation. Ludwig and von Kries also measured capillary blood pressure (28).

Blood gases, soon to be brought into the dynamics of the circulation, were actively under study. In 1859, Ludwig and Setschenow improved on the extraction methods of Magnus. Further improvement was made independently by Pflüger in his own laboratory. Earlier, Lothar Meyer, a student of Ludwig's in Vienna, had studied the combination of oxygen with hemoglobin in the blood (28).

As an indication of the continued interest of Ludwig's students in the circulation and related matters, it might be noted that more than half the papers in the Festschrift celebrating his seventieth birthday (1887) were on such subjects: Bohr of Copenhagen on the combination of hemoglobin with CO_2, Fano of Genoa on the tonus of the heart, Fick of Würzburg on phonographic methods, Fleischl of Vienna on the heartbeat, Gaskell of Cambridge on electric changes in heart muscle after vagus stimulation, Héger of Brussels on blood vessel activity, Hüfner of Tübingen on blood pigments, von Kries of Freiburg on velocity of fluids in tubes, Rubner of Marburg on daily variations in CO_2 output, and Wooldridge of London on blood clotting (64).

Propagation of the Pulse Wave and Velocity of Blood Flow

The description of Carl Ludwig's physiological institute and its activities should not obscure the obvious fact that many equally important observations were being made in this field during these years in other laboratories. Among the most significant were those having to do with the movement of blood in the periphery.

As Harvey had observed and recorded, ejection of blood by the ventricle dilates the aorta. This distention passes down the aorta and out its branches as a pressure pulse wave. Spallanzani, in 1773, proved this by surrounding the artery with a ring and noting the narrowing of the space between, with each systole; Poiseuille proved the same point with a plethysmograph (*91*).

The pulse wave is, of course, propagated much faster than the flow of blood. As early as 1825 the brothers Ernst Heinrich and Eduard Friedrich Weber measured this rate, and it was further studied by Korteweg, and by Moens, in 1870. The general relation was developed that the velocity of propagation is faster, for a given pressure rise, when the arterial volume change is small as related to its initial volume; the mathematical expressions differed in detail. A transformation of the Korteweg formula by J. C. Bramwell and A. V. Hill (*6*) is $V_p = 0.357 \sqrt{\Delta PV/\Delta V}$, in which V_p is the pulse wave velocity in meters per second; ΔPV the increment in pressure in mm. Hg, corresponding to ΔV, the increment in volume in cubic centimeters starting from V, the initial volume of the artery. This seemingly rigid dimensional approach from an easily measurable quantity, the pulse wave velocity, has caused many investigators to believe that the uptake of blood by the arteries and hence the stroke output of the heart can be predicted from the pulse wave velocity (*2*). This approach neglects the fact that the initial volume of the arterial bed is much more variable than is the absolute volume uptake per unit pressure increase and that this initial volume cannot be measured from one individual to another (*36*). It also neglects the fact that the viscous and resistant properties of the arterial wall play a large role in determining the pulse wave velocity but have little consequence in setting the total uptake by the end of systole (*79*).

It was recognized early that the movement of blood, the velocity pulse, was altogether different in form and nature from the pressure pulse. The estimates of Stephen Hales on speed of blood along the aortic column have been noted. Chauveau, the veterinary surgeon whose measurement of pulmonary vascular pressures was described in the preceding chapter, invented his "hemodromograph" in 1860. This was an instrument for recording the details of the velocity pulse by placing a tiny paddle in the axis of the stream in a cannula which was interposed in an artery (*7*). The movements of this paddle by an ingenious system of levers were transmitted to a tambour writing on a smoked drum. The record, semiquantitative in nature, foreshadows the details of quantitative records taken by means of modern electronic instruments showing rapid systolic flow, backflow during the filling of the aortic cusps, and slow undulating forward flow, gradually decreasing during diastole (*36*).

The generating force for peripheral flow, the pressure developed within the heart, was also measured by É. J. Marey and A. Chauveau, by direct intracardiac cannulation, as has already been mentioned (*67*).

An even simpler concept of blood flow velocity is the circulation time. Hering in 1829 showed that the blood stream will carry an injected foreign substance (potassium ferrocyanide) around the circulation from jugular to jugular in the horse in about 30 seconds (*47*). Vierordt, in 1858, making the same measurements in smaller animals, noted that the circuit seemed to be accomplished in each species in about the same number of heart beats. These circulation time measurements were neglected for some forty years; we shall come back to the subject again (*88*). The subject of blood pressure and its recording is reviewed in another chapter.

Thus, in brief, the last half of the nineteenth century up to about 1890 found a firm and adequate foundation being built for an understanding of the physiology of the heart, the mechanism of its pumping action, its regulation, and many of the characteristics of the contraction of cardiac muscle, as well as an appreciation of the control of the blood vessels. And yet, with all this wide range of new knowledge, there was obviously something lacking, namely, an integration or calculation which might bring one group of phenomena into quantitative relation with others. The pieces of the fabric were there, but there was little interest in putting them together. This is especially curious, since in other fields quantitative physiology was in full progress. Several of Ludwig's former students, such as Max Rubner in metabolism and Christian Bohr in blood-gas relations, were leading the way in quantitative studies and syntheses in their respective subjects.

The reason for this perhaps lies in the complexity of this branch of biology. The histologist describes a meshwork of interlacing anastomosing blood vessels with blood hurrying in complex patterns through this labyrinth. To describe such phenomena in general terms is difficult; to describe them in quantitative terms is almost impossible. The effect of nerve stimulation, producing as it does variations in heart rate, blood pressure, and other functions, which are in themselves highly variable in different biological preparations and in the same preparation under slightly different conditions, did not offer much temptation to a rigid quantitative outlook.

Some of the responsibility perhaps lay with Carl Ludwig himself. By his own admission, he was not interested in mathematics; his eager, dynamic nature led him rather to more observation and more experiment than to prolonged reflective thought upon quantitative biological interrelations.

Another trend that came into operation during the last half of the nineteenth century was the preoccupation of biologists with evolutionary hypotheses. The patterns of the heart and great vessels in embryology and in comparative anatomy are of great importance in evolutionary theory, and such studies may well have deflected interest that might otherwise have expressed itself in liters per minute and quantitation of evanescent pressure changes.

Output of the Heart

There was one man in his field during this era who devoted his major interest and effort to the precise quantitative analysis of physiological phenomena. This was Adolf Fick. Though known at the present time in physics chiefly for one generalization, and in physiology for another, Fick was a mathematician, physicist, and physiologist, a scientist who made many contributions in many fields (29). He was a quiet, earnest, scholarly man, deeply read in philosophy and literature as well as in science, one who did not publish his findings widely, nor exploit them. His influence on physiological thought, we believe, has been undervalued, and it may be of interest to know something more about the man and his work.

With a strong early bent toward mathematics, Fick was first educated for a university degree in mathematical physics at Marburg, but changed to medicine on the advice of an older brother. After taking his medical degree, he accepted a prosectorship with Carl Ludwig in Zurich in 1852, and was one of Ludwig's first students. They remained lifelong friends. Fick continued at Zurich for sixteen years, then was appointed to the chair of physiology in Würzburg, succeeding von Bezold. Here he continued for the rest of his active life. The faculty at Würzburg was a distinguished one, and Fick with his broad interests, had many friends: the anatomist Kölliker, the jurist Regelsberger, the pathologist Rind-

THE HEART

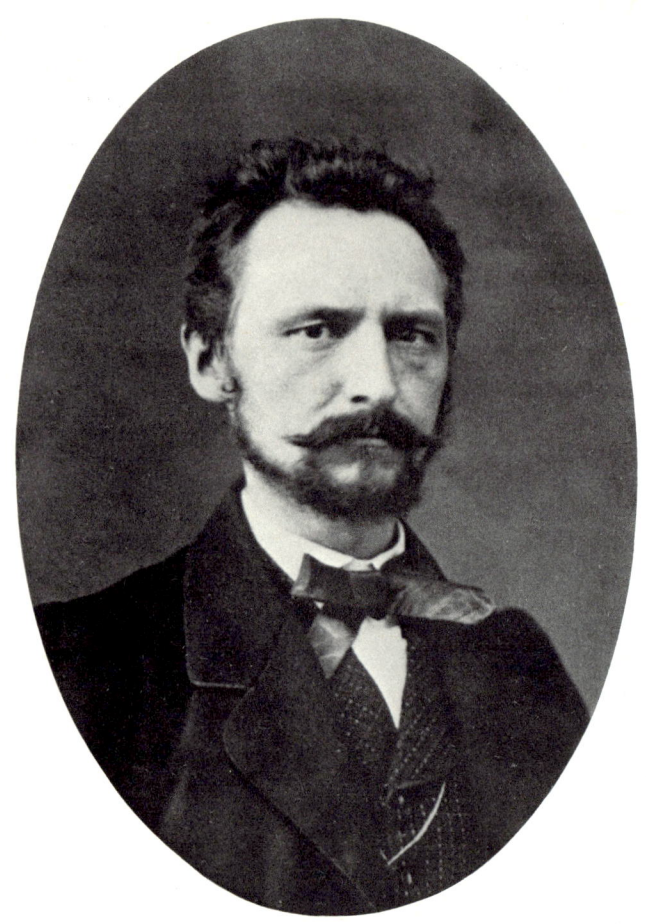

Figure 9. Adolf Fick (1829–1901).

fleisch, the clinicians Bergmann and Gerhardt, the chemist Wislicenus, and the physicists Clausius, Quincke, Kohlrausch, and Röntgen.

Fick achieved distinction as a physicist when he was quite young; his law of diffusion in fluids was published in 1855, when he was twenty-six years old (16). This was the statement of the general relation that diffusion is proportional to concentration gradient, a concept which he developed mathematically from Fourier's theory of heat equilibrium. Experimental proof of this was delayed for a quarter of a century, but Fick was undisturbed. The law was physically sound and logically correct, and for him this was enough.

In the year following, he published a 500-page book, *Medical Physics* (*17*). In this he considered a number of things with which he was later concerned as a physiologist: the mixing of air in the lungs, measurement of carbon dioxide output in man, the work of the heart, and the heat economy of the body.

THE OUTPUT OF THE HEART

A famous experiment in its day was the ascent of the Faulhorn by Fick and Wislicenus in 1865, which Fick undertook to test Liebig's theory that the energy of muscular exercise is derived from protein (*23*). Fick measured his own urinary nitrogen excreted during this ascent, and for six hours thereafter, and calculating the work expended on the ascent, found the minimum work to be more than two and one-half times the energy derivable from the protein metabolized. Liebig's theory was thus disposed of.

Fick's major experimental activity, extending over thirty years, was devoted to the physiology of muscular contraction. He demonstrated precisely and in various ways the relation between length of fiber and strength of contraction, with skillfully constructed experiments on isometric and isotonic contraction (*22*). This was the fundamental background of the studies of both skeletal and heart muscle in the ensuing decades; we shall return to this presently. Fick made extended calculations on energy and heat development in relation to muscular contraction and concluded that muscle is not a thermodynamic machine, but rather that chemical energy is directly transferred to mechanical energy.

Here was a man, then, who thought about physiology in quantitative terms, who was a good physicist and mathematician, and who was able to bring separate but related phenomena into quantitative formulation.

This was his achievement in the simple Fick principle for calculation of cardiac output: that the total oxygen absorbed per minute, divided by the uptake of oxygen into the blood per unit of blood flowing, i.e. the arteriovenous oxygen difference, gives the total blood flow through the lungs. A similar equation obviously obtains for CO_2 output and CO_2 arteriovenous differences.

This simple relation has more in it than would appear at first glance. It was the first physiological synthesis of the notion of blood flow and the notion of respiratory gas transport. In another relationship it was essentially the expression of the dilution principle for blood flow measurement: the faster the blood flow the less oxygen taken up per unit of blood flowing. The dilution principle is really the basis of most of the accepted methods of measuring the cardiac output and the flow of blood to organs and regions. Among these are foreign gas and injection (indicator dilution) methods, including clearance techniques for measuring blood flow through liver and kidney. It is hard to exaggerate the importance and widespread influence of the ideas which have evolved in close relation to the principle exemplified in the calculation which has since become known as the Fick principle.

The Fick principle was published in the brief proceedings of the Würzburg Physikalische-medizinische Gesellschaft for July 9, 1870 (20). (One cannot resist noting that the item in the proceedings immediately preceding Fick's communication announced the election of the young physicist, Wilhelm Röntgen, to membership in the society.) Here is the complete communication:

"Herr Fick had a contribution on the measurement of the amount of blood ejected by the ventricle of the heart with each systole, a quantity the knowledge of which is certainly of great importance. Varying opinions have been expressed on this. While Thomas Young estimated the quantity at about 45 cc., most estimates in modern textbooks, supported by the views of Volkmann and Vierordt, run much higher, up to 180 cc. It is surprising that no one has arrived at the following procedure by which this important value is available by direct determination, at least in animals. One measures how much oxygen an animal absorbs from the air in a given time, and how much CO_2 it gives off. One takes during this time a sample of arterial and a sample of venous blood; in both samples oxygen content and CO_2 content are measured. The difference of oxygen content gives the amount of oxygen each cubic centimeter of blood takes up in its passage through the lungs; and as one knows how much total oxygen has been taken up in given time, one can calculate how many cubic centimeters of blood have passed through the lungs in this time, or if one divides by the number of heartbeats during this time, how many cubic centimeters of blood are ejected with each beat. The corresponding calculation with CO_2 quantities gives a determination of the same value, which provides a control for the other calculation.

"Since for the demonstration of this method two gas pumps are needed, your reporter unfortunately is not in a position to communicate experimental data.

He will only give, therefore, a calculation of blood flow in man according to this method, based on more or less arbitrary data. According to the experiments of Scheffer in Ludwig's laboratory, dog's arterial blood contains 0.146 cc. oxygen per cc. (measured at 0°C. and 1 atm. pressure); 1 cc. of venous blood contains 0.0905 cc. oxygen. Each cc. of blood therefore takes up 0.0555 cc. oxygen in its passage through the lungs. Let us assume the same in man. Assume, further that a man absorbs in 24 hours 833 grams of oxygen. This will occupy a space of 433,200 cc. at 0°C. and 1 atm. pressure. According to this, 5 cc. of oxygen would be absorbed by the lungs of a man each second. In order to effect this absorption, 5/0.0555 cc. of blood must perfuse the lungs per second, that is, 90 cc. Assuming, finally, 7 systoles in 6 seconds, each systole would then eject 77 cc. of blood."

It was characteristic of Fick that having once published the principle, he was satisfied. This new concept, this physiological synthesis, was indubitably sound, and it was of no great concern to him whether full experimental proof came immediately, or waited a decade or two. But this does not mean that Fick himself stopped thinking about it, or stopped teaching it to his students. In his short textbook, or "compendium" of physiology, which ran through several editions, and which he must have used in his teaching, the Fick principle was very clearly set forth (*18*). He still did not have the A-V difference for man, but using again the value for the dog, and the total CO_2 output for man, a figure easily obtainable, he had in the textbook an estimate of $(270/5.8) \times 100 = 4.6$ liters per minute for the resting cardiac output of man.

There was a considerable hiatus between the enunciation of the principle and its experimental demonstration. In 1886 there was a short paper in the *Comptes rendus*, by Grehant and Quinquaud, describing measurements of the blood flow in dogs (*31*), and in 1898 a lengthy and detailed study was published by Zuntz and Hagemann of the cardiac output of the horse (*93*). Since the blood of the horse is slow to clot, these investigators were able to pass a tube down the jugular vein and into the heart to take samples of right atrial blood, just as Marey and Chauveau had passed their cardiac sound for registering pressure changes.

Nathan Zuntz brought much experience to his work. A former student in Pflüger's laboratory, he was an expert in blood gas analysis and had done pioneering work in the quantitative study of metabolic gaseous exchange as well as work in many other fields of physiology. In his later years he discovered the nitrous oxide method for measuring the cardiac output, of which more will be said presently. Measuring the oxygen consumption from the expired air and analyzing the arterial and right heart blood for oxygen, Zuntz and Hagemann calculated the cardiac output of the horse at rest, during exercise, and during digestion. The results were expressed to five figures in elaborate protocols.

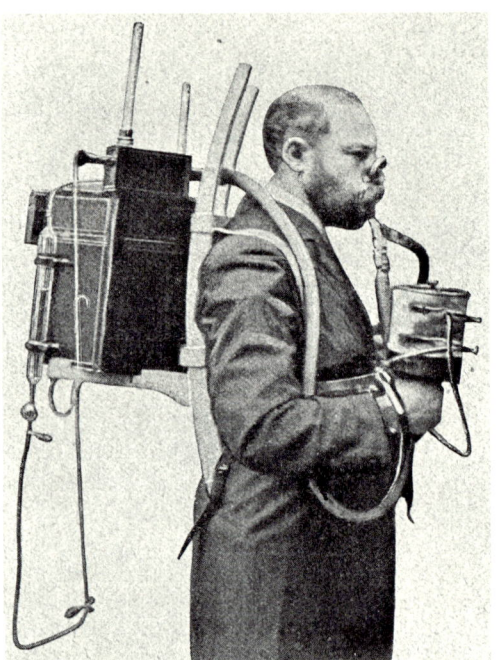

Figure 10. Nathan Zuntz (1847–1920) and his apparatus for collecting expired air.

This application of the Fick procedure by the direct analysis for oxygen of the mixed venous blood from the right heart was not pursued further for nearly thirty years. Zuntz and his collaborators were more interested in metabolism than in hemodynamics. Human physiology had not developed to this point, and the physiology of abnormal circulatory states, in clinical disease, had scarcely moved beyond the measurement of arterial blood pressure.

The important advance in experimental animal physiology in this field, during the last decade of the century, was that of Otto Frank on the dynamics of heart muscle contraction; this will be considered in the closing section of this chapter.

Measurements of Cardiac Output: "Indirect" and "Direct" Fick Methods

Interest in the measurement of cardiac output in the intact individual was finally reawakened by way of human physiology. Of the three measurements required by the Fick principle, the total respiratory gas exchange was easily obtained, and a sample of deeply expired or "alveolar" air gave a CO_2 tension approximating the arterial. The problem was to obtain some estimate of the gases in the blood entering the right heart, the mixed venous blood.

Loewy and von Schrötter in 1903 (60) had the ingenious idea that if one bronchus were blocked for a few seconds, the air distal to it would be in equilibrium with the incoming pulmonary arterial or mixed venous blood. A sampling of this trapped air should give the respiratory gas tensions of this blood. This was theoretically correct, providing that the subject was in a physiologically steady state, which, in this situation, would be highly doubtful. The difficulty of the procedure made the method impractical.

A simpler method of obtaining mixed venous values, by rebreathing gas mixtures out of a small bag until the blood coming into the lung was in equilibrium with the lung-bag system, was discussed in part of an extensive and now all but forgotten monograph, "Hämodynamische Studien," by J. Plesch in 1909 (74). His method was used on a series of normal and abnormal subjects. In the two decades that followed there were many modifications of this procedure and further attempts to measure cardiac output by this indirect Fick procedure. A brief critique of this method is in order.

While the arterial CO_2 value could be fairly well determined by measuring the alveolar CO_2 tension and applying this to a standard CO_2 dissociation curve, this measurement was soon obtainable directly by arterial puncture as well. The main problem was still the mixed venous CO_2 value. A partial simplification was suggested by Henderson and Prince (45), of having high oxygen concentration in the rebreathing mixture, so that the CO_2 equilibrium could take place with oxygenated blood, and the "oxygenated mixed venous tension" then plotted on the oxygenated CO_2 dissociation curve of blood. So far as the rebreathing procedure itself was concerned, its validity was conditioned as follows:

If the rebreathed CO_2 concentration from the bag was such that on *complete mixing* with the CO_2 in the residual lung volume, a close approximation of the mixed venous CO_2 tension resulted, and *if* exact equilibrium could then take place between air and incoming blood *before* extensive recirculation occurred (10–18 seconds) and before the *added* effort of deep breathing altered the resting values, *then* the expired sample after rebreathing would represent the mixed venous CO_2 tension.

As the above set of conditions implies, there were many sources of error, some of which were the following:

1. Incomplete equilibrium between CO_2 in lungs and in blood. Retarded mixture of bulk gases in the system, too little CO_2 added to the gas in the rebreathing bag, and the "disappearance" of CO_2 into pulmonary tissues other than pulmonary arterial blood were some of the factors preventing a clear-cut "mixed venous plateau" during rebreathing (37). With abnormal lungs, such as are found in emphysema, poor intrapulmonary mixing of gases made the method worthless.

2. Recirculation of blood before the procedure was complete. It was thought for some time that appreciable amounts of blood recirculated only after 30 seconds, whereas significant recirculation actually begins in 10–18 seconds. An error here would give cardiac output values that were too low.

3. Non-steady state of the subject at the time of the test.

4. Technical error. With a total CO_2 A-V difference in the range of 10 mm. Hg, or 4 volumes per cent, small errors of measurement made large errors in the cardiac output figure.

A further mistake that many were falling into at this time was one that might be called the "Fallacy of Good Checks." If a procedure was repeated, and consistent values obtained, this was taken as proof that the method was valid, whereas, in fact, the procedure was only repeating the same errors each time. A typical example was as follows: The subject rebreathed a mixture low in CO_2, and repeated this until a constant P_{CO_2} (partial pressure of CO_2 gas in the air) was obtained on successive rebreathings. This was accepted as the "mixed venous" value; but simple calculation could show that on each successive rebreathing, the residual air was diluting the mixture by a fixed amount,

THE OUTPUT
OF THE HEART

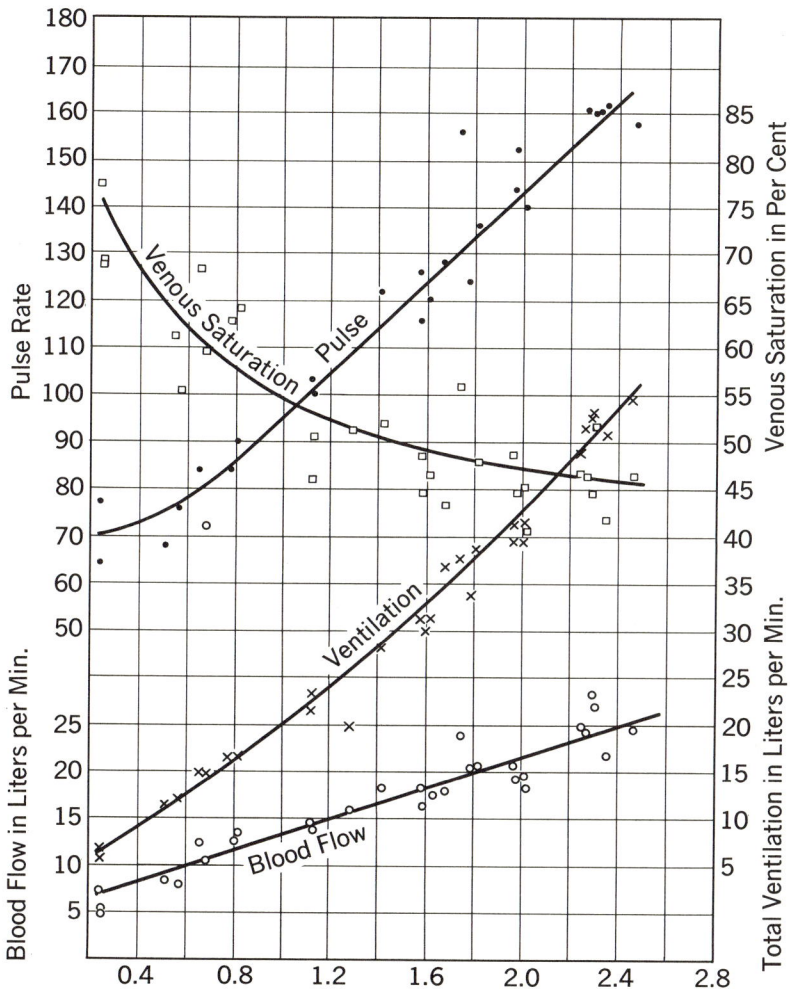

Figure 11. Relation between oxygen consumption, heart rate, ventilation, and cardiac output. These figures, obtained in the Harvard Fatigue Laboratory with the use of an indirect Fick method, compare well with later data using direct Fick procedures.

so that equilibrium with mixed venous blood was never achieved. This error gave cardiac output figures that were too high.

In spite of all these defects, the indirect Fick procedure in the hands of careful workers provided some valuable studies both in rest and exercise, with cardiac output values which subsequent work with more reliable methods has confirmed (43). There were many others whose results were erroneous.

It should be noted, also, that beginning in the 1920's, a number of studies of cardiac output in animals were carried out, using the direct Fick procedure by cannulation or puncture of the right heart, to investigate the effects of drugs, of hemorrhage and shock, etc.

Another method of cardiac output determination, and a very ingenious one, was introduced by Markoff, Müller, and Zuntz (68), and developed by Krogh and Lindhard in Copenhagen (59). It was based on the absorption into the pulmonary blood stream of an inhaled foreign gas, on the general principle that the faster the blood flow the more gas taken up. The gas used was nitrous oxide; the procedure was to inhale and rebreathe from a bag of nitrous oxide-in-air for about fifteen seconds, in order to achieve complete mixture, then partly exhale and sample, then hold for another eight seconds, then exhale and sample again. By simple equations, the nitrous oxide absorbed can be determined and, the solubility of the gas in blood being known, the blood flow can be calculated. But most of the sources of error in the indirect Fick methods are also in this, and in addition the procedure takes longer. Dye injection studies later showed that not only has recirculation begun by 10 to 18 seconds, but very shortly thereafter half to two-thirds of the blood is on its second round. With recirculation of foreign gas, less fresh gas can be taken up, and the cardiac output as measured is too small, as was in fact the case. But with the nitrous oxide method, in the hands of capable workers such as Krogh, Lindhard, and Liljestrand, although the absolute values of cardiac output were low, the changes noted in rest and various forms of exercise gave correctly the general course of physiological events (59, 57).

The dilution method used most widely in the late 'twenties and through the 'thirties was that of Grollman (32). He had found that acetylene was a nontoxic gas rapidly absorbed into the blood on inhalation, and he fashioned this into a cardiac output method analogous to that using nitrous oxide. His chief error again was the assumption that the circulation time in man was 20–30 seconds and he supported this by showing that rebreathing could be prolonged from 18 to 30 seconds without causing the calculation of output to change. He overlooked the fact that 18 and 30 seconds bracketed the time of the second circulation rather than the first, so that measurements could be too low without disagreeing (another example of the "Fallacy of Good Checks").

The actual average figure for normal cardiac output in man, as "standardized" by the Grollman method, was 2.2 ± 0.2 liters per minute per square meter of body surface—the so-called cardiac index. A large volume of work was carried out for a full decade, using this method, in normal and abnormal clinical states. Like the nitrous oxide method, it gave results normally in the right direction, but low (*32*). It was also insensitive: it failed, for example, to detect the higher cardiac output in the lying as compared with sitting and standing positions, which had already been discovered by the indirect-Fick rebreathing techniques.

At about this time also, evidence began to accumulate showing that the blood flow to the different organs of the body summated to figures much larger than the limits set by Grollman of about four liters per minute. It was shown in the late 'thirties and early 'forties that blood flow to the kidneys was 1.3 liters per minute, to the splanchnic area 1.5 liters, and to the brain and heart another 1.2 liters per minute, with blood flow to skeletal tissues, thyroid, adrenal, etc., still to be accounted for. These figures, since confirmed, add up to more than that allocated to the whole body by Grollman. The time was ripe for a new departure.

The solution to the use of the direct Fick principle for measuring cardiac output came from an unexpected source. A young surgical intern in Eberswald, Germany, Werner Forssmann, was seeking a safe method of administering medications directly into the chambers of the heart in order to treat emergencies such as cardiac arrest during operation. He introduced a catheter into a vein of his own arm and advanced the tip into the right atrium of his heart. Suffering no ill effect, he repeated the procedure in several subsequent experiments. In the note which he published in 1929 (*24*), reporting his experience, he commented that the procedure might be useful in physiological studies. Following this lead, several investigators in the next few years obtained mixed venous blood from the right atrium; arterial blood and oxygen consumption in the usual way, and so were able to measure cardiac output by the direct Fick principle. Cournand and his associates (*11*), beginning in 1941, carried out an extensive series of studies, using the catheterization technique. Their average figure for cardiac output in man at rest was 3.1 liters per minute per square meter of body surface (cardiac index), and this has been generally confirmed by others. They also made further progress in technique, showing first that the catheter could be left in place for protracted periods without harm, and second, that the tip could be advanced with safety into the right ventricle, and thence into the pulmonary artery. These developments led to experiments measuring volume flow combined with recordings of pressures and blood volume, thus providing a more complete hemodynamic study (*10*). Since the whole procedure was not only safe and painless but involved no active co-operation by the subject, it was applicable to the study of patients with various forms of circulatory and pulmonary dysfunction; such studies were undertaken by these and many other investigators. This, however, is beyond the scope of this discussion.

A particular emphasis of Cournand and his associates was that the determination of blood flow by the Fick procedure must be done during a steady state when the expiratory exchange represents the actual respiration of the cells, and respiratory gases are not going into or coming out of storage in the body—a major source of error in experiments involving acute hypoxia. Visscher and Johnson (*89*) have brought out a further consideration, that when flow changes as a result of the cardiac or respiratory cycle or as a result of sudden vasomotor or cardiac alterations, the mixed venous sample taken when the flow is changing does not represent the true average of oxygen content adequately, because it cannot be weighted to represent the greater volume during rapid flow. It represents the time average rather than the volume average which should be used in calculating the mean flow. These considerations make manifest a source of error in the Fick and in other dilution procedures which can be minimized by the maintenance of a steady state and by the recognition that venous samples should be taken in such a way that the rapid flow component is well mixed with the slow flow component before the stream reaches the sampling point. Thus the cyclic augmentation of the pulmonary stream in atrial septal defect should be determined by samples from the pulmonary artery rather than from the right atrium.

Measurement of Cardiac Output—The Indicator Dilution Method

During the years when cardiac output measurements were stylized about the procedures and results of Grollman, and it was held that the flow of blood should be within the rigid limits of 2.2 ± 0.2 liters per minute per square meter of body surface, a series of experiments was being performed by Hamilton, Moore, and Kinsman in Louisville which indicated that the cardiac output was half again as large; and thus in general agreement with the earlier indirect-Fick results. The experiments suggesting slow or nonmoving arterialized fluids in the lungs, outlined above, the constant increase in A-V CO_2 difference with rebreathing time, and the definitive proof that acetylene returns in the venous blood in a very short time to hinder foreign gas getting into the blood of the lungs, convinced these workers that it would be impractical to measure the cardiac output by means of respiratory procedures. They became interested in a technique which had been used in experimental animals but not in man, the injection method (*52*). This method has an interesting history.

In 1897 George Neil Stewart, formerly a student of the English physiologist William Stirling, and later professor of physiology at Western Reserve University, published a series of experiments on the circulation time (*88*). He gave an intravenous injection of salt solution, and then picked up the conductivity change in an artery when the salt solution arrived there. This was simple enough. Stewart, being a physiologist with imagination, then considered other possibilities: thinking that the most rapid circulation time was the average circulation time, he investigated the capacity of the vascular bed. He proceeded to use a continuous infusion of his indicator, arguing that the amount of dilution, when picked up on the arterial side, would be proportional to the size of the stream. Thus if the salt solution were run in at 5 cc. per second, and the analysis showed that the arterial blood had added to it 0.2 cc. of salt solution, there would be a blood flow of 5/0.2, or 25 cc. per second, or 1.5 liters per minute.

Henriques (*46*) made an important modification of this principle by showing that the calculation can be made just as accurately if the injection is made all at once instead of by a constant flow infusion. When this is done, the indicator (Henriques used thyocyanate) appears in the artery five or six seconds after injection into the right heart, and rises and falls in concentration during a period many times longer than the duration of the injection. His observations differed radically from the ideas of Stewart, who thought that the duration of the passage of altered blood was the same as the duration of the infusion and that the appearance time and mean circulation time were identical. The formula for

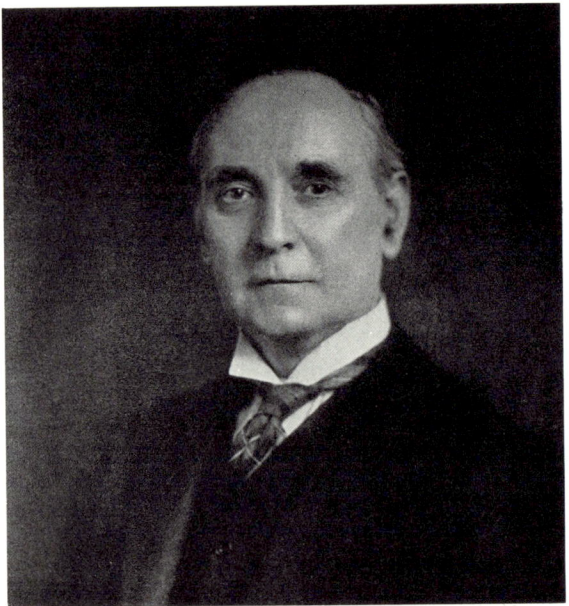

Figure 12. George Neil Stewart (1860–1930).

calculating the flow from the concentration curve resulting from instantaneous injection is $F = I/ct$. Thus the flow (F) is 3 liters in 30 seconds or 6 liters per minute if the injection (I) is 12 mg., the average concentration (c) is 4 mg. per liter, and the time of passage (t) is 30 seconds (Fig. 13).

The Louisville workers decided to follow the procedure of Henriques rather than that of Stewart. In modifying the procedure they

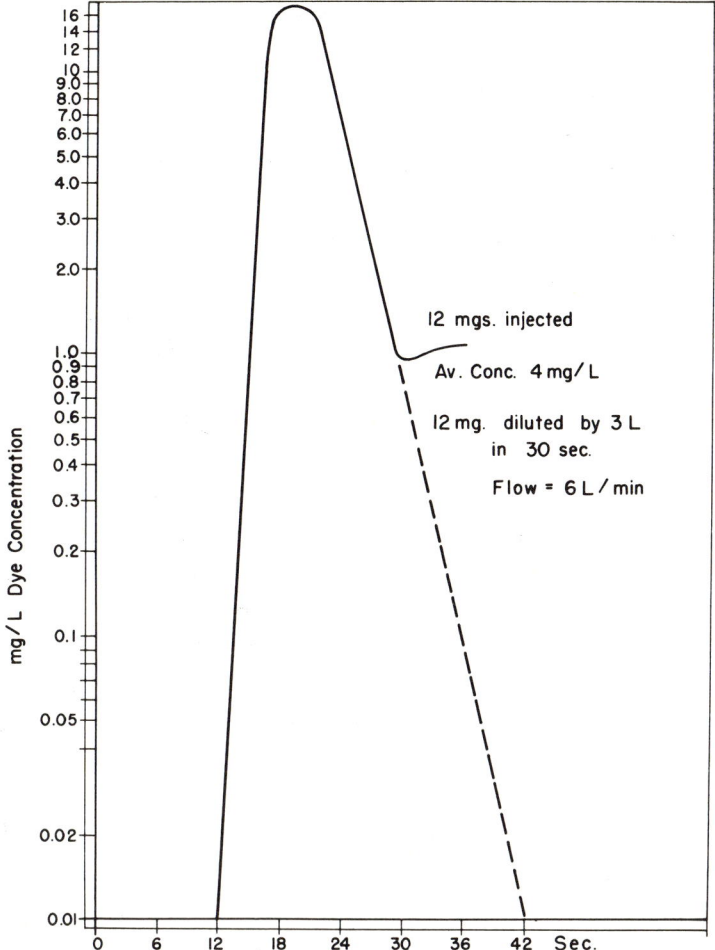

Figure 13. Dye dilution curve, concentration against time, used in dye dilution method of cardiac output determination.

showed that the indicator should be a substance that remained intravascular (such as vital red, or the blue dye T-1824) and that flows calculated from such dilution curves agreed quantitatively with measured flows in glass models, in perfused heart-lung systems, and with flows measured in normal dogs by means of the direct Fick procedure (70). In order to get a high order of agreement between measured and calculated flow in models which recirculate and in animals, it is necessary to base the calculation on an indicator which has not recirculated. The descending limb of the dye curve is nearly always exponential, a washout curve based on the washing out of dye from a volume which corresponds mathematically to an indeterminate fraction of the real volume of the system. It was hoped at first that the volume of the system could be calculated from the slope of the washout curve, but experiment showed that this was not possible.

However, prolonging the exponential downslope as a straight line on semilogarithmic coordinates enables one to plot the complete concentration curve of dye on its first circulation. From this curve it is possible to calculate the flow, and the circulation times, including the mean circulation time. This last quantity $MCT = \Sigma CT/\Sigma C$, where C and T are read from the curve at regular (i.e. one-second) intervals. The mean circulation time is of particular importance because the product of the mean circulation time and the flow equals the capacity of the stream bed between the point of injection (including temporally equivalent tributaries) and the point of sampling (including temporally equivalent branches). Experiments with models have shown that the true capacity of the bed equals the product of flow and mean circulation time even though the washout is greatly prolonged. If the flow can be measured from the average concentration, *ipso facto* the capacity of the active bed can be measured.

It was more than a decade before the validity of the dye dilution method came to be generally accepted. This was in part because the technique, with its many samplings, was a tedious one, and in part because the results obtained were not in accord with the then popular acetylene method. A number of studies carried out and published in 1932 are of interest, in view of later developments. Fifteen normal individuals under nonbasal conditions had cardiac indices averaging 3.9 liters, with stroke volumes of 40 to 60 cc.; seven cases of anemia were found to have high blood flows, and a series of cases of congestive heart failure had low blood flows (*38*).

In 1948 the original dye injection investigators (Hamilton, et al.) and members of the cardiac catheterization team (Cournand, et al.) joined forces and during the course of that summer, with members of the research force as subjects, carried out a rigorous series of simultaneous measurements with the dye method and with direct-Fick cardiac catheterization. The results were a triumph for collaborative study, showing remarkably good agreement with the two methods, both in rest and varying degrees of exercise (*40*).

The technical advances in methods of analyzing blood for the concentration of the indicator have contributed greatly to the increasing use of the injection method of measuring blood flow. The task set by the original method, involving as it did the analysis of twenty to thirty small blood samples, repelled many workers. These technical advances, continuously recording the optical density, the conductivity, or the radioactivity of blood drawn out of the arterial stream and passed through a sensitive recorder, simplified the method considerably. About 1950 it was shown that the dye T–1824 could be measured in a stream of fully oxygenated blood passed between a light source and a photoelectric cell (*92*).

The use of radioactive indicators depended at first upon the analysis of separate samples (tagged cells or plasma). Various apparatus have been designed so that a scintillation rate meter can be used on a stream of arterial blood withdrawn through the cuvette. Such a rate meter has also been collimated over the femoral artery or over the heart so that measurable curves can be traced. In brief, during the past decade and a half, the dilution methods have come into rapidly increasing use in the analysis both of normal and all sorts of abnormal circulatory patterns (such as those in congenital heart conditions). The review of these is beyond the scope of the present chapter (*12*).

Besides the dilution methods for measuring the circulation rate, we have methods by which the aortic stream may be measured volumetrically by the cardiometer (*55*), the rotameter (*62*), or by the recently perfected electromagnetic flowmeters (*53*). The last of these is especially important since, after the implantation procedure, one has essentially an intact animal.

The methods considered so far may be called primary methods, in that if reasonable assumptions be granted, they are direct measures of the cardiac output. Contrasted to these are methods which are best referred to as empiric methods, which achieve their validity from constants derived by comparison with a primary method. These have now been almost completely discarded in favor of the direct techniques. Two that are of historical interest may be mentioned: the estimation of stroke output from the pulse pressure, by Erlanger and Hooker (*14*); and the ballistocardiograph of Starr (*86*)—the estimation of cardiac output from the movement of the body resulting from the impacts imparted by the heart's systolic contraction. Although not a measure of cardiac output, the ballistocardiographic record shows a number of interesting differences in abnormal as compared with normal heart beats (*87*).

The Regulation of the Stroke Volume

The most important problem to which physiologists address themselves in studying the circulation is to understand, even partially, the mechanism by which the circulation is regulated. How can blood flow increase and decrease with shifting demands for oxygen transport and heat dissipation, changing sixfold or more and yet maintaining arterial and venous pressures within relatively narrow limits?

Obviously, two sets of regulatory arrangements are needed, one for the peripheral vessels, and the other for the heart. The vasomotor control of the circulation is the subject of a later chapter; we shall close this present discussion with an account of a few of the major steps in the development of knowledge of the regulation of the heart beat and stroke output.

Basic knowledge of the performance of heart muscle was derived in considerable part from earlier knowledge of the physiology of skeletal muscle. As we have seen, Adolf Fick was a leader in this latter field over a period of more than thirty years, beginning with his publication, *Untersuchungen über Muskel-Arbeit*, in 1867 (*19, 21, 22*). Blix, the Scandinavian physiologist, a former student of Fick's, made further observations on the relation between length of fiber and strength of contraction (*4*). Important studies on heart muscle contraction were made by Blasius (*3*), Marey (*66*), and Dreser (*13*), but it remained for Otto Frank to bring together and formulate some of the fundamental principles of atrial and ventricular contraction (*25*).

Like Adolf Fick, Frank in his early training devoted much time to mathematics and physics, and was accomplished in classical mechanics. He was one of the last students to work with Carl Ludwig, leaving Leipzig in 1894, the year before Ludwig's death, to join Voit in Munich.

He succeeded Voit as professor of physiology in 1908, a position which he held until his retirement in 1934. He died in 1944.

Frank's classic paper, "Zur Dynamik des Herzmuskels," has recently been translated into English by Chapman and Wasserman, and published in the *American Heart Journal* (26, 27). Frank used a small, simple, yet elegant preparation of the whole frog heart, perfused with diluted ox blood. He was able to fill or empty the heart chambers, and make continuous records throughout the cardiac cycle of pressures in various

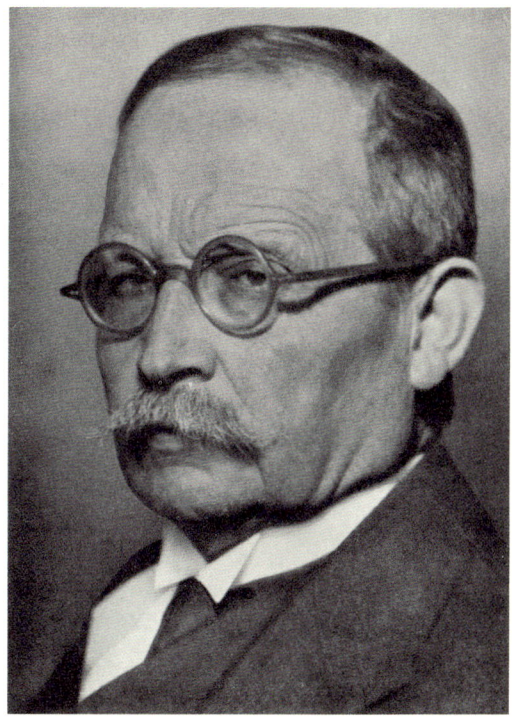

Figure 14. Otto Frank (1865–1944).

parts of the system, of volumes in the heart chamber (filling), and of volume output. He first studied the isometric contraction, allowing measured amounts of blood to enter the heart, then closing the aortic stopcock to prevent outflow. "I discovered the following law concerning the dependence of the form of the isometric pressure curve, on the initial tension. The peaks (maxima) of the isometric pressure curve rise with increasing initial tension (filling). (I call this part of the family of curves the first part.) Beyond a certain level of filling the pressure peaks decline (second part of the family of curves)." Then he defined the time relations of the curves more exactly. "Fick discovered the same law for skeletal muscle." "Fick arranged the peak values (maxima) of the individual curves as functions of the fiber lengths. I could proceed similarly if I could regard maximal tensions as functions of cardiac filling." But this Frank found experimentally difficult with his preparation, because he filled both atrium and ventricle, and with increased tensions the atrium often became overfilled with blood at the expense of the ventricle.

From this point, Frank examined isotonic ventricular contraction, the ventricle ejecting blood into a sort of elastic capsule; he then considered the whole process of normal contraction, analyzing the initial phase of isometric contraction against varying initial aortic pressures,

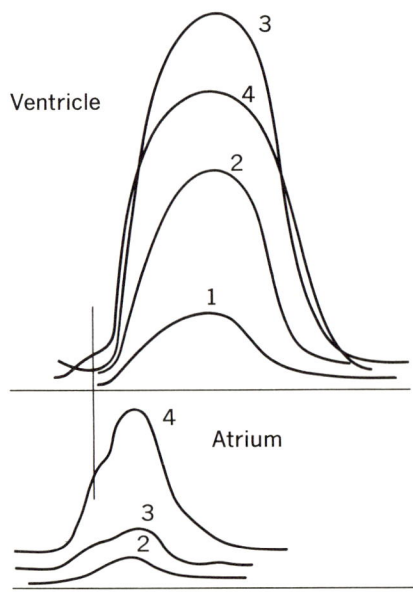

Figure 15. Pressure curves developed during systolic contraction, and subsequent relaxation, in the frog heart of Frank's preparation. It can be seen that, with increased filling pressure, there was increased systolic ejection pressure, up to a maximum (1 to 3), followed by a lesser systolic pressure as inflow pressure was further elevated (4).

as well as the ejection and relaxation periods. A number of other important observations were made; the increased speed of pressure build-up, or muscular contraction in early systole, with increased initial filling; and the presence of residual blood at the end of systole, this increasing with increased aortic resistance and increased diastolic filling.

The chief point here is that both Adolf Fick and Otto Frank were entirely familiar with the relation between muscle fiber and length and strength of contraction, the basis of the subsequent Starling's law; Frank only hesitated in regard to his particular experimental findings of fiber length and diastolic filling, because in his preparation he could not measure them accurately. Frank was aware of the contemporaneous work of Blix in Scandinavia, which also stressed the proportionate relation of fiber length to strength of muscular contraction.

More than fifteen years later, Ernest H. Starling, brilliant and distinguished professor of physiology at University College, London, undertook to study the same problem using the isolated perfused heart-lung of the dog, a preparation which he himself had perfected. This work was carried out in part at University College, aided by his associates, S. W. Patterson, H. Piper, and J. Markwalder, and in part in Professor Max Rubner's laboratory in Berlin (*69, 73, 72*).

This was a substantial series of experiments, well conceived and skillfully executed, moving steadily over a period of years to answer one question after another. The essential achievement was the measurement of ventricular volumes and ventricular stroke outputs, as the conditions of venous inflow and of aortic resistance were varied in successive experiments.

Starling expressed his final conclusion as follows:

"*The law of the heart is therefore the same as that of skeletal muscle, namely that the mechanical energy set free on passage from the resting to the contracted state depends on the area of 'chemically active surfaces,' i.e. on the length of the muscle fibre. This simple formula serves to 'explain' the whole behaviour of the isolated mammalian heart.*"

This disarmingly simple statement has proved to have all the virtues, and also certain of the vices, that might be expected from so sweeping a generalization; though actually the "vices" came more from too broad an extension of Starling's principle by his enthusiastic admirers, who neglected the conditions and qualifications of Starling's own statement.

As to the virtues, it is certainly true that within properly defined limits the heart does possess automatic regulation which depends upon the stretch response. A small increase in initial tension works a great increase in the diastolic size and in the force of contraction. As the initial tension is further increased in much larger measure, the increase in diastolic size and the increase in contractile force are minimal and the latter even begins to decline. Over the whole range, the contractile force, oxygen consumption, and work per beat in the isolated heart correlate more closely with diastolic size than with initial tension.

Starling's great merit was to put this stretch response in a clearly defined biological setting and to show how an animal can make use of it in meeting (within limits) its needs. Thus, if the arterial pressure is

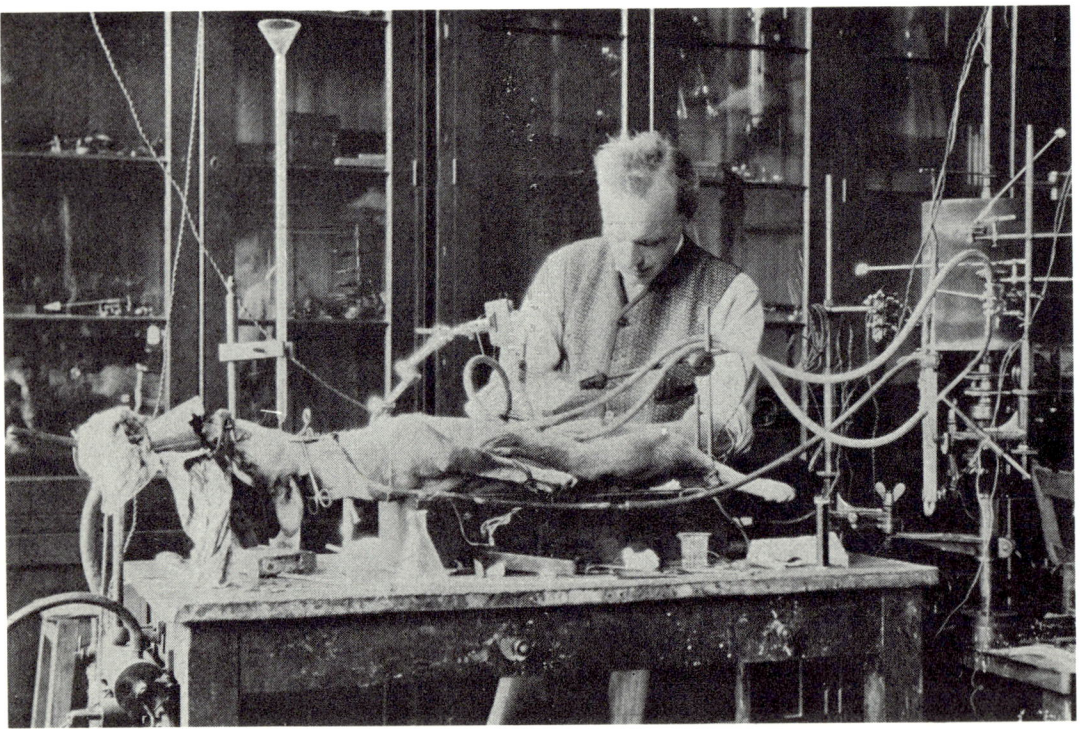

Figure 16. E. H. Starling at work on a dog experiment.

increased the ventricle empties less completely, while the residual blood is added to the diastolic filling and causes increased diastolic size. This, in turn, causes an increased contractile force which, if the task is not too great, enables the heart to do its increased job. Again, if the load upon the heart is increased by increasing the venous pressure and hence the inflow volume, the heart is directly filled to a size larger than before and contracts more strongly. Moreover, when the heart is overdistended it becomes weaker. The heart compensates for increased work or handicap by dilation within physiological limits, becomes decompensated by overdilation, and recompensates when the overdilation is abrogated. It is indeed a delightfully simple and elegant example of what might be called either cybernetics or homeostasis, whichever currently popular term one prefers; in which failure of the heart to perform its tasks leads automatically to increased size and that in turn leads to a great measure of work until a new balance is struck fitting the new task (*85*).

Starling's brilliant exposition of this thesis found acceptance among clinicians, who were becoming interested in the role of physiological mechanisms in disease, and were familiar with the enlarged weak hearts that would improve in performance when venous pressure was lowered by venesection or tourniquets. Physiologists were enthusiastic about Starling's law of the heart since it was derived from fundamental observations in pure science.

However, in neither skeletal muscle nor heart muscle is this response to stretching capable of accounting completely for the performance of a muscle in the intact body (*36*). Without the coordinating stimulus of the central nervous system skeletal muscle is quite inert. Without the coordinating stimulus of the central nervous system and the hormonal control governed by this system, the truly isolated heart seems to vary its pumping function between that of a heart in a normal resting animal and that of a heart in an animal moribund in the last stages of shock. It never reaches the scale of activity seen in the normal heart during moderate activity.

It had long been recognized and was well known to Starling that other factors than mere stretching were operating, even in the isolated heart, and much more in the heart of an intact organism. Epinephrine, for example, would cause the heart, at a given diastolic size, to pump

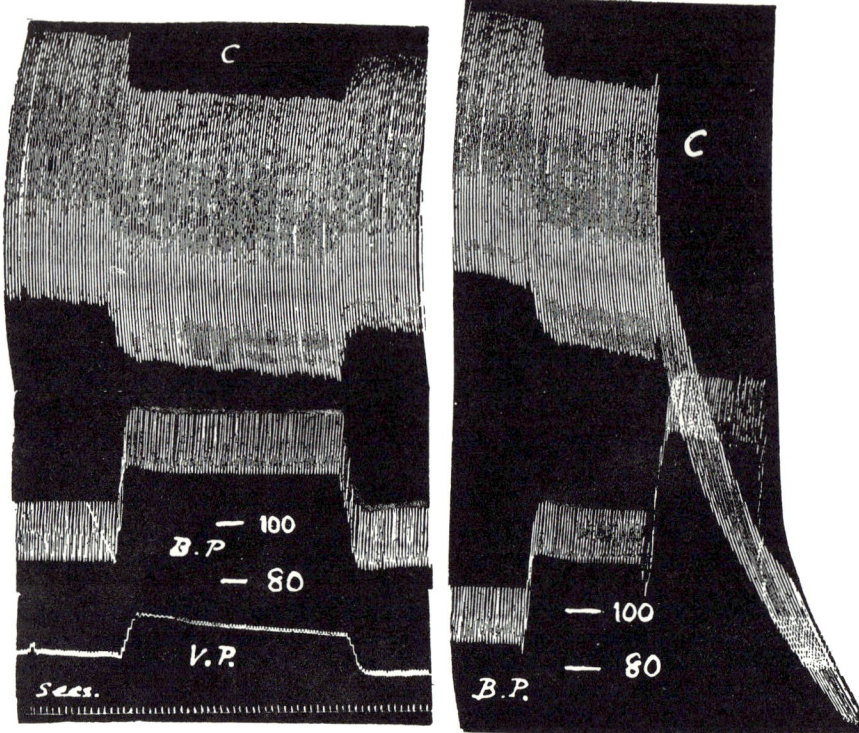

Figure 17. *Left:* Effect of increased arterial pressure on volume changes in the heart (volume increase shown by a downward deflection). *Right:* Effect of excessive arterial pressure rise. From Patterson, Piper, and Starling (*72*).

more blood and consume more oxygen in the process. Starling himself frequently referred to the loss of "tone," the deterioration of performance, in his heart-lung preparation. He was therefore not fully justified in claiming that the stretch response serves to explain the "whole behaviour" of the isolated mammalian heart. More recent work has shown a whole range or family of curves of filling-versus-output response with addition of epinephrine or with alteration in coronary blood flow (*82*).

Filling pressure, moreover, is a useful index to diastolic size only if the heart rate and ventricular stimulation are constant. When the heart is subject to normal regulation it is often seen that rapid hearts may be small when the venous pressure is high and slow hearts may be large when the venous pressure is low. Heart size is much more closely related to heart rate than to filling pressure (*61*).

The cardiometer cannot be used to measure size changes in the natural heart *in situ* because of the necessary surgery. Rushmer's diameter or circumferential gauges give an index to changes in heart size and can be used in the intact animal (*81*). The standard measure of whole heart size and contour has been the X ray. In recent years, angiocardiographic techniques have provided further definition. By direct injection of opaque media, atria and ventricles can be outlined separately.

These direct measures of cardiac size indicate that the heart when doing the most work is smaller than when its work is minimal. The mechanism by which this takes place is worth our attention.

In making adjustments in its pumping function, the most obvious and well-known response is a change in heart rate. This is reflexly produced and is of greatest importance in regulating heart size because it is uniquely related to heart size in the intact animal. Multiple correlation studies of such factors as stroke volume, stroke work, and filling pressure have shown that none of these were related to heart size when the influence of heart rate was statistically extracted (*39*). When the heart accelerates, and pumps more blood, it becomes smaller; when it slows, it fills more and becomes larger; changes in rate thus work against any application of the Starling law in the intact animal (*36*).

The reflexes that accelerate the heart increase the strength of its beat. Therefore, it empties more completely and becomes smaller even though it is doing more work than it would have done without this stimulation. This effect also works against the application of the Starling law in the intact animal (*36*).

The influence of parasympathetic stimulation is just the opposite. Vagus slowing causes the heart to fill to a larger size and to empty less completely so that the heart becomes larger while doing less work.

Normally the heart is under vagus restraint. The fact that the left ventricle in the resting animal contains large amounts of residual blood and hence is normally well filled is documented by the fact that when an arteriovenous fistula (*71*) is opened, the next beat ejects a double-sized stroke volume against the lowered aortic pressure. This could not happen if the blood were not already in the ventricle.

All these considerations mean that the reflex influences, to which the

THE HEART

normal heart in the intact animal is subject, ensure that, at rest, the venous return is adequate to fill the heart so well that there is residual blood left at the end of systole; it also ensures that it empties itself more completely, fills less completely, and becomes smaller when it beats rapidly under sympathetic stimulation.

Similar ideas are needed to explain observations on the size of the human heart. Liljestrand, Lysolm, and Nylin (58) recorded the work of about twenty authors, beginning in 1902 and ending with their own work in 1938, which shows that the acceleration and augmentation of heart beat which accompanies and follows exercise are not marked by an increase in heart size. The size of the heart is smaller during exercise than at rest in the supine position. This latter is its maximal size, according to these workers. It is hard to see how these results, reported by reliable observers and well documented, could have been so completely ignored. They ran counter to contemporary opinion, which misapplied the Starling principle and urged that the laboring heart must have a large diastolic size. The fact that the slow quiet heart was the larger was completely ignored for many years.

In the following paragraphs, we shall try to follow in detail the responses of the cardiovascular system in supplying an increased blood flow. It is now held that in the normal animal, as distinguished from the usual physiologist's preparation, the venous return is always ample to fill the heart and is hence not a key to the regulation of the cardiac output. On the other hand, the pumping action of the heart is regulated reflexly to maintain the arterial pressure within physiological limits despite the changes in flow. These changes in flow are the direct result of peripheral vasomotion in response to reflex and hormonal stimuli and to locally produced metabolic vasodilatory influences. The response as a whole serves to supply the demands for oxygen of the active tissues and to dissipate heat produced by the activity of the body.

It is a matter of everyday experience that when we anticipate strenuous effort, there is a recruitment of cardiovascular activity. The heart beats more quickly and strongly and in the excitement there is an increase in arterial pressure. Rushmer (81) has documented this in the dog. When the animal is placed on a treadmill, or even shown one, its heart accelerates, the systolic pressure increases, and the heart does more work. Its size and the pressure which fills it tend to decrease rather than to increase. These changes are augmented as treadmill running is started. At no time is there a significant increase in filling pressure or in diastolic size.

The heart is evidently responding to an increase in reflex stimulation organized by the higher centers and being implemented by a greater concentration of epinephrine and norepinephrine. The increase in arterial pressure is known to cause peripheral dilation as a result of reflexes from the baroreceptors. This action is augmented by the presence of epinephrine in the arterioles of the skeletal muscles so that at the onset of exercise, the circulation as a whole is augmented, the flow to the muscle increased, and that to the viscera relatively unchanged or possibly restricted, while the blood pressure is maintained at normal or slightly augmented levels. As the muscular activity starts, chemical stimuli cause a further dilation of arterioles in active organs and a further fall in peripheral resistance. The excitement and the baroreceptors keep the arterial pressure near normal levels, by augmented cardiac pumping, despite the low peripheral resistance. As the work reaches a steady state and the initial excitement passes off, the regulation of the circulation to meet the oxygen needs and to dissipate heat produced will probably become more automatic and less dependent on the intervention of higher centers. The arteriocardiac reflexes maintain physiological arterial pressure in spite of reduced peripheral resistance in active tissues. This means a greatly increased flow, adjusted so that arterial pressure remains within physiological limits. In describing the difference between the control of the respiration and the circulation, Rein (78) has enumerated and given experimental evidence for the operation of most of the factors given above.

It is often held that the venous return is an important factor in the regulation of the circulation rate. This is no doubt true in animal preparations subject to anesthesia and surgery, but the evidence given above indicates that there is an ample supply of blood in the heart itself and at its portals except in such abnormal conditions as severe hemorrhage or shock. The fact that normal animals can support very high outputs with little or no change in venous pressure testifies to the adequacy of mechanisms supporting venous return (muscular and respiratory venous pump, venomotor mechanism, etc.).

The preponderance of evidence points to the conclusion that the natural heart in the normal healthy body does not increase its diastolic size in order to increase its output of work or energy. Nevertheless, the Starling relationship probably plays an important role in augmenting the strength of the failing heart that has already utilized the nervous and hormonal resources that can be mobilized by reflex stimulation.

The Starling relationship also plays an important role in equalizing the output of the right and left ventricles, which have no intercommunicating reflexes, nor separate hormonal control. The necessity and nicety of the adjustment must be apparent when we realize that if each ventricle pumped slightly more or slightly less blood than the other the pulmonary bed would soon be either engorged or depleted of its blood (36).

Long before the Starling law was formalized, Henderson and Prince (44) showed that a minimum pressure must be transmitted through the lungs in order to fill the left ventricle. This also prevents the depletion of the lung blood volume. Moreover, an increased filling pressure will cause the left ventricle to dilate, strengthen its beat, and pump a larger volume than can be ejected by the right ventricle. Henderson and Prince held that this mechanism serves to prevent engorgement of the lungs. This general idea has been given detailed documentation (83).

Although other controls bypass Starling's law in the control of the work of the normal heart in the healthy body, it should be kept in mind that the heart is a muscular organ and that a full understanding of its working must encompass the effects of diastolic size, working at different levels of capacity and stimulation, as an important part of the background of myocardial physiology (36).

BIBLIOGRAPHY

1. Agricola, G. De re metallica. Tr. by H. C. Hoover and L. H. Hoover. New York, Dover Publications, 1950.
2. Bazett, H. C., F. S. Cotton, L. B. Laplace, and J. C. Scott. The calculation of cardiac output and effective peripheral resistance from blood pressure measurements with an appendix on the size of the aorta in man. Amer. J. Physiol., 113:312, 1935.
3. Blasius, W. Am Frosch-Herzen angestellte Versuche über die Herz-Arbeit unter verschiedenen innerhalb des Kreislaufes herrschenden Druck-Verhältnissen. Verh. phys.-med. Ges. Würzburg, 2:49, 1872.

4. BLIX, M. Die Länge und die Spannung des Muskels. Skand. Arch. Physiol. 3:295, 1891.
5. BOYLE, R. A Disquisition about the Final Causes of Natural Things. London, Taylor, 1688.
6. BRAMWELL, J. C., and A. V. HILL. The velocity of the pulse wave in man. Proc. roy. Soc. B, 93:298, 1922.
7. CHAUVEAU, A., G. BERTOLUS, and L. LAROYENNE. Vitesse de la circulation dans les artères du cheval d'après les indications d'un nouvel hémodromètre. J. Physiol. (Brown-Séquard), 3:695, 1860.
8. CLERKE, A. M. Galileo Galilei. Encyclopaedia Britannica (11th ed.), 11:406.
9. COLVIN, S. Leonardo da Vinci. Encyclopaedia Britannica (11th ed.), 16:444.
10. COURNAND, A. Measurement of the cardiac output in man using the right heart catherization. Description of technique, discussion of validity and of place in the study of the circulation. Fed. Proc. 4:207, 1945.
11. COURNAND, A., and H. A. RANGES. Catheterization of the right auricle in man. Proc. Soc. exp. Biol., 46:462, 1941.
12. DOW, P. Estimations of cardiac output and central blood volume by dye dilution. Physiol. Rev., 36:77, 1956.
13. DRESER, H. Ueber Herzarbeit und Herzgifte. Naunyn-Schmiedeberg's Arch. exp. Path. Pharmak., 24:221, 1887.
14. ERLANGER, J., and D. R. HOOKER. An experimental study of blood pressure and of pulse pressure in man. Johns Hopk. Hosp. Rep., 12:145, 1904.
15. FABRICIUS, H. De venarum ostiolis (1603). Reprinted in Opera Anatomica. Padua, Meglietti, 1625.
16. FICK, A. Ueber Diffusion. Ann. Phys., 94:59, 1855.
17. FICK, A. Die Medizinische Physik. Braunschweig, Vieweg, 1856.
18. FICK, A. Compendium der Physiologie des Menschen. Wien, Braumüller, 1860-91.
19. FICK, A. Untersuchungen über Muskel-Arbeit. Basel, Georg, 1867.
20. FICK, A. Ueber die Messung des Blutquantums in den Herzventrikeln. S.B. phys.-med. Ges. Würzburg, July 9, 1870.
21. FICK, A. Ueber die Aenderung der Elasticität des Muskels während der Zuckung, Pflüg. Arch. ges. Physiol., 4:301, 1871.
22. FICK, A. Mechanische Arbeit und Wärmeentwickelung bei der Muskelthätigkeit. Leipzig, Brockhaus, 1882.
23. FICK, A., and J. WISLICENUS. Ueber die Entstehung der Muskelkraft. Vjschr. naturf. Ges., Zürich, 10:317, 1865.
24. FORSSMANN, W. Die Sondierung des rechten Herzens. Klin. Wschr., 8:2085, 1929.

25. Frank, O. Zur Dynamik des Herzmuskels. Z. Biol., 32:370, 1895.
26. Frank, O. On the dynamics of cardiac muscle. Tr. by C. B. Chapman and E. Wasserman. Amer. Heart J., 58:282, 1959.
27. Frank, O. On the dynamics of cardiac muscle. Tr. by C. B. Chapman and E. Wasserman. Amer. Heart J., 58:467, 1959.
28. Franklin, K. J. A Short History of Physiology. London, Bale, 1933.
29. Frey, M. von. Adolf Fick: Gedächtnisrede. S. B. phys.-med. Ges. Würzburg. Nov. 14, 1901.
30. Galilei, Galileo. Dialogues concerning Two New Sciences. Tr. by H. Crew and A. de Salvio. New York, Macmillan, 1914.
31. Grehant, N., and C. E. Quinquaud. Recherches expérimentales sur la mesure du volume de sang qui traverse les poumons en un temps donné. C. R. Soc. Biol. (Paris), 36:285, 1886.
32. Grollman, A. The Cardiac Output of Man in Health and Disease. Springfield, Ill., Thomas, 1932.
33. Hales, Stephen. Encyclopaedia Britannica (11th ed.), 12:834.
34. Hales, S. Statical Essays. Vol. I. Vegetable Staticks. London, Innys and Manby, 1727.
35. Hales, S. Statical Essays. Vol. II. Haemastaticks. London, Innys and Manby, 1733.
36. Hamilton, W. F. The physiology of the cardiac output. Circulation, 8:527, 1953.
37. Hamilton, W. F., J. W. Moore, and J. M. Kinsman. Delay of blood in passing through the lungs as an obstacle to the determination of the CO_2 tension of the mixed venous blood. Amer. J. Physiol., 82:656, 1927.
38. Hamilton, W. F., J. W. Moore, J. M. Kinsman, and R. G. Spurling. Studies on the circulation. IV. Further analysis of the injection method, and of changes in hemodynamics under physiological and pathological conditions. Amer. J. Physiol., 99:534, 1932.
39. Hamilton, W. F., J. W. Remington, and W. F. Hamilton, Jr. Factors relating to heart size in the intact animal. Amer. J. Physiol., 163:260, 1950.
40. Hamilton, W. F., R. L. Riley, A. M. Attyah, A. Cournand, D. M. Fowell, A. Himmelstein, R. P. Noble, J. W. Remington, D. W. Richards, Jr., N. C. Wheeler, and A. C. Witham. Comparison of the Fick and dye injection methods of measuring the cardiac output in man. Amer. J. Physiol., 153:309, 1948.
41. Harvey, W. Epistola prima Paulo Marquarto Slegelio, Hamburgensis, April 7, 1651. In his Opera Omnia. London, Bowyer, 1766, p. 613.

42. HARVEY, W. Exercitatio anatomica de motu cordis et sanguinis in animalibus, with an English translation by C. D. Leake. Springfield, Ill., Thomas, 1928.
43. HENDERSON, L. J. Blood, a Study in General Physiology. New Haven, Yale University Press, 1928.
44. HENDERSON, Y., and A. L. PRINCE. The relative systolic discharges of the right and left ventricles and their bearing upon pulmonary congestion and depletion. Heart, 5:217, 1914.
45. HENDERSON, Y., and A. L. PRINCE. Application of gas analysis. II. The CO_2 tension of the venous blood and the circulation rate. J. biol. Chem., 32:325, 1917.
46. HENRIQUES, V. Über die Verteilung des Blutes vom linken Herzen zwischen dem Herzen und dem übrigen Organismus. Biochem. Z., 56:230, 1913.
47. HERING, E. Versuche, die Schnelligkeit des Blutlaufs und der Absonderung zu bestimmen. Z. Physiol. 3:85, 1829.
48. HOFF, H. E., and L. A. GEDDES. Graphic recording before Carl Ludwig: an historical summary. Arch. Inst. Hist. Sci., 12:3, 1959.
49. HOFF, H. E., and L. A. GEDDES. Graphic registration before Ludwig; the antecedents of the kymograph. Isis, 50:5, 1959.
50. HOFF, H. E., and L. A. GEDDES. The technological background of physiological discovery: ballistics and the graphic method. J. Hist. Med., 15:345, 1960.
51. JENKINS, E. Elizabeth the Great. New York, Coward-McCann, 1959.
52. KINSMAN, J. M., J. W. MOORE, and W. F. HAMILTON. Studies on the Circulation. I. Injection method: physical and mathematical considerations. Amer. J. Physiol., 89:322, 1929.
53. KOLIN, A., Electromagnetic blood flow meters. Science, 130:1088, 1959.
54. KROGH, A., and J. LINDHARD. Measurements of the blood flow through the lungs of man. Skand. Arch. Physiol., 27:100, 1912.
55. LAMMERANT, J. Le Volume sanguin des poumons chez l'homme. Bruxelles, Editions Arscia, 1957.
56. LIDDELL, H. G., and R. SCOTT. Abridged Greek-English Dictionary, Oxford, 1871. With an Appendix by G. R. Berry, New York, Hinds & Noble, 1901.
57. LILJESTRAND, G., and J. LINDHARD. Über das Minutenvolumen des Herzens beim Schwimmen. Skand. Arch. Physiol., 39:64, 1920.
58. LILJESTRAND, G., E. LYSOLM, and G. NYLIN. The immediate effects of muscular work on the stroke and heart volume of man. Skand. Arch. Physiol., 80:265, 1938.
59. LINDHARD, J. Untersuchungen über statische Muskelarbeit. Skand. Arch. Physiol., 40:145, 1920.

60. LOEWY, A., and H. VON SCHRÖTTER. Ein Verfahren zur Bestimmung der Blutgasspannungen, der Kreislaufgeschwindigkeit und des Herzschlagvolumens am Menschen. Arch. Anat. Physiol., Physiol. Abth., p. 394, 1903.
61. LOMBARD, W. P. The Life and work of Carl Ludwig. Science, 44:363, 1916.
62. LONGINO, F. H., and D. E. GREGG. Comparison of cardiac stroke volume as determined by pressure pulse contour method and by a direct method using a rotameter. Amer. J. Physiol., 167:721, 1951.
63. LOWER, R. De corde. Tr. by K. J. Franklin. In R. T. Gunther. Early Science in Oxford, v. 9, Oxford, 1932.
64. LUDWIG, C. Beiträge zur Physiologie: Carl Ludwig zu seinem siebzigsten Geburtstage gewidmet. Leipzig, Vogel, 1887.
65. MAGNUS, G. Ueber die im Blute enthaltenen Gase, Sauerstoff, Stickstoff, und Kohlensäure. Ann. Phys., n.s., 12:583, 1837.
66. MAREY, É. J. La circulation du sang à l'état physiologique et dans les maladies. Paris, Masson, 1881.
67. MAREY, É. J., and A. CHAUVEAU. Determination graphique des rapports du choc du cœur avec les mouvements des oreillettes et des ventricles. C. R. Acad. Sci. (Paris), 53:622, 1861.
68. MARKOFF, I., F. MÜLLER, and N. ZUNTZ. Neue Methode zur Bestimmung der im menschlichen Körper umlaufenden Blutmenge. Z. Balneol., 4:373, 409, 441, 1911.
69. MARKWALDER, J., and E. H. STARLING. On the constancy of the systolic output under varying conditions. J. Physiol. (Lon.), 48:348, 1914.
70. MOORE, J. W., J. M. KINSMAN, W. F. HAMILTON, and R. G. SPURLING. Studies on the circulation. II. Cardiac output determinations. Comparison of the injection method with the direct Fick procedure. Amer. J. Physiol., 89:331, 1929.
71. NICKERSON, J. L., D. C. ELKIN, and J. V. WARREN. The effect of temporary occlusion of arteriovenous fistulas on heart rate, stroke volume, and cardiac output. J. clin. Invest., 30:215, 1951.
72. PATTERSON, S. W., H. PIPER, and E. H. STARLING. The regulation of the heart beat. J. Physiol. (Lond.), 48:465, 1914.
73. PATTERSON, S. W., and E. H. STARLING. On the mechanical factors which determine the output of the ventricles. J. Physiol. (Lond.), 48:357, 1914.
74. PLESCH, J. Hämodynamische Studien. Z. exp. Path. Ther., 6:380, 1909.
75. POISEUILLE, J. L. M. Recherches sur la force du cœur aortique. Paris, Didot, 1828.

76. POISEUILLE, J. L. M. Recherches expérimentales sur le mouvement des liquides dans les tubes des très petite diamètres. Mem. Acad. Sci. (Paris), 9:433, 1846.
77. POWER, D'A. William Harvey. London, T. Fisher Unwin, 1897.
78. REIN, H. Die physiologischen Verknüpfungen von Atmung und Kreislauf. Fortbildungslehrgang. Bad Nauheim, v. 11, 1935.
79. REMINGTON, J. W., W. F. HAMILTON, and P. DOW. Some difficulties involved in the prediction of the stroke volume from the pulse wave velocity. Amer. J. Physiol., 144:536, 1945.
80. ROSEN, G. Carl Ludwig and his American students. Bull. Inst. Hist. Med., 4:609, 1936.
81. RUSHMER, R. F., and T. C. WEST. Role of autonomic hormones on left ventricular performance continuously analyzed by electronic computers. Circulat. Res., 5:240, 1957.
82. SARNOFF, S. J. Myocardial contractility as described by ventricular function curves; Observations on Starling's law of the heart. Physiol. Rev., 35:107, 1955.
83. SARNOFF, S. J., and E. BERGLUND. Ventricular function. I. Starling's law of the heart studied by means of simultaneous right and left function curves in the dog. Circulation, 9:706, 1954.
84. SINGER, CHARLES, E. J. HOLMYARD, A. R. HALL, and TREVOR I. WILLIAMS. A History of Technology. v. 3. From the Renaissance to the Industrial Revolution c. 1500–c. 1750. Oxford, Oxford University Press, 1956.
85. STARLING, E. H. The Linacre Lecture on the Law of the Heart given at Cambridge, 1915. London, Longmans, Green, 1918.
86. STARR, I., A. J. RAWSON, H. A. SCHROEDER, and N. R. JOSEPH. Studies on the estimation of cardiac output in man, and of abnormalities in cardiac function, from the heart's recoil and the blood's impacts; the ballistocardiogram. Amer. J. Physiol., 127:1, 1939.
87. STARR, I., and F. C. WOOD. Twenty-year studies with the ballistocardiograph. The relation between the amplitude of the first record of "healthy" adults and eventual mortality and morbidity from heart disease. Circulation, 23:714, 1961.
88. STEWART, G. N. Researches on the circulation time and on the influences which affect it. IV. The output of the heart. J. Physiol. (Lond.), 22:159, 1897.
89. VISSCHER, M. B., and J. A. JOHNSON. The Fick Principle: analysis of potential errors in its conventional application. J. appl. Physiol. 5:635, 1953.
90. WHITEHEAD, A. N. Science and the Modern World. New York, Macmillan, 1931.

91. WIGGERS, C. J. The Pressure Pulses in the Cardiovascular System. London, Longmans, Green, 1928.
92. WOOD, E. H. Special instrumentation problems encountered in physiological research concerning the heart and circulation in man. Science, 112:707, 1950.
93. ZUNTZ, N., and O. HAGEMANN. Untersuchungen über den Stoffwechsel des Pferdes bei Ruhe und Arbeit. Landw. Jb., 27 (Ergänz. Bd. 3), 1898.

III

Heart Muscle

ONE could hardly find a more appropriate introductory sentence for an essay on the contractility of the heart than the opening statement of Starling's Linacre Lecture (*126*):

"No one who has attempted to investigate the motions of the heart and to discover the secret of the manner in which it is able to regulate its activity according to the needs of the body as a whole, can avoid realizing the truth of the words with which Harvey commences his immortal treatise, On the Motion of the Heart and Blood: *'When I first gave my mind to vivisection, as a means of discovering the motions and uses of the heart, and sought to discover these from actual inspection, and not from the writings of others, I found the task so truly arduous, so full of difficulties, that I was almost tempted to think, with Fracastorius, that the motion of the heart was only to be comprehended by God.'"*

Such an admission of one's limitations will always impress itself upon the investigator mature enough to see the complexity of a complete and exhaustive "explanation" of vital phenomena, and he will strive toward more restricted objectives.

This essay will be restricted to certain basic aspects of the function and activity of the heart as a special muscle. Some of the topics, such as the molecular physiology of contraction, are modern, and an attempt will be made to trace their origins. Other problems are more classical, yet seem to have the habit of reappearing. For example, the staircase effect, discovered in 1871 by Bowditch (*9*), received little investigative attention for over half a century; but interest in it has suddenly revived due to the work by Szent-Györgyi and Hajdu (*41*), and it may turn out to be a way to penetrate the profound problem of the relation between stimulus and response.

Fundamental Aspects of Myocardial Contractility

Heart and other muscles may be said to be engines. They transform the energy of chemical reactions, "metabolism," into mechanical energy, often into work. The mechanisms whereby they accomplish this are much more obscure than those of man-made machines. Still, an important part of physiological, biochemical, and biophysical investigation is aimed at solving this riddle. There is no assurance that such a solution will ever be obtained, but it is a part of the optimism of science to keep up the effort.

The metabolic reactions in the living organism have often been compared with combustion and, in a similar fashion, comparisons have been made between muscles and combustion engines. In light of this analogy, it is of interest to consider the mechanism of an automobile motor, both from the "physiological" and from the "biochemical" standpoint. The ultimate contribution of the biochemist would be to identify the energy-yielding reaction by some equation describing the combustion of a mixture of lower hydrocarbons. To the physiologist, this would appear to be only a very peripheral piece of information, for it would stand in no relation to the specific performances of the different parts of the machine, and would not explain how these latter become engaged in a sequence of translocations whereby force and motion are produced.

Would this comparison also imply that the biochemical analysis of the contractile machinery in myofibrils, which has played such a prominent role during the last generation, will always stay on the outside of the real fundamental problems? Not at all, because there is an essential difference. In the combustion engine the moving parts are macroscopic; they are propelled by the forces generated by large populations of chemically reacting molecules, but do not interact with these individually in any way. In fact, the linkage between the machinery and the fuel is entirely nonspecific, since the hydrocarbons can be replaced by alcohol or ether or wood distillate, or could even, after relatively minor adaptations in the engine, be replaced by steam or compressed air. In contractile tissues, on the other hand, both the energy-yielding processes and the motions of the engine occur on the same scale of molecular dimensions, and the linkage between them is undoubtedly of a topochemical nature, meaning that an engine-molecule reacts with a fuel-molecule in order to cause either shortening or sliding or whatever motion forms the basis of contractility. Hence, chemical mechanisms lie right at the heart of the problem, although we cannot take it for granted that the kind of chemistry involved is already known to us. Similar considerations apply to the profound and barely investigated question as to what sets off and terminates these mechanisms, that is, what is the link between stimulation and contraction; and, for that matter, what is stimulation? We shall continue to expect, therefore, further periods of investigation in which workers with different interests approach these problems differently; anticipating, at the same time, that the deeper we penetrate, the less distinction there will be between chemistry, physics, and physiology.

There are a few fundamental physical concepts which it will be useful to review. In order not to be caught up in a discussion of first principles, we shall take the concepts of mass, length, and time for granted, reminding ourselves only that these concepts, no matter how rigorous the physical definitions we attempt to give them, are in large measure derived from personal physiological and psychological experience. Mass is always associated with matter, and length divided by time gives velocity (*111*). We know that to impart velocity to, that is, to accelerate, a mass, we have to do something with our muscles that is associated with some feeling of strain. This sensation is possible for skeletal muscles which are equipped with certain proprioceptors; no such sensation occurs each time the heart gives velocity to a mass of blood. This is our image of the concept of force, and the physical definition of force is that which accelerates a mass: $f = m \times \text{acceleration} = m \times l \times t^{-2}$. We also observe that there are forces in nature outside our muscles; this we judge by the fact that we can match or balance these with the force of our muscles. A stone in midair falls because it is accelerated by another force, gravity, which we can oppose and balance by holding the stone in our hands by muscular effort. We can also lift a stone with our muscles, meaning that we displace the point of action of a force in, or opposite to, the direction of its action. This we call work: $w = f \times l = ml^2t^{-2}$. Finally, work performance per unit of time is called power: $h = w/t = ml^2t^{-3}$. A careful and profound analysis of natural phenomena by such workers as Rumford, Mayer, Helmholtz, and Joule has revealed that work is closely related to other quantities in nature into which it can be transformed, and vice versa, one of which is heat. Collectively, these forms are called energy, which has the same dimensions as work. While all forms of energy can be completely converted into heat, the possibility of transformation of heat into other forms of energy is subject to very definite limitations defined by the science of thermodynamics, notably by its second law.

Transformations of energy are common play in living organisms. In fact, this is really all they seem to aim at, and while these transformations may take special forms that appear purposeful to the discerning mind, from the thermodynamic viewpoint the whole of living nature is nothing but an extremely complicated and fanciful way of turning the energy of sunlight into heat, a feat that could be accomplished much more simply by absorbing the radiation directly into the earth.

We shall not pursue this argument, but instead recall the first law of thermodynamics, which states that in all the processes of nature energy is never created or destroyed, but is always quantitatively transformed from one form into another. Besides mechanical work and heat, some other forms of energy should be listed. Potential mechanical energy is possessed by virtue of its position in some field of forces; it can change this into work, heat, or kinetic energy by changing its position, e.g. by falling down if the potential energy was due to gravitation. Kinetic energy is that possessed by a body due to its motion; it equals $(1/2)\ mv^2$. Chemical energy is encountered in the course of chemical reactions. When two substances A and B react to form C and D, and heat is produced in the course of this reaction, it is obvious that energy is liberated in the process and can in principle also be liberated or obtained in forms other than heat. Conversely, it would require an input of energy to drive the reaction in the direction $C + D \to A + B$, and such a process, by an extension of the original meaning of the word, would be called chemical work. Changes in energy are also related to the differential distribution of substances, e.g. it would require osmotic work to concentrate all of a solute into one corner of a solution, and once brought there it would again spontaneously spread out by diffusion. Electrical energy is yet another manifestation of energy; a direct conversion of chemical into electrical energy takes place in an electrochemical element. In contractile tissues, we presume that there is a direct conversion of chemical into mechanical energy in a "mechanochemical element," the nature of which has eluded us so far.

When a process such as a chemical reaction is conducted in a way such that all its energy appears as heat (this usually does not require special arrangements, but occurs by itself), this amount of heat measures the total energy effect of the reaction, ΔH, which is the difference between the energy content (strictly, the "heat content" or enthalpy) of the reactants and the products: $\Delta H = H_{C,D} - H_{A,B}$. Not all of this energy is necessarily released in a form that is convertible into work. There may be fundamental reasons, related to the concept of entropy S, which require that some fraction of the energy exchange must take place in the form of heat. I have called this "obligatory" heat production (96, 97); only the remainder, the free energy ΔF, is available for work: $\Delta F = \Delta H - T\Delta S$. This entropy factor may cause the free energy to be larger than ΔH, in which case more work would be available and the system would cool off; or, conversely, the free energy is less and obligatory heat is produced. Imperfections in the machine may create a situation in which not all of the ΔF is utilized, and any losses so caused would also appear as heat; this I have called "dissipative" heat production.

While the first law of thermodynamics is usually formulated more or less in the form given above, it must be stressed that, by implication, the law contains more than the usual statements define explicitly. The transformation of one form of energy into another should not merely be accounted for from a bookkeeping point of view, but there should be channels or mechanisms which make these transformations possible physically. As Lewis and Randall (77) have said, "it would not satisfy the conservation law if one system were to lose energy, and another system, at a distance therefrom, were simultaneously to gain energy in the same amount." If an amount of energy were suddenly to appear on Earth by no physical mechanism, the law would not be satisfied by the fact that somewhere in the universe the same amount had disappeared, unless a mode of transfer were demonstrable; on the contrary, the energy law would have been violated twice. What is true on the cosmic scale is equally true within cellular or even molecular dimensions. This touches a problem which caused considerable difficulty to biochemists earlier in this century, when observations seemed to show that some endergonic, hence not spontaneously occurring, reactions could be driven through coupling with exergonic reactions. As long as the driving and the driven reaction seemed to have nothing in common there was no clear mechanism whereby one reaction could cause another one to occur against its natural direction. Some forty years ago, von Euler postulated that such coupling could occur if both reactions were catalyzed by the same homogeneous catalyst. While this explanation would now be regarded as out of touch with the facts, it did nevertheless indicate an entirely correct appreciation of the nature of the problem. Nowadays we know that such coupling takes place by means of "high-energy" substrates such as ATP, which participate in both reactions, and which cause the endergonic reaction to appear as a result of several exergonic ones. For example, observations might indicate that the synthesis of phosphocreatine from creatine and phosphate, a reaction which cannot take place spontaneously because its equilibrium is entirely oriented toward the splitting of phosphocreatine, can occur when coupled, e.g. with the oxidation of phosphoglyceraldehyde. Although this oxidation process would supply enough energy to cover the former reactions from the bookkeeper's point of view, still the first law of energetics would not be satisfied unless a mechanism should exist to make their coupling possible. There is no single homogeneous catalyst to promote all these reactions at once; rather, each one of them is caused by one or more separate specific enzymes. The solution finally found was that in the process of the oxidation of phosphoglyceraldehyde there is a synthesis of adenosine triphosphate (ATP). (In fact, there are two such syntheses, one linked with the oxidation step to phosphoglyceric acid (PC), and another one if this substance is further converted to phosphopyruvic acid which can react with adenosine diphosphate (ADP) to form ATP and pyruvate.) ATP, in turn, can react with creatine to form PC and ADP. Hence, the mechanism of coupling has been explained by the occurrence of $ATP \rightleftharpoons ADP$ as a common substrate between the driving and the driven reaction, and only catalytical amounts of this common substrate are needed to effect the coupling. This type of explanation emerged from that great period in biochemistry in the 1930's, when the pathways of glycolysis and fermentation were clarified by Embden, Meyerhof, Warburg, Parnas, and C. F. and G. T. Cori, and the concepts of the high-energy phosphate bonds were systematized by Lipmann and Kalckar. Such a coupling mechanism has general validity to explain the occurrence of nonspontaneous endergonic chemical reactions. However, the common substrate need not be ATP, it may be an acyl-coenzyme-A or something else, and in principle it does not even have to be a small-molecular substance but may be a reactive group of an enzyme itself. Osvaldo Cori and his associates (*18*) have recently reported that transphosphorylation between phosphopyruvate and creatine in muscle extracts may occur without any ATP; if this result were shown to be independent of any common substrate, the range of possible coupling mechanisms would be considerably extended.

This approach to the coupling between two biochemical reactions implies, then, that an exergonic reaction can cause the occurrence of an endergonic one, if there is a high-energy intermediate which is common to both reactions in the form of a joint substrate such as ATP or possibly in the form of a high-energy grouping on an enzyme. Can we invoke similar mechanisms when the problem is not the change of one form of chemical energy into another, but into mechanical work? Can this be accomplished by obtaining the energy of the driving reaction in the form of heat, and then utilizing it by the principles of a heat engine? There is a convincing reason why this cannot, or cannot generally, be the case. The efficiency of a heat engine (the fraction of the heat input that can be transformed into work) can be calculated on theoretical grounds, and is found to depend on the difference in absolute temperature between the warmer (T_2) and the colder (T_1) reservoir: $\varepsilon = (T_2 - T_1)/T_2$. There are cases in which the efficiency of biological work engines is known to be quite high, e.g. 40 per cent for the initial processes in skeletal muscle (*54*). The efficiency of heart muscle is equally high, about 25 per cent under optimal conditions. To achieve such an efficiency in a heat engine would require very great differences in temperature; for instance, even if the cold reservoir were at 0°C. (and it could hardly be lower), T_2 would have to amount to some 200°C. Such temperatures are entirely incompatible with the properties of living matter, and completely out of the range of any temperatures ever detected. Hence, this mode of energy transfer does not seem to be utilized, certainly not in contractile tissues.

Due in part to conversations with Dr. D. E. Atkinson at U.C.L.A.

and Dr. D. R. Wilkie at University College, London, I have become convinced that the physiological use of the term "efficiency" is really quite limited: when used in its engineering sense, as above, the term has a strict theoretical meaning only for the case of a heat engine. For a chemodynamic engine, the formula would become $\varepsilon = w/\Delta H$, and this has no theoretical foundation at all. Instead, one might choose a "free-energy efficiency" $\varepsilon' = w/\Delta F$, and this would have the descriptive value of indicating what fraction of the theoretically possible work is actually obtained; it still does not mean anything more than that. However, this criticism does not aim at abolishing the physiological use of the term efficiency. Since for an over-all metabolic process such as respiration, ΔH and ΔF are approximately equal, the same numerical value applies reasonably well to both cases, and the concept is of use in expressing at what "cost" a certain physiological activity is performed. But if we try to become more sophisticated and apply the concept, e.g. to a partial reaction of the initial phase of contraction, the theoretical meaning becomes more doubtful.

The statement that a contractile tissue cannot act as a heat engine should not be misunderstood to mean that no part of its action can resemble one, since the calculation applies only to an entire cycle. In a steam engine, for example, the work is done by the expansion of the heated system, and this half of the cycle is not specifically dependent on any temperature difference. We could have a reservoir of a compressed gas at room temperature, and get all its free energy in the form of work (while cooling the gas or the surroundings) by letting it escape through a suitable machine. But, once the gas was gone, we would be faced with the problem of the reverse part of the cycle, and this would reintroduce the limitations unless it were accomplished, e.g. by direct chemodynamic coupling.

We should furthermore emphasize that, while our technical heat engines are based upon the use of some gas or vapor as the working substance, which would seem to be unbiological, the possibilities are not restricted to this. The physiologist Wöhlisch (155, 156) has made a great scientific contribution in showing that there are features in the statistical behavior of large molecules that obey laws perfectly analogous to the gas laws. With further developments introduced by K. H. Meyer, et al. (82, 85) the following picture emerges (Fig. 1). A macromolecule consists of many individual parts which have more or less flexible linkages. Statistically, it is most unlikely that all these links should be so oriented as to have all molecules stretched all the time. Rather, they will assume average configurations known as random coils, which are shorter than stretched chains. It will be understood that, if all the chains were stretched at one time, their approach to the coiled condition would be perfectly analogous to the expansion of a compressed gas, both being caused by a trend toward the most probable configuration. The elasticity of rubber and of elastic tissue are explained on this basis, and indeed the stretching of rubber, like the compression of a gas, causes warming,

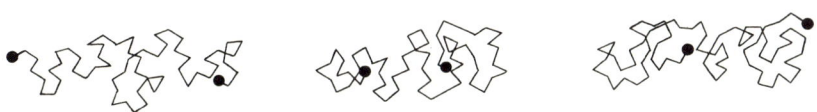

Figure 1. Schematic representation of a flexible chain molecule in the entirely extended configuration (top) and in three randomly kinked forms (bottom).

and its shortening gives rise to cooling. The thermodynamics of these processes, for "ideal rubberlike materials," has been worked out by Wöhlisch (*155, 156*), Wiegand and Schneider (*148, 149*), and others, and is perfectly analogous to the thermodynamics of an ideal gas (*112*).

It appears, furthermore, that mechanisms of this nature may lend themselves to patterns of mechanochemical and topochemical coupling not commonly found in more conventional systems. This may be illustrated by the investigations on fibers made from macromolecular polyelectrolytes, e.g. strips of a mixed polymer of polyvinyl alcohol and polyacrylic acid (*71, 63*):

$$---CH_2-CHOH-CH_2-\underset{\underset{COO^-}{|}}{CH}-CH_2-CHOH-CH_2-CHOH-$$

$$-CH_2-CHOH-CH_2-CHOH-CH_2-\underset{\underset{COO^-}{|}}{CH}-CH_2---$$

In the charged condition, i.e. in alkaline solution, such chain molecules will tend to be stretched because of electrostatic repulsions between the negative groups. Deionization of these by acidification removes this elongating influence, and the molecules will tend to coil. Such strips were shown to be capable of performing repeated work cycles by alternate acidifications and alkalizations. The "efficiencies" obtained were very low, partly for avoidable reasons. Greater perfection was obtained by Katchalsky (62) with a model of polymetacrylic acid, with which he studied a reversible work cycle in which complete reversible transfer of the chemical energy can be obtained.

There are many reasons why such models may not apply to the problems encountered in muscle contraction, yet it is obvious that as the first examples of mechanochemical coupling their study is of great importance.

The concepts outlined above have had a great influence on our thinking on the possible mechanisms of mechanochemical coupling. Obviously, here was a mechanism of which living tissues with their polypeptide chains might well avail themselves. Yet, let us observe that no proof or demonstration was ever given that it is operative and, as will be shown further on, the results of modern electron microscopy point in an entirely different direction. The fact that a certain physicochemical mechanism is discovered during our lifetime, and assumes considerable technical importance, is no argument whatsoever that this is the mechanism of life, just as it is beyond belief that the inhabitants of some distant planet began to send us flying saucers coincident with the development of our interest in the subject.

In the light of these considerations it is worth inquiring whether in contractile tissues the shortening process may be due to a spontaneous entropy mechanism rather than accepting that it is caused by direct coupling with the energy-supplying process. The latter had always been considered as the obvious possibility until Ritchie (116) developed the view that contraction may be a triggered spontaneous event, and that active effort only enters into relaxation in order to load up the system again. This new viewpoint was a significant innovation, although the facts heralded as experimental proof were really not conclusive, since they were based on the mistaken notion that chemical events have a high, while physical ones have a low, temperature coefficient. With or without proof, the new idea caused such a widespread "Aha!" sensation among physiologists that many seemed, and still seem, to assume that nature must employ this roundabout way of doing things. The decision between pre- and post-energization mechanisms, or contraction- versus relaxation-coupling, awaits further experimental work. Although there can be no unanimity until the contraction mechanism is completely elucidated, the weight of evidence is much in favor of contraction coupling, unless one makes additional, and rather arbitrary, assumptions. We shall leave this problem for the moment.

One important feature which distinguishes contractile tissues from some engines is in the kind of "work" which they perform. This feature can be reproduced in model systems. For example, one such model would be that of an automobile held stationary on a grade not by means of the brake but by continuously running the engine with the clutch loosely coupled. This distinction appears to have confused physiologists a great deal, although the matter is really quite simple. We have previously defined "work" as the displacement of a force against its direction. This might consist of the lifting of a weight against the force of gravity, and physiologically we associate this with muscular effort and eventually fatigue. We know, however, that merely to hold up a weight also involves effort and likewise leads to fatigue, yet no work is performed; indeed, we might have hung the weight from a tree with a rope, or placed it on a chair, and no one would have tired. The explanation is that it takes energy to activate muscle, but that this state of tension quickly declines and has to be re-established by a new input of tension. Or, more correctly perhaps, it requires power to maintain active tension in muscle, while it does not do so to maintain tension in a rope. In fact, no power is required (or very little, some being involved in the maintenance of the live tissue) to hold resting tension in a muscle, but active tension is something that has to be established and re-established all the time, at a cost of energy. The amount of power required to maintain tension depends on a property of the muscle which is called its economy. The economy of skeletal muscle is poor, that of smooth muscle high; that of cardiac muscle might probably be called intermediate, although the concept is not strictly applicable since the heart does not maintain tension by tetanic contraction. So, although we exert effort and generate power when holding a weight or maintaining a posture, we do not perform work.

Since work is a well-defined physical concept, with which we should not tamper, a term is needed to indicate the other phenomenon. The term "physiological work" being both cumbersome and inaccurate, I believe that "effort," already used above, would fill the bill. A more sophisticated interpretation could be developed by the application of steady-state thermodynamics, but this will not be attempted on this occasion.

In summary, then, the heart and other contractile tissues appear as engines which convert the chemical energy of metabolism into the potential energy of tension or into work by shortening. In the following section we shall consider some of the mechanical properties of these tissues, without reference to the intricate mechanisms of the contractile process.

The Heart as an Engine

In this section we shall accept as a fact that muscular tissues can be in either a resting or an active state, disregarding the manner in which this active condition is brought about. This would be like considering the fiber as a variable spring that alternates between low and high tensions for a given length, without establishing the cause and mechanism of this change. Although this comparison becomes grossly incorrect when considering the energetics and dynamics of the matter, for strictly mechanical descriptions it will do (*48, 49*). Conversely, we may regard the fiber as a spring which assumes different lengths at the same tension. The question as to whether muscular activity is primarily a tendency toward shorter length or toward greater tension may be quite meaningful, but seems to be unanswerable at the moment.

To return to the definition of work: a muscle performs work when it shortens, while displacing a load, against the direction of its vector; e.g. when lifting a weight against the force of gravity, or when accelerating an inert mass. When the load is constant, the work is simply the product of force and distance: $w = f \times l$. When the load is variable, and a function of the shortening that has already occurred, its magnitude at any moment should be properly considered: $w = \int f \, dl$. The load can be a function of l in several ways, e.g. directly because of the properties of the lever systems upon which the muscle acts, in which case the relation between f and l would be quite invariable. Or the relation may be more involved, as in the case of the circulation where the aortic pressure increases as the heart empties, but where other variables that are not, or are only indirectly, dependent on the momentary degree of systole come into play. The work of the heart, too, may be looked upon as a product of force and distance: the former being the blood pressure times the cross sectional area of the vessel, the latter being the distance over which an element of blood is propelled. But since this distance equals the propelled volume divided by the cross section of the vessel, so that the cross section cancels, the familiar formula $w = pv$ is obtained, or, more accurately, $w = \int p\, dv$, in view of the variability of p during the cardiac cycle. (It is perhaps not superfluous to remark that the appearance of the product pv in this formula is completely unrelated to the fact that a similarly written product happens to be constant in the case of ideal gases.) To this pv factor, the factor $(1/2)\, mv^2$ is added to account for the acceleration of the mass m of the blood. As explained in the textbooks, the factor $(1/2)\, mv^2$ is relatively small, indeed negligible, at low degrees of cardiac work, but becomes more sizeable when the minute volume increases and the increased velocity becomes prominent. Mathematically, the relation between work and volume change in a cavity can be defined by considering the element of work performed by each surface element, as is done in physical thermodynamics in defining volume work (28), but such a treatment has not yet been applied to the heart—and may not contribute much.

Considerable physiological insight can be gained by an elementary consideration of the work that can be performed by a stretched spring. Assume that this obeys Hooke's law of the proportionality between force and extension, and that a load of 10 arbitrary units causes a stretch by 10 units of length. Assume that the spring has been lengthened to this extent (Fig. 2), and that now weights of 10, 9, 8, . . . 1, 0 units are attached to it before release. With a load of 10 units, there will be no shortening and no work. Without load, there will be maximal shortening, but again no work. With intermediate loads, the relation between load, shortening, and work can be tabulated and is shown in Fig. 3, illustrating that the work curve is a bell-shaped optimum curve, maximal work being obtained at half the maximal load. A similar if somewhat distorted curve will be found for muscular

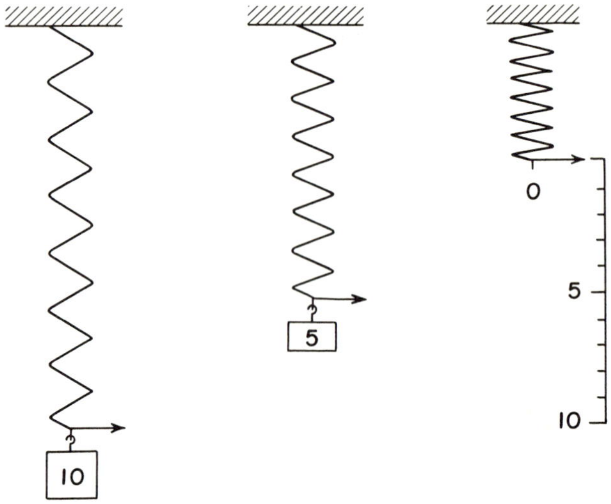

THE HEART

Figure 2. Shortening and work performance by a spring previously stretched over a distance of 10 units by 10 units of load, which is then released with 10, 5, and 0 units of load, respectively.

tissues. The distortion arises from the nonlinear relationship between length and tension in active muscle. The curve represents, therefore, a simple mechanical law; not, as I have heard in classroom teaching, a physiological regulation.

The work so obtainable still does not represent the total free energy of the stretched spring, because in the initial stage of shortening a heavier load could have been lifted, while after the mid-point further shortening against lighter weights could have occurred. Clearly, the maximal work could be obtained if at each stage of shortening the spring would be opposed by a load just equal to its tension. Fundamentally, maximal work in thermodynamics is, after all, defined as the work theoretically obtainable when the system throughout the process goes through a sequence of equilibrium states. This maximal work can be found (Fig. 4) from the length-tension diagram of the spring as the surface under the line, since $w_{max} = \int f \, dl$. In the case of a rectilinear length-tension diagram, this maximal work is twice that obtainable with an optimal constant load.

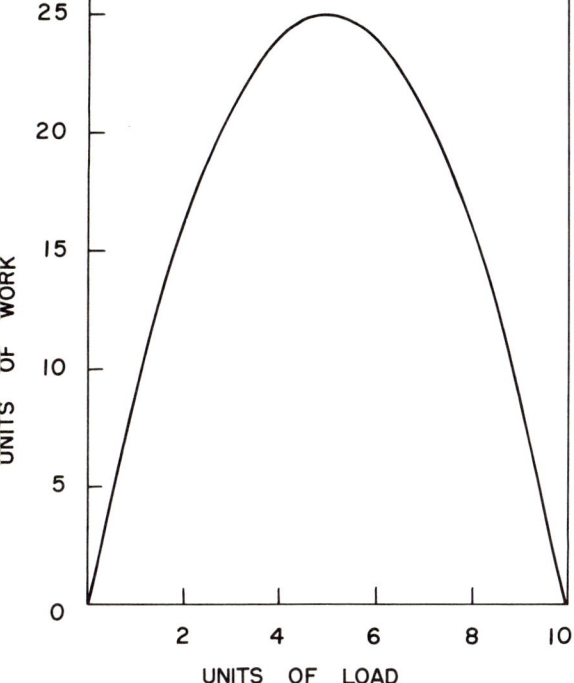

Figure 3. Work obtainable from a stretched spring, as in the case of Fig. 2.

No work is obtained at load zero (because no force is displaced) or at load 10 (because there is no shortening). Maximal work occurs at an intermediate value of the load, where the product of force × distance assumes its greatest value.

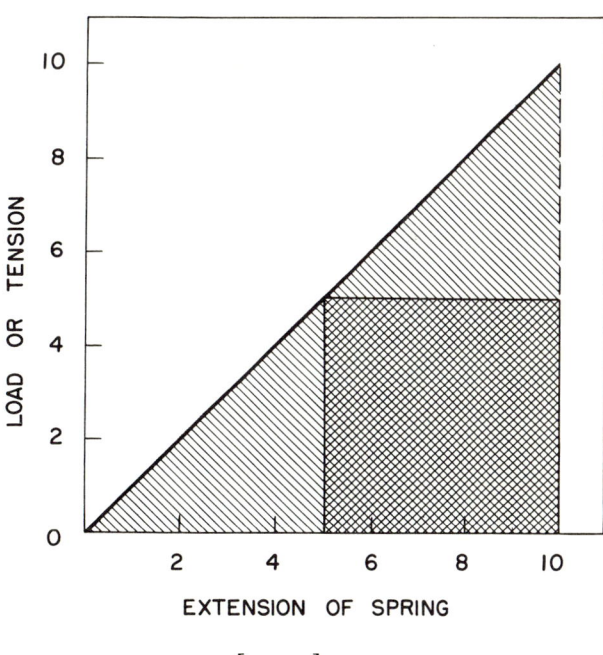

Figure 4. Length-tension diagram of the spring in the experiment of Fig. 2.

The total area under the curve (lightly shaded) indicates the maximal work which can be obtained by lifting a variable load always equal to the force exerted at a particular length. The doubly shaded area indicates the work obtainable "isotonically," by lifting a constant weight, as in the case of load 5 in Fig. 2.

THE HEART

The length-tension diagram of muscular tissues is less simple than that of a body with Hookean extensibility. For resting skeletal muscle, it is given by the curve R in Fig. 5. A similar curve for cardiac muscle appears in Fig. 6. The nature of the elastic process may be different from case to case, but the following points are important. In the region of relatively small extensions, the tension increases with a rise in temperature, hence the elasticity is anomalous (since bodies usually tend to extend when heated) or rubber-like (*84, 156*). This type of elasticity may be explained in terms of the disorienting effect of Brownian motion upon molecular elements. Thus, muscle at moderate extensions displays thermokinetic elasticity, but at greater stretches there is an inversion point and elasticity becomes "normal." One may ascribe the thermokinetic component to the contractile structure and the normal one to the sarcolemma and connective tissue, but there is no unanimity on this point.

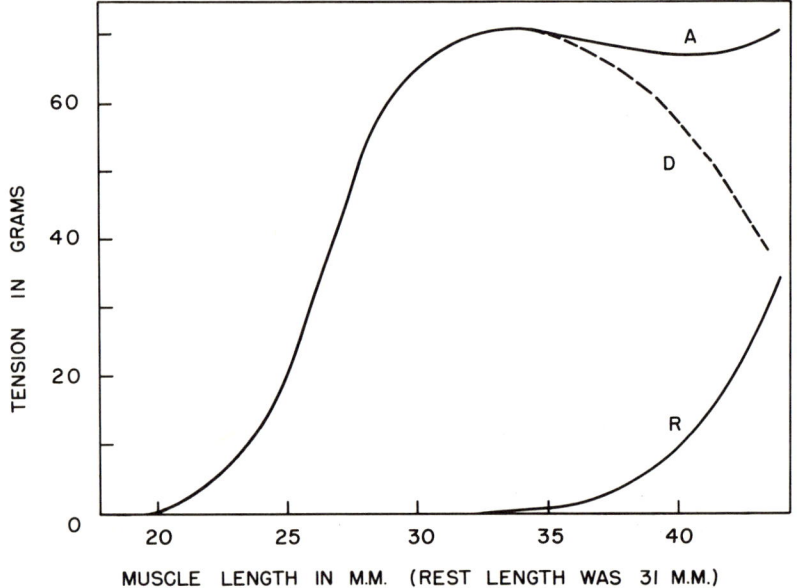

Figure 5. The length-tension diagram of skeletal muscle, based upon the measurements of Wilkie on a frog sartorius muscle. R = resting tension; A = total active tension of the tetanized muscle; D = the difference between A and R, corresponding to the actively developed tension in response to stimulation. The cross section of the muscle was probably about 2 mm.².

What appears to be a good experimental argument is that both skeletal (*157*) and heart muscle (*158*) display a negative thermal expansion coefficient at low extension and a positive coefficient at high extension only when living. In dead muscle, in which the participation of the living contractile apparatus is perhaps eliminated, or in which, alternatively, it is in a condition of rigor, the thermal expansion coefficient is positive throughout. In contraction, which is, by definition, a property of the contractile component, the muscle appears to change into a structure with a normal temperature-elasticity relationship (*53, 3, 4*).

Active skeletal muscle shows a length-tension diagram as in curve *A* of Fig. 5. There is considerable variability and hysteresis in such curves, and one does not always reach the same point "isometrically" and "isotonically." However, by careful experimentation, Wilkie (*153*) has minimized these variations, and the curve of Fig. 5, taken from his

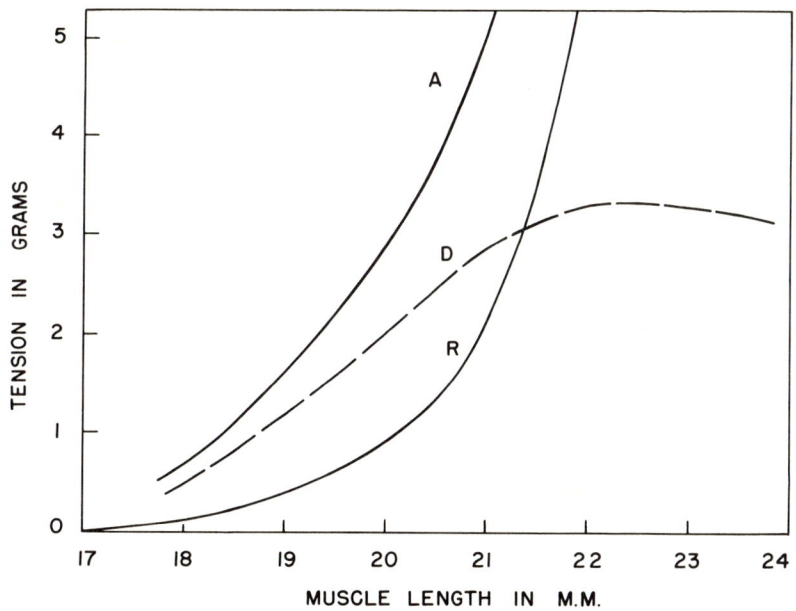

Figure 6. The length-tension diagram of cardiac muscle, based upon the measurements of Abbott and Mommaerts on a cat papillary muscle. A, R, and D as in Fig. 5. The cross section of the muscle was 1.8 mm.², approximately the same as in the case of Fig. 5, but the developed tension is much less.

work on the frog sartorius muscle stimulated tetanically, may be fairly representative for skeletal muscle. One of its features is that, above a certain extension, the active tension decreases with lengthening before increasing again. This is more easily understood if looked upon in the following way: the total tension of the active muscle, curve A, is the sum of the resting tension R and the actively developed tension D. The latter follows a bell-shaped curve (obtained in practice by subtracting R from A), which shows how the tension developed depends on the length of the contractile structures. The fact that a certain length of these is optimal for the development of tension will eventually be explained in terms of the molecular mechanism of contractility, but can now be done in descriptive terms. Whether the total tension curve A does or does not show a decline depends on how the addition of R and D happens to come out. An important addition to this argument may be found in the measurements of Ramsey and Street on single isolated muscle fibers (*114*). These are not contaminated by connective tissue and, apart from possible structures within the myofibril, the parallel elasticity is now confined to the sarcolemma. Consequently, the resting tension is minimized, and the declining force at greater extension becomes so pronounced as to reflect predominantly the length-response curve of active contraction, upon which resting tension is superimposed only at great stretch. It has also been observed by E. Weber (*143*) that at very great extension, muscle may "relax" upon stimulation, an observation known as "Weber's paradox."

Of direct importance is the fact that the optimal length for the development of tension is approximately the point of natural length, slightly more than the resting length of zero tension. Since most skeletal muscles do not shorten or stretch very appreciably in the body, they work at this optimal point and change their tension but little in activity. Large sections of the length-tension diagram might therefore be termed unphysiological, or we should rather say un-functional, since they are still of eminent theoretical importance.

The work that a muscle can perform is illustrated in Fig. 7, which again emphasizes that the maximal work obtainable is represented by the surface under the active-length-tension diagram between the lengths over which shortening occurs. If a constant load were lifted, the work would be represented by the cross-hatched area. If the muscle were preloaded with this same weight, its length would increase and a much greater amount of work would be done. Whether the muscle is pre- or after-loaded, the same types of considerations about the optimal load for the most work at constant load apply as for the spring (Fig. 3). But, since the length-tension diagram is not linear, the curve is not symmetrical and calculable but must be found empirically. Similarly, the work obtainable with a constant load will not be exactly half the maximal work.

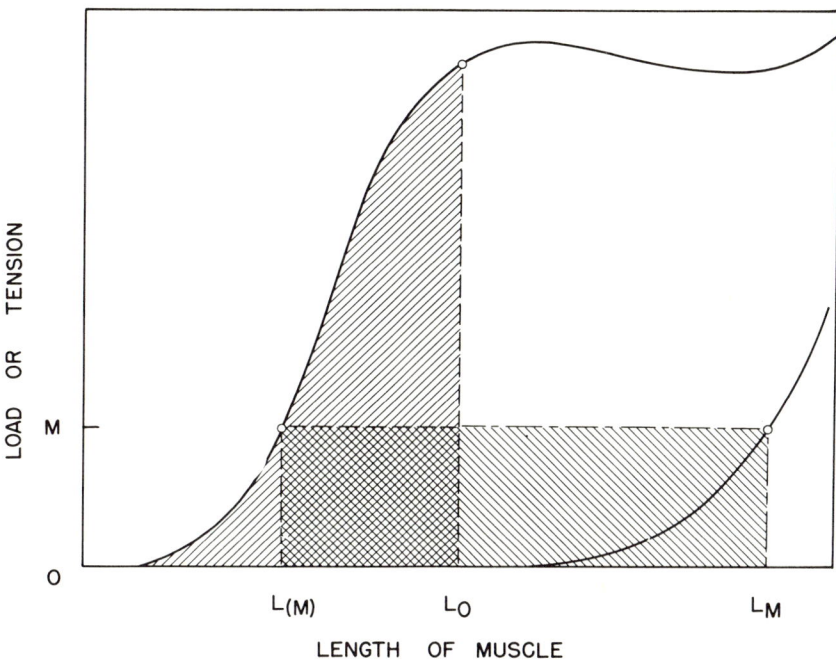

Figure 7. The work obtainable from active muscle, derived from consideration of the length-tension diagram, as in Fig. 4. When stimulating at the resting length L_0, the maximal obtainable work is represented by the shaded surface of the approximately triangular area under the diagram. When isotonic work is done upon a load of the value M, applied by afterloading, the work is represented by only the doubly shaded area between $L_{(M)}$ and L_0. If the same load is applied by preloading, the larger amount of work given by the rectangle between $L_{(M)}$ and L_M is obtained. But the part of this rectangle corresponding to the area underneath the length-tension diagram of the resting muscle represents work which was first done upon the muscle to stretch it.

While, as stated, the maximal work cannot be realized with a constant load, it would be possible to obtain it by letting the load decrease as the muscle shortens, so that at all times the load is just in equilibrium with the exerted muscle force. Variation of the load per se is not convenient (although it could be accomplished by magnetic pull equalized to the muscle tension through a servosystem); instead, we can vary the leverage. This could be accomplished by constructing a variable lever, where the muscle pulls constantly over a pulley but the load arm varies by means of a curved surface over which the connecting thread runs.

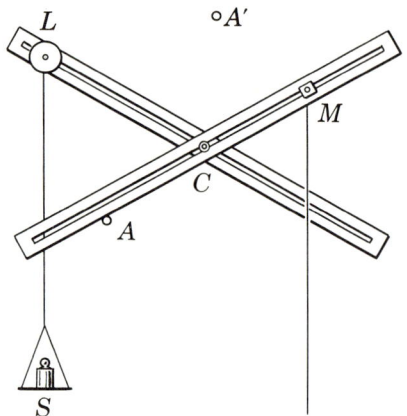

Figure 8. The tipping lever of A. Fick.

This curved surface must be cut to correspond exactly to the length-tension diagram. However, it is not practical to do this for each new muscle. More convenient, although more approximate, is Fick's tipping lever (*33*) also used by Meyerhof (*86*), in which the leverage of the muscle improves during shortening. By adjusting the position of the major weight *M* (various adjustable counterweights are not shown) and the distance of action *d*, one can adjust the lever so as to approach maximal work reasonably well. Although these instruments give only crude approximations to reversible work (a better way of going about the problem is by means of the Levin-Wyman ergometer (*76*)), the designs are of major physiological importance: in general because the muscles of the body have variable leverage and in particular because the myocardium changes its mechanical advantage during contraction. It is clear that mechanical advantage permits the displacement of greater forces only at the expense of smaller displacements; but the point is that without favorable leverage the force could not be displaced at all.

Although the efficiency with which work at constant load is performed cannot be predicted, some of its variations can. For, clearly, when no work is performed—whether the load is zero or is too heavy to be lifted—the efficiency is also zero. Between these two extremes, the course of the efficiency-load curve must conform to the work-load curve if the energy mobilized by the muscle is constant, and will be distorted but still similar to this curve when the energy output (as is the case) is influenced by work and shortening (a curve is shown in Fig. 9B; see Hill (51) for actual examples).

Another mechanical characteristic of muscles is the force-velocity relation, to which we shall return in a later section, but which is given here (Fig. 9A) as an empirical description. It will be seen that this curve may be used to transform a load coordinate into a velocity coordinate, and hence to obtain (Fig. 9C) the relation between efficiency and velocity of shortening (51). This curve shows that there is a certain velocity of shortening at which work is performed optimally. It is believed that this optimal velocity is a constant characteristic of a given muscle when the usual parameters, such as temperature and medium, are kept unaltered.

For the heart, such fundamental mechanical properties have been studied less extensively and not along quite the same lines. For a strict comparison with skeletal muscle, we would require measurements on heart muscle strips, which have been little investigated (79). Our own recent measurements (2) on the papillary muscle of the cat heart seem to provide the best illustration (Fig. 6). Compared to the diagram of skeletal muscle (Fig. 5) there are several differences. The diagram for resting cardiac muscle is not strikingly different from that of skeletal muscle. If our papillary muscles and Wilkie's frog sartorius may be considered as typical examples, a comparison of the extensibilities would show that the resting extensibilities in the two cases are of quite the same order of magnitude, (about 3 grams per mm.^{2} cross section for a 30 per cent stretch) but that the active tension developed in the heart is markedly less.

However, this resting extensibility does not only depend on the muscle substance and sarcolemnar material, but also on the amount of admixed connective and other inert tissues. Strict comparisons, therefore, would only be meaningful for isolated fibers, provided that these could be obtained without any alteration of the mechanical properties.

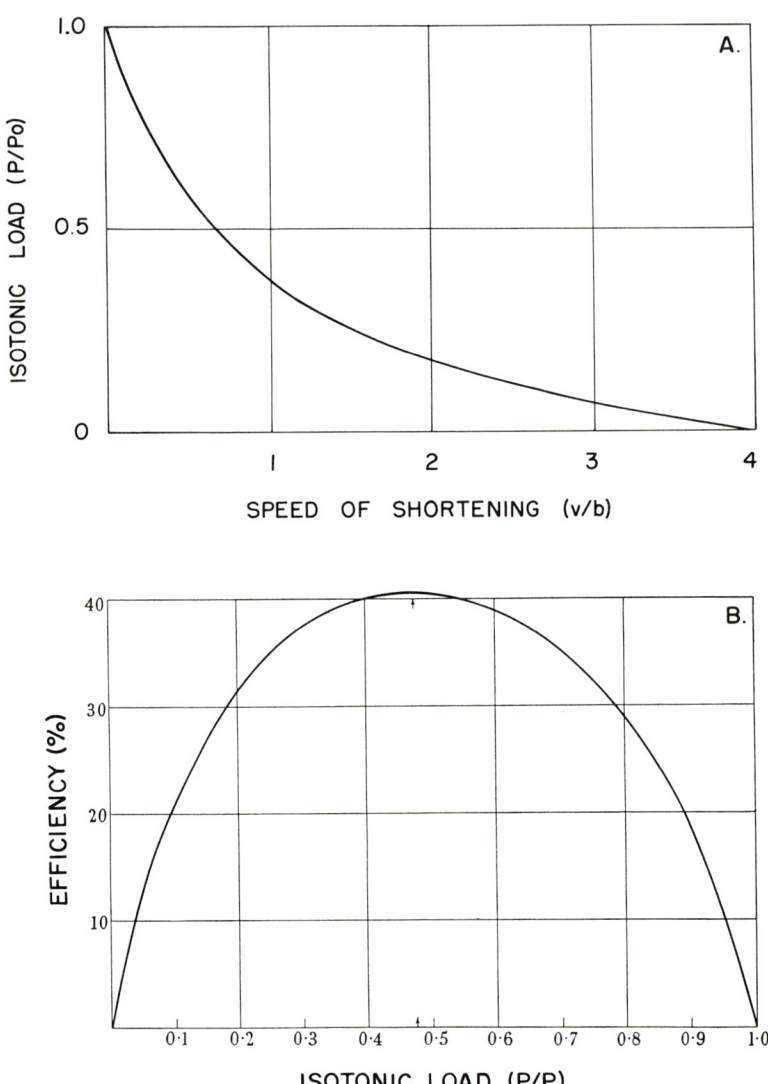

Nor would this question be simple to investigate even then, since the extensibility should be studied in the complete absence of any active tonus. Finally, it should be realized that cardiac muscle has no rigidly defined resting or natural length which can be assumed unquestionably as the point of origin for our considerations.

More marked differences can be noted in the active (A) and developed (D) tensions. In skeletal muscle, the latter has a fairly sharp peak, at lengths approximately equal to the resting or natural length. Such muscle can develop its maximal force from a length at which the resting tension is zero, and this active force does not vary greatly with moderate variations of length in either direction from the starting

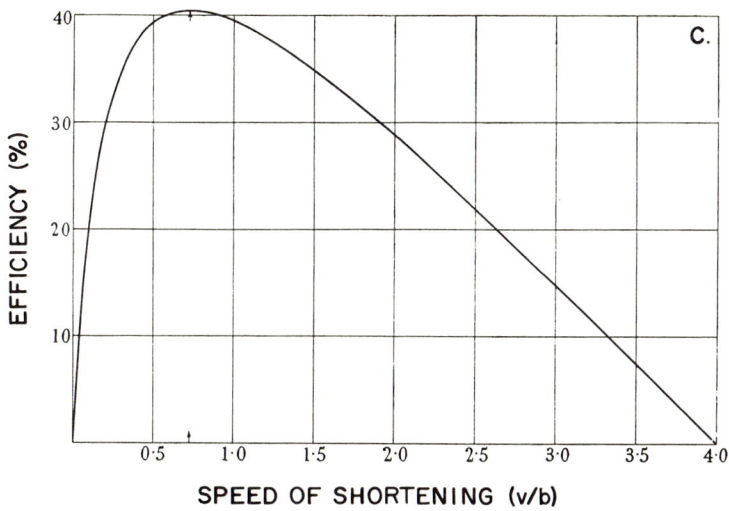

Figure 9. Relation between various mechanical properties of muscle (frog sartorius). A = force-velocity relation, discussed in the text. The ordinate gives the load in proportion to the maximally exerted force, the abscissa the speed of shortening in proportion to the constant b in the Hill equation. B = the efficiency-load relation. This is based upon measurements of the efficiency at various loads, but the general nature of this curve can be understood by comparison with Fig. 3, since, obviously, when no work is performed the efficiency is zero, and the efficiency is likely to be maximal about at the point the work is maximal. C = the efficiency-velocity relation. This can be determined experimentally (see Hill, 1939), but it is instructive to see that it can also be derived from A and B by simple coordinate transformation.

point. In the heart, the active tension is small when the resting tension is zero; it becomes considerable only at great extensions when resting tensions are also large. The curve of the developed tension continues to increase and reaches its broad optimum only at great extension. A decline of force at greater extension does not occur, as a rule. Finally, the magnitude of the developed tension is less. In skeletal muscles, active tensions of 1 to 5 kg. per cm.² cross section are the rule (54). In the papillary muscle we have only observed some 200 grams per cm.². We shall see below that such forces suffice for the required cardiac performance.

While such investigations on the "linear" mechanical properties of cardiac muscle are of fundamental importance, it is of more direct functional significance to study the relation between pressure and volume of the intact heart chambers. The classical investigations in this

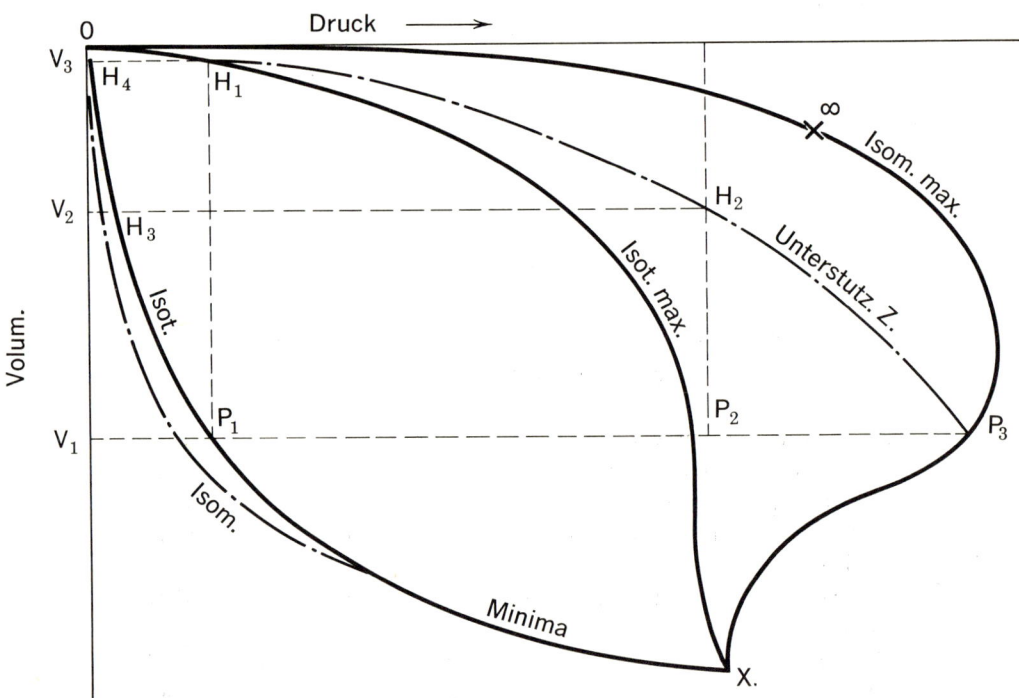

Figure 10. Relation between pressure and volume of the intact heart according to O. Frank (38).

field are those of Frank (*37, 38*), Starling (*126*), and Patterson, et al. (*110*). The diagrams given by these authors are graphs of the pressure-volume relation analogous to the tension-length graph. The published figures of that period differ from those given above in that a lesser contractile force at greater extension is evident, and strong or even maximal tension is displayed while the resting pressure is still low. Both Frank and Starling emphatically stress the analogy between heart and muscle, especially with regard to the effect of diastolic filling, corresponding to resting fiber length, upon work performance (see below). However, it has not been brought forward until recently that when the filling of the heart increases, the stretching of its fibers differs in a characteristic way from that of a muscle.

The connections between the laws for the length-tension relation in a linear muscle and for the volume-pressure relation in a hollow organ are not as generally known as they should be; these connections have been well exposed in Burton's recent essay (*13*). They are expressed by Laplace's law, which was first applied by Woods (*159*) to the problem of the pressure in hollow organs. Two quantities have to be distinguished. The first of these is the pressure, P, which is expressed in dynes per cm.^{2} surface. The second is the tension, F, to be exerted over a cm. by the wall. This tension can be most easily visualized, according to Burton, by imagining an arbitrarily directed cut of 1 cm. length in the wall, and regarding the tension as the force pulling the two edges of the cut apart. If r_1 and r_2 are the principal radii of curvature at a point in the wall, the relation is

$$P = F[(1/r_1) + (1/r_2)].$$

Simple formulas hold for certain special cases, for example,

$$P = 2F/r, \text{ and } P = F/r$$

for a sphere and a cylindrical tube, respectively. These equations indicate that, to contain the same pressure, a large vessel will exert a greater wall tension and hence will need a stronger wall. Or, in other words, the wall of a small cavity has a better leverage upon the pressure.

Now a heart has a complicated shape, and the curvature of the wall differs greatly at various places. Assuming the mechanical properties of the musculature to be identical throughout, greater tension requirements must be met by a greater wall thickness. Woods performed measurements on human hearts and found the product of the wall thickness and the factor $[(1/r_1) + (1/r_2)]$ to be constant throughout the various regions of each ventricle, and to be about six times as high in the left ventricle as in the right, in accordance with the difference in pressure.

On the basis of this theory, it becomes possible to calculate the muscle force which must be developed in the cardiac wall to produce the arterial pressure. For the human heart, Burton finds this value to be about 500 grams per cm.^{2} of cross sectional area of muscle. This is well below the 2 kg. per cm.^{2} we have become accustomed to regard as typical for skeletal muscle. Our own measurements on cat heart muscle, quoted above, gave only 200 grams per cm.^{2} of active tension, and this may well relate to the better leverage in small hearts with shorter radii of curvature. Of course, nature might also have chosen to use thinner walls, and perhaps she has, in other animals.

It is pertinent to consider the relationship between the size of the heart and the degree of diastolic filling and dilatation. Important theoretical considerations along this line by Burch, et al. (*12*) were made without knowledge of Laplace's law, but arrived at virtually the same principles. Only the general problem will be sketched. When a heart becomes dilated to twice its normal linear dimensions, the tension in the cardiac wall, as defined, would become doubled to maintain the same pressure, but quadrupled for the same amount of muscle since the circumference has doubled too (*13*). This steeply increasing mechanical disadvantage must undoubtedly be an important contributory factor in heart failure. That it is not even worse is due to the shallow course of the length-tension diagram of cardiac muscle (Fig. 6). If the diagram were like that of skeletal muscle in Fig. 5, each dilatation would set off a self-reinforcing expansion of fatal nature.

Among the most important implications of the mechanical properties of the heart is the regularity which has become known as Starling's "Law of the Heart" (*110, 126*). Although the presentation by Starling in his Linacre Lecture is largely responsible for the currency of the principle, the preliminary contributions of Howell and Donaldson (*57*) and of Frank (*37, 38*) should be recalled. Also, several subsequent investigations such as those by Wiggers, Straub, Katz, and Krayer (*151, 97*) helped to crystallize the principle.

The essential features are contained in Starling's words. After having described experiments in which the work of the heart is enhanced by increased peripheral resistance and by increased venous inflow, respectively, he concluded:

"Now here are two conditions in which the work of the heart is increased and in which this organ adapts itself by increasing the chemical changes in its muscle at each contraction to the increased demands made upon it. It is evident that there is one factor which is common to both cases, and that is the increased volume of the heart when it begins to contract. So that we may make the following general statement. Within physiological limits the larger the volume of the heart, the greater are the energy of its contraction and the amount of chemical change at each contraction."

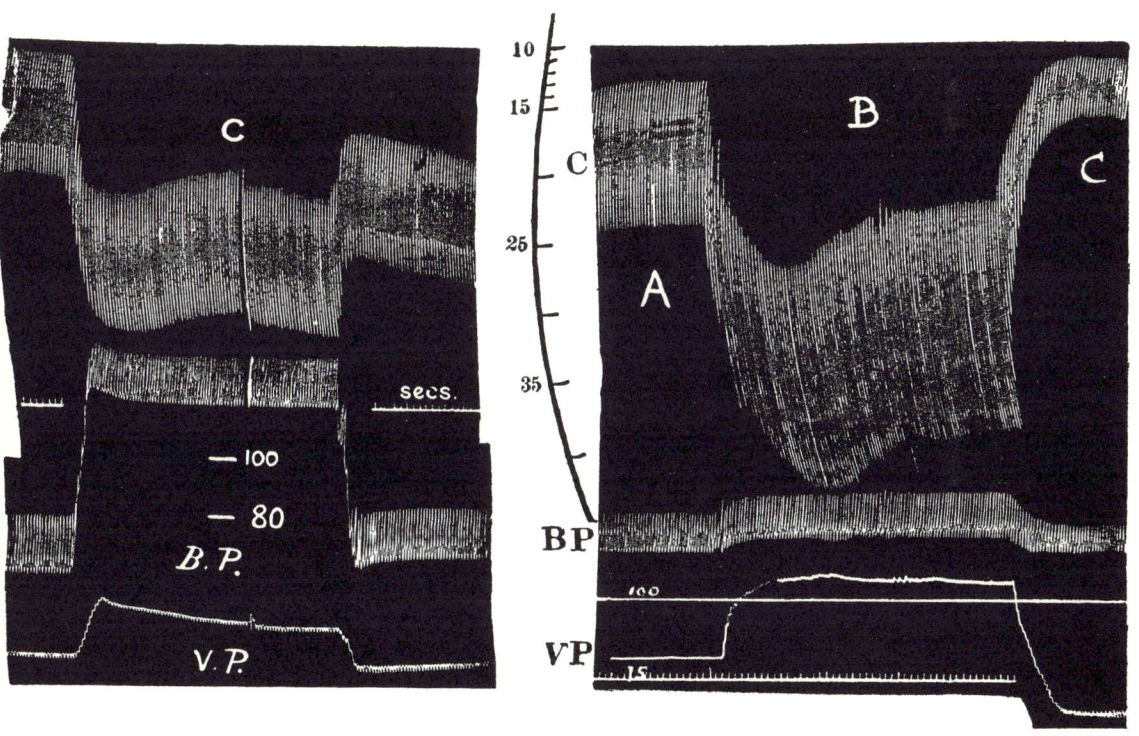

Figure 11. Left: Effects of rise of arterial resistance on the volume of the heart. C: cardiometer tracing; B.P.: arterial pressure; V.P.: venous pressure. *Right:* Effect of alteration in venous supply on volume of the heart.

Returning again to an analogy with a "linear" muscle, there is a way in which Starling's law may be clearly explained, based upon an analogy made by Henderson, et al. (*47*) between the work of the heart and that of a muscle acting upon a work-cumulating device known as Fick's work adder (*33*). This analogy was used by Patterson, Piper, and Starling (*110*). In such a device the muscle lifts a heavy load arranged with a toothed wheel and ratchet; in this way, lengthening occurs under the influence of a light weight only, so that no work is done upon the muscle during relaxation. The analogy is that cardiac diastole too takes place with the light "load" of diastolic filling (apart from the important question, discussed by Brecher (*11*), of the possibility of actual ventricular suction). The heavy load and, by analogy, the systolic arterial pressure are applied by afterloading, but preloaded stretching depends on the diastolic load. The physiological variables determine which part of the tension-length diagram (as in Fig. 7) is operative, and so determine the amount of work performed.

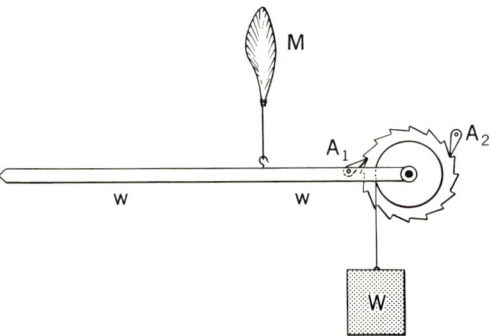

Figure 12. Fick's work adder. The muscle M after contraction is extended simply by the weight of the lever *w*. When it begins to contract, the arm on the lever catches in the ratchet wheel so that the weight W is drawn up, W being supported by the arm A_2, so that the muscle after excitation cannot raise the weight W until its tension is equal to that of the weight. As soon as it has completed its contraction and begins to relax, the weight W is taken off it (cf. closure of aortic valves) and it is then extended by the small weight of the lever (pressure of inflowing blood). It is evident that the length of the muscle before it begins to contract depends on the weight of the lever, i.e. on the diastolic load. The extent to which it will contract depends on the tension aroused in it when it contracts and the amount of the weight W which it has to overcome.

The physical difference between linear and volume work, in the sense of Laplace's law, modifies these relations quantitatively, but in one respect they introduce a difference not recognized by earlier authors (*13*). When diastolic filling increases very much, it is found that cardiac work decreases again, and the heart is now "decompensated." This was previously ascribed to decreasing contractile strength at overoptimal fiber length, but we have raised some question as to what extent this occurs in the heart. The additional and perhaps overwhelming cause is the one just alluded to, namely that a dilated heart works at a greater mechanical disadvantage (*12*), so that decompensation would occur even if the active contractile strength were not diminished.

A most fundamental extension was given by Starling and Visscher (*127*), who discovered that with the increasing work the metabolism of the heart increases as well. Here too, we shall leave the detailed discussions of current problematics to another section, but, instead, discuss some of the fundamental relations between work, metabolism, and energy mobilization, as investigated for skeletal muscle.

We may introduce this by presenting a dilemma that became manifest around 1922 (*48*). By that time, the foundations had been laid by A. V. Hill's myothermic studies on the energy liberation during muscular contraction (*48, 49, 50*). It is clear that, when a muscle is made to contract isometrically, no work is performed at all, so that the initial heat set free during its contraction is a measure of the total energy liberated; no matter what specific forms this energy may have had, it appears as heat under the circumstances of this measurement. Let its quantity be I. Conversely, we can estimate the work which the muscle so stimulated could have performed from its length-tension diagram as in Fig. 7. This quantity was found to be closely equal to I, so that the mechanical efficiency of such a muscle would have been about 100 per cent, sometimes even more. This is surprising, but not impossible. Yet, when well-designed efforts were made to determine the optimal efficiency experimentally, the 100 per cent figure was not nearly approached. Indeed, only about 50 per cent could be reached even with refined techniques (*50*). This remained a most puzzling situation until Fenn made a fundamental discovery (*30, 31*): an isometrically stimulated muscle liberates a certain energy as heat; a muscle performing work produces about the same heat, but does work in addition. Hence,

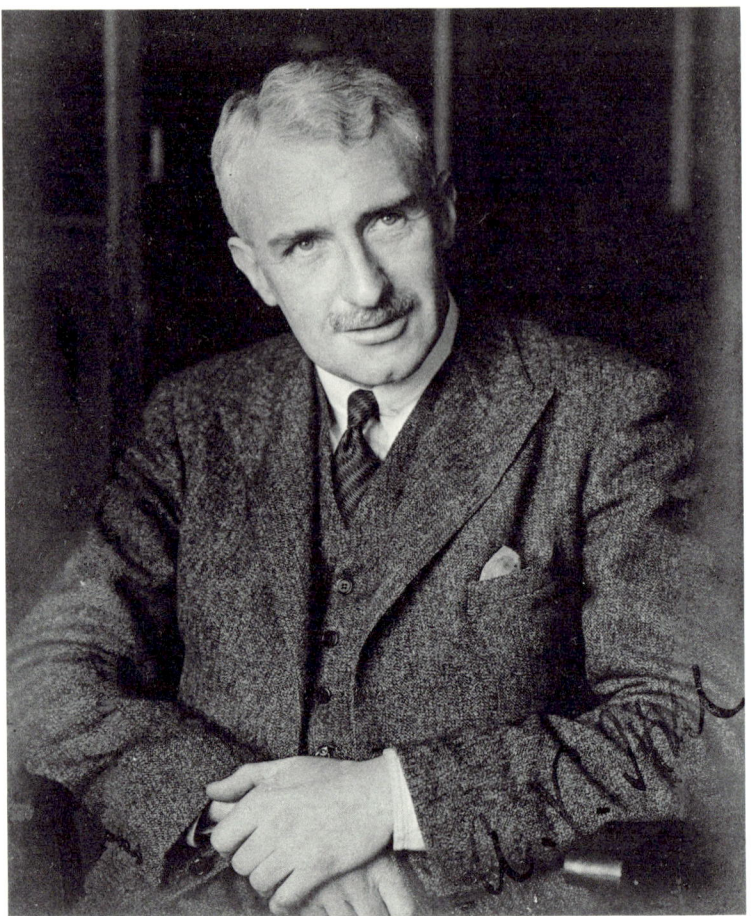

Figure 13. Archibald Vivian Hill (1886–   ).

the total energy generated increases when work is to be done. It is clear that the solution of the above problem lies here. The possible work and the isometric initial heat are about the same, which seems to be a coincidence unless it has a deeper reason that has eluded us. The working muscle mobilizes more energy, and so displays the smaller efficiency. In his classical investigation of 1938 (*50*), Hill extended Fenn's work, and found that in general the mobilized energy falls into three categories: activation or maintenance heat (a constant, although it is dependent on the length of the muscle and other circumstances), shortening heat (proportional to the extent of shortening, x), and work: $E = A + ax +$

work. The paper, furthermore, contains the first allusion to the fact that when a contracting muscle is stretched, there is a diminution of heat production. This problem, when approached biochemically, may turn out to be of great interest.

Evidently, the facts disclosed by Hill are also the basis of the Starling relationship between work and metabolism, but insufficient direct information is available on the subject to warrant further discussion. Nor is it feasible to make predictions, since quantitatively, the relations in the heart may be quite different from those in muscle. For one thing, its resting metabolism is much higher. Also, it is uncertain whether a temporal separation exists between initial and delayed heat, although that should not fundamentally affect the treatment of this problem. An important field of investigation lies fallow here, although, as our own preliminary explorations indicate, it is a very difficult one technically.

The last remaining problem may also be introduced by means of a dilemma from the early 1920's (48). In the attempt to find the optimal efficiency, and in order to circumvent the difficulty of eliciting maximal work in a lever system, measurements were made of work done upon a flywheel. Let us first consider a flywheel with several grooves along which strings can be run, so that pulling the strings will accelerate the wheel. The kinetic energy obtained by the wheel equals $q\omega^2$, in which q is the momentum of inertia and ω is the angular velocity. If the same mass M is allowed to turn the wheel along these different grooves, by falling over a constant distance h, it will drop slower or faster, depend-

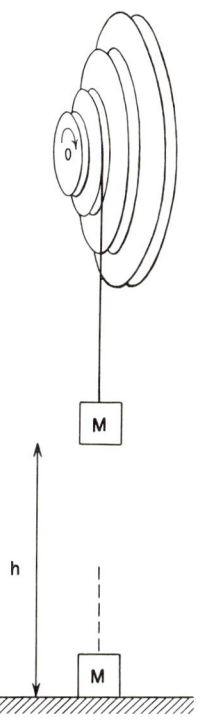

Figure 14. Performance of work upon a flywheel by a falling weight (as an example of a constant force).

The potential energy of the load, Mh, is conferred onto the flywheel to give it kinetic energy $(1/2)q\omega^2$. Depending on whether the load pulls over a large or a small pulley, its velocity of fall will differ, but $(1/2)q\omega^2$ is always the same since Mh is the same. The same could be done with a stretched spring. If, instead of accelerating the wheel with a weight or with a spring, the experiment is repeated with muscle, it is found that more work is done when the muscle contracts slowly, (working on the small pulley) than when the muscle contracts rapidly (working on the large pulley of the flywheel). This was the first indication of the existence of a fundamental force-velocity relation for muscle.

ing on the leverage. However, in each case, the flywheel will reach the same rotational velocity because the work results from the same potential energy Mh: $Mh = (1/2)\, q\omega^2$. In other words, a constant force displaced over the same distance imparts the same kinetic energy to a flywheel, no matter how long (depending on its leverage) it has to act.

Now when similar experiments were done with human arm muscles or with a frog muscle acting upon an inertia lever, it was found that the velocity did have an effect. Fast contraction gave little work, and as the velocity of shortening was decreased progressively, increasing amounts of work were obtained up to a maximal value. This can only mean that, unlike the preceding experiments with constant masses, the force was not constant. Although not formulated in this manner initially, this demonstration provided the first indication that the faster the shortening, the less the force that a muscle can develop.

The specific formulation of this relationship as a fundamental property of muscle, the force-velocity relation, was made by Fenn and Marsh (32) and by Hill (50). There is as yet no theory to predict the form of the relationship, and several formulas have been proposed to fit the data. We shall use Hill's formula, which has the advantage of showing a connection with energetics, although others may turn out to be more accurate: $(P + a)v = (P_0 - P)b$, in which P is the load, P_0 the maximal tension, and a and b are constants. Constant b is a velocity, while a has the dimensions of a force. We can write the left hand as a sum of two powers: Pv the rate of work, and av the rate of other energy liberation. It is found that the term a in this equation usually equals the factor a of the shortening heat.

Why should there be a force-velocity relation at all? If a stretched spring were permitted to shorten under different loads, its shortening would show an accelerated course and be determined entirely by the relation $F = (dv/dt)m$. Without load, shortening would be infinitely fast, apart from the slight effects of accelerating the spring's own mass, and internal friction. Shortening muscle, on the other hand, contracts more slowly, and even without load still assumes a finite characteristic velocity. Originally, this was ascribed to friction from an internal viscosity, but more and more doubts have been cast on this view. We now think instead, although vaguely, in terms of a topochemical rate-process which determines the speed of shortening. This is not as complete a change of viewpoint as it might seem. The theory of such a rate process will undoubtedly have to account for motions of particles crossing energy-barriers, and, after all, viscosity involves similar phenomena. However, we now suspect that there are fundamental connections between the rate of liberation of energy and topochemical factors of position. These connections may involve not only the rate but also the amount of energy liberated, and so eventually explain the Fenn effect. My current measurements on chemical changes in working and shortening muscles suggest that a direct chemical basis exists for these relations: the breakdown of definite amounts of high-energy phosphate in a series of twitches seems to be correlated with activation and work. Although experimentally more difficult than measurements of heat, this approach may in time allow a further penetration into the nature of the underlying phenomena.

Excitation and the Concept of the Active State

Although the possible contractile mechanisms will be discussed subsequently in terms of molecular mechanisms, we should realize that considerable insight has been gained into these problems from purely mechanical experimentation. This insight stems largely from the Hill school, beginning with the study of Gasser and Hill (39) in 1924 and reaching full development in recent years (52, 55, 117, 152, 153).

Basic to the mechanical approach is the view that muscle consists of contractile and elastic components in series (76, 50). The existence of these can be discerned clearly in Wilkie's experiment in which a muscle is tetanized isometrically, and is then suddenly released under a certain load (154). The resultant shortening occurs in two phases: the first is practically instantaneous, and represents the shortening of the series elasticity in a manner analogous to that of a released spring (see Fig. 2); the second is slower and involves the shortening of the contractile component according to the force-velocity relation.

We can now derive qualitatively what happens during the development of an isometric twitch. As may be seen in the dashed curve at the far left of Fig. 15, the development of tension is nearly instantaneous, and it persists for a time at a plateau of full intensity. However, in order to exert this tension macroscopically, the force of the contractile elements has to be transmitted through the elastic elements. To this end, the elastic elements have to be stretched, and this implies shortening of the contractile elements in accordance with the force-velocity relation. Thus, the actual course of the externally measurable tension in Fig. 15 is determined by these delays and so assumes the familiar appearance of a twitch. It is likely that the active state will decline before the tension has achieved its full value, and so the twitch will decline again.

There are three major experimental devices with which information about the active state may be gained. The first (Fig. 15) is simply that of tetanization, by which time is allowed for the full development of the active state and its intensity measured directly. The second (Fig. 16) is Hill's method of rapid stretches (52): if soon after the stimulus a stretch is applied which is just sufficient to extend the series elasticity by the

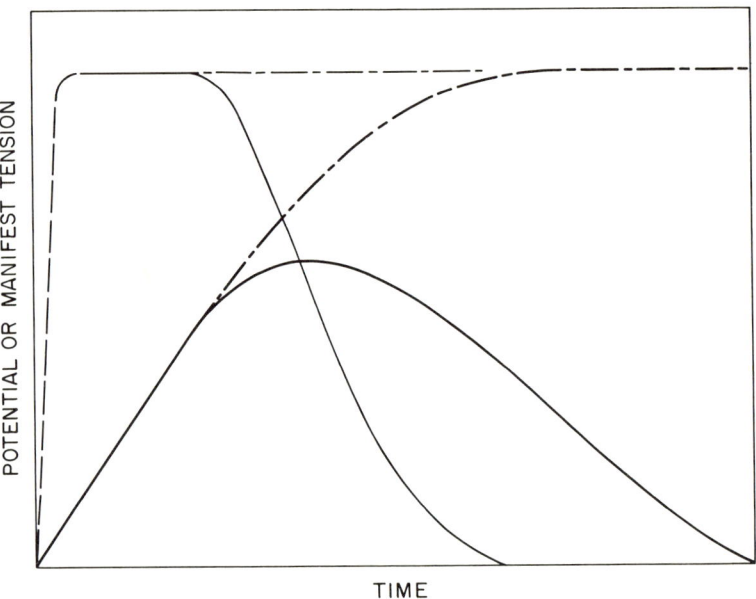

Figure 15. The concept of the active state. As indicated by the light curve on the far left, the fundamental mechanical activity reaches its full intensity shortly after stimulation, remains at a constant plateau for some time, and then declines. Measurable tension (heavy curve) lags behind the fundamental process and will usually not have reached the full value of the latter when this already declines. However, by tetanization the duration of the plateau can be prolonged, and tetanic tension reaches the full intensity of the active state (dot-dash curves).

required amount, the full amplitude of the active state will be manifest. The third (Fig. 17) is Ritchie's method for determining the decline of the active state (117), which involves the extension of the muscle for

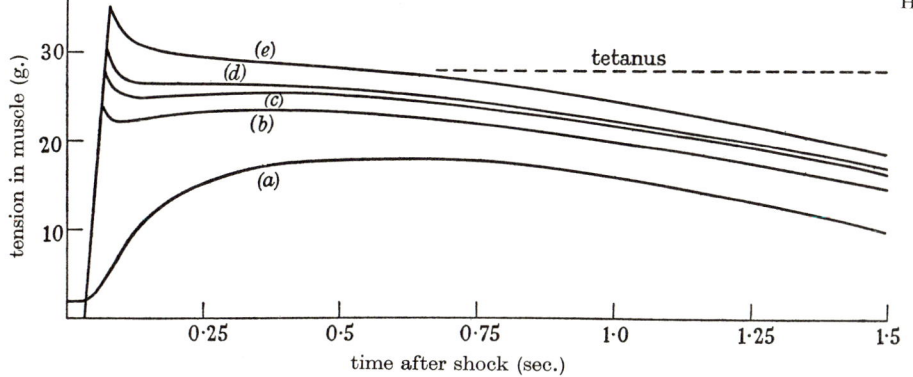

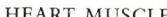

Figure 16. Effect of stretching a muscle various amounts at the same moment shortly after a maximal shock. Toad's sartorius 0°C. 62 mg., 36 mm. under 1.7 g.; latent period 32 msec.; 30 g. tension equivalent to 1.8 kg./cm.². Stretch started in (b), (c), (d), and (e) 34 msec. after, and in (a) 70 msec. before, the shock. Stretches as follows: (a) 4.3 mm., (b) 3.9 mm., (c) 4.3 mm., (d) 4.7 mm., (e) 5.1 mm. Final stretched length 36 mm. throughout. Broken line, final level of tension in isometric tetanus at length 36 mm.

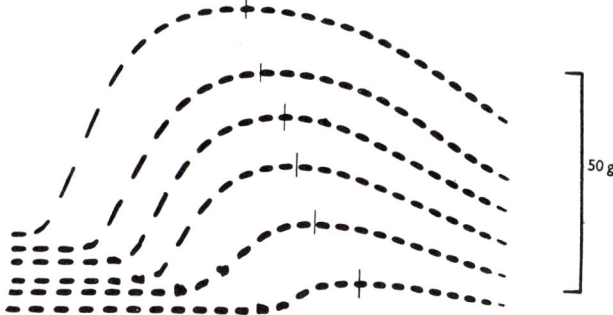

Figure 17. Records of tension/time curves of frog's sartorius at 0°C. Standard length: 37 mm.; weight: 129 mg. Top record is ordinary isometric twitch at standard length. Subsequent records have been preceded by quick releases of about 3 mm. to the standard length timed at about 10, 40, 60, 100, and 175 msec. after the stimulus. The vertical bars mark the peaks of the contraction curves. Tension calibration: 50 g. The tetanic tension was 75 g.

varying periods after a stimulus and then its sudden release to contract over a short distance.

Using such methods, the English workers have described different aspects of muscle function, including the relationship between the duration of the active state and the strength of contraction: it is clear from Fig. 14 that a lengthened duration will permit a stronger twitch, and vice versa. However, this relationship is not invariable, since, during anaerobic fatigue, when the duration of the active state is prolonged rather than shortened, the intensity of contraction is decreased (*99*).

The important contributions from the Hill school have had remarkably little influence on cardiac physiology, probably because of the differences between their refined mechanical and myothermic techniques and those used for cardiovascular research in the intact animal or even isolated hearts. An effort to combine these two approaches has been made in my laboratory using the isolated papillary and trabecular carneae preparations (*2, 10*). This program is designed not merely to copy the work on skeletal muscle, but to study problems which are specific for the myocardium. It may be illustrated by our analysis of the staircase effect.

The staircase effect was described in 1871 by the young American physiologist Bowditch (*9*) who went to study in Ludwig's great physiological laboratory, one of the leading scientific centers of the time. Subsequent investigations, especially Woodworth's (*160*), helped to define the phenomenon: when, after a prolonged rest, an excised myocardial preparation is stimulated at regular intervals, the initial contraction is weak, but the vigor of the following contractions increases with every stimulus to a value which is characteristic for the preparation. The record of the phenomenon has the appearance of ascending stairs, hence the name. It may be noted parenthetically that Bowditch's German publication employs the word "Treppe," a word which has since appeared often in the English literature. Although there is no more justification for this usage than for calling yeast "Hefe," one would have peace with this enrichment of our scientific dictionary if it were not for the widespread ignorance about the origin, spelling, and pronunciation of the word.

There are several variants of the staircase phenomenon, including a number of possibly related effects such as post-extrasystolic potentiation or the potentiation in the first twitch or so after a period of rest. The phenomenon is not restricted to cardiac muscle, but among skeletal muscles ordinarily used in laboratory investigations it does not appear strikingly. Perhaps it is more pronounced in muscles which, like the heart, contract rhythmically over long periods of time, and in which, therefore, rhythmicity and its alteration is a functionally meaningful parameter.

Although the subject has been considered often since 1871, there has been little gain in understanding beyond that afforded by the pioneer investigations. In due time, of course, it became ascribed to the presence of a "substance." A more useful, and perhaps profound, insight came with the proposition that "each contraction temporarily leaves a

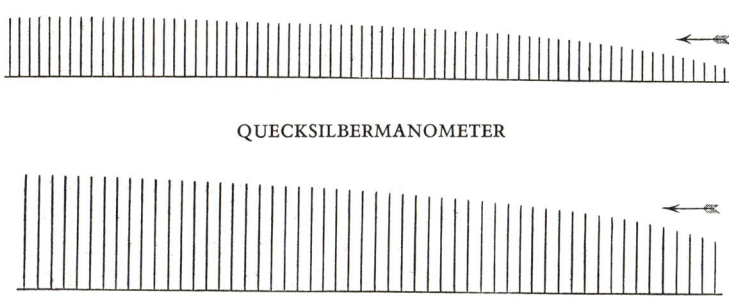

QUECKSILBERMANOMETER

WASSERMANOMETER

War vor dem Beginn einer in etwa 4 bis 6 Secunden Intervall aufeinander folgenden Reihe von immer gleich intensiven Reizen die Herzspitze mehrere Minuten hindurch in vollkommener Ruhe gewesen, so löst diese eine Folge von Zuckungen aus, wie sie in den Holzschnitten IX u. X wiedergegeben ist. Die Autographen sind von zwei verschiedenen Herzen geschrieben; IX arbeitete in ein Quecksilber- X in ein Wassermanometer.

Die erste Zuckung, welche nach einer Pause von Minuten langer Dauer hervorgerufen wird ist also die kleinste, und jede folgende nimmt an Umfang zu, jedoch in der Weise, dass mit der steigenden Zahl der Zuckungen der Zuwachs kleiner und kleiner wird bis er endlich ganz verschwindet; von nun an besitzen die hintereinander auftretenden Zuckungen denselben Umfang. Wir wollen eine so beschaffene Reihe von Zuckungen unter dem Namen einer Treppe zusammenfassen.

Figure 18. The staircase effect, as observed by Bowditch (1871) on frog heart after a prolonged rest.

condition favorable to the next contraction"(*20*). Recently, the problem was taken out of the scientific attic by Szent-Györgyi's (*137*) and Hajdu's (*41*) work, which culminated in the theory that during rest the muscle accumulates an excessive amount of K-ions; during each contraction some of the excess is lost so as to maintain a somewhat lower stationary level which is, in turn, determined by the frequency of stimulation. A lively dispute rages now about the generality and validity of this interpretation.

However, besides the problem of the nature of the "favorable condition," we also have the problem of the manner in which the contractile apparatus responds to it. Our analysis (*2, 10*) has shown, so far, that potentiation is not caused by a prolongation of the active state. It is true that there are circumstances of altered ionic composition of the medium (*105*), as well as cases of negative staircase, where the time course of the twitches suggests that a negative inotropic change is brought about by a shortened active state. But, the typical staircase and post-extrasystolic potentiation are not caused in this way. Instead, they are correlated with a shift in the force-velocity of shortening. Whether this is caused by a direct change in the fundamental constant of the Hill equation, or primarily by an increased intensity of the active state, has not yet been established because of unexpected (but not unsurmountable) experimental roadblocks.

Bowditch's paper contains another classical contribution, one that is contained in a single sentence. It is the "all-or-none principle," which states that a stimulus is either insufficient to excite the heart, or else excites it to the full extent. This concept was subsequently elaborated upon by Ranvier (*115*), who called it the "heart's motto." It contradicts in no way the immense range of responses the heart may manifest upon stimulation. It merely states that such variations cannot be brought about by varying the stimulating impulse; on the contrary, once a propagated impulse occurs, it elicits the maximal activation possible under the "circumstances." Thus, the act of stimulation may be likened to pulling the trigger of a gun; either one does or does not pull it hard enough to fire the cartridge. But the size of the cartridge and the strength of its charge may still be varied. The principle, if properly formulated, is of general validity, applying equally well to conduction in nerve and to contraction of skeletal muscle. Apparent exceptions may be encountered in local-non-propagated stimuli, but the principle was enunciated not to cover these, but propagated stimuli only.

One apparent exception of great interest, because it led to the recognition of a new type of potentiation, was recently discovered by Whalen (*147*). When, in a regularly stimulated myocardial preparation, the strength of the stimulus is increased greatly, there develops gradually a strong potentiation of the muscular contraction, which declines gradually when regular threshold stimulation is resumed. This phenomenon is ascribed to the stimulation of adrenergic nerve endings within the myocardium. An even more striking demonstration of the same phenomenon was accomplished by stimulating the preparation by a train of brief impulses applied once during the refractory period of the muscle (*10*). These two phenomena, according to the time course of their decay, are identical, but are totally different from staircase and post-extrasystolic potentiation.

When considering the "all-or-none principle," the question arises whether the magnitude of the mechanical response and the release of energy are conditioned, in part, by the stimulus itself; it would also be of interest to know what parts of the mechanical events are directly determined by variations in some quantitative characteristic of the excitation process other than the strength of the external stimulus. Recent evidence, gained in this laboratory by Dr. Brady, suggests that the duration of the active state is directly determined by the duration of the plateau of the action potential: the membrane event switches the active state on and off. So far, however, we have not recognized any direct influence of the membrane event either upon the intensity of the active state or upon the force-velocity relation. Similar attempts to unravel the fundamental relations between excitation and mechanical activity are now under way in several quarters (*56, 146*). It would be premature, at this point, to appraise these efforts.

Metabolism and Molecular Mechanisms

The statement that cells and organs satisfy their energy needs by metabolism is of general validity, but there are great differences in what this energy is used for. Many organs, many whole organisms indeed, seem to have little else to do than to carry out chemical reactions. For many a microbe, apart from the constant process of multiplication, life seems to have no other horizon than the production of ethanol, acetic acid, or hydrogen sulphide. In the human body, the liver is such an organ; its task seems to be exclusively that of acting as a versatile chemist. For example, it extracts carbohydrates from the portal blood and lactate from the systemic blood—especially after intense exercise—and converts these substances into glycogen. This glycogen is slowly reconverted to glucose, according to needs elsewhere in the body. The liver also receives various donors of ammonia which it feeds into the ornithine-citrulline-arginine cycle, to form the end product, urea. This latter sequence, up to the formation of arginine, is an example of a series of reactions which does not occur spontaneously, and which, according to principles indicated earlier, must therefore proceed by coupling with other, exergonic reactions. But the only point of importance is whether the reactions do or do not go in a certain direction; the direction can be expressed just as well descriptively, in terms of equilibrium constants, as in terms of energy. Indeed, considerations about energy become most significant when the transformation of one form of energy into another is the point of inquiry.

Tissues such as the liver (and organisms such as numerous immobile microbes) which seem to devote themselves exclusively to the practice of chemistry, have still other activities, including turnover, regeneration, and growth. But these too are of a chemical nature, although on a very special and organized level. Such purely chemical activities also occur in tissues which are concerned primarily with functions other than metabolism, e.g. contraction. And even where the over-all task of metabolism is to provide energy for mechanical activity, only a few of the many reactions are immediately associated with that ultimate act. The others represent transformations of a preparative chemical nature, designed to bring the right substances to the right places. Hence, large parts of metabolism are not involved directly in energy transformations.

A second form of cellular activity, which is also presumed to be of universal occurrence, is the maintenance of a cellular ionic composition different from that of the medium. In irritable cells, the release of potassium and the influx of sodium ions, and presumably several other migratory processes, are a fundamental part of the phenomena known as stimulation or the conduction of impulses. I am not familiar with systematic knowledge on the occurrence of such ionic shifts in tissues other than the "irritable" sensory, conducting, or motoric effector cells. However, studies on the erythrocyte have shown that even decaying red blood cells devote part of their chemical activity to the maintenance of such concentration gradients. The preservation of concentration gradients by chemical activity represents the osmotic counterpart of the "effort" in the upkeep of mechanical tension in muscle. In both instances, the distribution of ions could be kept up forever without any flux of energy, merely by "closing the door," i.e. by rendering the membrane impermeable. Indeed, such impermeability had been tacitly assumed until it was shown that even ions that do not take part in sudden shifts still permeate gradually (65, 45). It appears that a condition of total impermeability is simply not compatible with cellular life. This problem clearly has an energetic aspect: the dissipation of a concentration gradient proceeds spontaneously with an increase in entropy; its reversal requires work. In many cases, e.g. in the uptake of anions by plant cells, a definite fraction of the respiratory metabolism can be shown to be associated with such ionic movements (73). In excitable animal cells, it appears that in many situations the dominant process exists of an active expulsion of Na^+, associated with retention of K^+ to preserve electrical neutrality: the Na-pump hypothesis. Although this process must also involve an output of energy, the underlying mechanism remains obscure. Indeed, the stage of investigation has not yet passed much beyond the level of assuming the existence of a transporting substance, called "Na-pumpate"—hardly an acceptable scientific solution! In tissues that specialize in the generation, transformation, or conduction of stimuli, these ionic shifts and the underlying chemical mechanisms constitute the main occupation of the cells. In contractile tissues too, they are an essential activity, but energetically this is inconspicuous compared to the vast transformation of energy associated with the mechanical activity itself. The energy output involved in a nerve impulse is of the order of microcalories per gram (1), while contractile activity is associated with magnitudes a thousand times as great. Considering, however, that the events of stimulation occur in thin cellular membranes, the magnitude, per element of volume, of an elementary act of stimulation may be fully as great as that of an act of contraction.

The third form of transformation of energy is the generation of the mechanical energy of contraction, and it is this process which will receive our main attention. We have already noted that, unlike man-made machines, the interaction between the energy-supplying substance and the machinery takes place in molecular dimensions, and that undoubtedly the coupling between metabolism and contraction is of a topochemical nature.

Biological analysis on the molecular level is relatively old and was practiced actively and aggressively by the great botanist Nägeli toward the middle of the nineteenth century under the name *Molekularphysiologie* (*104*). There was much of a prophetic nature in his work; indeed, until the advent of modern macromolecular chemistry (*83*, *128*) and of the molecular viewpoint in protein chemistry (*131*), the successors of Nägeli were occupied with the elucidation of the structural basis for accurate biological application of his concepts. Currently, "molecular biology" has become very important, but is restricted somewhat one-sidedly to mechanisms of biosynthesis and heredity, as shown by a definition in *Time* magazine: "An esoteric kind of biochemistry that deals with the large molecules that control the growth and reproduction of living organisms." The term "molecular physiology" seems to have disappeared, until I revived it in the title of a book on the contraction mechanisms in muscle (*89*). The molecular physiology of contraction will be considered after a discussion of cellular metabolism.

Cellular Metabolism

The association between "life" and some form of chemical change, often of a fermentative or putrefactive nature, has long been recognized. Similarly, the close relation between life and the processes of oxidation attracted attention early, and became susceptible to definition after the discovery of oxygen and the recognition of the true nature of oxidation. The famous investigation of Lavoisier and Laplace (*74*) drew an accurate comparison between combustion in a flame and in an animal. For a long time, it was believed that oxidation took place only in the lungs, but our current concept, that such metabolisms occur in all parts of the body, became established in the first half of the nineteenth century. The relation between oxidation and fermentation was recognized by Pasteur, who spoke of fermentation as "la vie sans l'air," thereby recognizing aerobic and anaerobic modes of life as alternate possibilities.

The basis for the modern insights in cellular metabolism were largely contributed early in the present century by Wieland (*150*) and especially by Warburg (*142*), whereas the elaboration of some of their results to a unifying concept encompassing the whole of living nature is to a large measure due to Kluyver and Donker in their famous essay "Die Einheit in der Biochemie" (*68*). Wieland, in his analysis of organic-chemical oxidations, recognized that only in a minority of cases could these be considered, as the name would imply, as a combination with oxygen. Instead, a vast number of examples had to be regarded primarily as a removal of hydrogen instead of an addition of oxygen. According to this view, the hydrogen is transferred to a hydrogen acceptor, which can be oxygen, but can also be something else. For example, the oxidation of succinate to fumarate is a dehydrogenation and not primarily an oxygenation, and it can proceed with a variety of hydrogen acceptors, A:

$$\begin{array}{c} COOH \\ | \\ CH_2 \\ | \\ CH_2 \\ | \\ COOH \end{array} + A \longrightarrow AH_2 + \begin{array}{c} COOH \\ | \\ CH \\ \| \\ CH \\ | \\ COOH \end{array}$$

Even cases in which a combination with oxygen does seem to take place were, upon closer analysis, formulated as consisting of a primary hydration followed by dehydrogenation, e.g. the oxidation of aldehydes:

$$RC{=}O\!\!\diagdown_{H} + H_2O \longrightarrow \left[RC\diagup^{OH}_{\diagdown H\ OH} \right], + A \longrightarrow AH_2 + RC\diagup^{OH}_{\diagdown\!\!\diagdown O}$$

Similar mechanisms also occur in biological oxidations, e.g. the oxidation of alcohol to acetate by acetic acid bacteria, which, according to

[169]

Wieland (*150*), could proceed without oxygen if other hydrogen acceptors, such as methylene blue, were available:

$$C_2H_5OH + A \longrightarrow CH_3 \cdot CHO + AH_2$$
$$CH_3 \cdot CHO + A + H_2O \longrightarrow CH_3 \cdot COOH + AH_2$$

According to Kluyver and his co-workers (*67, 68, 69*) such a consideration can be applied fruitfully to nearly all metabolic reactions since these, except for cleavage reactions, involve inter- or intra-molecular hydrogen transfers. Such a generalization would now be considered too broad, since many other categories of group transfers (e.g. transacetylation) have been recognized. However, as a first attempt at order in an unclassified multitude of reactions, Kluyver's concept was of enormous significance. The main addition we shall have to make concerns the role of phosphate.

Warburg's contributions originally centered on the question of the mechanism by which oxygen, the final hydrogen or electron acceptor, enters cellular metabolism (*141*). These culminated in the assumption of a respiratory enzyme, *Atmungsferment*, which, by brilliant indirect experiments, was identified as an ironporphyrin-containing enzyme. The discovery by Keilin (*64*) that such substances can be detected in a variety of living cells led to the recognition of several such pigments, called cytochromes. The oxidation catalysis consists of one of these cytochromes being oxidized in turn by another, until one of them, cytochrome oxidase, i.e. the original *Atmungsferment*, reacts with oxygen. On the other side of the respiratory chain, the dehydrogenation of substrate molecules by cytochrome is mediated by codehydrogenases and flavoproteins, likewise discovered primarily by Warburg. An interesting sidelight in the growth of ideas is the resolution of the differences between the original Warburg and Wieland views by the unique experimental contributions of Warburg.

One additional point to explain, beyond the single steps in the dehydrogenation of metabolites, e.g. from lactate to pyruvate, is the complete oxidation of such molecules to CO_2 and H_2O. The key to this understanding lies in two main experimental approaches. The first was that of A. Szent-Györgyi (*132*), who discovered that metabolites such as succinate, fumarate, malate, and oxaloacetate actually have a catalytic role in the main pathway of cell respiration. The second, based upon an important investigation by Martius and Knoop (*81*) on the oxidation of citric acid, was that of H. A. Krebs (*70*), who recognized that the above-named metabolites are all members of a cycle, into which oxidizable matter enters by combination with oxaloacetate to form citrate—whereupon in one go-around oxaloacetate is reformed and the substrate molecule is converted to CO_2 and H_2O. The mechanism of the entry of the oxidizable matter into the cycle in the form of an acetylgroup was elucidated by Lipmann's work on coenzyme A or coacetylase (*78*), a key factor in many group transfers which, incidentally, owed its discovery, in part, to the work of Nachmansohn and Berman (*103*) on the acetylation of choline in nerve tissue. The formation of transferable acetyl groups, in turn, requires thiamine pyrophosphate and lipoic acid.

Such oxidative mechanisms, however, do not act directly upon nutrient molecules, such as glucose, but act instead upon split products formed through pathways common to both respiration and anaerobic fermentation or glycolysis. In animal tissues, these splitting reactions usually lead to lactate, in microbes sometimes to alcohol and CO_2 or to a variety of other products. The formulation of these reactions involved the efforts of many investigators, including Harden (*44*), Kluyver (*67*), Embden, Deuticke, and Kraft (*25*), Meyerhof and his collaborators (*87, 88*), Parnas (*109*) and C. F. and G. T. Cori (*16*). A summary of the major pathways is given in Fig. 19, which indicates that, while our brief remarks were directed especially at the metabolism of carbohydrates, the metabolism of lipids and amino acids employs the same common pathway of oxidation after different initial reactions.

We may ask why nature has to employ such a multitude of individual reactions in order to accomplish a relatively simple oxidation or splitting reaction. Why, for example, does it take a series of half a dozen flavoproteins and ironporphyrin proteins to oxidize a molecule of reduced diphosphopyridine nucleotide? I remember vividly the incredulity with which the first insights into the complicated reaction sequences were received in the 1930's. One might suppose that these sequential reactions related to the piecemeal liberation of the large energies of reaction. This is correct, but in terms of chemical mechanisms it begs the question. The essential additional feature is the participation of

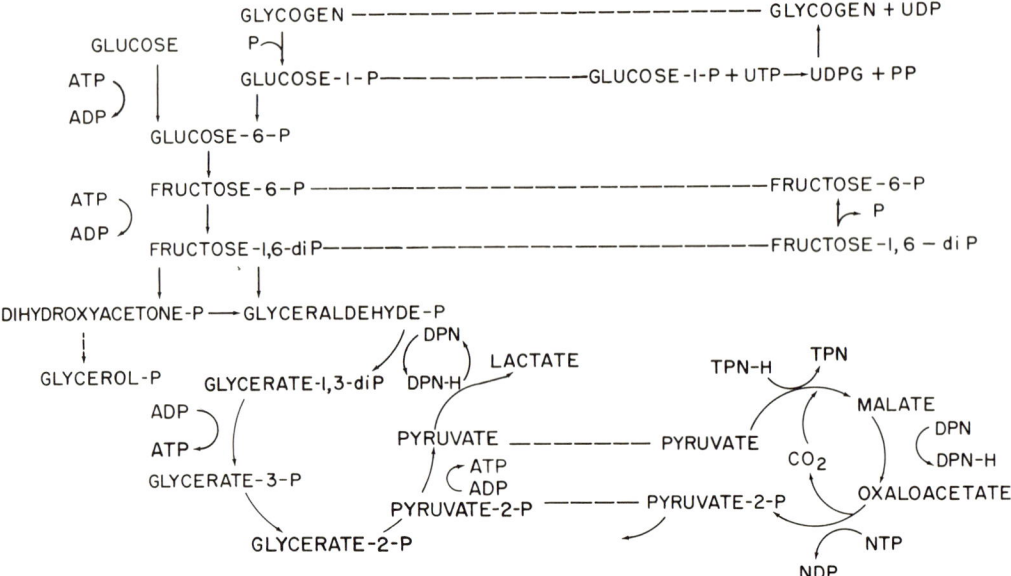

Figure 19. LEFT SIDE EQUATIONS: Scheme of the major reactions involved in the glycolysis of glycogen or glucose to lactic acid, somewhat simplified by the omission of a few transient coenzyme-substrates.

The arrows are drawn in the direction of the lactate formation, but, in principle, most of the reactions are reversible. There are, however, four sites where the reversal requires special mechanisms. In two of these, the formation of fructose diphosphate, and of glucose-6-phosphate from glucose, the reversal is simply brought about by a phosphatase (which, in the latter case, does not occur in muscle but in liver). The other cases require special cycles, given in the equations on the right.

RIGHT SIDE EQUATIONS: Scheme of the special mechanisms presumably employed in the reversal of glycolysis for the purpose of the reconversion of lactate to glycogen.

Upper: The UDPG cycle for the formation of glycogen. Although the phosphorylase reaction is readily reversible, the formation of glycogen would require a concentration of glucose-1-phosphate that never occurs in muscle; instead, a pathway employing uridine diphosphoglucose (UDPG) is assumed to occur.

Lower: The Utter cycle for the formation of phosphopyruvate. The reaction: phosphopyruvate + ADP → pyruvate + ATP is not demonstrably reversible. The cycle involves the incorporation and re-elimination of CO_2, and utilizes another nucleotide triphosphate (ITP or GTP) instead of ATP; presumably, it is driven by the difference in energy between the oxidation of TPN-H and the reduction of DPN at the prevailing concentrations.

phosphate in these intermediary reactions. Let us illustrate this first for the glycolytic pathway.

When glycolysis starts from glycogen by means of the phosphorylase reaction, the primary product is not glucose but glucose-1-phosphate, which is converted into glucose-6-phosphate. If it starts from glucose, the first step is the formation of glucose-6-phosphate in the hexokinase reaction. This key-substance is converted into fructose-6-phosphate, which is further phosphorylated to fructose-1,6-diphosphate. From there on, all reactions continue to involve phosphorylated compounds until phosphopyruvate is dephosphorylated prior to its reduction to lactate or its complete oxidation in the Krebs-cycle. This participation of phosphate in fermentation reactions had been known ever since the pioneer observations of Harden and Young (*44*), but its meaning was not appreciated except in vague terms related to the "labilization" or "activation" of the intermediates. For a more correct understanding we have to introduce a new substance and a new concept.

The substance is adenosine triphosphate (ATP), a nucleotide discovered in the early 1930's and immediately recognized as an essential coenzyme in phosphorylation processes (*89*). It was also found that upon hydrolysis of ATP a relatively large amount of heat is liberated (although the original estimates of approximately 10,000 calories per mole were somewhat excessive, they were qualitatively correct), and it was estimated that the free-energy effect of its splitting is likewise high. On the basis of such considerations, Lipmann (*78*) derived his concept of high-energy phosphate compounds, of which ATP is the prototype; these substances contain phosphate in such bonding that its hydrolysis releases an unusually large amount of free energy. Although Lipmann's concepts have been criticized, largely on account of the difficulty in formulating the nature of the high-energy bond, they afford a useful basis for further conceptualization and investigation.

Returning to the glycolytic pathway, let us consider the formation of pyruvate. Were this to originate from glyceric acid, the higher energy of the latter would be dissipated as heat. However, the equilibrium reactions involved in the conversion of phosphoglycerate to phosphopyruvate, which entail insignificant changes in energy, are characterized by the acquisition of high-energy properties by the phosphate radical of the phosphopyruvate instead of the low-energy character of the phosphoglycerate. Hence, the energy change in the reaction glycerate → pyruvate, when conducted with the phosphorylated compounds, is preserved in the energy-rich phosphate of the pyruvate. It can now be used to form ATP from adenosine diphosphate (ADP), the only way in which phosphopyruvate can be metabolized further. This part of glycolysis, then, accounts for the formation of ATP, two moles for every mole of hexose which is metabolized. Another two moles are formed in the oxidation of phosphoglyceraldehyde to phosphoglycerate, by a somewhat more complex mechanism involving the actual uptake of inorganic phosphate. In all, four moles of ATP are formed in the fermentation of one mole of glucose. However, one mole of ATP had to be expended to make fructose-1,6-diphosphate from fructose-6-phosphate, since this phosphorylation requires ATP to drive it and will not occur spontaneously with inorganic phosphate. Similarly, the phosphorylation of glucose requires ATP, but that of glycogen does not, sufficient energy being contained in its glycosidic linkages to permit spontaneous formation of glucose-1-phosphate. Hence, the glycolysis of one mole of glucose leads to a net production of two moles of ATP, and that of one glucose equivalent of glycogen to three moles. The result is that a large part of the enthalpy and free-energy effects of glycolysis is invested in the synthesis of the high-energy compound. It takes only one further imaginative step, partly based upon what will be said below on the cell's use of ATP, to conclude that it is the very purpose of glycolysis to synthesize ATP, and that nature employs this particular tortuous pathway for a simple fission reaction in order to employ intermediates which lend themselves to effect this synthesis.

A similar conclusion has emerged from the study of respiration. The pioneer investigations of Belitzer and Tsibakova (6), Runnström, et al. (120), Engelhardt (26), and Kalckar (60, 61), established that oxidative reactions also involved the uptake of inorganic phosphate. Subsequent investigations, e.g. by Ochoa (107), showed that ATP is formed and that the oxidative phosphorylation accompanying the respiratory oxidation of substrates leads to the formation of fixed proportions of high-energy phosphate (P:O ratios). Some of these phosphorylation reactions, like the formation of one ATP in the oxidation of α-ketoglutarate to succinate, are substrate-linked and are not fundamentally different from the reactions encountered in glycolysis. However, most phosphorylations are not of this nature, but are linked with the individual oxidation steps in the codehydrogenase-flavoprotein-cytochrome series. The mechanisms of these steps are not yet elucidated, but the study of them is in active progress and constitutes one of the most profound chapters in contemporary biochemistry (*75, 14, 125*). In keeping with the much greater energy obtainable from oxidation than from fermentation, e.g. of glucose, many more than two molecules of ATP are obtainable by oxidation—as many as forty.

In Fig. 19 (left equations), it has been assumed that the pathway proceeds from glycogen to lactate, as is the case when glycolysis is called upon by activity or anaerobiosis. Since all, or nearly all, the component reactions are equilibrium reactions, it has long been assumed that the reversal of glycolysis (as occurs in muscle during the recovery phase and mainly in the liver as a part of the Cori cycle for the resynthesis of glycogen) merely proceeds by running through the same reactions in the opposite way, somehow steered by the energy of respiratory metabolism. This explanation, which was never satisfactory, has been invalidated by the demonstration of several reaction steps, both reversible and irreversible (Fig. 19), which proceed by separate pathways. Regarding the major reversal cycles (*140, 46, 118*), we can only defer further discussion until more is known about the physiological mechanisms that direct metabolism into one channel or another.

As will be explained in greater detail in the next section, it seems likely that ATP is also the substance which is utilized by cells for miscellaneous activities which require energy. At least, ATP is very close to those fundamental activities. We might symbolize this in the following cycle:

$$\text{CONTRACTILE AND OTHER CELLULAR ACTIVITIES} \quad \left(\begin{array}{c} \text{ATP} \leftarrow \\ \rightarrow \text{ADP} \end{array}\right) \quad \text{RESPIRATION OR GLYCOLYSIS}$$

This diagram emphasizes the way nature uses its multitude of metabolic reactions. The proposition that the stepwise, rather than explosive, release of energy requires individual stages of reaction entails the prospect that each of these many reactions could require a separate mechanism for mechanochemical coupling (restricting ourselves to contractile functions) in order to make its contribution. Such a complex arrangement has been circumvented by funneling every reaction into the production of ATP so that only the participation of the latter in cellular activities has to be taken into account. In a remarkably farsighted book (*132*), Szent-Györgyi pictured nucleotides as the energetic coinage of the cell. This is indeed a proper comparison: the role of ATP in cell metabolism is much like that of money in commercial relations.

ATP is not the only high-energy phosphate. Aside from the fact that there are other nucleotide triphosphates (cytosine-, guanosine-, inosine-, uridine-, and other triphosphates; adenosine tetraphosphate; and who knows what more), there is also a group of substances which gave rise to the formation of phosphate under the conditions of the Fiske-Subbarow reaction with acid molybdate. This turned out to be phosphocreatine (*34*). Later, phosphoarginine was discovered in certain invertebrate muscles, but this substance, although acid-labile, is actually stabilized by molybdate. Several other substances have been discovered in invertebrate animals, with varying labilities toward molybdate. Nowadays, one would not define these substances in terms of their behavior in a chemical test, but would instead characterize them biologically as a group of substances occurring in tissues which can, under the influence of tissue enzymes, donate their phosphate group to ADP. For creatine phosphate the enzyme creatine kinase or creatine phosphoryltransferase has been crystallized and well characterized, but in most other instances this identification has not yet been accomplished. Often, the phosphagen content of a muscular tissue is considerable, e.g. in the frog sartorius muscle there may be up to 25 micromoles of phosphocreatine per gram, as compared to 5 micromoles of ATP. This proportion has led to the widespread belief that phosphagens act as a storehouse for the replenishment of ATP. But one wonders if there is not a more direct and fundamental role for them.

There are certain regularities in the distribution of various metabolic activities throughout the cell. The oxidative-phosphorylative enzyme systems seem to be located in their entirety within the mitochondria, presumably in an organized pattern (*75, 40*). By contrast, the glycolytic enzymes are apparently soluble and cytoplasmic; so are many other enzymes, including the one for the transfer of phosphate between phosphocreatine and ATP. The reactions for the mechanochemical transfers must, of course, be fibrillar. It is likely, then, that ATP diffuses back and forth between the mitochondria or the sarcoplasm where it is made, and the fibrils, where it is used. This explanation may suffice if the diffusion paths are sufficiently short, i.e. of the order of a micron or so.

There are great differences between the relative intensities with which the several types of metabolism can occur. The speed of utilization of ATP is, in general, not known from direct observations, but several estimates (*89*) have indicated that it may be of the order of a micromole or less per gram per minute at rest, and up to a thousand times more during full activity (varying, of course, with the intensity and the economy of the activity). Since metabolism is directed toward the restitution of the utilized ATP, we have to inquire whether it can do so fast enough, and, if not, what consequences result. There is no difficulty in accounting for the observed rates of energy production in terms of the simultaneous metabolism; in fact, these are of exactly the same orders of magnitude when expressed in the same units, e.g. as calories per gram per minute. How a metabolic rate can be converted into a power (rate of energy production) is known from the empirical calibration of metabolism by animal calorimetry. The direct measurement of energy production by calorimetry, on the other hand, may require some explanation. In particular, if a fraction of the metabolic energy is used for the performance of some mechanical, osmotic, or chemical work, it might be argued that this part of the energy cannot appear as heat and will therefore escape detection. Therefore, such measurements are designed so that mechanical energy is dissipated into heat (e.g. by isometric contraction). Since osmotic work usually reverts to heat by processes of diffusion, the only possible exception could be the endergonic synthesis of chemical substances. But biocalorimetry has always taken care to account for such processes separately (*138*). Let us use the events in muscular contraction, as studied by A. V. Hill, as an example.

During the contraction process itself the initial heat appears. This heat consists of the changes in enthalpy of whatever chemical processes occur; these processes may do work during activation but eventually this work reverts to heat. If actual work is done, a corresponding fraction will not appear as heat during contraction, but will manifest itself during relaxation when the returning load does an equal amount of work upon the muscle substance. If, by special experimental design (or in the normal physiological course of events) this return does not take place, a corresponding amount of heat is indeed missed, but it is accounted for in the work which is performed. Let the total initial energy be E_I. To give it a definite chemical connotation, let us ascribe it to the splitting of phosphocreatine; this is undoubtedly an oversimplification, but one which may apply approximately under certain circumstances.

In the recovery process, we observe the delayed heat, corresponding to the energy E_D. This is the balance between the change in the enthalpy of respiration (E_R) minus the enthalpy of the resynthesis of phosphocreatine or whatever else has been used in the initial events ($-E_I$). Hence, $E_R = E_I + E_D$, and the total energy E_R corresponds to the heat effect of respiration. The circumstance of approximately equal E_I and E_D is related to the fact that the energetic yield of aerobic phosphorylation is about 50 per cent.

The necessary equality between metabolic intensity and the production of energy applies both to conditions of rest and of activity, but the intensities in these two states can differ vastly. In fact, I have estimated (89) that the transition from rest to maximal activity involves an acceleration of metabolism of up to a thousandfold. In the heart the change may be less dramatic because its "resting metabolism" (however that may be approached) is much greater than that of voluntary muscle, undoubtedly because the heart never rests and therefore has no provision for an efficient resting metabolism. Yet, here too there is a great metabolic activation commensurate with increased performance (29). Accepting as a physiological fact that stimulation leads to activity and to the release of energy, what mechanisms are available to explain the activation of metabolism which is needed to cover this heightened expenditure of energy?

There is one fundamental mechanism which, to many biochemists, seems to be all we need for an explanation. It is the principle, clearly demonstrated in experiments such as those of Rabinowitz, et al. (113), Lardy and Wellman (72), and Siekevitz and Potter (123), that, since phosphorylation of ADP to ATP is an obligatory part of respiration and glycolysis, metabolism can only proceed at a rate permitted by dephosphorylation of the ATP which is formed in this way. Indeed, certain phenomena in muscle metabolism can well be investigated from that point of view (*15*). Yet, there is some doubt whether this is the only possible explanation. In living muscle, for example, there is no significant increase in ADP during many forms of exercise, even though these are accompanied by increased glycolysis or respiratory metabolism.

There is one special regulatory mechanism which, although its applicability cannot yet be evaluated, may be of great interest. Investigations in C. F. Cori's laboratory (*16*, *17*) have disclosed that phosphorylase can occur in two forms, a and b, of which only the former is active under physiological conditions (i.e. in the absence of adenylic acid). Cori has noted that the fraction present in the a-form varies with the condition of muscle and has seen the possibility that at rest there is so little active phosphorylase as to limit the rate of glycolysis. Our current investigations with the method of instantly freezing a resting muscle confirm this hypothesis, since in resting muscle only about 25 per cent or so of the enzyme is active, but its activity increases promptly upon stimulation. This would not be enough to limit glycolysis, but the reaction may be further restricted by the prevailing low phosphate level. How the activation is accomplished is a problem in itself, but the results may indicate that, at rest, metabolism is throttled at the very beginning of the reaction chain, and, during stress, glycolysis is started by promoting the breakdown of storage glycogen. This mechanism is obviously of use mainly for muscles with intermittent activity, because a storage nutrient can answer only a transient demand. Yet, even the heart, although always active, will have periods of greater and lesser metabolic need, and may initiate its adjustments in ways akin to those employed in intermittently working muscles.

These are not the only possibilities, in fact, there is a fundamental resemblance between our problem and the mechanism of that other metabolic regulation, the Pasteur effect, for which many theories have been discussed (*21*). For the time being, we do not know the answer.

While physiological-chemical studies on muscle have traditionally emphasized the metabolism of carbohydrates, it would be a mistaken notion to assume that this is always the only fuel of muscle. Anaerobically it is, since only carbohydrate is involved in glycolysis. But aerobically in steady state activity, it may not be. Such measurements as have recently been performed indicate that lipid oxidation is predominant under those circumstances. But, to the extent that this too proceeds via the citric acid cycle, our considerations are still valid.

Molecular Physiology

The relation between form and function in biology has been discussed in many contexts and from many angles (*139, 66, 8*). Usually, these discussions consider structures that are visible macroscopically, or at least microscopically. It was realized early, however, that the problem does not stop at the limits of microscopic visibility, because structure obviously exists beyond the limits of optical resolution imposed by the wavelength of visible light. Indeed, it became apparent, or rather it was assumed, that the true mysteries of life are to be found on the other side of this limit. In part, this awareness stemmed from the recognition that even microscopic structures seem to have certain full attributes of living systems. This insight also reflected a consequence of our tendency to pursue our questions further and further in the same direction: if a heart contracts because its cells do, if the cells contract because the myofibrils do, if the fibrils contract because the sarcomeres do, then what makes the sarcomeres contract? To quote dePourtales in *La Pêche miraculeuse*: "How unfortunate," he said, "that we have not a long series of lives at our disposal, for we find universe within universe the further we explore, like those Japanese lacquer boxes that you buy in Port Said, the smallest of which is so tiny that you can't open it at all." "It was precisely in the last and most infinitesimal cell that the truth of all things lay concealed."

This last sentence is a perfect definition of the aims of molecular physiology. Yet there is one pitfall: while looking for the mechanism of life in smaller and smaller structures, while going from sarcomeres to filaments to molecules of myosin and actin, to mero- and protomyosins, hence to peptide units and single atoms, we will lose the secret of life somewhere en route. In fact, we started to lose it when we disrupted the organization of the cell. Obviously, then, our atomistic approach is not entirely truthful.

Aside from these philosophical restrictions, it is clear that certain important parts of the biological events take place at a level between the microscopic and the macromolecular, which, for nonbiological systems, Ostwald called "Die Welt der vernachlässigten Dimensionen" (*108*).

In this world, we deal with the macromolecules of protein, of such dimensions that they present a huge surface area while at the same time invalidating our macroscopic concepts of surfaces; we deal with topochemical reactions between sites on these molecules and small molecules and ions; we deal with problems of intermolecular forces, of factors of shape, and of intermolecular arrangements as in liquid crystals, tactoids, and coacervates; and with the problem of local reactions which influence more remote parts of the same molecule.

At the molecular level of the "form and function" problem we must also start with morphological descriptions; at this level, morphology is intricately bound to chemical identification. The early history of this subject has largely been that of the application of the polarization microscope (*121*). In brief, these studies suggested that muscle possessed a submicroscopic filamentous structure which was arranged longitudinally with respect to the direction of the myofibrils: submicroscopic refers to the width of the filamentous elements; their lengths are of the order of microns, but they are too thin to be seen. This situation remained somewhat vague until the momentous publications by von Muralt and Edsall in 1930 (*101*, *102*), which contained the observation that a muscle protein, myosin, shows the phenomenon of flow birefringence. A body shows birefringence (i.e. light transmission when held between crossed polarizers) (*95*) when it has some internal anisotropy with respect to its refractivity. This phenomenon is common in crystals where it has no special molecular-morphological connotation. In biological systems, however, the occurrence of the phenomenon is usually associated with anisometric (e.g. filamentous) particles. Solutions of the latter, as occur in extracts of the muscle protein, myosin, will not show birefringence because of the random arrangement of the constituents. When orientation is effected, birefringence will appear; such orientation by means of flow in a solution is possible when the particles are very long so as to follow the streamlines without suffering major derangements by thermal movement. The result of von Muralt and Edsall thus indicated that myosin consists of long particles obviously suited for making up the filamentous structure of the sarcomere. Soon afterwards, Weber (*144*) and Noll and Weber (*106*) announced the preparation of myosin filaments, and a complete polarization-optical study that demonstrated the fundamental similarity of the filaments and of muscle.

Having recognized the structural protein, the next great event was the disclosure of how it might interact with energy-yielding metabolism, by Engelhardt and Ljubimova (*27*), who discovered that myosin has enzymatic activity and catalyzes the splitting of ATP. We seemed then to have a fibrous enzyme molecule, able to capture the energy of the reaction it catalyzes and to turn it into shortening, tension, or work. Further developments have taken us away from this simple and satisfying view, but even so it represented a great breakthrough.

The limitations of this attractive hypothesis were apparent: the anisotropy of myosin and its ATPase activity were facts, everything else was conjecture. But a new field for experimentation had been opened. The first explorations were done by the Needhams and their group (*19*). Their work suggested alterations in the myosin molecule by its interaction with ATP; but, fascinating as this work was, it did not bring striking demonstrations comparable to those of A. Szent-Györgyi (*5*).

The first contribution by Szent-Györgyi was the recognition that preparations of myosin were variable, a situation ascribed to the simultaneous occurrence of two proteins: myosin proper and actin, which combines to form a complex, actomyosin (myosin + actin → actomyosin). ATP, added to actomyosin solutions, reverses the process and causes dissociation of the complex as long as it is in solution. In the gel state, on the other hand, other reactions occur, and these were first demonstrated with threads prepared in Weber's manner from actomyosin. These threads were found to contract when, in the appropriate salt medium (about 0.18 molar with respect to potassium, 0.01 molar with respect to magnesium ions), ATP was added. Subsequently, the experiment was refined by the development of an "actomyosin fiber" made without ever dissolving and disorganizing the actomyosin, i.e. by removing most of the other constituents through extraction with glycerol at low temperature. These threads (*135*) become thicker with shortening, can raise weights, and can develop about the same tension as the muscles from which they are derived, while the precipitated actomyosin threads, by virtue of their lack of internal cohesion and orientation, shrink in all directions and show plastic stretch when loaded. A fairly extensive literature has developed around the behavior of these threads (*136, 145*), and we shall return to some aspects of this topic later.

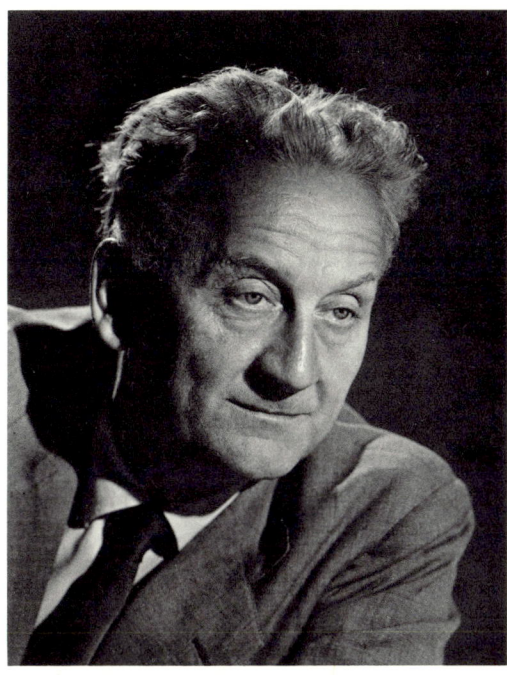

Figure 20. Albert Szent-Györgyi (1893–   ).

It will be realized that, while the discovery of myosin and of ATPase initially gave rise only to interesting hypotheses, we have now reached the stage of actual experimental demonstrations which do not leave much room for skepticism. Szent-Györgyi's discovery prompted many investigations, of which we shall consider a few (*89, 133–136*).

The ATPase activity of myosin has become the subject of a most extensive, but disappointing, literature. Disappointing because on the one hand no well-substantiated views have yet resulted to indicate how this splitting reaction, or the enzyme-substrate combination which precedes it, can give rise to the transfer of energy and the phenomena of contraction. Disappointing also, because the literature on this subject has become so erratic and complex as to be quite useless. The acidity, the concentrations of potassium, sodium, magnesium and calcium ions and of substrate; the specificity of the substrate; the presence of activators and of inhibitors; and the properties of myosin versus actomyosin; all cause innumerable variations, and the effect of each factor is drastically modified by almost any other factor. The introduction of enzyme-kinetic analyses in the description of these influences has not made matters any simpler. There is simply nothing sensible that one can conclude from this; yet some day these facts will have to be entered into a more synthetic picture.

Actin is fully as interesting a protein as is myosin. As described by its discoverer, Straub (*129, 130*), it can occur in a globular and in a polymerized or fibrous form. In the absence of salt, the former (G-actin) occurs, and polymerization is initiated by adding salt. Throughout these reactions ATP has to be present, because without it actin becomes inactivated. The process of polymerization involves a stoichiometric breakdown of ATP to ADP, one molecule for each actin molecule entering into the fibrous polymer (*90–93*). More recently, it has begun to emerge that this strict stoichiometric coupling is a limiting case; we can also have polymerization without coupled nucleotide breakdown. The polymer, if not aggregated sidewise, forms long chains or strands of G-actin molecules, the latter having a molecular weight of about 60,000.

Myosin itself has an anisometric molecule, and is often regarded as rod-shaped although this has not been proven. If it is, it has a length of 1600 Angstrom units and a molecular weight of about 480,000. These rod-shaped particles attach themselves to the actin filaments in the formation of actomyosin; in solutions or during the extraction of muscle, they do this in a random, crisscross manner since there is no organizing influence. In vivo, undoubtedly, there is orientation. In fact, as we shall see below, there is such an elaborate organization that it is doubtful whether we can speak of "actomyosin" in the living muscle fibril at all.

Szent-Györgyi's extracted fiber preparations have been studied by others, especially Weber and Portzehl (*145*). Unfortunately, much remains to be learned about the mechanisms involved in the contraction of these fibers. It can be defended equally well that their contraction is caused by a simultaneous splitting of ATP (*143*) or that it is caused by the combination between ATP and myosin prior to its splitting. Of particular interest was the discovery by Marsh (*80*) and Bendall (*7*) of a relaxation factor which can cause the reversal of the contraction of the fiber preparations. Subsequent work has suggested

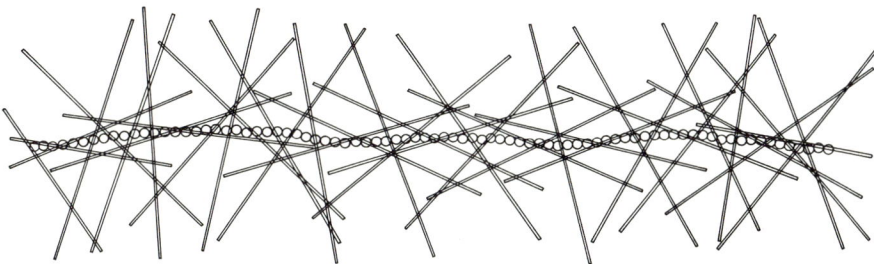

Figure 21. Diagram of the molecular structure of an actomyosin micell in solution. The myosin molecules (here represented as straight rods) are randomly attached to an actin filament composed of globular units polymerized end to end. There is, approximately, one myosin molecule (length 1600 Angstroms, mol. wt. 420,000) for every two actin monomers (mol. wt. 60,000).

that this reversal phenomenon is partly associated with the presence of an enzyme restoring the hydrolyzed ATP (such as myokinase, creatine kinase, or pyruvate kinase), but it also requires a specific particulate factor (*23*) which is related to the in vivo relaxation in some obscure way. The relaxation factor was originally discovered in connection with the reversal of certain post-mortem changes, and there is no clear proof that it participates in the contraction cycle. Therefore, considerable work is needed before the possibilities raised by Szent-Györgyi's experiment are fully realized.

Concerning the structural basis on the submicroscopic level, a great deal has been learned from electronmicroscopy, to which a sequence of pioneers (*42, 119, 22*) has contributed with increasing technical perfection, till the contemporary work of Hanson and Huxley (*43*), Huxley (*58*), and Sjöstrand (*124*). As a result of this work, and of supporting

THE HEART

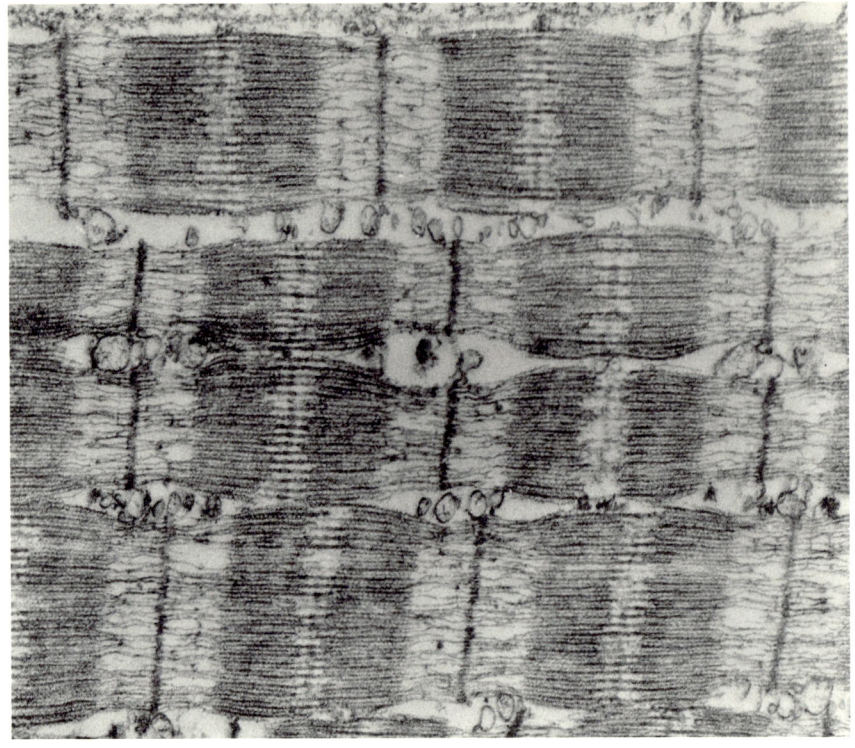

Figure 22. Extremely thin section of striated muscle.
Clearly visible are the dense A-bands, bisected by H-zones; and the lighter I-bands, bisected by Z-lines.

studies mainly by interference microscopy but also by X-ray diffraction, one accepts that the sarcomere is built up of two sets of interdigitating rods, thinner actin rods running from the Z band into the A band up to the limit of the H zone, and heavier myosin rods which extend over the full length of the A band. Contraction is ascribed to a sliding motion of the actin rods inward into the A regions. This picture is convincingly supported by the best of electronmicroscopy, yet there are some reservations which might be offered. First, there seems to be difficulty in confirming that the A rods are made of myosin. It is rumored that application of fluorescent antibodies against H- and L-meromyosin, respectively, suggests these proteins to be in different areas of the A band, which would not be compatible with our general knowledge. Here we can only await further developments. Second, it is mainly the structure of resting (or, more precisely, rigor mortis) muscle which has been investigated electronmicroscopically; the events during contraction in life are only inferred, although on plausible grounds, from interference microscopy. Third, most of this work is done upon glycerol-extracted fiber preparations, which have the great advantage of sharpening the structures by elimination of much of the soluble proteins; however, pictures obtained from fixed living muscle are not entirely in accord, and it remains to be decided whether the differences in appearance arise from technical difficulties or from real differences between the living and the post-mortem preparations.

If, in one form or another, the picture of sliding particles is maintained and confirmed, we will have to develop our theories of the mechanism of contraction in accordance with this model. This will not be easy, because there are no clearly applicable inorganic models; in order to make a start, one might find analogies in the behavior of liquid crystals. Several active experimenters in the field of contractility take a dim view of the numerous theories or hypotheses that are constantly being offered. Certainly there is no justification for designing mechanisms when the major facts are entirely unknown.

The major weakness of the entire problem at this moment seems to be the lack of connection between the biochemical and structural work on the one hand and the activities of living muscles on the other. We know that actin can polymerize and depolymerize and react with ATP: we know that actin and myosin can associate and dissociate; we know that myosin can combine with ATP and split it, and that during this enzyme-substrate combination its interaction with actin is modified. We do not know whether, when, or to what extent, each of these phenomena occurs in living tissues. To approach this complex of problems we developed a method of instantaneously freezing a muscle at a given moment of activity (98). However, the problems of identifying the molecular-morphological situation fixed within the frozen tissue are formidable, and little headway has been made.

The freezing method has been applied intensively to one particular problem, but the result has not brought undivided happiness. When trying to demonstrate the breakdown of ATP in the course of a twitch (93, 94, 35, 36), an absolutely negative result was obtained. This result was entirely unanticipated in view of the strong biochemical evidence upon which the assumed role of ATP is based. If this result is final, it will have an immense impact upon our fundamental beliefs in the whole field of contractility. However, there are still several reasons why these experiments may be misleading, and so it is wisest again to postpone judgment until we know more about the subject. More recently, our work has begun to demonstrate phosphocreatine breakdown regularly in some muscles, but the exceptions have not yet been explained.

Some Afterthoughts

Having dealt at some length with the experimental, and sometimes the historical, origin of some of the concepts of importance for the understanding of the contractility of the heart, perhaps we should notice how varied and heterogeneous these concepts are. As far as understanding specific aspects of myocardial function, it is obvious that only direct observations on the heart can lead us to an answer. But to elucidate the fundamental mechanisms of contractility, the investigator has recourse to contractile materials other than heart muscle. As the preceding discussions have indicated, except for the investigation of respiratory enzymes, where heart muscle has frequently been the tissue of choice, studies on muscle have been done largely with skeletal muscle. This lopsidedness has two main reasons, one valid and the other invalid. The valid reason is that, for many experimental approaches, skeletal muscles (such as the frog sartorius for refined mechanical and myothermic measurements, and rabbit leg muscles for biochemical preparative work) have decided technical advantages. The invalid reason is that cardiac physiology has often developed in close relation to clinical problems and through the special techniques of hemodynamic research, while muscle physiology has been more inclined to develop its own methods. How fruitful an attempt at cross-fertilization can be is indicated by our current experience with the fundamental mechanical properties of the isolated mammalian papillary muscle preparation (2, 10).

Unexpectedly, perhaps, for an essay of this nature, no attempt has been made to present a theory of the mechanism of contractility. I might quote a remark made in 1926 by Einthoven to his visitor, C. J. Wiggers: "The truth is all that matters; what you or I may think is inconsequential." Like photosynthesis, which as early as 1917 could boast dozens of different "theories" concerning its mechanism (*122*), contraction has also appealed traditionally to the imagination, and has often invited speculation among workers who were not involved directly in its experimental investigation. It is often said, of course, that hypotheses have the value of leading to new experiments. But is it necessary for new experiments, first to form hypotheses with strong emotional attachments? I should like to compare the work of the experimenter with that of a taxonomist who sets out to establish the identity of an unknown plant: he does not start with formulating a hypothesis like the assumption that it might be *Strelitzia regina*, or *Chara nodosa*; he follows, instead, a path of dichotomous choices, without prejudice, which eventually leads him to the answer. Of course, the experimenter working in virgin fields has no dichotomous system in front of him, and no guaranteed result at the end. But is not the formulation of well-formulated questions better than that of hypothesis? I remember my first meeting with A. V. Hill in which I said I had a theory of contraction. He looked at me with amusement and said: "Oh yes? I never had one." Of course, the emotional needs of individual investigators are different, and it takes all kinds of people to assure scientific progress. But, in my opinion, a "theory of contraction" is not even in sight. Nor do I feel the need for one particularly, since there are so many good questions all around us. From questions and answers we build structures of thought. "These are our cathedrals" (*77, page vii*).

BIBLIOGRAPHY

1. ABBOTT, B. C., A. V. HILL, and J. V. HOWARTH. The positive and negative heat production associated with a nerve impulse. Proc. roy. Soc. B, 148:149, 1958.
2. ABBOTT, B. C., and W. F. H. M. MOMMAERTS. A study of inotropic mechanisms in the papillary muscle preparation. J. gen. Physiol., 42:533, 1959.
3. AUBERT, X. Le couplage énergetique de la contraction musculaire, Editions Arcsia, Brussels, Belgium, 1956.
4. AUBERT, X. La thermo-élasticité du muscle en contracture iodoacétique. Arch. int. Physiol., 61:116, 1953.
5. BANGA, I., T. ERDÖS, M. GERENDAS, W. F. H. M. MOMMAERTS, F. B. STRAUB, and A. SZENT-GYÖRGYI. Myosin and muscular contraction. Stud. Inst. med. Chem. Szeged, 1, 1942.

6. BELITZER, V. A., and E. T. TSIBAKOVA. The mechanism of phosphorylation as related to respiration. Biokhimija, 4:516, 1939.
7. BENDALL, J. R. Further observations on a factor (the "Marsh" factor) effecting relaxation of ATP-shortened muscle-fibre models, and the effect of Ca and Mg ions upon it. J. Physiol., (Lond.) 121:232, 1953.
8. BÖKER, H. Einführung in die vergleichende biologische Anatomie der Wirbeltiere. Jena, Fischer, 1935.
9. BOWDITCH, H. P. Ueber die Eigenthümlichkeiten der Reizbarkeit, welche die Muskelfasern des Herzens zeigen. Ber. math. -phys. sächs. Ges. Wiss., Leipzig. 13:652, 1871.
10. BRADY, A. J., B. C. ABBOTT, and W. F. H. M. MOMMAERTS. Inotropic effects of trains of impulses applied during the contraction of cardiac muscle. J. gen. Physiol., 44:2, 1960.
11. BRECHER, G. A. Venous Return. New York, Grune & Stratton, 1956.
12. BURCH, G. E., C. T. RAY, and J. A. CRONVICH. Certain mechanical pecularities of the human cardiac pump in normal and diseased states. The George Fahr Lecture. Circulation, 5:504, 1952.
13. BURTON, A. C. The importance of the shape and size of the heart. Amer. Heart J., 54:801, 1957.
14. CHANCE, B., and G. R. WILLIAMS. The respiratory chain and oxidative phosphorylation. Advanc. Enzymol., 17:65, 1956.
15. CHANCE, B., and C. H. CONNELLY. (In preparation).
16. CORI, C. F. Enzymatic reactions in carbohydrate metabolism. Harvey Lect., 61:253, 1946.
17. CORI, C. F. Regulations of enzyme activity in muscle during work. In Henry Ford Hospital. International Symposium on Enzymes, p. 573. New York, Academic Press, 1956.
18. CORI, O., A. TRAVERSO-CORI, M. LAGARRIGUE, and F. MARCUS. Enzymic phosphorylation of creatine by 1:3-diphosphoglyceric acid. Biochem. J., 70:633, 1958.
19. DAINTY, M., A. KLEINZELLER, A. S. C. LAWRENCE, M. MIALL, J. NEEDHAM, D. M. NEEDHAM, and S.-C. SHEN. Studies on the anomalous viscosity and flow-birefringence of protein solutions. III. Changes in these properties of myosin solutions in relation to adenosinetriphosphate and muscular contraction. J. gen. Physiol., 27:355, 1944.
20. DALE, A. S. The staircase phenomenon in ventricular muscle. J. Physiol. (Lond.), 75:1, 1932.
21. DICKENS, F. Anaerobic glycolysis, respiration, and the Pasteur effect. In J. B. Sumner, and K. Myrbäck, Eds. The Enzymes, 2:624. New York, Academic Press, 1951.

22. DRAPER, M. H., and A. J. HODGE. Studies on muscle with the electron microscope. I. The ultrastructure of toad striated muscle. Aust. J. exp. Biol. med. Sci., 27:465, 1949.
23. EBASHI, S. A granule-bound relaxation factor in skeletal muscle. Arch. Biochem., 76:410, 1958.
24. EGGLETON, P. The place of phosphagen in muscle biochemistry. Ergebn. Enzymforsch., 3:227, 1934.
25. EMBDEN, G., H. J. DEUTICKE, and G. KRAFT. Über die intermediären Vorgänge bei der Glykolyse in der Muskulatur. Klin. Wschr., 12:213, 1932.
26. ENGELHARDT, W. A. Ortho- und Pyrophosphat im aeroben und anaeroben Stoffwechsel der Blutzellen. Biochem. Z., 227:16, 1930.
27. ENGELHARDT, W. A., and M. N. LJUBIMOWA. Myosin and adenosinetriphosphatase. Nature, 144:668, 1939.
28. EPSTEIN, P. S. Textbook of Thermodynamics. New York, Wiley, 1937.
29. EVANS, C. The physiology of plain muscle. Physiol. Rev., 6:358, 1926.
30. FENN, W. O. A quantitative comparison between the energy liberated and the work performed by the isolated sartorius muscle of the frog. J. Physiol. (Lond.), 58:175, 1923.
31. FENN, W. O. The relation between the work performed and the energy liberated in muscular contraction. J. Physiol. (Lond.), 58:373, 1924.
32. FENN, W. O., and B. S. MARSH. Muscular force at different speeds of shortening. J. Physiol. (Lond.), 85:277, 1935.
33. FICK, A. Mechanische Arbeit und Wärmeentwicklung bei der Muskelthätigkeit. Leipzig, Brockhaus, 1882.
34. FISKE, C. H., and Y. SUBBAROW. Phosphocreatine. J. biol. Chem., 81:629, 1929.
35. FLECKENSTEIN, A., J. JANKE, G. LECHNER, and G. BAUER. Zerfällt Adenosintriphosphat bei der Muskelkontraktion? Pflügers Arch. ges. Physiol., 259:246, 1954.
36. FLECKENSTEIN, A., J. JANKE, R. E. DAVIES, and H. A. KREBS. Contraction of muscle without fission of adenosine triphosphate or creatine phosphate. Nature, 174:1081, 1954.
37. FRANK, O. Zur Dynamik des Herzmuskels. Z. Biol., 32:370, 1895.
38. FRANK, O. Die Grundform des arteriellen Pulses. Erste Abhandlung. Mathematische Analyse. Z. Biol., 37:483, 1899.
39. GASSER, H. S., and A. V. HILL. The dynamics of muscular contraction. Proc. roy. Soc. B, 96:398, 1924.
40. GREEN, D. E. Fatty acid oxidation in soluble systems of animal tissues. Biol. Rev., 29:330, 1954.

41. HAJDU, S., and A. SZENT-GYÖRGYI. Action of DOC and serum on the frog heart. Amer. J. Physiol., 168:159, 1952.
42. HALL, C. E., M. A. JAKUS, and F. O. SCHMITT. An investigation of cross striations and myosin filaments in muscle. Biol. Bull., 90:32, 1946.
43. HANSON, J., and H. E. HUXLEY. The structural basis of contraction in striated muscle. Symp. Soc. exp. Biol., 9:228, 1955.
44. HARDEN, A. Alcoholic Fermentation. 4th ed. New York, Longmans, Green, 1932.
45. HARRIS, E. J. Transport and Accumulation in Biological Systems. London, Butterworths, 1956.
46. HAUK, R., and D. H. BROWN. Preparation and properties of uridinediphosphoglucose-glycogen transferase from rabbit muscle. Biochim. biophys. Acta, 33:556, 1959.
47. HENDERSON, Y., M. McR. SCARBROUGH, and F. P. CHILLINGWORTH. The volume curve of the ventricles of the mammalian heart, and the significance of this curve in respect to the mechanics of the heart-beat and the filling of the ventricles. Amer. J. Physiol., 16:325, 1906.
48. HILL, A. V. Muscular Activity. Baltimore, Williams & Wilkins, 1926.
49. HILL, A. V. Adventures in Biophysics. Philadelphia, Univ. Pennsylvania Press, 1931.
50. HILL, A. V. The heat of shortening and the dynamic constants of muscle. Proc. roy. Soc. B, 126:136, 1938.
51. HILL, A. V. The mechanical efficiency of frog's muscle. Proc. roy. Soc. B, 127:434, 1939.
52. HILL, A. V. The abrupt transition from rest to activity in muscle. Proc. roy. Soc. B, 136:399, 1949.
53. HILL, A. V. The "instantaneous" elasticity of active muscle. Proc. roy. Soc. B, 141:161, 1953.
54. HILL, A. V. The design of muscles. Brit. med. Bull., 12:165, 1957.
55. HILL, A. V., and L. MACPHERSON. The effect of nitrate, iodide and bromide on the duration of the active state in skeletal muscle. Proc. roy. Soc. B, 143:81, 1954.
56. HODGKIN, A. L., and P. HOROWICZ. The differential action of hypertonic solutions on the twitch and action potential of a muscle fibre. J. Physiol. (Lond.), 136:17P, 1957.
57. HOWELL, W. H., and F. DONALDSON, JR. Experiments upon the heart of the dog with reference to the maximum volume of blood sent out by the left ventricle in a single beat, and the influence of variations in venous pressure, arterial pressure, and pulse-rate upon the work done by the heart. Philos. Trans. Pt. I:139, 1884.

58. HUXLEY, H. E. The double array of filaments in cross-striated muscle. J. biophys. biochem. Cytol., 3:631, 1957.
59. HUXLEY, H. E. The contraction of muscle. Sci. Amer., 199 (Nov.): 66, 1958.
60. KALCKAR, H. Phosphorylation in kidney tissue. Enzymologia, 2:47, 1937.
61. KALCKAR, H. The nature of phosphoric esters formed in kidney extracts. Biochem. J., 33:631, 1939.
62. KATCHALSKY, A. Solutions of polyelectrolytes and mechanochemical systems. J. Polymer Sci., 7:793, 1951.
63. KATCHALSKY, A. Polyelectrolyte gels. Prog. Biophys. 4:1, 1954.
64. KEILIN, D. On cytochrome, a respiratory pigment, common to animals, yeast, and higher plants. Proc. roy. Soc. B, 98:312, 1925.
65. KERR, S. E. Studies on the inorganic composition of blood. III. The influence of serum on the permeability of erythrocytes to potassium and sodium. J. biol. Chem., 85:47, 1929.
66. KLAAUW, C. A. VAN DER., ed. Forma et Functio. Folia Biotheoretica I. 1936.
67. KLUYVER, A. J. The Chemical Activities of Micro-organisms. London, University of London Press, 1931.
68. KLUYVER, A. J., and H. J. L. DONKER. Die Einheit in der Biochemie. Chem. Zelle Gewebe, 13:134, 1926.
69. KLUYVER, A. J., and C. B. van NIEL. The Microbe's Contribution to Biology. Cambridge, Harvard University Press, 1956.
70. KREBS, H. A. The tricarboxylic acid cycle. In D. M. Greenberg, Chemical Pathways of Metabolism, 1:109. New York, Academic Press, 1954.
71. KUHN, W., and B. HARGITAY. Muskelähnliche Kontraktion und Dehnung von Netzwerken polyvalenter Fadenmolekülionen. Experientia, 7:1, 1951.
72. LARDY, H. A., and H. WELLMAN. Oxidative phosphorylations: role of inorganic phosphate and acceptor systems in control of metabolic rates. J. biol. Chem., 195:215, 1952.
73. LATIES, G. G. Respiration and cellular work and the regulation of the respiration rate in plants. Survey biol. Prog. 3:215, 1957.
74. LAVOISIER, A. L., and P. S. DE LAPLACE. Mémoire sur la chaleur. Mém. Acad. Sci. (Paris), p. 355, 1780.
75. LEHNINGER, A. L. Oxidative phosphorylation. Harvey Lect., 49:176, 1953–54.
76. LEVIN, A., and J. WYMAN. The viscous elastic properties of muscle. Proc. roy. Soc. B, 101:218, 1927.
77. LEWIS, G. N., and M. RANDALL. Thermodynamics and the Free Energy of Chemical Substances. New York, McGraw-Hill, 1923.

78. LIPMANN, F. Metabolic generation and utilization of phosphate bond energy. Advanc. Enzymol., 1:99, 1941.
79. LUNDIN, G. Mechanical properties of cardiac muscle. Acta physiol. scand., Suppl. 20, 1944.
80. MARSH, B. B. The effects of adenosinetriphosphate on the fibre volume of a muscle homogenate. Biochem. biophys. Acta, 9:247, 1952.
81. MARTIUS, C., and F. KNOOP. Der physiologische Abbau der Citronensäure. Vorläufige Mitteilung. Hoppe-Seyl. Z. physiol. Chem., 246:I, 1937.
82. MEYER, K. H., and C. FERRI. Sur l'élasticité du caoutchouc. Helv. chim. Acta, 18:570, 1935.
83. MEYER, K. H., and H. MARK. Der Aufbau der Hochpolymeren organischen Naturstoffe auf Grund molekular-morphologischen Betrachtungen. Leipzig, Akademische Verlagsgesellschaft, 1930.
84. MEYER, K. H., and E. R. PICKEN. The thermoelastic properties of muscle and their molecular interpretation. Proc. roy. Soc. B, 124:29, 1937.
85. MEYER, K. H., G. VON SUSICH, and E. VALKÓ. Die elastischen Eigenschaften der organischen Hochpolymeren und ihre kinetische Deutung. Kolloid Z., 59:208, 1932.
86. MEYERHOF, O. Die Energieumwandlungen im Muskel. V. Mitteilung. Milchsäurebildung und mechanische Arbeit. Pflügers Arch. ges. Physiol., 191:128, 1921.
87. MEYERHOF, O. Die chemischen Vorgänge im Muskel und ihr Zusammenhang mit Arbeitsleistung und Wärmebildung. Berlin, Springer, 1930.
88. MEYERHOF, O. Über die Intermediarvorgänge der enzymatischen Kohlehydratspaltung. Ergebn. Physiol., 39:10, 1937.
89. MOMMAERTS, W. F. H. M. Muscular Contraction, A Topic in Molecular Physiology. New York, Interscience, 1950.
90. MOMMAERTS, W. F. H. M. The molecular transformation of actin. I. Globular actin. J. biol. Chem., 198:445, 1952.
91. MOMMAERTS, W. F. H. M. The molecular transformation of actin. II. The polymerization process. J. biol. Chem., 198:459, 1952.
92. MOMMAERTS, W. F. H. M. The molecular transformation of actin. III. The participation of nucleotides. J. biol. Chem., 198:469, 1952.
93. MOMMAERTS, W. F. H. M. Is adenosine triphosphate broken down during a single muscle twitch. Nature, 174:1083, 1954.
94. MOMMAERTS, W. F. H. M. Investigation of the presumed breakdown of adenosine-triphosphate and phosphocreatine during a single muscle twitch. Amer. J. Physiol., 182:585, 1955.

95. Mommaerts, W. F. H. M. Flow birefringence. In S. P. Colowick and N. O. Kaplan. Methods in Enzymology, 4:166, New York, Academic Press, 1957.
96. Mommaerts, W. F. H. M. Metabolism of the heart. In Cardiology, an Encyclopedia of the Cardiovascular System, vol. 1, 2-19. New York, Blakiston Division, McGraw-Hill, 1959.
97. Mommaerts, W. F. H. M., and G. L. Langer. Fundamental concepts of cardiac dynamics and energetics. Ann. Rev. Med., 14:261, 1963.
98. Mommaerts, W. F. H. M., and M. O. Schilling. Interruption of muscular contraction by rapid cooling. Amer. J. Physiol., 182:579, 1955.
99. Mommaerts, W. F. H. M., and R. Summit. Unpublished observations, 1957.
100. Mommaerts, W. F. H. M., W. J. Whalen, and B. C. Abbott. (In preparation 1959).
101. Muralt, A. L. von, and J. T. Edsall. Studies in the physical chemistry of muscle globulin. III. The anisotropy of myosin and the angle of isocline. J. biol. Chem., 89:315, 1930.
102. Muralt, A. L. von, and J. T. Edsall. Studies in the physical chemistry of muscle globulin. IV. The anisotropy of myosin and double refraction of flow. J. biol. Chem., 89:351, 1930.
103. Nachmansohn, D., and M. Berman. Studies on choline acetylase. III. On the preparation of the coenzyme and its effect on the enzyme. J. biol. Chem., 165:551, 1946.
104. Nägeli, K. W. Micellartheorie. Ostwald's Klassiker der exakten Wissenschaften No. 227. Leipzig, Akademische Verlagsgesellschaft, 1928.
105. Niedergerke, R. The "staircase" phenomenon in the frog's ventricle and the action of calcium. J. Physiol. (Lond.), 128:55P, 1955.
106. Noll, D., and H. H. Weber. Polarisationsoptik und molekularer Feinbau der Q-Abschnitte des Froschmuskels. Pflügers Arch. gen. Physiol., 235:234, 1934.
107. Ochoa, S. Efficiency of aerobic phosphorylation in cell-free heart extracts. J. biol. Chem., 151:493, 1943.
108. Ostwald, W. Die Welt der vernachlässigten Dimensionen. Dresden, Steinkopf, 1915.
109. Parnas, J. K. Der Mechanismus der Glykogenolyse im Muskel. Ergebn. Enzymforsch., 6:57, 1937.
110. Patterson, S. W., H. Piper, and E. H. Starling. The regulation of the heart beat. J. Physiol. (Lond.), 48:465, 1914.
111. Porter, A. W. The Method of Dimensions. London, Methuen, 1933.

112. PRYOR, M. G. M. The rheology of muscle. In A. Frey-Wyssling, Ed., Deformation and Flow in Biological Systems. New York, Interscience, 1952.
113. RABINOWITZ, M., M. P. STULBERG, and P. D. BOYER. The control of pyruvate oxidation in a cell-free rat heart preparation by phosphate acceptors. Science, 114:641, 1951.
114. RAMSEY, R. W., and S. F. STREET. The isometric length-tension diagram of isolated skeletal muscle fibers of the frog. J. cell. comp. Physiol., 15:11, 1940.
115. RANVIER, L. A. Leçons d'anatomie générale faites au Collège de France. Année 1877–78. Paris, Baillière, 1880.
116. RITCHIE, A. D. Theories of muscular contraction. J. Physiol. (Lond.), 78:322, 1933.
117. RITCHIE, J. M. The effect of nitrate on the active state of muscle. J. Physiol. (Lond.), 126:155, 1954.
118. ROBBINS, P. W., R. R. TRAUT, and F. LIPMANN. Glycogen synthesis from glucose, glucose-6-phosphate, and uridine diphosphate glucose in muscle preparations. Proc. nat. Acad. Sci. (Wash.), 45:6, 1959.
119. ROSZA, G., A. SZENT-GYÖRGYI, and R. W. G. WYCKOFF. The electron microscopy of F-actin. Biochim. biophys. Acta, 3:561, 1949.
120. RUNNSTRÖM, J., A. LENNERSTRAND, and H. BOREI. Oxydation und Phosphatbindung im Hämolysat der Pferdeblutkörperchen. Biochem. Z., 271:15, 1934.
121. SCHMIDT, W. J. Die Doppelbrechung von Karyoplasma, Zytoplasma und Metaplasma. Berlin, Borntraeger, 1937.
122. SCHROEDER, H. Die Hypothesen über die chemischen Vorgänge bei der Kohlensäure-Assimilation. Jena, Fischer, 1917.
123. SIEKEVITZ, P., and V. R. POTTER. Intramitochondrial regulation of oxidative rate. J. biol. Chem., 201:1, 1953.
124. SJÖSTRAND, F. S., and E. ANDERSSON. The ultrastructure of skeletal muscle myofilaments. In First European Regional Conference on Electron Microscopy, Stockholm, 1957. Proceedings. p. 204. New York, Academic Press, 1957.
125. SLATER, E. C. The constitution of the respiratory chain in animal tissues. Advanc. Enzymol., 20:147, 1958.
126. STARLING, E. H. The Linacre Lecture on the Law of the Heart. London, Longmans, Green, 1918.
127. STARLING, E. H., and M. B. VISSCHER. The regulation of the energy output of the heart. J. Physiol. (Lond.), 62:243, 1927.
128. STAUDINGER, H. Organische Kolloidchemie, 3. Aufl. Braunschweig, Vieweg, 1950.
129. STRAUB, F. B. Actin. Stud. Inst. med. Chem. Szeged, 2:3, 1942.

130. STRAUB, F. B. Actin II. Stud. Inst. med. Chem. Szeged, 3:23, 1943.
131. SVEDBERG, T., and K. O. PEDERSEN. The Ultracentrifuge. Oxford, Clarendon Press, 1940.
132. SZENT-GYÖRGYI, A. Studies on Biological Oxidation and Some of its Catalysts. Leipzig, Barth, 1937.
133. SZENT-GYÖRGYI, A. Chemistry of Muscular Contraction, 1st ed. New York, Academic Press, 1947.
134. SZENT-GYÖRGYI, A. Nature of Life, a Study on Muscle. New York, Academic Press, 1948.
135. SZENT-GYÖRGYI, A. Free-energy relations and contraction of actomyosin. Biol. Bull., 96:140, 1949.
136. SZENT-GYÖRGYI, A. Chemistry of Muscular Contraction, 2nd ed. New York, Academic Press, 1951.
137. SZENT-GYÖRGYI, A. Chemical Physiology of Contraction in Body and Heart Muscle. New York, Academic Press, 1953.
138. TAMIYA, H. Le bilan matériel et l'énergetique des synthese biologiques. Paris, Hermann, 1935.
139. THOMPSON, D'A. W. On Growth and Form. Cambridge, The University Press, 1942.
140. UTTER, M. F., and K. KURAHASHI. Mechanism of action of oxalacetic carboxylase. J. biol. Chem., 207:821, 1954.
141. WARBURG, O. Ed. Ueber die katalytischen Wirkungen der lebendigen Substanz. Berlin, Springer, 1928.
142. WARBURG, O., Ed. Wasserstoffübertragende Fermente. Berlin, W. Saenger, 1948.
143. WEBER, E. Muskelbewegung. In R. Wagner. Handwörterbuch der Physiologie III/2. Braunschweig, Wieweg, 1846.
144. WEBER, H. H. Der Feinbau und die mechanische Eigenschaften des Myosinfadens. Pflügers Arch. ges. Physiol., 235:205, 1934.
145. WEBER, H. H., and H. PORTZEHL. Kontraktion, ATP-Cyclus und fibrilläre Proteine des Muskels. Ergebn. Physiol., 47:369, 1952.
146. WEIDMANN, S. Elektrophysiologie der Herzmuskelfaser. Bern, H. Huber, 1956.
147. WHALEN, W. J. Apparent exception to the "all or none" law in cardiac muscle. Science, 127:468, 1958.
148. WIEGAND, W. B. Tendencies in rubber compounding. Trans. Inst. Rubber Ind., 1:141, 1925.
149. WIEGAND, W. B., and J. W. SCHNEIDER. The rubber pendulum, the Joule effect, and the dynamic stress-strain curve. Trans. Inst. Rubber Ind., 10:234, 1934.
150. WIELAND, H. On the Mechanism of Oxidation. New Haven, Yale University Press, 1932.

151. WIGGERS, C. J. Determinants of cardiac performance. In his Circulatory Dynamics, Physiologic Studies. New York, Grune & Stratton, 1952.
152. WILKIE, D. R. Facts and theories about muscle. Progr. Biophys., 4:288, 1954.
153. WILKIE, D. R. The mechanical properties of muscle. Brit. med. Bull., 12:177, 1956.
154. WILKIE, D. R. Measurement of the series elastic component at various times during a single muscle twitch. J. Physiol. (Lond.), 134:527, 1956.
155. WÖHLISCH, E. Untersuchungen über elastische thermodynamische, magnetische und elektrische Eigenschaften tierischer Gewebe. Verh. phys.-med. Ges. Würzburg, N.F. 51:53, 1928.
156. WÖHLISCH, E. Die kautschukartige Elastizität, ihr Wesen und ihre biologische Bedeutung. J. prak. Chem., N.F. 180:217, 1942.
157. WÖHLISCH, E., and H. G. CLAMANN. Quantitative Untersuchungen zum Problem der thermoelastischen Eigenschaften des Skelettmuskels. VIII. Mitteilung. Über tierische Gewebe mit Faserstruktur. Z. Biol., 91:399, 1931.
158. WÖHLISCH, E., and F. RENK. Die thermoelastischen Eigenschaften der Herzmuskulatur. Pflügers Arch. ges. Physiol., 240:753, 1938.
159. WOODS, R. H. A few applications of a physical theorem to membranes in the human body in a state of tension. J. Anat., 26:362, 1892.
160. WOODWORTH, R. S. Maximal contraction, "staircase" contraction, refractory period, and compensatory pause, of the heart. Amer. J. Physiol., 8:213, 1902.

IV

Coronary Circulation and Cardiac Metabolism

ANGINA pectoris was described clinically as long ago as the first century A.D., when Lucius Annaeus Seneca (*86*), the Roman stoic philosopher, faithfully recorded the symptoms of his own disease; but an understanding of the physiology of the coronary circulation, or even an appreciation of its clinical importance, was not achieved for another seventeen hundred years.

CORONARY CIRCULATION

Similarly, until modern concepts of bodily heat and energy exchange were established, at the end of the eighteenth and beginning of the nineteenth centuries, there could be no knowledge of the metabolism of the heart.

But the ancients were greatly concerned about such matters as the heating and cooling of the body, and the source of body heat. In some systems, such as the Egyptian, the Aristotelian, and the Galenical, the heart was considered to be a chief agent in this process, as this organ was also believed to be the center of life and understanding, the "seat of the soul."

In the present chapter, I shall begin with a brief account of the earliest known descriptions of the heart, in Egyptian writings, then turn to Greek and Roman ideas on "innate heat"—the ancient counterpart of our modern concepts of metabolism; and then on to the medievalists and the Renaissance.

Egypt: The Beginnings

Probably the earliest record of knowledge of the heart that we now possess is contained in the Edwin Smith Surgical Papyrus (*39*). This remarkable document is a seventeenth-century B.C. editing of a much

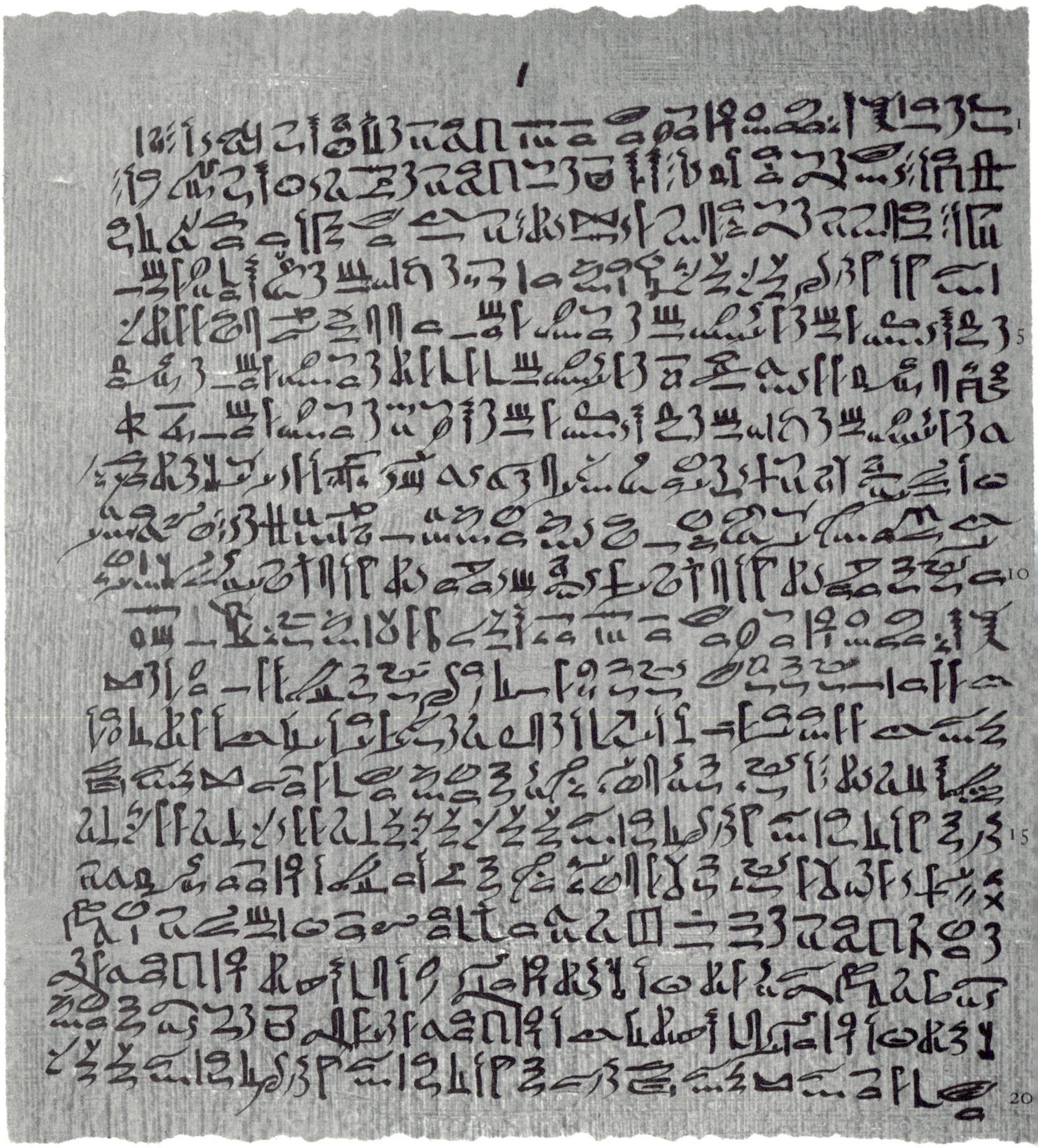

Figure 1. A page from the Ebers papyrus.

earlier (2500–3000 B.C.) writing. In discussing a case of head injury the surgeon related the peripheral pulse to the activity of the heart, commenting that the observation of the pulse was undertaken "in order to know the action of the heart." This is historically a rather notable statement when we consider that the significance of the pulse was apparently not known to Hippocrates, twenty centuries later, either as an index of heart action or as an index of disease states generally. The significance of the pulse was rediscovered by a subsequent generation in the school of Cos.

The heart and the great vessels leading from it were described in several of the ancient papyri (although the coronary vessels were not), and the primary importance of the heart was recognized. In the Ebers Papyrus (70), just as in the later Aristotelian system, the heart was considered to be the seat of consciousness, as well as character. In the well-known picture in the Book of the Dead, the heart is placed in one pan of a balance, and the emblem of truth in the other.

The complex regulations for embalming prescribed that the heart be left *in situ*, and never removed with the other organs. As stated in some of the Egyptian religious texts, the welfare of the dead man was safeguarded, "if his own true heart is with him."

The studies of mummified Egyptian hearts, the presence of coronary artery calcification, atheroma, and other changes, as developed by Sir Marc Ruffer (82) at the turn of the century, is of great interest but not within the scope of this discussion.

In practical medicine, the Egyptian writings were frequently confused, since the physicians were also the priests, and the clinical art was inextricably mixed with magic, legend, hierarchical tradition, and all the sacrificial and occult practices of the time. A clinical cure by the Egyptian priesthood had to be a divinely contrived miracle. Also, there could be no error: the priest always had to be right. In the Westcar Papyrus, now in the Berlin Museum, there is a series of popular stories of the wonders worked by magician-priests for the entertainment of the pharoahs of the pyramid age. As Dawson (24) pointed out, it is characteristic of the magician in all times that he should have more than one string to his bow. Thus in the medical papyri we find numerous alternative prescriptions, and in the texts on magic, alternative spells are provided for every sort of sickness or calamity. In such documents it is impossible to sift fact from fraudulence, religious dogma, or pure fiction.

The Heart and "Innate Heat": Aristotle and Galen

The development of knowledge of the heart and circulation from the Greeks to Galen has been reviewed in the first chapter. It is sufficient to note here that neither Greeks nor Romans were aware of the significance of the coronary circulation.

The Greek concept of metabolism in general was well expressed by Aristotle (*21, 2*). "Animation and the possession of vitality are necessarily associated with heat. . . . In whatever region of the body and in whatever organ the principle of heat is primarily located, there also must be the original vital principle of nutrition." Aristotle wrote of the "fire of nature" and suggested that "nature kindles the nutritive function in this fire." He said, "in the heart there is a continual accession of liquids from the nourishment; and their expansion by heat extending to the walls of the organ causes its pulsations. There is an incessant ingress of fluids to supply the substance of the blood elaborated in the interior of the heart." The dominant idea in Aristotle's physiology of metabolism was the innate vitality operating through the agency of animal heat. Respiration furnished the cooling influence to dampen this vital heat. "The animal organism in all cases requires a cooling influence on account of the kindling of the principle of fire within the heart" (*21, 2*). In animals with both heart and lungs, this was supplied by the act of inspiration.

In the Aristotelian system, heat was thus a driving force and the heart was a kindling place of this animal heat. Of the two processes of metabolism, i.e. digestion and the actual utilization of foods by means of oxidation, the Greek school was familiar only with the first. The Hippocratic essay on nutriment (*104*) says "power of nutriment reaches to all parts of the body, to bone, to sinews, to veins, to arteries, to muscle, to membranes, etc." and "it reaches also to heat, breath, and moisture."

Whether the great advances of the Alexandrian school under Herophylos and Erasistratos extended beyond anatomy and physiology to metabolism remains a question. Erasistratos (*91*) is said to have experimented with a "respiration calorimeter": this consisted of a jar in which a fowl was confined, and measurements were made of the weight of the animal and its food, and of its excreta, before and after digestion. There is apparently no record of "respiration" or heat exchange. Nonetheless, it seems clear enough that Erasistratos was thinking about metabolic processes, and was thus more than a thousand years ahead of his time. Probably because of their keen perception and their reluctance to speculate on the basis of isolated observations, the members of the Alexandrian school were little concerned with Aristotle's ideas on the nature of vital spirits. It was not until Galen that these speculations were revived and dogmatized. For him, the heart became again the center of organic life, the immediate residence of the animating principle, "the source and as it were, the fireplace of the innate heat by which the living organism is directed and controlled" (*104*).

A reappraisal of Galen's actual doctrine has been presented in Chapter I, and his contributions are reviewed again in Chapter VII.

Medieval Medicine: Galenical Stagnation

Medieval medicine was not altogether without value, and should receive some credit for sustaining ancient doctrines, even if it did not progress beyond them. It is true that medical authoritarianism, just as much as ecclesiastical authoritarianism, stifled new thought; more will be said on this presently. But medicine was still a substantial and respected profession throughout the Middle Ages, and the training of the good physician was by no means casual.

In the school of Salerno in southern Italy (*51, 68*), which was the center of medical teaching for nearly three hundred years (A.D. 900–1200), candidates were required to be at least twenty-one years of age, to have studied "logic" for three years, and medicine and surgery for five years, before being admitted to an examination; and to have studied anatomy for another year before practicing surgery. Dissection was carried out, in the true Galenical tradition, on the pig. Arabic medicine, and probably much of Greek and Roman medicine, were brought to Salerno by Constantine of Africa about A.D. 1050. Textbooks at the school included certain of the writings of Aristotle, Hippocrates, Galen, and Avicenna.

Salerno was a center for practical therapy as well as theory, and patients went there from all parts of Europe. The school declined after 1200, and Paris and Bologna then became the leading medical centers. There was probably a store of practical medical and surgical knowledge in these schools, and a resourceful physician could do much for his patients: prescribing opiates, purgatives, mercurials, encouraging the simple rules of health as set forth in the Regimen Sanitatis Salernitanum; wounds washed with strong urine, or wine and honey, with the skillful and, one hopes, sparing use of the knife and the cautery, and even at times an effective letting of blood.

But this is undoubtedly too favorable a picture. Even practical medicine was riddled with quackery, magic, "astrology," and humbug, and medicine as a science could not even begin. There was no experimentation, and it was heresy even to question the hallowed writings of the ancients.

The successful physician of the fourteenth century was well described by Geoffrey Chaucer (17):

> "*With us ther was a Doctour of Phisyk,*
> *In al this world ne was ther noon him lyk*
> *To speke of phisik and of surgerye;*
> *For he was grounded in astronomye.*
> *He kepte his pacient a ful greet del*
> *In houres, by his magik naturel. . . .*
> *He knew the cause of everich maladye,*
> *Were it of hoot or cold, or moiste, or drye,*
> *And where engendred, and of what humour;*
> *He was a verrey parfit practisour.*"

—with more, of a less flattering character, on his profitable deals with his apothecaries, his fine clothes, and his liking for gold, and the sly notation that "his study was but little on the Bible."

A typical example of a medieval professor was Mondino de' Luzzi (*87*), who held the chair of medicine at the University of Padua in 1315 and was the author of the first comprehensive anatomy text. He was one of the first after Galen to write on the heart. In his chapter dealing with this organ he explains its crucial form by the fact that it is the source of animal heat and "because a pyramidal form is the specific figure belonging to the principle of heat." The main function of the auricles is that of relieving the ventricles by dilatation "when an unusual quantity of blood is produced in the body of spirits in the left ventricle." He explains the greater thickness of the walls of the left ventricle by stating the blood in the right side of the heart is heavier than the spirits in the left, the "parietes" (walls) of the organ on the left side are thicker, to counterbalance the weight of the blood on the right. The work of Mondino affords a good criterion of the scientific status of Europe during the late Middle Ages and the early Renaissance. The teachings of Galen were accepted without reservation, and although anatomy was studied, the spirit of the time forbade any interpretation of findings that may have been in disagreement.

Berengario da Carpi (4), professor of Bologna, who lived two centuries after Mondino, interpreted the pyramidal form of the heart by stating that the point of the organ is small because this part, lying in contact with the walls of the chest, is more likely to be injured during its movements and "consequently the smaller it is, the less injury will be received." He mentions the report that men have sometimes been born with the heart covered with hair, on which account they were braver than other people. The entrance and exit of blood and spirits by the different orifices, the filtration of blood through the septum into the left ventricle, the passage of air for the generation of vital spirits through the arteria venalis (pulmonary vein) to the heart, and the discharge of fuliginous vapors into the lung by the same channel were all given in the Galenical tradition, without modification.

Andreas Vesalius, Discoverer and Crusader

It is hard to believe that Vesalius could have published *De humanis corporis fabrica* less than thirty years after the writing of Berengario's work. But no less astonishing was the reactionary state of all medicine in his day. Consider the time: this was the high tide of the Renaissance, and the whole of Christendom was in ferment—political, intellectual, religious—and expanding boundlessly in space and in thought. This was the age of Erasmus and Luther, of Henry the Eighth, Francis the First, and Charles the Fifth, of Agricola and Copernicus, of François Rabelais and Benvenuto Cellini, of Holbein, Leonardo da Vinci, Michelangelo, and Titian. Christopher Columbus and Vasco da Gama had died only a few years before. In the year 1536, when Vesalius left Paris, Jacques Cartier, voyaging along the shores of Canada, named the great river of the north, and claimed a continent for the King of France; and in that

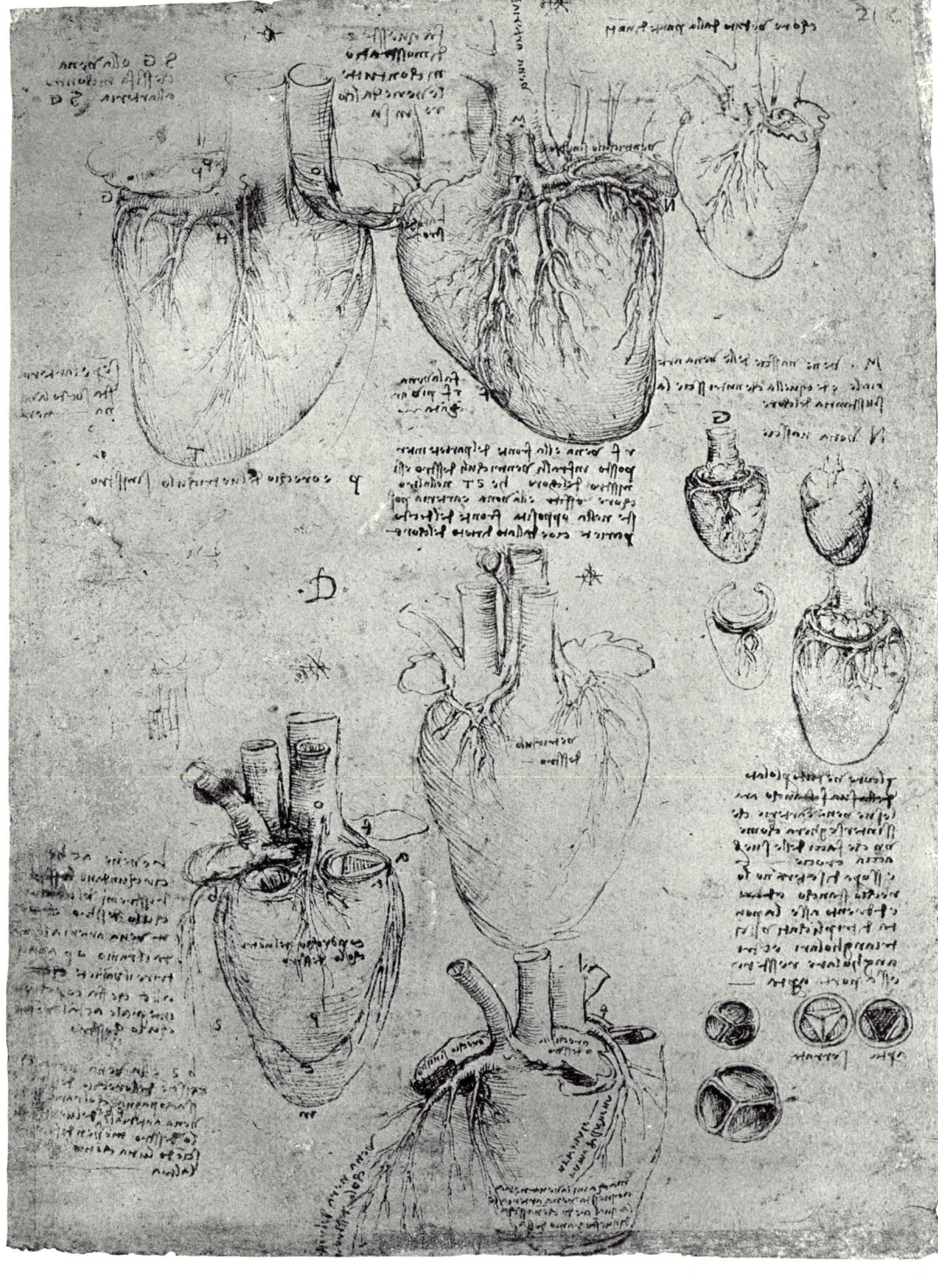

same extraordinary year, under the banner of a still mightier sovereign, Cortez with his handful of conquistadores completed his incredible conquest of Mexico, and Pizarro fought and destroyed the army of the Incas in Peru.

All the world was reaching into the unknown, discovering new lands and new ideas, but in the midst of it medicine slumbered on, in ignorance, complacency, and superstition, a thousand years behind the times. Jacobus Sylvius in Paris and Matthaeus Curtius in Bologna were still lecturing by the book, still confined within the incomplete and imperfect texts of Galen, Aristotle, Hippocrates, and Avicenna. Even the arrival of new and authentic Greek manuscripts from the East served only to intensify the backward search into antiquity.

To move or even stir this extraordinary inertia, there was needed a man with mind and character at once clear-sighted, objective, forceful, and contentious, someone who could find the truth by careful observation and experiment, who would challenge authority without equivocation, who would bring medicine into contact with the vibrant, imaginative, tumultuous, artistic, intellectual forces of the day, and who would attract and inspire young students to continue the work with the same zeal and in the same spirit. This was the immense achievement of Andreas Vesalius, all accomplished within a span of seven years.

To evaluate this achievement, one must know something of the life of this extraordinary man (*83*). Born in Brussels in 1514 of a well-to-do family with a long medical tradition, Vesalius studied first at the University of Louvain, and transferred to Paris in 1533. There he came under the influence of a number of the most distinguished physicians of his day, including Johann Guinther of Andernach, the philosopher-physician Jean Fernel, and Jacobus Sylvius. The last was so ardent and unswerving a Galenist that he held that any structure found in contemporary man that differed from Galen's description must be due to a degeneration in the human species since Galen's golden day. Instructed in and at first subscribing to Galenical doctrine, Vesalius also had the intense desire to examine and dissect the human body with his own hands. He frequented the gibbets, cemeteries, and charnel houses, made

Figure 2. Drawing of the heart and coronary vessels by Leonardo da Vinci (1452–1519).

THE HEART

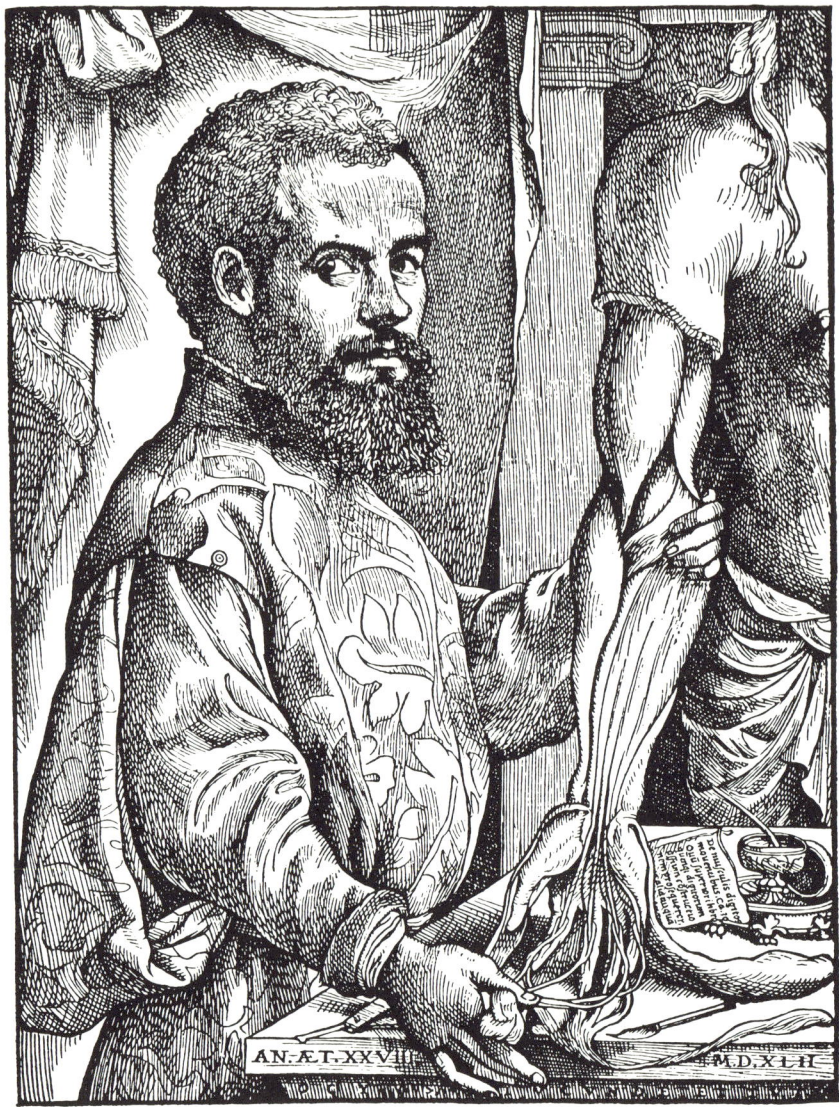

Figure 3. Andreas Vesalius (1514–64). A portrait by Jan Stefan Kalkar, Vesalius's friend and illustrator.

off with whatever bones or other parts he could lay his hands on, and studied them avidly. In 1536 he returned to Louvain, published a classical thesis on the Ninth Book of Rhazes, and, much more exciting, was appointed to conduct the first human dissection that had been permitted in that city for nearly a generation.

The next year he journeyed to Padua, continued his studies, visited the sick under the guidance of Montanus, and received his doctorate of medicine, "with highest distinction," on December 5, 1537. On the following day he was nominated by the Venetian Senate as Professor of Surgery. He was then twenty-three years old.

"With characteristic energy," wrote Saunders and O'Malley (*83*), "the young and ambitious Professor of Surgery began his academic duties ... with a success which exceeded all expectations. The sight of a Professor descending from his academic chair to dissect and demonstrate personally on the cadaver was something entirely novel. Students, physicians, and men of learning crowded his classes. Many came to dispute the statements of this brash young man only to be convinced by ocular demonstration."

In 1959 a remarkable book was published which illuminates the character of Vesalius and gives a vivid picture of his teaching. This is the exact translation (*45*), by Ruben Eriksson, of notes taken by a German student, Baldesar Heseler, an eyewitness of "Andreas Vesalius' First Public Anatomy at Bologna, 1540." The manuscript, written on parchment, was discovered recently, as part of a larger collection, in the Royal Library in Stockholm.

It seems that Vesalius came in 1540 as a visiting professor to Bologna and gave twenty-six demonstrations on human cadavers—practically all of them hanged criminals, of whom there appeared to be then an unlimited supply. The professor of "theoretical" anatomy at Bologna was Matthaeus Curtius, an arch-Galenist. Frequently Curtius had given his lecture before Vesalius began, and from time to time Curtius stayed on, and the sharp and even angry interchanges between the two are among the most entertaining passages in Heseler's notes. Heseler was a thorough German and he wrote down everything. Here are some examples.

"*[Vesalius is demonstrating the muscles of the abdomen.] Here Curtius remarked that this, however, was not Galen's opinion. No, Domine, he said, even if that is not Galen's opinion we shall however demonstrate here, that in fact it is so.*

THE HEART

"*[Vesalius is about to demonstrate the azygos vein in the thorax.] When the lecture of Curtius was finished, Vesalius, who had been present and heard the refutation of his arguments, asked Curtius to accompany him to the anatomy. For he wanted to show him that his theory was quite true. Therefore he brought Curtius to our two bodies. Now, he said, excellentissime Domine, here we have our bodies. We shall see whether I have made an error. Now we want to look at this and we should in the meantime leave Galen, for I acknowledge that I have said, if it is permissible to say so, that here Galen is in the wrong, because he did not know the position of the vein without pair [azygos] in the human body, which is the same today just as it was in his time. Curtius answered smiling, for Vesalius, choleric as he was, was very excited: No, he [Curtius] said, Domine, we must not leave Galen, because he always well understood everything, and, consequently, we also follow him. Do you know how to interpret Hippocrates better than Galen did? Vesalius answered, I do not say so, but I show you here in these bodies the vein without pair, how it nourishes all the lower ribs, except the two upper ones.*"

This quotation is perhaps overlong, but nothing could be more important than this proof at first hand that, for the first time in a thousand years, a man stood up and challenged medical authority on the basis of experimental fact, got furiously angry about it, and would not give ground. This was Vesalius's greatest service to medicine and to mankind. This evidence should dispel all comment such as Zilboorg's, in his so-called "psychological" study of Vesalius (*107*), that "he was no fighter," that his criticism of Galen was "cautious and almost hesitant," etc.

It was not that Vesalius despised Galen. Indeed, in his writings he repeatedly protested that he venerated the Prince of Physicians as much as anyone; but he considered him human and not infallible, and when he, Vesalius, proved Galen wrong, he said so.

It would carry this digression even further afield to review the successive publications of Vesalius, culminating in the great *Fabrica* of 1543; his relationship with Jan Stefan van Kalkar, who drew the earlier Tabellae Sex (Six Tables) from which Vesalius taught during his early years at Padua (*83*); the question of whether it was Kalkar himself who made the drawings for the *Fabrica*, or some other person or persons in the school of Titian, where Kalkar was studying; and the interesting question, brought forward by Singer (*88*) and by Edelstein (*25*), of the entire relationship of Vesalius with the great artists and schools of artists in the northern Italy of his day.

One can only emphasize again the vast achievement of the five years that culminated in the *Fabrica*; the time and energy spent in dissection, observation, and recording, and the equally colossal task of writing, organizing, illustrating, printing, and publishing.

CORONARY CIRCULATION

To return to the coronary circulation, one can say that while Vesalius did not greatly stress this part of human anatomy, he certainly did not

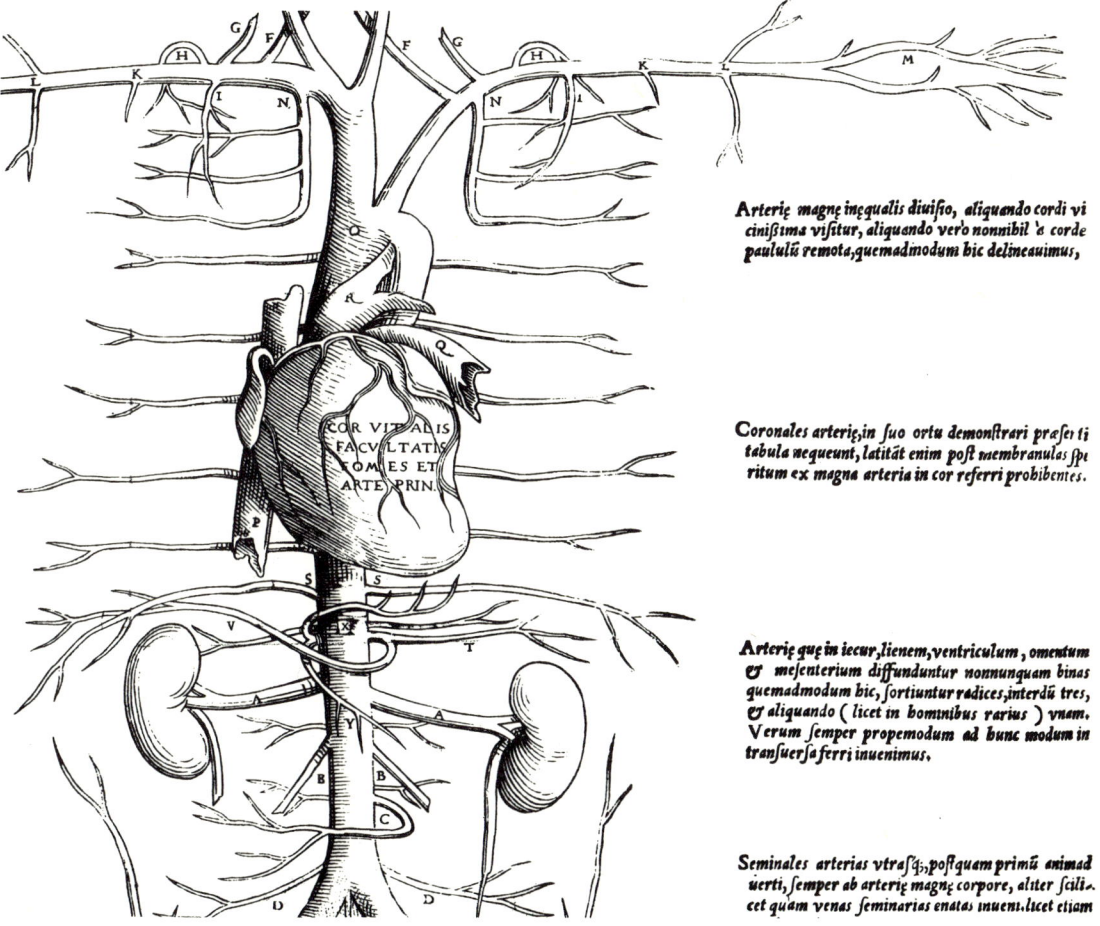

Figure 4. The coronary vessels, as drawn in the "Six Tables" of Vesalius and Kalkar, from which Vesalius taught during his early years as professor of anatomy in Padua. (*93*).

THE HEART

neglect it, and his descriptions are accurate. Here is a vivid passage from Heseler's account, as he watched Vesalius dissect a human heart (*45*):

"*I saw the wall in the middle which separates the two ventricles of the heart. I saw also the nerves leading from the brain to the heart, likewise the vein encircling the heart which runs from the liver in order to nourish the heart.*"

Since the Galenical theory still prevailed, that blood flowed from the liver to nourish all the organs, the coronary vein (from the liver via coronary sinus and vena cava) was obviously more important than the coronary arteries.

But these, also, are carefully described, perhaps most succinctly in the third of the Six Tables of 1538 (*93*), of Vesalius and Kalkar, in which the heart is shown with the coronary vessels coursing over its surface, and with the following note in the margin: "The coronary arteries at their origin cannot be demonstrated in the present table, because this origin is hidden behind the little membranes [valves] which prevent the [vital] spirits from flowing backward from the great artery [aorta] into the heart." The sixth book of the *Fabrica* (*92*) describes all this again, but with no further discovery of importance.

As many have noted, the classical point on which Vesalius differed with Galen—that he could not find, with a fine probe, the "perforations" in the interventricular septum—might well have led him to the conclusion that all the blood must flow from right ventricle to left through the lungs. But there was no time, in those few crowded years in Padua, for him, or for anyone, to have moved from a description of structure to a deliberate contemplation of function.

It is difficult to make a just appraisal of the action of Vesalius in leaving Padua and joining the service of Charles the Fifth so soon after the publication of the *Fabrica*. The sequence of events can be simply told (*83*). The manuscript and wood blocks of the *Fabrica*, and of the smaller *Epitome*, were taken from Venice to Basel in the summer of 1542, and Vesalius himself followed a few months later, to see to the proofreading and other tasks connected with the printing and publishing of the great work. The first copies were ready in August 1543, and it is recorded that Vesalius journeyed to Speyer and presented a special copy to the Emperor, Charles the Fifth. It is not improbable that even at this time Vesalius was negotiating to join the emperor's service as one of the imperial physicians. He was already known as one of the great surgeons, as well as anatomists, of his time, and he apparently prized the one distinction as much as the other.

The publication of the *Fabrica* created a great stir throughout Europe, as evidenced by the numerous copies that were made and published in various countries. Anatomy from this moment became Vesalian anatomy. But the reaction of the conservatives, the Galenists, was prompt, and they were savage in their opposition. His old teacher Jacobus Sylvius demanded Vesalius's recantation of his heresy (*83*).

On his return to Italy, Vesalius found his former student Realdus Columbus already lecturing in his place (*83*). Vesalius recorded in a subsequent letter that he burned his manuscripts as he prepared to leave Padua, but whether this was because of his disappointment over the reception of his great work, or simply as a part of a decision already made to give up his academic position, is not clear. It may be that the opposition of the Galenists during all his years in Padua had made his place there a difficult one. One strong friend, Duke Cosimo of Pisa, strove mightily to persuade Vesalius to accept the chair at that University, even writing an appeal to the emperor, but the answer was no, and in the summer of 1544 Vesalius joined the emperor's forces in the war that had by then broken out between France and Spain. It is interesting that at the first encounter, before the walls of Saint-Dizier, Vesalius was the surgeon for the Spanish side and Ambröise Paré for the French. Thenceforth Vesalius passed from scientific history, except for his revision of the *Fabrica* for a second edition, some ten years after the first.

There is no need to give more than a passing word to the melancholy end of the Vesalian saga: the fifteen years of devoted service to the Emperor Charles, up to the latter's voluntary abdication in 1556; the unhappy years with Philip II; the arousal of his old scientific ardor by a letter from his former student and now his successor in Padua, Gabriel Fallopius; his journey to Jerusalem, with a brief stop in Venice; and his untimely death on his return voyage across the Aegean, in 1564.

Fallopius was succeeded at Padua by Hieronymus Fabricius, who in turn was the teacher of William Harvey. This part of our history has been reviewed in the second chapter.

The Coronary Arteries: Harvey, de Vieussens, Morgagni

There is no doubt that Harvey realized the role of the coronary arteries in the nutrition of the heart, since he wrote (*40*), "besides, if the blood could permeate the substance of the septum, or could be imbibed from the ventricles, what use were there for the coronary artery and vein, branches of which proceed to the septum itself, to supply it with nourishments." We need not concern ourselves with the arguments concerning the priority of Caesalpinus versus Harvey, but we must stress that at the close of the sixteenth century the heart was still considered the seat of vitality, the source of animal heat, the laboratory of vital spirits and of arterial blood. The knowledge of metabolism—or to use a less confining term, nutrition—was equally primitive. For example, it was thought that nutrition was supplied by the venous blood, while the arterial blood supplied the tissues with vitality and heat. Thus we have the peculiar situation of two systems of blood vessels, both carrying blood from the periphery but not returning it to the heart. Harvey's findings dispelled these notions. While the source of animal heat was still incorrectly assigned, the orderly flow of blood for the nourishment of the tissues was established and the coronary circulation was recognized as nourishing the heart muscle, including the septum.

Harvey's scientific antagonist, Jean Riolan (*79*), carefully dissected the coronary vessels and confirmed the findings of Vesalius and Fallopius on their origin, but he did not associate them with the nutrition of the heart as Harvey had done. As we have seen in Chapter II, Riolan rejected the idea of the circulation of blood through the lungs, considered the liver still as the organ of blood formation, and believed in the passage of blood through the interventricular septum. He believed with Descartes that the heart admits and expels only one or two drops of blood at each pulsation. Obviously, with this concept of the circulation he could not have been aware of the true role of the coronary arteries which he so carefully dissected.

Thus, we see that at the end of the seventeenth century, the coronary circulation had been described and its function had been recognized. Vesalius may be considered as the end of one era and Harvey as the beginning of a new one.

Before embarking further on a discussion of the seventeenth and eighteenth centuries, we must examine the general trends which had led to a predominantly mechanical interpretation of nature (*84*). These trends are expressed in the Copernican and Cartesian theories, and culminate in those of Newton.

Copernicus (1473–1543), as a mathematician, made it his purpose to discover a more rational system of the courses of the heavenly bodies. He had complete confidence in the mathematical order of nature. Kepler (1571–1630) spent his life searching for the relations between the forces of the solar system. Exploiting the precise astronomical instruments of his master Tycho Brahe (1546–1601), he was able to create broad generalizations and to verify them by mathematical calculations. Galileo (1564–1642) was complimentary to Copernicus. He could "listen only with greatest repugnance when the quality of unchangeability is held up as something pre-eminent and complete in contrast to variability" (*84*). He set forth the outlines of the dynamics of motion, pointing thereby to the concept of a universal law in nature. Descartes (1596–1650) popularized the mathematical interpretation of nature. To him, and to his disciples all over Europe, space or extension became the fundamental reality. Newton (1642–1747) stands at the end of this distinguished line. He too subjected "the phenomenon of Nature to the laws of mathematics" (*66*). He operated on the principle that every event in nature is to be explained by reasoning from mathematical principles; experiments were necessary to check the interpretation of nature. And, to him, "Nature does nothing in vain, and more is in vain when less will serve; for Nature is pleased with simplicity and affects not the pomp of superfluous causes."

So far as the coronary circulation is concerned, after William Harvey there was a pause for a full century. Stephen Hales studied many things, but never inquired into the special function of the coronary vessels.

One of the first to study the effect of ligation of the coronary arteries was Pierre Chirac (*18*). He noted that ligation resulted in cardiac standstill. He and his greater contemporary, Raymond de Vieussens, were bitter enemies. The scientific ranks of the two men were strikingly different. Chirac, an arrogant and pompous man, was a powerful member of the faculty of Montpellier; Vieussens never even became a member of the faculty. But, according to Senac (*85*), "Chirac and de

THE HEART

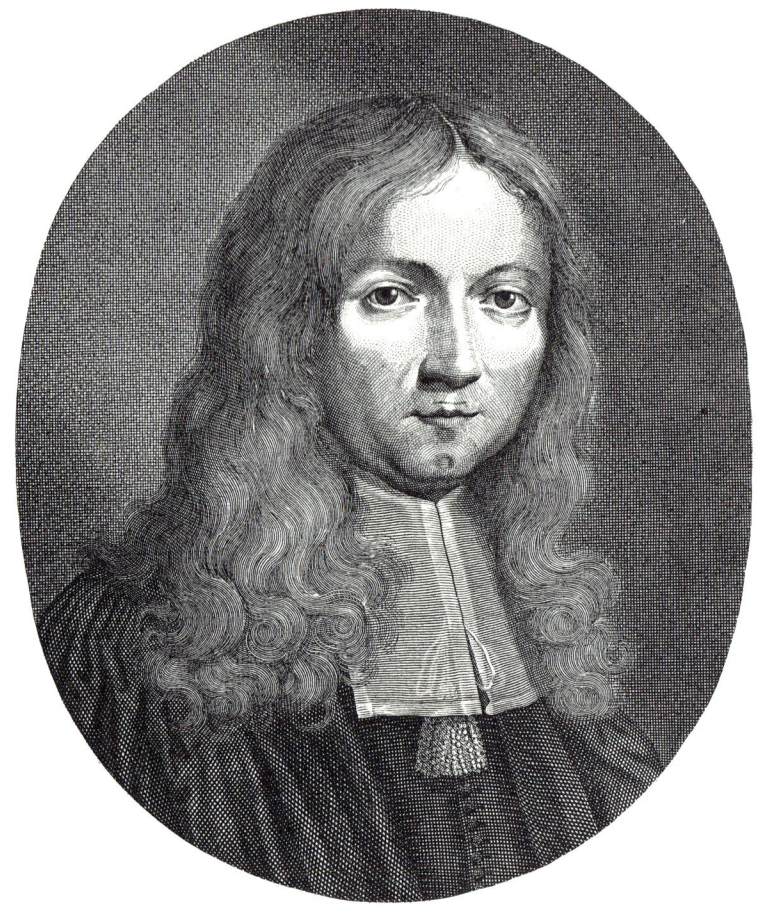

Figure 5. Raymond de Vieussens (1614–1715).

Vieussens have written after Lower on the structure and movements of the heart; here then are two treatises written on the same subject by two men who had always been animated by hatred of one another; their different standing in the public esteem no longer deceives us."

Of the many advances made by Vieussens (*48, 93*) in the knowledge of the anatomy of the heart, the one he himself esteemed most was his discovery of the so-called third circulation which takes place through the vessels which have since been mislabeled Thebesian. Vieussens was a superb clinical observer and a competent pathologist, but his interpretations were clouded by the Cartesian prejudices of his time. His discovery of the vessels which opened on the inner surface of the ventricles was fundamental to Descartes's view (1662) that a ferment in the heart continuously re-energizes it. But, as Lower stated subsequently (1669) (*60*), "those, moreover, who claimed the existence of such a ferment in the heart should have known the source from which it is continuously replenished. For, if they say that the coronary arteries distributed through the heart, pour a certain juice into its ventricle, they should notice that the inner membrane of the ventricle is so impervious that it allows nothing to penetrate into its cavity; as is clear when one forcibly injects the arteries with some dye."

More than two years after the work of Vieussens had appeared, Thebesius took up the same subject. But as Senac said (*85*) "he showed more self-assurance than good faith in his dissertation; if he mentions de Vieussens, it is as a writer who, following the steps of Broen, has been hunting for the source of imaginary ferment as deposited in the

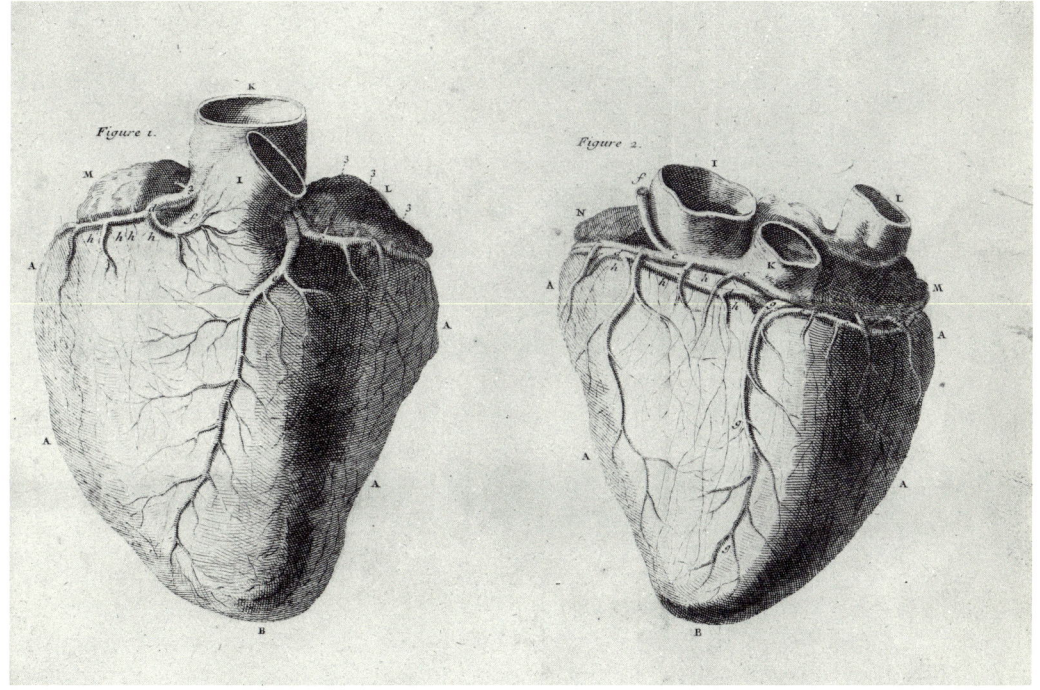

Figure 6. The heart as drawn by de Vieussens.

little cavities between the columns." Nevertheless, Thebesius was forced at last by the very words of Vieussens to admit that this writer had discovered vessels opening onto the inner surface of the ventricles; he tried, therefore, only to render obscure the expression of his rival.

The pathologic state of the heart in angina pectoris was recognized by Morgagni in 1707. A student of the works of Vesalius at sixteen, in his subsequent work he elevated pathologic anatomy to its proper position in the medical sciences. In 1761, he published his famous *De sedibus et causis morborium* (*64*), a masterpiece of clinical pathological description. Written in the form of letters, *De sedibus* contains the clinical and pathological descriptions of approximately seven hundred cases. In his twenty-fourth letter he described the case of a patient who was brought to the hospital at Padua because of an incarcerated hernia, and subsequently died:

"As I examined the internal surfaces of the heart, the left coronary artery appeared to have been changed into a bony canal from its very origin to the extent of many fingers breadth, where it embraces the greater part of the basis. And part of that very long branch, also, which it sends down upon the anterior surface of the heart, was already become bony to so great a space as could be covered by three fingers placed transversely."

The British Clinicians: Angina Pectoris

The important contributions to the knowledge of the coronary circulation, especially the manifestations of its disturbance in disease, were made by the great English clinicians of the eighteenth century, John Hunter, Jenner, Parry, Heberden, Fothergill, Marshall Hall, and Allan Burns. There were two main groups, one around Hunter, with Jenner and Parry, the other around Fothergill and Heberden. These men, working "with the spirit and technique of original investigators" (*44*), in the course of tending the sick recorded their careful observations, and controlled their bedside opinions by the revelations of the autopsy. Occasionally, they even supplemented observation by simple experiment. They were able to define coronary heart disease, clarify its symptoms, and demonstrate the anatomical changes at autopsy.

Except for Burns, these men were predominantly observers rather than "physiologists" or "clinical investigators." They had at their dis-

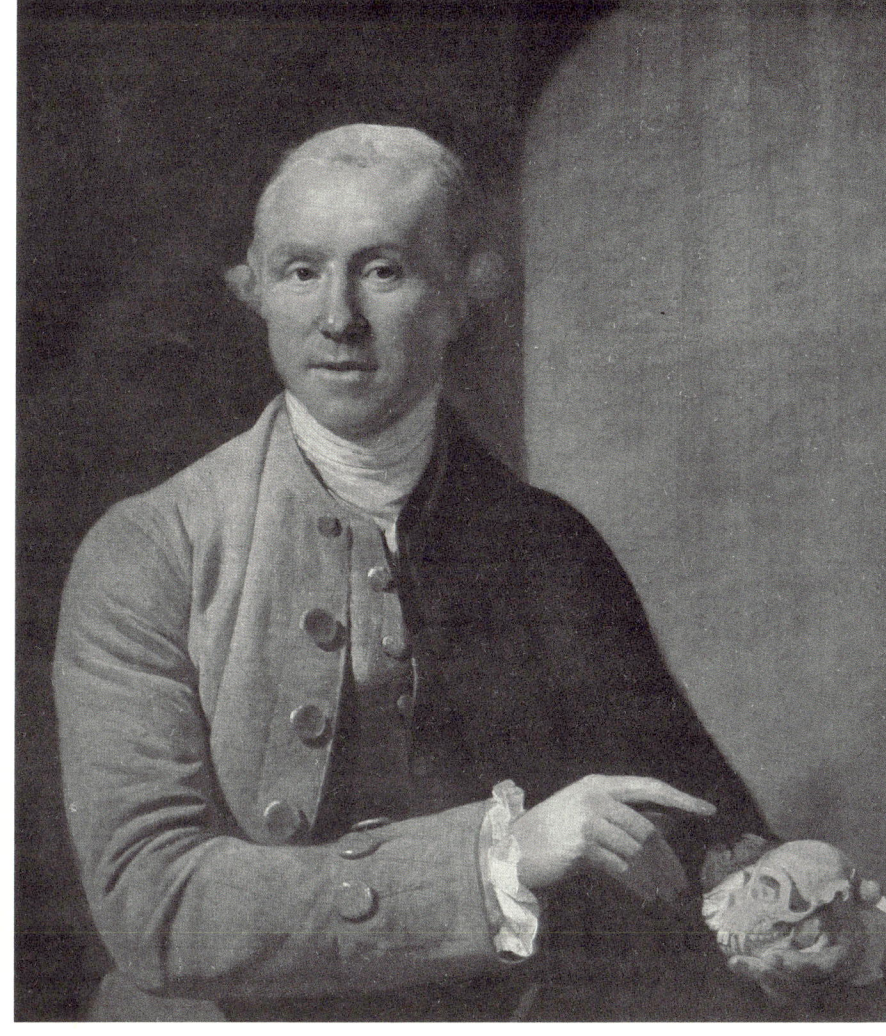

Figure 7. John Hunter (1728–93).

posal the patient and his signs and symptoms, but little access to animal experimentation nor skill in experimental method. Physiological studies on the coronary circulation were still at least a hundred years in the future.

The story of John Hunter is well known, and remains a landmark in medical history (46). At the age of forty, he began to suffer from recurring attacks of what is now known as angina pectoris. His brother-in-law described these attacks as follows:

". . . there was a pain in the stomach and it was a sensation peculiar to those parts and became so violent that he tried change of position to procure ease. He sat down, then walked, laid himself down, then sat upon chairs, but could find no relief. He then called his physician, who could not find any pulse. Being afraid of death soon taking place if he did not breathe, he produced a voluntary act of breathing by working his lungs by power of the will."

Hunter died during an attack which was provoked by a Hospital Board meeting.

"On October 16, 1793, when in his usual state of health, he went to St. George's Hospital and meeting with some things which irritated his mind and not being perfectly master of the circumstances, he withheld his sentiments in which state of restraint he went to the next room and turned around to Dr. Robertson, one of the physicians of the hospital, gave a deep groan and dropped down dead."

At autopsy, performed by Jenner, there was intense "ossification of the coronary arteries."

Parry wrote a book entitled *Syncope Anginosa* (71) which was based on cases similar to that of John Hunter. He carefully observed several individuals suffering from "syncope anginosa" and correlated their clinical symptoms with autopsy findings. An outstanding feature of the book is its logical reasoning as to the disordered physiological process that could induce such attacks. Parry paid more attention to the suddenness of the attack of weakness "due to the loss of strength of the heart muscle" than to the pain; the latter was to become a prominent feature in Heberden's description of angina pectoris. The probability exists that Parry included some cases of coronary thrombosis in the category of angina pectoris. As he reported in one instance, "the inner surface of the coronary arteries was found crusted over with a lymphatic exudation not very dissimilar to the matter which forms on the inside of the trachea in croup." This might well have been a case of coronary thrombosis.

It remained for Heberden (41), on the basis of more than a hundred cases, to draw a remarkably accurate clinical picture of what he called angina pectoris. This great clinician, however, had no conception of the

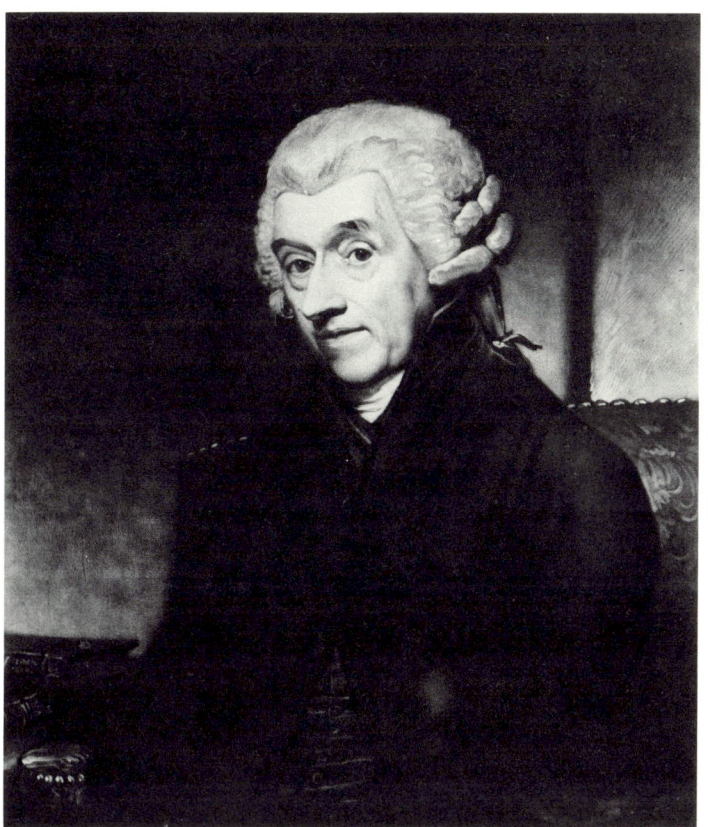

Figure 8. William Heberden (1710–1801).

relation between chest pain and coronary artery disease. This is in marked contrast to Jenner and Parry, who were well aware of the connection between coronary arteriosclerosis and angina pectoris. In his "Commentaries on the History and Cure of Disease," in chapter 70, devoted to "Pectoris Dolor," Heberden describes the symptoms of angina pectoris: "they who are afflicted with this disease, are seized while they are walking (more especially if it be uphill, and soon after eating) with a painful and most disagreeable sensation in the breast which seems as if it would extinguish life if it were to increase or to continue; but the moment they stand still, all this uneasiness vanishes." He makes a special point of his finding that the pain may be localized in various places. He says that males are more liable to this disease,

THE HEART

especially such as have passed their fiftieth year. He also mentions that later on the pain will appear not only when the persons are walking, but when they are lying down, especially if they lie down on the left side.

"Angina pectoris, as far as I have been able to investigate, belongs to the class of spasmodic, not of inflammatory complaints. For, in the first place, the access and recess of the fit is sudden. Secondly, there are long intervals of perfect health. Thirdly, wine and spirituous liquors and opium afford considerable relief. Fourthly, it is increased by disturbances of the mind. . . . Sixthly, in the beginning, it is not brought on by riding on horseback or in a carriage as is usual in diseases arising from scirrhus or inflammation. Seventhly, during the fit the pulse is not quickened. Lastly, its attacks are often after the first sleep; which is a circumstance common to many spasmodic disorders."

He ended this remarkable chapter by stating, "I know one who set himself a task of sawing wood for half an hour every day, and was nearly cured. In one also, the disorder ceased of itself. Bleeding, vomiting and purging, appear to me improper."

Fothergill, a great admirer and friend of Heberden's, carefully examined the hearts of patients who died with the symptoms and signs which Heberden had described (29). Based on this experience, he predicted that future dissections in such cases would reveal the substance of the heart to be affected. His prediction was borne out by a subsequent autopsy on a man of sixty-three who died with typical angina of effort. The autopsy, performed for Fothergill by John Hunter, disclosed that, "the two coronary arteries from their origin to many of their ramifications upon the heart were become one piece of bone."

Allan Burns deserves a special place in this illustrious group of Englishmen (43). He was an original investigator and a man who fearlessly rejected traditional authority. But the main reason for giving him a prominent space in this chapter is that he was the first imaginative experimentalist to deal with the coronary circulation. At fourteen he began to study medicine, and at sixteen he took upon himself the sole direction of the dissecting rooms of his elder brother, John Burns, who at that time was an extramural lecturer on anatomy and surgery at Glasgow. He excelled not as lecturer but as demonstrator and dissector. Not having a university degree, Burns had to gain his experience as a physician and surgeon chiefly by attending and studying the patients of his brother and of his friends. He accumulated drawings which were subsequently used to prepare his books on the diseases of the heart, on the blood vessels, and on surgical anatomy. When he was twenty-three, he accepted the invitation of the Empress Catherine of Russia to go to St. Petersburg as director and surgeon of a hospital. But he soon returned home to take up again the lectures on anatomy and surgery. Burns died in 1813 at the age of thirty-one, probably of a ruptured appendix. Shortly before his death Burns commissioned Granville Sharp Pattison to publish his works. Those interested in strange personalities in medicine should consult Herrick's delightful description of the life and character of this physician (*43*).

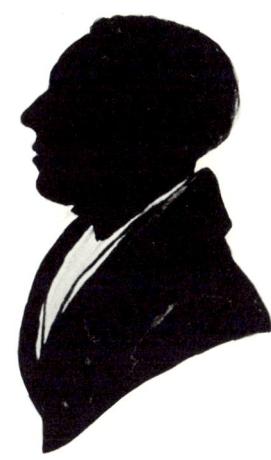

Figure 9. Allan Burns (1781–1813).
This silhouette is the only known representation of Burns.

Burns's book, *Observations on Some of the Most Frequent and Important Diseases of the Heart*, was published in 1809 (*16*). Chapter 7 is of special interest.

"*By a series of well related cases, Parry established the regular history of the disease* [angina pectoris] *and by fair induction from a series of accurately performed dissections he confirms his opinion respecting the cause of this affection;*

which, I think, he has incontrovertibly proved to originate from some organic lesion of the nutrient vessels of the heart. In all the patients who have died of syncope anginosa, where the body has been carefully examined, the coronary arteries have either been found ossified or cartilaginous. [*He then goes on to state,*] *the heart, like every other part, has particular vessels set apart for its nourishment. In health, when we excite the muscular system to more energetic action than usual, we increase the circulation in every part, so that to support this increased action, the heart and every part has its power augmented. If, however, we call into vigorous action a limb, around which we have with a moderate degree of tightness, applied a ligature, we find then that the member can only support its action for a very short time; for now its supply of energy and its expenditure do not balance each other; consequently, it soon, from a deficiency of nervous influence in arterial blood, fails and sinks into a state of quiescence. A heart, the coronary vessels of which are cartilaginous or ossified, is in nearly a similar condition; it can, like the limb, begirt with a moderately tight ligature, discharge its functions so long as its action is moderate and equal. Increase, however, the action of the whole body and along with the rest, that of the heart, and you will soon see exemplified the truth of what has been said; with this difference, that as there is no interruption to the action of the cardiac nerves, the heart will be able to hold out a little longer than the limb. If a person walks fast, ascends a steep hill or mounts a pair of stairs, the circulation in a state of health is hurried, and the heart is felt beating more frequently against the ribs than usual. If, however, a person with the nutrient arteries of the heart diseased in such a way as to impede the progress of the blood among them, attempts to do the same, he finds that the heart is sooner fatigued than the other parts are, which remain healthy. . . . By these exciting causes, applied to a person in whom nutrient arteries of the heart are diseased, an alarming fit of illness is induced. The heart is overpowered with blood accumulated in its cavities, it struggles with its load, but cannot free itself; the right ventricle ceases to propel the blood in due quantity into the pulmonary vessels, a sense of suffocation ensues, and an indescribable anxiety and oppression result from the accumulation of blood about the chest."*

It is not within the scope of this chapter to include detailed biographies and sketches of all who contributed to the clinical knowledge of coronary artery disease. Instead, attention will be paid only to those who helped to formulate new concepts concerning the coronary circulation. Thus, such outstanding clinicians of the eighteenth and nineteenth centuries as Hodgson, Corvisart, and Laënnec will only be afforded passing mention. Corvisart, the colorful physician of the first Napoleon, in his well-known book, *Essai sur les maladies et les lesions organiques de cœur et des gros vaisseaux (20)*, made no mention of angina pectoris and refers to the coronary arteries in a very cursory fashion; this despite the fact that he must have had access to Allan Burns's, Heberden's, and Parry's contributions. The great Laënnec paid only scant attention to the coronary arteries (53). It is peculiar that he failed to mention sclerosis of the coronary arteries in his autopsy reports. Hodgson of Birmingham (44) recognized the connection between coronary arteriosclerosis and heart disease, but did not stress this subject.

Heat and Energy Exchange: Lavoisier to Helmholtz

Antoine Laurent Lavoisier has been vividly portrayed in the first chapter, and the discovery of respiratory gas exchange described. But his work is also the cornerstone of the science of metabolism as applied to the whole body. Lavoisier did not fear to indulge in philosophy, although he separated his philosophy distinctly from the description of his experiments. Thus, he wrote in the preface of *Traité Élémentaire de Chimie* (56):

"We think only through the medium of words . . . languages are true analytical methods . . . algebra which is adapted to its purpose to every species of expression is the most simple, most exact, and best manner possible, it is at the same time a language and an analytical method . . . the art of reasoning is nothing more than the language well arranged. . . . We must trust to nothing but facts: these are presented to us by nature and cannot deceive. We ought, in every instance, to submit our reasoning to the test of experiment, and never to search for truth but by the natural road of experiment and observation. . . . [And, he continued] I am thoroughly convinced of these truths, I have imposed upon myself, as a law, never to advance but from what is known to what is unknown; never to form any conclusion which is not an immediate consequence necessarily flowing from observation and experiment; and always to arrange the facts and the conclusions which are drawn from them in such an order as shall render it most easy for beginners in the study of chemistry thoroughly to understand them."

THE HEART

Through ingenious experiments, Lavoisier first discovered the true importance of oxygen, to which he gave its present name after first calling it "eminently respirable air." He made extensive use of an ice calorimeter which had been first described by Laplace. He used this calorimeter to investigate the heat liberated by an animal, correlating this with the amount of oxygen consumed. In performing these experiments, using sparrows and later guinea pigs, Lavoisier found that the "eminently respirable air" was exhausted by respiration and replaced by fixed air, that is, oxygen was taken up by the animal and replaced by carbon dioxide. Lavoisier and Laplace found that the amount of oxygen consumed by the animal was greater than the amount of carbon dioxide produced, or to use Lavoisier's words, "that the fixed air was less than would correspond to the amount of eminently respirable air." He further found that the amount of oxygen consumed was greater when the animal was kept at low temperatures and it rose during ingestion of food and after body movements. However, he never advanced beyond his initial concept that combustion of material takes place in the lungs. This notion was dispelled soon after Lavoisier's death by the demonstration that the heat actually developed in the lungs was far less than would occur if carbon and hydrogen were burned in the lungs.

Lavoisier established the fact that oxygen is closely connected with metabolism, that metabolism is some kind of combustion, and that, as a result of combustion, heat develops. Although he appreciated the relationship between oxygen and metabolism and tried to find the relationship between heat production and metabolism, his experiments along this line were unsuccessful.

In the eighteenth century the ideas of Newton's world machine ruled the scientific minds of Europe and caught the imagination of the intellectual classes. The nineteenth century reacted against the age of reason and, with the pendulum swinging in the opposite direction, became the century of romanticism; the emotional rather than the rational was emphasized (*100*). This century also saw further battles between the lower classes and the rising forces responsible for industrialization. It is useless to speculate whether the transition from the age of reason to the age of romanticism was a step backward or forward. Modern man certainly has carried both packs on his back without too much discomfort. Romanticism, as Randall stated (*75*) is "an emphasis on the less rational side of human nature. It is the voicing of the conviction that life is broader than intelligence and that the world is more than what physics can find in it." It is certainly interesting that the advance of modern atomic physics, although not swinging the pendulum completely back toward Newtonism, has at least effected a balance between the attitudes of the eighteenth and nineteenth centuries.

Several separate scientific revolutions took place during the nineteenth century. The first was the theory of evolution; its impact on biological thinking was immediate. This idea, formulated in 1859, has influenced and permeated biology, philosophy, and religion alike. Because of it, biological sciences have come to regard all events as passing, developing, and nonstatic. The events of evolution are as disorderly as the medieval neoplatonic systems were orderly. Instead of a logical sequence, one finds events irregular, dying out in one direction, while gathering speed and momentum in another.

The second revolution began with the work of the obscure Austrian monk, Gregor Mendel, who formulated the laws of heredity; this was at first much less spectacular, but its subsequent effects have been just as great.

The third stemmed from a concept that was indispensable for the study of metabolism; this concept is embodied in the law of the conservation of energy formulated by Mayer and Helmholtz. As Helmholtz stated (*84*),

"*The last decades of scientific development have led us to the recognition of a new universal law of all natural phenomena, which from its extraordinarily extended range, and from the connection which it constitutes between the natural phenomena of all kinds, even the remotest times and the most distant places, is especially fitted to give us an idea of the character of the natural sciences. This law is the law of the conservation of force; it asserts that the quantity of force which can be brought into action in the whole of Nature is unchangeable, and can neither be increased nor diminished.*"

A fourth revolution was the development of bacteriology. This new science, associated with the names of Pasteur and Koch, also introduced profound changes in medicine. Indeed, according to Herrick (*44*), "these great advances in this new field, together with those in endocrinology and the discovery of the X ray by Roentgen, relegated the coronary arteries and their diseases to a secondary place in medicine."

Coronary Blood Flow: Experimental Pathology

The correlation between coronary artery disease and fatty changes of the cardiac muscle was recognized by Sir Richard Quain, who published a book on fatty diseases of the heart in 1850 (74). In it he distinguished two forms under which fat may be involved in cardiac disease, (a) so-called fatty growth of the heart, which he described as fat found in the heart fibers in the form of oily matter in cells, and (b) fatty degeneration of the heart's muscle. He devoted considerable space to what he called fatty degeneration arising chiefly from a local modification of nutrition: "I have seen the coronary arteries extremely ossified going directly to the only part of the heart affected.... This connection between fatty softened heart and obstructed arteries suggests an analogy with softening of the brain, in which a like condition of the vessel is known to exist." Quain must have mistaken the scar formation in heart muscle for fatty degeneration. But at least he noticed the connection between changes in the heart muscle and occlusion of the coronary arteries.

The work of Marshall Hall and that of John Erichsen are of greater interest because they represent the beginnings of experimental pathology. Hall entered Edinburgh University as a medical student in October 1809, and by 1811 he had been elected senior president of the Royal Medical Society of Edinburgh. As a practitioner of medicine he expressed the belief that sudden death was often due to arrest of the coronary circulation. He outlined plans for testing this notion by animal experiments (37). This suggestion was taken up by Erichsen (27), who posed the problem in the following way: "The question, then, is to determine what effect that arrest of the coronary circulation would have upon the action of the heart." To answer this question, Erichsen ligated the coronary vessels of dogs. He observed that the average duration of the ventricular action, after ligation of the coronary vessels, was 23.5 minutes. He stated that the "bearing of these results on the immediate cause of death in some diseases of the heart is sufficiently obvious." Any circumstance that may interfere with the passage of the blood through the coronary arteries, either directly as in ossification of the "coats of

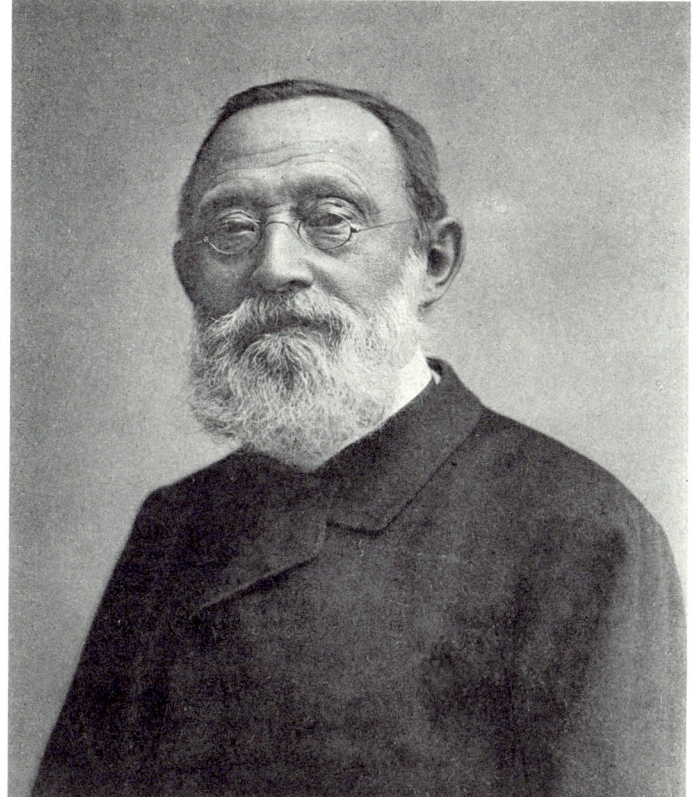

Figure 10. Rudolf Ludwig Karl Virchow (1821–1902).

those vessels, or indirectly, by there being insufficient blood sent out of the left ventricle, as in cases of extreme obstruction or regurgitant disease of the aortic or mitral valves, may occasion the fatal event."

These early attempts to investigate the role of the coronary circulation were followed and greatly expanded by the German school of experimental pathology of the second half of the nineteenth century. The outstanding men in this field were Rokitansky and Virchow. Curiously, neither of the two showed any direct interest in the role of the coronary circulation despite the availability of a large autopsy material. However, they introduced methods and approaches which ultimately were to have a profound influence on the experimental pathology of the heart and the coronary vessels. Virchow's paper in

1845 on thrombosis and embolism (*94*) certainly laid the foundations for the later studies of his pupils, particularly of Cohnheim.

Julius Cohnheim contributed a great deal to the understanding of the role of the coronary arteries (*19*). He was the recognized master of experimental pathology of his time, and his studies, together with those of his contemporaries, von Bezold and Panum, must be considered as the first on the coronary circulation in which physiological measurements were employed. Von Bezold investigated the influence of ligation of

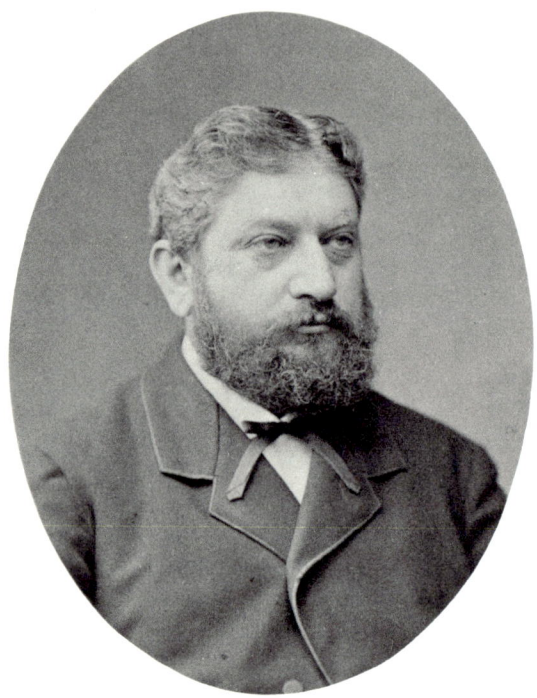

Figure 11. Julius Friedrich Cohnheim (1839–84).

the coronary arteries on cardiac activity (*5*). He found that ligation of the left coronary artery of the rabbit slowed the heart rate after about 10 to 20 seconds; after periods of 145 to 150 seconds, the rhythm became more irregular. Cohnheim also quotes Panum (*69*), who embolized the coronary arteries by means of injection of powder, wax, oil, and India ink. Despite complete injection of all visible coronary arteries, the pulsations of the heart continued for five minutes. Thereafter, however, pulsations of the left atrium continued to beat regularly but at a slower rate; not until seventy-five minutes after the injection did the activity of the left ventricles come to a halt.

On such experimental evidence, Cohnheim propounded his well-known hypothesis that the coronary arteries normally are end-arteries, that is, vessels without anastomoses. This view has been confirmed recently by Wiggers (*102*), who found in the dog that the collateral channels between the coronaries, if they do exist, are of no use in protecting against the consequences of acute coronary artery occlusion. How else could one explain the hypodynamic effects, the incidence of fibrillation, and the immediate diminution in contractility of the affected area of the heart muscle? In other words, if an extensive collateral circulation has not developed prior to the total occlusion the muscle in the affected zone is not likely to survive.

Cohnheim supported his observation that ligation of the left coronary arteries leads to immediate cessation of the heart beat and death of the animal by reference to clinical material (*19*):

CORONARY CIRCULATION

"If a man regularly goes after his business without edema or shortness of breath, without other signs of congestion, and then dies suddenly, this proves that up to this moment the heart has functioned sufficiently and that if death has been due to paralysis of the heart, something new had to be added by means of which the ability of the heart to work has been eliminated."

Cohnheim also performed experiments on the dog; these involved cannulation of the carotid, femoral, and pulmonary arteries, and in several instances the cardiac cavities. The fitted cannulae were connected to manometers for the recording of blood pressure. For the first 30 to 40 seconds after the left coronary artery had been ligated, no effect was noticeable. After the first minute, irregularities of cardiac activity appeared. Cardiac arrest with collapse of arterial blood pressure then ensued. After the arrest had lasted for about 10 to 20 seconds, "extremely lively peristaltic fibrillatory movements were noticed which persisted for 40 to 50 seconds or even longer; the atria meanwhile pulsated regularly." Cohnheim stated that these fibrillatory movements do not raise arterial blood pressure.

Cohnheim and Schultheiss-Rechberg (*19*) examined the possibility that the consequences of ligating a coronary artery arose from a lack of oxygen. This prospect, however, appeared to them unlikely since oxygen deprivation of the whole animal had quite different results. Cohnheim concluded, therefore, that a poison is released in heart muscle after coronary occlusion. He conceived this poison to be produced "metabolically" under the influence of cardiac contractions. Under ordinary conditions, these toxic substances could not exert their influences since they would be carried away by the blood stream. However, if the coronary circulation were to be interrupted, the toxins would accumulate in the heart muscle; and, once their concentration had increased sufficiently, they would produce slowing and irregularity of the heart rate as well as a sudden and irreversible paralysis of both cardiac ventricles.

Thus, Cohnheim, von Bezold, and Panum began the modern studies of the physiology of the coronary circulation in their laboratories of experimental pathology.

By the end of the nineteenth century, the pathologic and to some extent the clinical consequences of coronary occlusion had been clearly defined by others with similar interests: Weigert, Ziegler, and von Leyden. Weigert, in his article on pathological processes connected with coagulation (*98*), clearly describes a myocardial infarct; his great

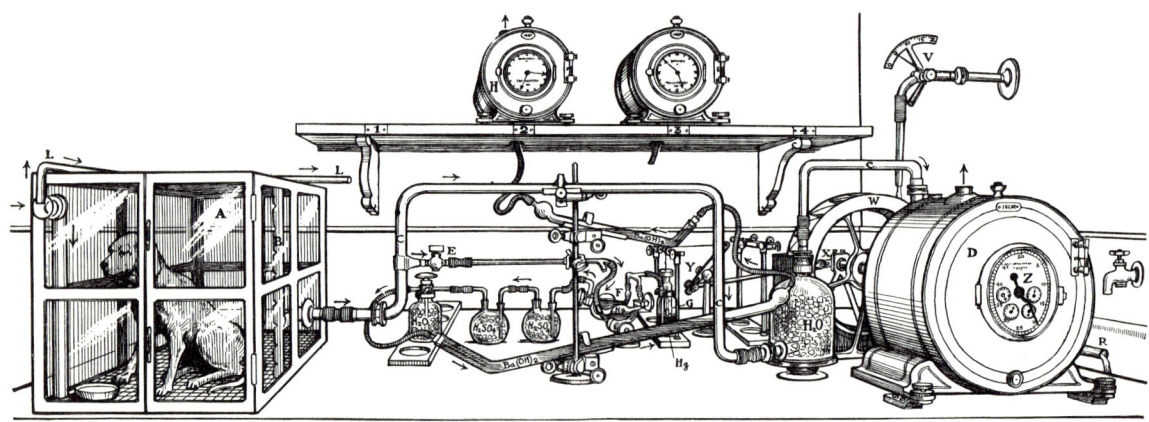

Figure 12. Respiration apparatus of Pettenkofer and Voit.

contribution was his appreciation that occlusion of the coronary artery can occur gradually:

"If the occlusion occurs gradually and in the absence of collateral circulation, producing chronic changes, a slow atrophy and destruction of the muscle fibers without damage to the connecting tissue can be observed. . . . The disappearing muscle fibers are then replaced by connective tissue."

Ziegler (*106*) coined the term *myomalacia cordis* as describing the "peculiar softening of the muscle of the heart, consequent on arterial anemia [ischemia]." Von Leyden (*57*) wrote a comprehensive clinical treatise on sclerosis of the coronary artery in which he distinguished between acute, subacute, and chronic occlusions.

Metabolism of Tissues: Voit and Rubner

The science of metabolism, following the pioneer discoveries of Lavoisier, was established during the nineteenth century. The rapid development of biochemistry stimulated metabolic studies on many organs, including the heart. In 1850, Regnault and Reiset (*77*) accurately determined the amount of oxygen consumed and of carbon dioxide expired by an animal in a closed chamber. Subsequently, Pettenkofer and Voit (*72*) not only performed similar studies on man but also estimated, from the nitrogen excretion and the carbon contained in expired air, what kinds of substances had been metabolized in the body and the oxygen equivalents of these substances. They thereby established that the consumption of oxygen and the utilization of substrate are interdependent, and that the relations between the amount of oxygen absorbed and carbon dioxide released depends on the same factor. In addition, Voit (*95*) showed that "metabolism was not proportionate to the oxygen supply . . .; also that the metabolism of the tissues, through its oxygen requirements and its carbon dioxide production, changes the condition of the blood and thereby regulates the respiration."

Finally, Rubner, a pupil of Voit and of Ludwig, developed an animal calorimeter, by means of which oxygen consumption and carbon dioxide production could be measured continuously, while simultaneously the amount of heat produced by the animal could be determined (*84*). The results, published in 1894, were a triumphant demonstration of the validity of the law of conservation of energy: the amount of heat calcu-

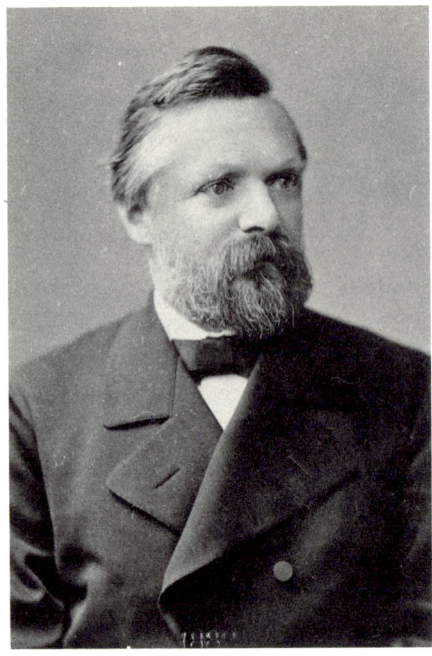

Figure 13. Carl von Voit (1831–1908).

lated by Rubner as the quantity that should have been derived from the metabolism of the dog was the same amount actually given off to the calorimeter. "*Ex nihilo nihil fit.*" Voit, at the turn of the century (95), clearly foresaw the application of these findings to tissue metabolism:

> "*The unknown causes of metabolism are found in the cells of the organism. The mass of these cells and their power to decompose materials determine the metabolism . . . if the power of the cells to metabolize is not exhausted by the protein furnished, then carbohydrates and fats are destroyed up to the limit of the ability of the cells to do so. From this use of material arise physical results, such as work, heat and electricity which we can express in heat units. This is the power derived from metabolism. . . . the requirements for energy cannot possibly be the cause for metabolism any more than the requirement for gold will put it into one's pocket. Hence, the production of energy has a very definite upper limit, which is afforded by the ability of the cells to metabolize. If the cells will metabolize no more, then further increase of work ceases even in the presence of direct necessity.*"

The door had indeed been opened for the great advances in cellular metabolism of modern times.

Measurements of Coronary Blood Flow

The problem of the relationship between cardiac contraction and coronary blood flow has been investigated since the middle of the nineteenth century. Brücke (15) believed that the opening and closing of the aortic valve is an important factor in the regulation of the coronary blood flow. Rebatel (76), working on this problem in horses and mules, summarized his results in 1872 as follows:

"In the very moment after the aortic valves have opened and the blood courses into the aorta, blood is ejected with violence into the opening of the coronary artery; this represents the first wave of blood entering the vessels. The elevation and the rapidity of both the speed and the rise of pressure demonstrate the rapidity of this wave and its coincidence with the aortic pulsation. Entrance of blood into the smaller vessels during systole is much more difficult. With diastole, the capillaries which have been empty of blood as a result of systolic compression, fill again from the larger coronary vessels. This represents the second weaker wave."

Newell-Martin and Sedgwick in 1882 registered graphically the blood pressure in the carotid artery and in a branch of the left coronary artery of the dog (65). They summarized their experiments as follows: "We find that whether arterial pressures be high or low, every feature of the carotid pulse occurs simultaneously in the coronary." They denied that the semilunar valves interrupt the coronary circulation, but they were of the opinion that during ventricular diastole blood flowing into the coronary arteries aids in distending the flaccid heart.

The experiments of Newell-Martin and Sedgwick as well as those of Rebatel suggested that blood enters the coronary arteries during diastole, as well as during systole. Klug, in 1876 (50), had observed that in the rabbit during cardiac diastole the vessels in all layers of the cardiac muscle appeared to be full of blood. This was particularly conspicuous at the apex; during systole, however, both superficial and deep coronary vessels appeared empty.

Much of what has been accomplished in the study of the physiology of the coronary circulation in the past sixty years has been the result of

CORONARY CIRCULATION

refinements in technique. Hemodynamic determinations depend primarily on accurate measurement of blood pressure and flow. The recording of pressure has been accomplished by the construction of optical or, more recently, of electrical manometers. The measurement of flow has been a more difficult undertaking.

In 1895, Bohr and Henriques (*14*), working at the Physiological Laboratory at the University of Copenhagen, tried to measure the rate of coronary blood flow by creating a preparation in which the aortic outflow could be assumed to equal the coronary flow. The so-called "irrigation coefficient" (cc. blood flow per 100 gm. of heart muscle per minute), an expression which bedeviled many articles on the coronary circulation of this period, was found by these investigators to be about 36 cc. Markwalder and Starling (*61*) later took issue with these results and concluded that the coronary blood flow is considerably greater. Using the heart-lung preparation as a feeder for a second heart, they found that "the coefficients of irrigation are much higher than those which Bohr and Henriques obtained and in all probability may be taken as about 60% of the weight of the heart per minute." Thus, in a heart weighing 100 grams, the coronary blood flow should be about 60 cc. We know now that these values, although true for the heart-lung preparation, are much lower than those found in unanesthetized dogs (*90*). In 1899, Langendorff introduced his preparation for the perfusion of the coronary arteries through the aorta and made numerous determinations of the coronary blood flow (*54*). A landmark in the study of the coronary blood flow was the development by Morawitz and Zahn in 1914 of a method for collection of blood from the coronary sinus (*63*); this method permitted the determination of the rate of coronary flow *in situ*. Their method was based on the earlier paper by Meyer in which a superficial vein of the heart was cannulated and the flow determined in the open chest animal. But as Morawitz says, "In Meyer's procedure the animal is losing blood continuously and blood volume can be maintained only with difficulty." Morawitz and Zahn's method was based on direct catheterization of the coronary sinus with a "Tampon Kanule." This was a double lumen catheter with one lumen communicating with a rubber balloon which could be inflated in the coronary sinus to prevent reflux of blood from the right atrium. Morawitz and Zahn, like many later investigators, debated whether or not the coronary sinus drains a constant fraction of the arterial inflow. It has since been established by experiments on the dog heart beating *in situ* that under a great variety of conditions the relationship of the coronary sinus outflow to left coronary inflow is remarkably constant. As Gregg says (*33*), "In no instance would a significant change in left or total coronary inflow have been incorrectly indicated by the corresponding coronary sinus outflow."

After Morawitz and Zahn, methods were devised which involved the use of the bubble flow meter and electromagnetic recording devices. These required opening the chest of the animal. But, in recent years, the combination of catheterization of the coronary sinus with the nitrous oxide method of blood flow measurement has made it possible to measure coronary blood flow in the intact dog and even in unanesthetized human subjects (*49, 10*). It is true that intubation of the coronary sinus in man is a lengthy procedure, involving many precautions. Certainly, a simpler approach would be highly desirable. But even if such a simple procedure could be conceived, catheterization of the coronary sinus would still remain a prerequisite for the study of human myocardial metabolism, in order to obtain the necessary blood samples for chemical analyses.

Langendorff's preparation also provided some fresh insights into the *nature* of the coronary blood flow (*54*). He measured the venous outflow from the cat heart and found that it increased during systole. Coronary arterial blood pressure and coronary inflow were also measured by means of a cannula inserted into the aorta. The fluctuations in pressure in the cannula were supposed to reflect resistances within the coronary vascular system. He reported that the stream velocity has two peaks during each cardiac cycle. The first corresponds to systole, the second to diastole. He held that during isometric contraction, the inflow of blood into the large coronary artery increases but outflow from the vessels is impossible due to muscular contraction; that during the ejection period, coronary inflow is diminished but the "squeezing out effect" of the blood on the cardiac veins is increased; that during isometric relaxation, inflow into the large coronary vessels recurs, but there is no outflow "because it takes time for these vessels to empty themselves"; finally, that during the period of slow ventricular filling the inflow is again increased but there is no outflow because the coronary sinus is closed. It is remarkable how close these views are to present concepts concerning the phasic nature of the coronary blood flow.

It is now generally accepted that with the onset of isometric contraction the rate of flow into the left coronary artery diminishes abruptly (Fig. 14). Thereafter, a record of blood flow shows a progressive decline to below the zero line and evidence of backflow. With the onset of ejection from the ventricles and the rise of aortic pressure, backflow diminishes and is rapidly converted to forward flow which reaches a maximum shortly before the peak of the aortic pressure curve. It then declines, leveling off during the latter part of systole. Coincident with the closure of the aortic valves and the onset of isometric relaxation, the inflow again rapidly augments and thereafter gradually declines with the diastolic fall of aortic pressure (*33*).

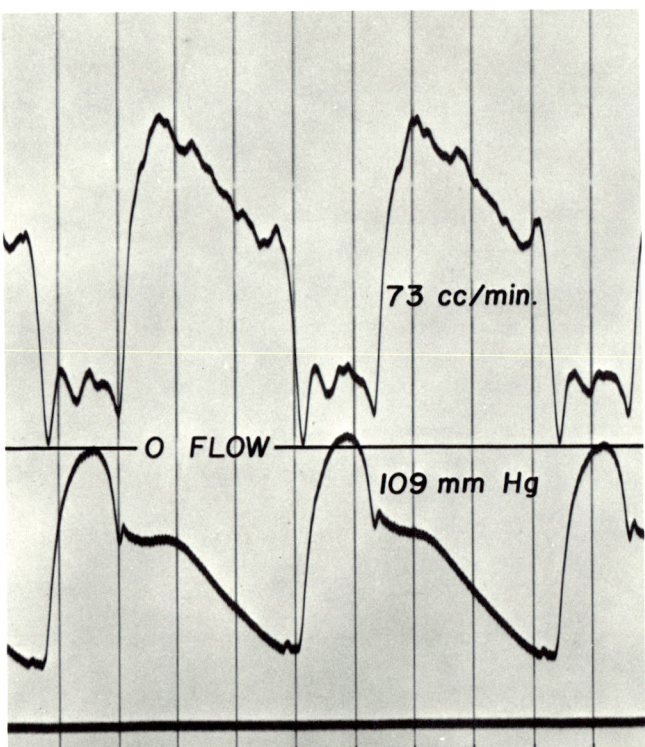

Figure 14. Time course of blood flow through the coronary system in the dog. *Above:* a tracing of the volume flow of blood through the coronaries; *below:* the aortic pressure curve.

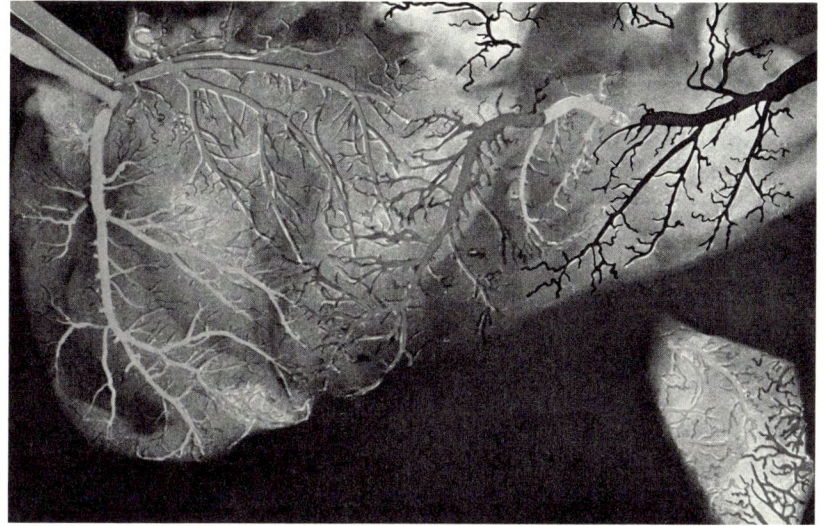

Figure 15. The coronary arteries, as demonstrated by injection.

CORONARY CIRCULATION

Problems of collateral circulation of the heart have also been investigated extensively during the last fifty years. Along this line it is pertinent to recall Cohnheim's insistence that the coronary arteries are end-arteries and Wigger's conclusion that coronary collaterals, if they exist at all, are of little physiological importance following a fresh occlusion of a coronary artery (*102*). In recent years, it has become clear that useful collateral vessels must develop as intercoronary arterial anastomoses. Anastomoses between the coronary vessels and the cardiac chambers, such as the vessels of Vieussens and Thebesius, are of no real import. The anatomist has lent a helping hand to the understanding of the collateral circulation. Gross (*34*), basing his technique on that of the German anatomist Spalteholz, utilized roentgenographic visualization of the coronary arteries following the injection of a barium sulfate gelatin mixture into the coronary arteries. The use of this technique, however, was complicated by the need for stereoscopy to interpret the roentgenograms thus prepared. This disadvantage was overcome by Blumgart, Zoll, Freedberg, and Gilligan (*12*), who substituted lead phosphate agar for the barium sulfate gelatin. Their method permits unrolling of the injected but still unfixed heart. Using this technique, they found that

[239]

collateral vessels develop in a variety of conditions, foremost among them coronary occlusion.

The role of the vessels of Vieussens and Thebesius have also been subjected to considerable scrutiny. Here we must return briefly to the eighteenth century. Almost fifty years after the first descriptions of these vessels by Thebesius and Vieussens, Haller (*38*) described "still more and smaller veins in the heart, whose little trunks being very short cannot easily be traced by dissection and these open themselves by an infinite number of oblique small mouths, through all the numerous sinuosities observed on the surface of the right and left ventricle." John Abernethy (*1*) in 1798 published a comprehensive treatise on the Thebesian vessels. He stated that when the ventricles of cadavers were opened, the foramina Thebesii not only appeared numerous and large but also were distended with a different colored wax which had been injected into the coronary arteries and veins. Bochdalek, in 1868, published the results of his observations on the Thebesian foramina of the auricles (*13*). He found mouths of small vessels in the auricles as well as in the ventricles. The foramina varied considerably both in number and size. Bochdalek concluded "that the greater number of small openings on the inner surface of the right as well as the left auricle, which from early times have borne the name of foramina Thebesii, represent the mouth of little veins that, often uniting into larger vessels, course with many branches through the auricular wall." In 1880 Langer published the report of his research on the foramina Thebesii of the human heart (*55*). By means of an injection technique, he demonstrated not only that foramina existed in all the cavities of the heart but also that communications existed between the coronary vessels and each of the four cardiac cavities. He concluded that the foramina Thebesii of the ventricles were not, as occasionally happens in the auricles, in direct communication with the coronary veins, but that they had their own separate capillary supply. In no case did he observe valves in relation to these openings. Pratt (*73*), by means of injections of water, of normal saline, and of defibrinated blood at constant pressures, demonstrated direct connection between the vessels of Thebesius and the coronary veins. The foramina Thebesii were shown to be connected with the smaller coronary veins by fine branches; the finest ramifications remained uninjected. Pratt was unable to "discover anything more free than a capillary connection between the vessels of Thebesius and the coronary arteries." He discussed at great length the role of these vessels in the nutrition of the heart, and came to the conclusion that "there can be no doubt of the genuinely nutritive character of the phenomena observed." He said that in cardiac arrest and ventricular fibrillation the nutrition through the vessels of Thebesius and the coronary veins may work to great advantage.

Wearn in 1928 presented evidence for the existence of direct, non-capillary connections between the coronary arteries and the chambers of the heart (*97*). He also demonstrated communications between the larger coronary arteries and the Thebesian veins and the drainage of myocardial capillaries into the Thebesian veins. Finally, he showed that "under certain conditions" as much as 90 per cent of the arterial flow escaped via the Thebesian vessels; during gradual closure of the orifices of the coronary arteries, the Thebesian vessels supplied the heart muscle with sufficient blood to maintain an efficient circulation. Wearn was careful to distinguish between the performance of the beating and the arrested heart. "In a beating heart, in the absence of dilation, the capillaries were filled and the Thebesian flow was greatly diminished. But in hearts in which the left ventricle did not beat, the capillaries were very imperfectly injected in contrast to the other chambers which were beating."

Within recent years, studies on the coronary circulation through the arrested heart have gained in importance because of the advent of surgery on the arrested heart. A study by Reynolds, Bing, and Kirsch (*78*) disclosed marked differences between the vascular pattern of the arrested and the beating heart. For example, in normal hearts erythrocytes move in capillaries with their flat sides apposed to the muscle fibers. In arrested and arrested-perfused hearts, the occurrence of this arrangement decreased with time: the erythrocytes become round, or if close together, are packed in geometric shapes. Capillaries of arrested hearts are generally larger than those of normal hearts and are often ruptured. These changes have been interpreted as evidence of weakening of connective tissue in the arrested heart.

The role of the Thebesian vessels in the blood supply to the heart is, however, by no means settled. It is likely that anastomoses do exist between the Thebesian veins, the coronary veins, and the coronary sinus.

But there is, as yet, no convincing evidence that the blood can pass freely from the cavities of the heart into the coronary arteries at any stage of the cardiac cycle, no matter how low the pressure falls in the arteries.

Metabolism of the Heart

The final chapter in the recognition of coronary artery disease was long delayed. It will be recalled that during the seventeenth and eighteenth centuries and also part of the nineteenth century, clinical-pathological studies provided important clues to the role of the coronary arteries in the production of angina pectoris. The subsequent work of the great English clinicians of the eighteenth century as well as that of the German and French pathologists and clinicians of the nineteenth century did not tell the final story. The final recognition of the clinical syndrome associated with coronary artery disease came in 1912 when James B. Herrick published his first paper on the clinical features of obstruction of the coronary arteries (*42*). One of Herrick's great achievements was his emphasis that the disease can be chronic and need not be immediately fatal.

Once the clinical picture was understood, and refined physiological methods became available, the circulatory alterations of coronary occlusion could be investigated thoroughly. Wiggers and his school supplied the fusion of physiological and clinical thinking about coronary occlusion (*102*). Their studies revealed that the coronary vessels are functional end-arteries as demonstrated by the fact that within 60 seconds after coronary occlusion the myocardial area affected by the obstruction no longer shortened during the period of systolic ejection but, instead, expanded brusquely during isometric contraction. This school also showed compensatory mechanisms by means of which dynamic conditions of the heart can be restored to normal if the remaining myocardium is in good responsive condition.

During the present century, there has been an ever-increasing interest in the metabolism of the heart (*28, 103, 6*). The modern science of intermediary metabolism can be traced to the work and ideas of Lavoisier, Liebig, Voit, Pettenkofer, Pasteur, and their followers. But the idea of the universality of biological events is a recent one. It has been recognized that basic features of the energy-producing mechanisms are ident-

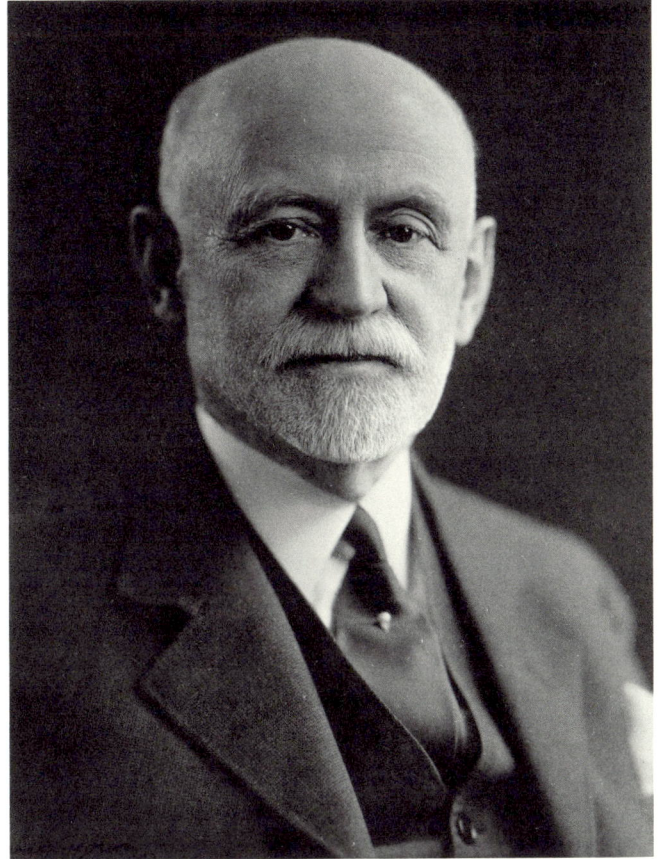

Figure 16. James B. Herrick (1861–1954).

ical or very similar in different types of organisms and organs. Energy-producing mechanisms were probably formed at a very early stage in the evolution of living matter. It is probably the lack of biological organization at this lower level that accounts for the fact that individual organs do not differ appreciably in the fundamental processes of energy production. But they do differ in the manner in which the energy is utilized or liberated (6). Energy production takes place primarily in mitochondrial systems of the cell in which a series of enzymes converts the bulk of the oxidative energy which is released into another form of chemical energy. The efficiency of this conversion is over 60 per cent. The dynamo for energy production is the tricarboxylic cycle, in which the energy released in various oxidative processes is harnessed to high-energy phosphate systems (ATP). This ATP (adenosine triphosphate) represents the link between energy production and energy utilization, since it constitutes the junction between the synthesis of the pyrophosphate bonds of ATP and the specific form in which the energy is utilized by the individual organs. While energy production, therefore, does not differ from species to species, energy utilization and liberation do vary greatly from organ to organ. The contractile proteins of skeletal and heart muscle represent the wheel of the engine driven by the dynamo of energy production. In them, energy is utilized for active work.

The ideas of intermediary metabolism can be briefly summarized (6). The over-all process involves the oxidation of foodstuffs to carbon dioxide and water. The original foodstuff is carried through a large series of intermediary reactions in which energy is absorbed and liberated. All foodstuffs can participate to varying degrees in this process of energy production. Most of the energy is derived from oxidative processes within the tricarboxylic or citric acid cycle. The catalytic enzyme systems within this energy dynamo are beautifully organized within units of the cell, known as mitochondria. They are the instruments by which the principal foodstuffs are burned and by which the chemical energy released is transformed into other forms of energy. One of the most fascinating aspects of modern biochemistry is the close association of cellular function and cellular structure on a molecular basis. As Green stated (32), "the problems of biochemistry are closely interwoven with cell particulates."

I have no intention of conveying the idea that these biochemical concepts are the final word on tissue metabolism. The painful writing of this chapter has convinced me that one should avoid at all cost the spirit conveyed in Galen's statement, that "it is certainly no small advantage that we enjoy living at the present day with the medical arts already brought to such a perfection." But biochemistry is certainly advancing at a more rapid rate than experimental physiology and much faster than classical anatomy.

The early work on cardiac metabolism was summarized in Tigerstedt's textbook of forty years ago, on the physiology of the circulation (*91*). After describing the effect of inorganic ions on the heart, he dealt with the effect of proteins and amino acids on cardiac contractility; however, studies on the myocardial utilization of amino acids were not then available, with the exception of an Italian paper which denied the utilization of amino acids by the heart. It was apparently Locke and Rosenheim (*58*) who first demonstrated myocardial utilization of glucose. The utilization of fat by the heart was not suspected until it was shown in the heart-lung preparation that the respiratory quotient of the heart was usually below one. Indeed, not until 1954 was it recognized that the heart prefers fatty acids to any other substrate (*11*).

The oxygen consumption of the heart has been studied in the frog heart perfused with electrolyte solution, in a wide variety of heart-lung preparations, in heart muscle slices, and in heart muscle homogenates. Little wonder that the results are divergent. Kronecker, in 1878, had maintained that the oxygen content of the perfusate had no effect on cardiac activity (*52*). Hearts of cold-blooded animals which were frequently employed need relatively little oxygen. It is surprising how often data from cold-blooded hearts are still cited in the modern literature as standard values! Winterstein first studied the survival time of the mammalian heart after complete ischemia (*105*). He found that the isolated mammalian heart died in four to twenty-five minutes when completely deprived of oxygen. The most recent work in this field, as stated by Katz in 1945 (*47*), emphasizes that "mechanical efficiency is not constant when increased work produced by increasing blood pressure is compared with that produced by increasing cardiac output. Oxygen consumption definitely increases when work is augmented by increasing blood pressure; it is slightly increased, unchanged or even decreased when work is increased by elevating cardiac output."

The advent of the heart-lung preparation resulted in a host of studies on the metabolism of the isolated heart. There is little doubt in my mind that the general applicability of these results is limited. Many ingenious modifications of the heart-lung preparation have been devised, but these models are uncertain bases for generalizations. There is no substitute for an organ working in its natural environment. Yet there is some virtue in isolating it. For example, cardiac efficiency is markedly diminished in the heart-lung preparation; it is unlikely that the basis for the diminished cardiac efficiency is purely mechanical. It is much more probable that the separation from the whole organism produces specific changes in the perfusion fluid which leads to this "spontaneous failure."

The deficiencies of the classical heart-lung preparation become particularly conspicuous in studies of the gaseous metabolism of the heart (*28*). The average oxygen usage of the *isolated heart* is only 5 ml. of oxygen/100 grams/minute; that of the *heart in situ* of unanesthetized dogs is at least three times as large. The reduction of the work of the heart in these preparations is even greater; thus, according to Evans (*28*), their mechanical efficiency is "more often about 5%"; on the other hand, the mechanical efficiency of the beating dog's heart, corrected for the oxygen consumption of the arrested heart, is 37 per cent, and it is 39 per cent in man (*90*). It is surprising that despite the obviously unnatural state of the heart-lung preparation, the metabolic data show close agreement with those obtained from the intact heart *in situ*: the respiratory quotient is below unity, suggesting usage of substances other than glucose; glucose, pyruvate, lactate, and ketone bodies are also utilized by the isolated heart; and although there is no evidence that the isolated heart can utilize amino acids, the human heart *in situ* is able to extract them from the blood.

Myocardial Metabolism in Man

The desirability of studying cardiac metabolism in the normally beating heart *in situ* is obvious. It is true that studies performed on the whole heart *in situ* suffer from the disadvantage that, unlike those in heart muscle slices of homogenates, the catalytic systems cannot be individually explored; but these experiments have the advantage that they are carried out on the whole organized system under physiological conditions. Briefly, the method consists in sampling of blood from the coronary sinus by means of a catheter, in measuring the myocardial extraction and usage of oxygen and various substrates, and in establishing the amount or quantity of oxygen which each individual metabolite contributes to the oxidative metabolism of the heart. Coronary flow is measured by means of the nitrous oxide method originally devised for measurement of the cerebral circulation (*10*). This is described further in a later chapter. These new techniques have made possible an investigation of the factors which regulate the energy requirements and expenditure of the human heart *in situ*.

It has been shown that in man the coronary blood flow averages 77 ml. per 100 grams per minute (*8*). In the anesthetized dog the coronary blood flow per unit of heart muscle is greater. In fact, an inverse relationship exists between the left ventricular flow per 100 grams and the total weight of the left ventricle. Smaller left ventricles have a relatively higher flow per unit of weight than larger ones. It is probable that the rate of coronary blood flow and of cardiac oxygen consumption per unit of cardiac tissue are related to the surface area. It is generally accepted that metabolic rate is a function of the ratio of surface area to body weight. As ventricular weight varies directly with body weight, the proportion of left ventricular weight to body weight is the same in small animals as in large animals. Since the ratio of surface area to left ventricular weight is higher in smaller animals, the cardiac metabolism per unit of weight is increased.

In severe anemia (below 6 grams of hemoglobin), the coronary blood flow is greatly increased; in these individuals the oxygen extraction by the heart muscle is so complete that the coronary venous blood contains less than two volumes per cent of oxygen (*26*). With the first line of defense, the oxygen extraction, thus lost, the heart must rely entirely on an increase in flow in order to satisfy its metabolic requirements. Because of the fact that even under normal conditions 75 per cent of the oxygen presented to the myocardium is removed from the blood, the heart is almost entirely dependent on changes in coronary flow to supply its oxygen demands.

Thus, it is primarily the coronary flow which responds to the oxygen needs of the heart. A number of workers have shown that it is alterations in blood pressure rather than in cardiac output which result in increased myocardial uptake of oxygen, through increased coronary blood flow. An increase in heart rate has similar effects, although tachycardia, in paralleling coronary flow, does not change myocardial oxygen consumption per beat (*6*). The heart also appears to be more efficient at slower than at faster rates. The effect of a sudden increase in mean aortic pressure on myocardial oxygen consumption and coronary flow suggests that the work of the heart, or more specifically, the work it performs in overcoming the resistance of the arterioles, is one of the more

CORONARY CIRCULATION

important of the factors which determine the usage of oxygen by the heart.

In addition to these dynamic factors, there are others in which the demands of the heart are regulated at the cellular level; myocardial anoxia, anemia, and thyrotoxicosis belong in this group (6, 7). It is true that in these conditions secondary alterations in cardiac work occur, but the main demand for oxygen originates within the cell itself. Gorlin and his associates (31) have used the ratio of myocardial oxygen consumption per second of systolic contraction to the work per minute in order to differentiate the influence of hemodynamic and non-hemodynamic factors on myocardial oxygen consumption. Any deviation from the normal ratio suggests that non-hemodynamic factors influence myocardial oxygen consumption. Regardless of where or how the primary demand for increased oxygen uptake originates, it is met by changes in aortic perfusion pressure and in the duration of diastole and of systolic inflow time, and by alterations in coronary vascular resistance.

Consequently, drugs influencing coronary circulation can act primarily by changing cardiac work or by altering the cellular demands for oxygen. Nitroglycerin, for example, doubles myocardial oxygen usage and coronary flow in normal individuals without changing left ventricular work. As a result, left ventricular efficiency per 100 grams decreases markedly. Since the ratio of myocardial oxygen consumption to work of the heart doubles, the changes in myocardial oxygen consumption appear not to be the result of alterations in hemodynamics, but rather of increased demands for oxygen on the cellular level. This is consistent with the concept that the various nitrites increase oxygen utilization by uncoupling of oxidative phosphorylation.

It remains for us now to bring up to date our present knowledge of myocardial metabolism (6). The history of the science of metabolism as illustrated in this essay has shown the way. As Voit states, "The unknown causes of metabolism are found in the cells of the organism. The mass of these cells and their powers to decompose materials determine the metabolism." There are two approaches currently available to study metabolism at the cellular level: (1) coronary sinus catheterization which allows in vivo studies without impairing the activity of the organ, and (2) the procurement of specimens of heart muscle that depict the end results of metabolic events. Each method has its obvious advantages and disadvantages.

Using the coronary sinus catheterization, we have shown that the human and dog heart utilize considerable quantities of fatty acids, ketone bodies, and amino acids as well as glucose, pyruvate, and lactate (7). It has also been shown for the human heart that both myocardial glucose usage and extraction are functions of the arterial glucose concentration: at blood sugar concentrations of below 80 mg. per cent,

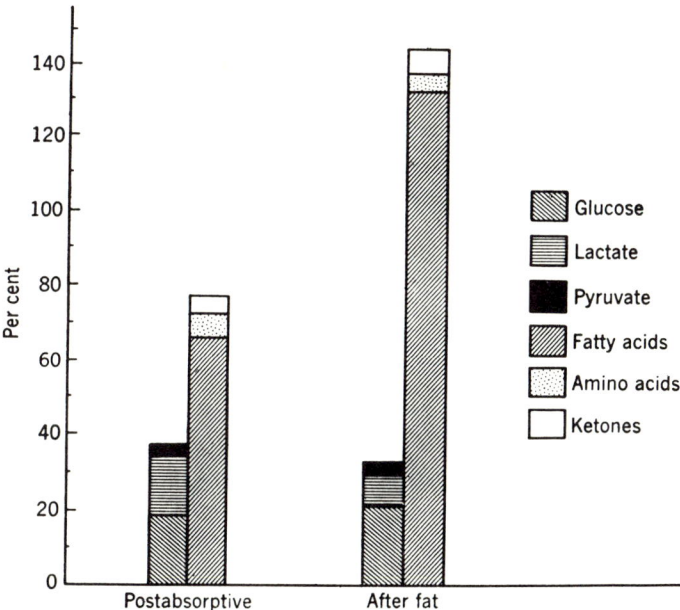

Figure 17. Cardiac metabolism: increase in consumption of fatty acids by the heart after a high fat meal.

the coronary arterial-venous glucose difference is less than 4 mg. per cent; as the arterial glucose concentration increases, the myocardial extraction rises rapidly, until at blood concentrations above 110 mg. per cent, the extraction of glucose appears to have reached its maximal value. As in the case of glucose, myocardial utilization of lactate depends upon its arterial concentration. At normal blood concentration, glucose and lactate are used by the human heart in approximately equal amounts. Pyruvate is also utilized by the human heart, but the concentrations in blood as well as the myocardial utilization of this metabolite are small.

If complete oxidation of these metabolites is assumed, the total aerobic metabolism of carbohydrates in man and dog can apparently account only for approximately 35 per cent of the total myocardial oxygen extraction. This calculation suggests that the heart also utilizes non-carbohydrate material as fuel. Consistent with this view is the demonstration that the human and dog heart can utilize considerable quantities of fatty acids, ketone bodies, and amino acids; myocardial usage of fatty acids is particularly pronounced after a meal rich in fat and it is likely that the heart stores fatty acids after an increase in the level of circulating fatty acids (3, 11). More recent studies have disclosed that the principal lipid fraction of plasma concerned with the transport and metabolism of fatty acids is the non-esterified free fatty acid fraction of the plasma (FFA), and that the heart uses considerable amounts of FFA. But even though the heart can extract fairly large amounts of FFA, even in the fasting state FFA accounts for less than half of the myocardial extraction of the total fatty acids (TFA) (30, 3).

Significant differences exist between the free fatty acid composition of arterial and coronary sinus blood (3). The proportion of oleic acid in coronary sinus blood is lower than that in arterial blood, demonstrating a high degree of extraction. In both man and dog, the percentage of palmitic acid in coronary sinus blood is higher than that in arterial blood, and in the dog the proportion of stearic acid is also higher in coronary sinus blood, demonstrating a low rate of myocardial uptake. Thus, although the percentage of an individual free fatty acid may be greater in coronary sinus than in arterial blood, the level of this free fatty acid can still be lower as a result of its myocardial extraction. Therefore, the human as well as the dog heart extracts all individual fatty acids analyzed. However, there exist significant differences in the rate of myocardial uptake of individual free fatty acids. This is indicated by the relatively larger percentage of myocardial extraction of oleic acid.

Oleic acid is also released to a larger extent by subcutaneous adipose tissue; the percentage of myocardial extraction of palmitic and stearic acids as well as their release from adipose tissues are low (80). These observations suggest different turnover rates of individual free fatty acids. Although there are several possible explanations for the different rates of myocardial uptake of individual free fatty acids, it is likely that a preferential uptake of oleic acid by the heart muscle exists.

The aerobic metabolism of ketones accounts for approximately 5 per cent of the total myocardial oxygen extraction. In contrast to the heart-lung preparation, the human and the dog hearts *in situ* extract considerable quantities of amino acids from the coronary blood. After infusion of amino acids, as much as 40 per cent of the total cardiac oxygen consumption can be accounted for by aerobic metabolism of amino acids; a 20 per cent increase in the arterial concentration of amino acids produces a disproportionate increase in the myocardial extraction of 245 per cent.

Thus, the results obtained in the beating human heart *in situ* show that fatty acids, and particularly esterified fatty acids, contribute more to myocardial energy requirements than does any other substrate. In addition to fatty acids, the heart can utilize glucose, pyruvate, lactate, ketones, and amino acids.

Myocardial metabolism in diseases of the heart has also been investigated with the cardiac catheter (22). For example, in subjects with diabetes mellitus, the myocardial usage of carbohydrates is reduced and the utilization of non-carbohydrate material is increased; the ability of the diabetic human and dog heart to utilize lactate is conspicuously decreased. The utilization of fatty acids and of ketone bodies is also greater than in non-diabetic hearts. Insulin increases the myocardial utilization of fatty acids and ketones, but does not affect the myocardial usage or extraction of glucose despite a decrease in the blood sugar. These results imply that insulin causes a relative increase in myocardial utilization of glucose. The hormone appears to fail to correct the metabolic defect responsible for diminished myocardial lactate usage. Although the results obtained on the diabetic heart *in situ* demonstrate a great variety of metabolic defects, it is unlikely that these diffuse changes in energy production affect the energy utilization of the heart. It seems valid to conclude that the fundamental importance of diabetes in cardiology lies in its relation to coronary vascular disease.

Studies in patients with congestive heart failure as a result of arteriosclerotic, hypertensive, and valvular disease have revealed no particular disturbance of energy production (7). In addition to normal myocardial usage of substrates, patients with compensated or decompensated heart disease have normal coronary blood flow and normal myocardial oxygen usage *per weight* of heart muscle despite increased diastolic heart size. Since the failing heart during exercise can increase its oxygen uptake, there appears to be no impediment to the delivery of oxygen to the myocardium. Digitalis preparations also do not affect coronary blood flow or myocardial oxygen consumption in the normal or failing human heart, although they sometimes do affect potassium efflux from the heart. In addition, there is no significant effect of lanatoside-C on the utilization of myocardial substrates despite improvement of the work capacity of the failing heart. Relative lack of high-energy phosphate due to rapid deterioration or insufficient formation from normal oxidation must still be considered. However, no changes in the levels of ATP or creatine phosphate in chronic congestive failure have been reported in dogs with induced valvular disease. Furthermore, oxidative phosphorylation in mitochondria obtained from hearts of guinea pigs in chronic congestive failure is normal.

In most instances in which disturbances in energy production were present, heart failure was produced by localized ischemia resulting from ligation of the coronary arteries. It is important to differentiate between failure resulting from anoxia and its resulting metabolic changes on the one hand, and failure resulting from hypertensive, valvular, and long-standing arteriosclerotic heart disease on the other (23).

By exclusion, the evidence points therefore to the organs of energy utilization, the contractile proteins, as the site of myocardial derangements in heart failure resulting from hypertensive, arteriosclerotic, and valvular disease. Certain advances have been made within recent years to define this defect. For example, actomyosin bands prepared from failing human hearts appear to possess diminished contractility; it has also been demonstrated that there exist differences in certain physical chemical properties of myosin. However, because of the difficulties in the preparation of myosin, there is no uniform opinion on the chemical properties of myosin obtained from failing hearts.

Recent observations by Meerson and Zayats (62) have given certain clues to possible metabolic causes of alterations in contractile proteins of failing heart muscle. These workers found definite disturbances in protein synthesis in the myocardium during experimental heart failure and considered this to be an important factor in the development of failure. Apparently the loss of cardiac contractility is connected with a disturbance of the normal process of protein synthesis in heart muscle. The cause for diminished protein synthesis may be prolonged anoxia with reduced ATP synthesis, or more likely a deficiency of DNA, the latter brought about by relative increase in the size of cytoplasmic as compared to nuclear mass.

In contrast to these conditions which belong to the "non-metabolic" type of heart failure, there is a type of metabolic heart failure which results from anemia, anoxia, hyperthyroidism, and thiamine deficiency, and which may be found in the isolated heart of the heart-lung preparation.

The pattern of the effect of anoxia and ischemia on the heart muscle is well defined (23). There occurs a diminution in glycogen and high-energy phosphate, while the level of glucose-6-phosphate (G-6-P) increases. The ratio of phosphorylase a/b probably decreases. Under these conditions the enzyme phosphofructokinase becomes the rate-limiting enzyme. Even brief anoxia, as present during angina pectoris and localized anoxia during myocardial infarction, leads to demonstrable glycolysis as evidenced by increased lactate levels in coronary sinus blood. Consequently, cardiac failure occurring as a result of anoxia is initiated by deficiencies in energy production. In heart failure from severe anemia, there is increased cardiac output and tachycardia. Because of the decreased blood oxygen capacity, the myocardial oxygen extraction falls. However, the coronary blood flow rises markedly and the total myocardial oxygen consumption may be higher than in the normal person.

The effect of anoxia is particularly conspicuous in ventricular tachycardia and fibrillation. In ventricular tachycardia and fibrillation the activity of malic acid dehydrogenase in coronary sinus blood is elevated, and there is a diminution in cardiac glycogen, a slight rise in glucose-6-phosphate, a marked elevation in lactic acid, and a temporary increase in phosphorylase-a activity. When, however, in ventricular and atrial fibrillation and ventricular tachycardia the coronary circulation is maintained, no alterations in carbohydrate intermediates and phosphorylase-a activity are observed.

The changes in myocardial metabolism in shock are also primarily the result of myocardial anoxia (26). This was suggested by Wiggers on the basis of pressure and volume curves obtained from dogs during various phases of hemorrhagic shock (101). He and his co-workers proposed that deterioration of myocardial expulsive power resulting from anoxia may contribute to circulatory failure and that this myocardial depression is responsible for the irreversible shock during the normovolemic phase of hemorrhagic shock. During hemorrhagic shock in dogs, coronary blood flow diminishes during both oligemic and normovolemic phases. Myocardial oxygen usage declines. Many of the changes observed during the hypovolemic phase of hemorrhagic shock persist after re-transfusion of blood. The myocardial extraction

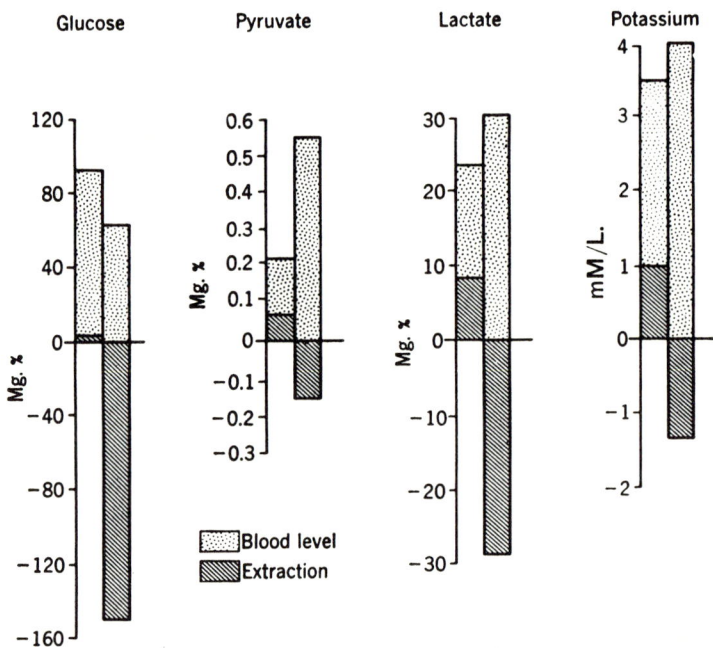

Figure 18. Cardiac metabolism: effects of ventricular fibrillation on glucose, pyruvate, lactate, and potassium extraction by the heart. Columns on the left are control values; on the right, values found during ventricular fibrillation. The concentrations of these metabolites in coronary venous blood exceed those in arterial blood during ventricular fibrillation, indicating elimination rather than absorption.

of lactate and pyruvate remains diminished while blood glucose levels fall to normal with increases in the blood volume. Thus, the essential change in myocardial metabolism in hemorrhagic shock is the result of myocardial anoxia resulting from diminished coronary flow. The heart participates in the general pattern of tissue anoxia as occurs in shock. The question has been asked as to whether the irreversibility of shock is related to or even caused by permanent myocardial changes in heart muscle. It does appear likely that myocardial anoxia produces irreversible changes in shock such as a fall in ATP, in phosphocreatine, and in glycogen; however, these metabolic events occur under the influence of anoxia in most body tissues. The irreversibility of shock, therefore, appears to be the dynamic expression of irreparable damage to metabolic processes produced by prolonged tissue anoxia.

The alterations in myocardial metabolism observed during experimentally produced coronary embolization and myocardial infarction also follow the pattern of myocardial anoxia (23). There is an almost immediate diminution in myocardial extraction of pyruvate and lactate. While these metabolic changes are reversible, they lead to changes in plasma enzyme activity associated with pathological events that take place many hours after coronary arterial embolization. Thus, the peak of plasma enzyme activity in the dog occurs twenty-four hours after embolization and is correlated with the height of coagulation necrosis of the myocardium.

As mentioned above, there are certain types of heart failure in which definite metabolic derangements in the heart muscle are present (22). Anemia and anoxia have already been discussed. In hyperthyroidism, it appears that the coronary blood flow, the myocardial substrate utilization, and the oxygen consumption are all increased. Myocardial oxygen utilization returns to normal following remission of thyrotoxicosis. The underlying metabolic disturbance may be sought in the action of the thyroid hormone which results in "uncoupling" of oxidative phosphorylation, leading to inefficient energy conservation; under these conditions more oxidation of substrates is required to produce the same amount of high-energy phosphate. Heart mitochondria are particularly susceptible to the effects of the hormone. It is therefore to be expected that high-energy phosphate compounds in these conditions are reduced in the heart muscle.

THE HEART

Thiamine deficiency resulting in beriberi affects primarily the nervous tissue, usually as a peripheral polyneuritis, and the heart. Beriberi heart disease has been produced in various laboratory animals by thiamine-deficient diet. Olson has studied the in vitro metabolism of cardiac muscle obtained from rats and ducks fed thiamine-deficient diets (*67*). Under these conditions, he was able to show that the rate of pyruvate utilization by slices of thiamine-deficient rat and duck ventricle was significantly reduced. There was also a relationship between the pyruvate disappearance and thiamine content of the ventricle. Apparently pyruvate utilization in these preparations did not fall until the thiamine content was reduced from a normal value of about 10 micrograms per gram to about 2.5 micrograms per gram. Hackel, Goodale, and Kleinerman (*36*), using coronary sinus catheterization, found that the coronary arteriovenous difference and total utilization of pyruvate in thiamine-deficient dogs were maintained within normal limits. However, the threshold for utilization of pyruvate was increased significantly, and the coefficient of its extraction was diminished. Apparently myocardial lactate extraction was inhibited more than pyruvate.

It is likely that in beriberi the heart participates in the general metabolic defect induced by thiamine deficiency. In contrast to heart failure resulting from arteriosclerotic, hypertensive, or valvular disease, beriberi heart disease is the result of deficient energy production.

In spontaneous failure of the isolated heart in the heart-lung preparation, the efficiency of the heart is greatly diminished (from 3 to 17 per cent as compared to 25 per cent for the heart *in situ*). This decline in mechanical efficiency of the isolated heart comes immediately after isolation of the organ; it is not the result of a diminution in fuel supply of the perfusate but depends upon continuity between the heart and the rest of the organism. Apparently inclusion of liver and spleen increases myocardial efficiency primarily by diminishing the myocardial oxygen consumption. The inclusion of these organs has no effect on the work of the isolated heart. Experiments undertaken in the author's laboratory reveal that the diminution in myocardial efficiency may be a consequence of the lack of catecholamines and acetylcholine in the perfusion fluid. By inclusion of liver and spleen in the perfusion circuit of the heart-lung preparation, these substances are added to the perfusion fluid, and the myocardial efficiency increases.

The feasibility of measuring coronary blood flow and cardiac metabolism simultaneously suggests an entirely new potentiality in cardiac research, namely, the use of the heart as a tool in the study of organ transplantation. As is well known, one of the most significant of recent advances in the medical sciences has been the knowledge gained in the mechanisms that govern homograft immunity (9). It has become apparent that transplantation immunity resulting in the rejection of the homograft is the result of antigens from the graft, which, on reaching the reticulo-endothelial system, stimulate the production of humoral antibodies. This immunity can be transferred from animal to animal by means of lymphoid cells prepared from the lymph nodes or spleen of a sensitized animal. The general concept of transplantation immunity and tolerance has mostly been gained from experiments on transplanted skin. These transplants afford the advantage that they are technically easy to carry out, but they have certain disadvantages. For example, alterations in metabolism of the graft that parallel the cellular changes are difficult to measure.

The transplanted heart, on the other hand, which permits precise measurement of organ blood flow, as well as the study of tissue metabolism, offers an ideal opportunity to analyze the alterations that accompany the onset of homograft immunity. Already, studies on the homografted heart have not only given information on mechanisms of homograft immunity but they have also shown possible new avenues for investigation of myocardial metabolism in general. One of the most interesting findings on the homografted heart has been the discovery that despite the presence of glycolysis, the enzymes and coenzymes concerned with the respiratory chain are still intact. This has been illustrated by the fact that the difference in oxidation-reduction potential between coronary arterial and venous blood is positive, in contrast to negative differences in potential as calculated from blood perfusing hearts in which the coronary circulation had been interrupted or impaired. Apparently, as first shown by Gudbjarnason (35), it is possible by means of the measurement of oxidation-reduction potentials in arterial and coronary vein blood to obtain information on the integrity of the respiratory chain; likewise, one can determine the absence or presence of glycolysis by the appearance of lactate and pyruvate in coronary vein blood and by the calculation of the percentages of glucose-oxygen extraction ratios.

Thus, it has been shown that homograft rejection results in increased cell permeability, which leads to loss of enzymes and coenzymes from the cell. There is a causal relationship between enzyme loss and metabolic function. Apparently, permeability changes of the cell play a primary role in the mechanism of the metabolic changes of the homografted heart.

The validity of present concepts on the coronary circulation and on cardiac metabolism will be tested during the centuries to come. It appears to the writer that there will be an increasing tendency to move away from studies on isolated artificial models and to concentrate on investigations of the whole human heart *in situ*. This will depend on the development of new experimental tools. It is here that our sister sciences, chemistry and physics, will have to lend a helping hand.

BIBLIOGRAPHY

1. ABERNETHY, J. Observations on the foramina Thebesii of the heart. Philos. Trans., p. 103, 1798.
2. ARISTOTLE. Opera omnia, Graece et Latine, cum indice nominum et rerum absolutissimo. Paris. Firmin-Didot, 1874–1889.
3. BALLARD, F. B., W. H. DANFORTH, S. NAEGLE, and R. J. BING. Myocardial metabolism of fatty acids. J. clin. Invest., 39:717, 1960.
4. BERENGARIO DA CARPI, G. A Short Introduction to Anatomy. (Isagogae breves.) Tr. by R. L. Lind. Chicago, University of Chicago Press, 1959.
5. BEZOLD, A. VON, and E. BREYMAN. Veränderungen des Herzschlages nach dem Verschlusse der Coronarnerven. Untersuchungen physiol. Lab. Würzburg. 1. Heft:288, 1867.
6. BING, R. J. The metabolism of the heart. Harvey Lect., 50:27, 1954–55.
7. BING, R. J. Metabolic activity of the intact heart. Amer. J. Med., 30:679, 1961.
8. BING, R. J., J. D. CHOUDHURY, G. MICHAL, and K. KAKO. Myocardial metabolism. Ann. intern. Med., 49:1201, 1958.
9. BING, R. J., A. CHRYSOHOU, S. CHIBA, and P. L. WOLF. Metabolic, histologic, and histochemical aspects of the homografted heart. Trans. Ass. Amer. Phys., 74:318, 1961.

10. BING, R. J., M. M. HAMMOND, J. C. HANDELSMAN, S. R. POWERS, F. C. SPENCER, J. E. ECKENHOFF, W. T. GOODALE, J. H. HAFKENSCHIEL, and S. S. KETY. The measurement of coronary blood flow, oxygen consumption, and efficiency of the left ventricle in man. Amer. Heart J., 38:1, 1949.
11. BING, R. J., A. SIEGEL, I. UNGAR, and M. GILBERT. Metabolism of the human heart. II. Studies on fat, ketone, and amino acid metabolism. Amer. J. Med., 16:504, 1954.
12. BLUMGART, H. L., P. M. ZOLL, A. S. FREEDBERG, and D. R. GILLIGAN. The experimental production of intercoronary arterial anastomoses and their functional significance. Circulation, 1:10, 1950.
13. BOCHDALEK, V. Zur Anatomie des menschlichen Herzens. Arch. Anat., p. 302, 1868.
14. BOHR, C., and V. HENRIQUES. Ueber die Blutmenge, welche den Herzmuskel durchstromt. Skand. Arch. Physiol., 5:232, 1895.
15. BRÜCKE, E. VON. Der Verschluss der Kranzschlagadern durch die Aortenklappen. Wien, Gerold, 1855.
16. BURNS, A. Observations on Some of the Most Frequent and Important Diseases of the Heart; an Aneurism of the Thoracic Aorta; on Preternatural Pulsation in the Epigastric Region; and on the Unusual origin and distribution of some of the Large Arteries of the Human Body. Edinburgh, Bryce, 1809.
17. CHAUCER, G. Works, vol. 4. The Canterbury Tales. Ed. by W. W. Skeat. Oxford, Clarendon Press, 1900.
18. CHIRAC, P. De motu cordis adversaria analytica. Monspelii, Martel, 1698.
19. COHNHEIM, J., and A. VON SCHULTHEISS-RECHBERG. Ueber die Folgen der Kranzarterienverschliessung fur das Herz. Virchows Arch. path. Anat., 85:503, 1881.
20. CORVISART, J.-N. Essai sur les maladies et les lesions organiques du cœur et des gros vaisseaux. Paris, Migneret, 1806.
21. DALTON, J. C. Doctrines of the Circulation; A History of Physiological Opinion and Discovery, in Regard to the Circulation of the Blood. Philadelphia, Lea, 1884.
22. DANFORTH, W. H., F. B. BALLARD, K. KAKO, J. D. CHOUDHURY, and R. J. BING. Metabolism of the heart in failure. Circulation, 21:112, 1960.
23. DANFORTH, W. H., and R. J. BING. The heart in anoxia and ischaemia. Brit. J. Anaesth, 30:456, 1958.
24. DAWSON, W. R. The Beginnings: Egypt and Assyria. New York, Hoeber, 1930.
25. EDELSTEIN, L. Andreas Vesalius, the humanist. Bull. Hist Med., 14:547, 1943.

26. EDWARDS, W. S., W. E. REBER, A. SIEGEL, and R. J. BING. Coronary blood flow and myocardial oxygen consumption in hemorrhagic shock. Surg. Forum, 4:505, 1953.
27. ERICHSEN, J. E. On the influence of the coronary circulation on the action of the heart. Med. Gazette, n.s. 30:561, 1842.
28. EVANS, C. L. The metabolism of cardiac muscle. Rec. Advanc. Physiol., 6:157, 1939.
29. FOTHERGILL, J. A Complete Collection of the Medical and Philosophical Works, with ... Life and ... Notes. Ed. by J. Elliot. London, Robinson, 1782.
30. GORDON, R. S., and A. CHERKES. Unesterified fatty acids in human blood plasma. J. clin. Invest., 35:206, 1956.
31. GORLIN, R., N. BRACHFELD, C. MACLEOD, and P. BOPP. Effect of nitroglycerin on the coronary circulation in patients with coronary artery disease of increased left ventricular work. Circulation, 19:705, 1959.
32. GREEN, D. E. Studies in organized enzyme systems. Harvey Lect., 52:177, 1956–57.
33. GREGG, D. E. Coronary Circulation in Health and Disease. Philadelphia, Lea and Febiger, 1950.
34. GROSS, L. The Blood Supply to the Heart; in Its Anatomical and Clinical Aspects. New York, Hoeber, 1921.
35. GUDBJARNASON, S., and R. J. BING. The redox-potential of the lactate-pyruvate system in blood as an indicator of the functional state of cellular oxidation. Biochim. biophys. Act., 60:158, 1962.
36. HACKEL, D. B., W. T. GOODALE, and J. KLEINERMAN. Effects of thiamin deficiency on myocardial metabolism in intact dogs. Amer. Heart J., 46:883, 1953.
37. HALL, M. On the Mutual Relations between Anatomy, Physiology, Pathology and Therapeutics, and the Practice of Medicine. The Gulstonian Lectures for 1842. London, Baillière, 1842.
38. HALLER, A. VON. First Lines of Physiology. Tr. from the Correct Latin Edition. 1:75. Edinburgh, Elliot, 1786.
39. HAMBURGER, W. W. The earliest known reference to the heart and circulation. The Edwin Smith Surgical Papyrus, circa 3000 B.C. Amer. Heart J., 17:259, 1939.
40. HARVEY, W. Exercitatio anatomica de motu cordis et sanguinis in animalibus. Tr. by C. D. Leake. Springfield, Ill., Thomas, 1928.
41. HEBERDEN, W. Commentaries on the History and Cure of Diseases. Boston, Wells and Lilly, 1818.
42. HERRICK, J. B. Clinical features of sudden obstruction of the coronary arteries. J. Amer. med. Assn. 59:2015, 1912.
43. HERRICK, J. B. Allan Burns: 1781–1813: Anatomist, Surgeon, and Cardiologist. Bull. Soc. med. Hist., 4:457, 1935.

44. HERRICK, J. B. A Short History of Cardiology. Springfield, Ill., Thomas, 1942.
45. HESELER, B. Andreas Vesalius' First Public Anatomy at Bologna, 1540; an Eyewitness Report. Tr. by R. Eriksson. Uppsala, Almqvist & Wiksells, 1959.
46. HUNTER, J. A treatise on the blood, inflammation, and gun-shot wounds. To which is prefixed a short account of the author's life, by his brother-in-law, Everard Home. London, Richardson, 1794.
47. KATZ, L. N. Analysis of the several factors regulating the performance of the heart. Physiol. Rev., 35:91, 1955.
48. KELLETT, C. E. The life and work of Raymond de Vieussens. Ann. med. Hist., 3rd ser. 4:31, 1942.
49. KETY, S. S., and C. F. SCHMIDT. The determination of cerebral blood flow in man by the use of nitrous oxide in low concentrations. Amer. J. Physiol., 143:53, 1945.
50. KLUG, F. Zur Theorie des Blutstroms in der Arteria coronaria cordis. Zbl. med. Wiss., 14:133, 1876.
51. KRISTELLER, P. O. The School of Salerno. Bull. Hist. Med., 17:138, 1945.
52. KRONECKER, H. K., and McGUIRE, J. Ueber die Speisung des Froschherzens. Arch. Anat. Physiol., Physiol. Abt., p. 321, 1878.
53. LAËNNEC, R. T. H. A Treatise on the Diseases of the Chest in which They are Described According to Their Anatomical Characters. Philadelphia, Weber, 1823.
54. LANGENDORFF, O. Zur Kenntniss des Blutlaufs in den Kranzgefässen des Herzens. Pflüg. Arch. Physiol., 78:423, 1899.
55. LANGER, L. J. Die Foramina Thebesii im Herzen des Menschen. S.B. Akad. Wiss., Wien, Math.-Naturw. Kl. 3. Abt., 82:25, 1880.
56. LAVOISIER, A. L. Traité élémentaire de chimie, présenté dans un ordre nouveau, et d'après les découvertes modernes. 3rd ed. Paris, Deterville, 1801.
57. LEYDEN, E. VON. Ueber die Sclerose der Coronar-Arterien und die davon abhängigen Krankheitszustände. Z. klin. Med., 7:459, 1884.
58. LOCKE, F. S., and O. ROSENHEIM. The effect of certain sugars on the isolated mammalian heart. J. Physiol. (Lond.), 31:XIV, 1904.
59. LOCKE, F. S., and O. ROSENHEIM. Contributions to the physiology of the isolated heart. The consumption of dextrose by mammalian cardiac muscle. J. Physiol. (Lond.), 36:205, 1907.
60. LOWER, R. De corde. In R. T. Gunther. Early Science in Oxford, v. IX. Tr. by K. J. Franklin. Oxford, 1932.
61. MARKWALDER, J., and E. H. STARLING. A note on some factors which determine the blood-flow through the coronary circulation. J. Physiol. (Lond.), 47:275, 1913.

62. MEERSON, F. Z., and T. L. ZAYATS. Changes in the intensity of protein synthesis in the myocardium during compensatory hyperfunction of the heart. Bull. exp. Biol. Med. (Engl. ed.), 60:678, 1960.
63. MORAWITZ, P., and A. ZAHN. Untersuchungen über den Coronarkreislauf. Dtsch. Arch. klin. Med., 116:364, 1914.
64. MORGAGNI, G. B. De sedibus et causis morborum per anatomen indagatis. Venice, Ex Typographia Remondiniana, 1761.
65. NEWELL-MARTIN, H., and W. J. SEDGWICK. Observations on the mean pressure and the characters of the pulse-wave in the coronary arteries of the heart. J. Physiol. (Lond.), 3:165, 1882.
66. NEWTON, I. Philosophiae Naturalis Principia Mathematica. 3rd ed. London, Innys, 1726.
67. OLSON, R. E., O. H. PEARSON, O. N. MILLER, and F. J. STARE. The effect of vitamin deficiencies upon the metabolism of cardiac muscle in vitro. I. The effect of thiamine deficiency in rats and ducks. J. biol. Chem., 175:489, 1948.
68. ORDRONAUX, J. Code of Health of the School of Salerno. Philadelphia, Lippincott, 1870.
69. PANUM, P. L. Experimentelle Beiträge zur Lehre von der Emboli. Virchows Arch. path. Anat., 25:308, 1862.
70. PAPYRUS, EBERS. Tr. by C. P. Bryan. London, Bles, 1930.
71. PARRY, C. H. Collected Works, vol. I. London, Underwood, 1825.
72. PETTENKOFER, M. VON, and C. VOIT. Untersuchungen über den Stoffverbrauch des normalen Menschen. Z. Biol., 2:459, 1866.
73. PRATT, F. H. The nutrition of the heart through the vessels of Thebesius and the coronary veins. Amer. J. Physiol., 1:86, 1898.
74. QUAIN, R. On fatty diseases of the heart. Med. Chir. Trans., 33:120, 1850.
75. RANDALL, J. H., JR. The Making of the Modern Mind; a Survey of the Intellectual Background of the Present Age. Boston, Houghton Mifflin, 1940.
76. REBATEL, F. Recherches expérimentales sur la circulation dans les artères coronaires. Thèse (§ 288), Paris, 1872.
77. REGNAULT, V., and J. REISET. Recherches chimiques sur la respiration des animaux des diverses classes. Ann. Chim. Phys. 26, 299, 1849.
78. REYNOLDS, S. R. M., M. KIRSCH, and R. J. BING. Functional capillary beds in the beating, KC1-arrested and KC1-arrested-perfused myocardium of the dog. Circulation Res., 6:600, 1958.
79. RIOLAN, J. Encheiridium anatomicum et pathologicum. Paris, Meturas, 1648.
80. ROTHLIN, M. E., and R. J. BING. Extraction and release of individual free fatty acids by the heart and fat depots. J. clin. Invest., 40:1380, 1961.

81. RUBNER, M. Die Quelle der thierischen Wärme. Z. Biol., 30:73, 1894.
82. RUFFER, M. A. On arterial lesions found in Egyptian mummies (1580 B.C.–A.D. 525). J. Path. Bact., 15:453, 1911.
83. SAUNDERS, J. B. DE M., and C. D. O'MALLEY. The Illustrations from the Works of Andreas Vesalius of Brussels. Cleveland, World Publishing, 1950.
84. SEDGWICK, W. T., and H. W. TYLER. A Short History of Science. New York, Macmillan, 1918.
85. SENAC, J. B. DE. Traité de la structure du coeur, de son action et de ses maladies. 2nd ed. 2 vols. Paris, Barbon, 1777.
86. SENECA, L. A. Opera, Epist. 55, Basileae, 1529. (Quoted by C. Allbutt. Diseases of Arteries and Angina Pectoris, vol. 2, p. 319. London, Macmillan, 1915).
87. SINGER, C. The Fasciculo de Medicina, Venice, 1493. In Monumenta Medica, vol. II. H. E. Sigerist, Ed. Florence, Lier, 1925.
88. SINGER, C. A Short History of Anatomy and Physiology from the Greeks to Harvey. 2nd ed. New York, Dover, 1957.
89. SINGER, C., E. J. HOLMYARD, A. R. HALL, and T. J. WILLIAMS. A History of Technology, vol. III. Oxford, Oxford University Press, 1957.
90. SPENCER, F. C., D. L. MERRILL, S. R. POWERS, and R. J. BING. Coronary blood flow and cardiac oxygen consumption in unanesthetized dogs. Amer. J. Physiol., 160:149, 1950.
91. TIGERSTEDT, R. A. A. Die Physiologie des Kreislaufes. vol. I. 2nd ed. Berlin, De Gruyter, 1921.
92. VESALIUS, A. De humani corporis fabrica libri septum. Basileae, Oporini, 1543.
93. VESALIUS, A., and J. S. KALKAR. Tabulae anatomicae. Venice, D. Bernardi, 1538.
94. VIRCHOW, R. Thrombose und Embolie, Gefässentzundung und septische Infection. In his Gesammelte Abhandlungen zur wissenschaftlichen Medicin. Frankfurt, Meidinger, 1856.
95. VOIT, C. Das Isodynamiegesetz. Münch. med. Wschr. 49:233, 1902.
96. VOIT, C., and M. VON PETTENKOFER. Untersuchungen über den Stoffverbrauch des normalen Menschen Z. Biol., 2:465, 1886.
97. WEARN, J. T. The role of the Thebesian vessels in the circulation of the heart. J. exp. Med., 47:293, 1928.
98. WEIGERT, C. Ueber die pathologischen Gerinnungsvorgänge. Virchows Arch. path. Anat., 79:87, 1880.
99. WEIZSACKER, V. VON. Stoffwechsel und Wärmebildung des Herzens. In Handbuch der normalen und pathologischen Physiologie, 71:689. Berlin, Springer, 1926.

100. WHITEHEAD, A. N. Science and the Modern World. New York, Macmillan, 1930.
101. WIGGERS, C. J. The Pressure Pulses in the Cardiovascular System. New York, Longmans, Green, 1928.
102. WIGGERS, C. J. The functional consequences of coronary occlusion. Ann. intern. Med., 23:158, 1945.
103. WIGGERS, C. Physiology in Health and Disease. 5th ed. Philadelphia, Lea and Febiger, 1949.
104. WINSLOW, C. E. A., and R. R. BELLINGER. Hippocratic and Galenic concepts of metabolism. Bull. Hist. Med., 17:12, 1945.
105. WINTERSTEIN, L. Ueber die Säuerstoffatmung des isolierten Säugetierherzens. Z. allg. Physiol., 4:333, 1904.
106. ZIEGLER, E. Lehrbuch der allgemeinen und speciellen pathologischen Anatomie für Arzte. Jena, Fischer, 1881.
107. ZILBOORG, G. Psychological sidelights on Andreas Vesalius. Bull. Hist. Med., 14:562, 1943.

V

Electrocardiography

ELECTROPHYSIOLOGY was created within the science of electricity rather than physiology. In this chapter we shall begin with an account of the early history of electricity, describe the first observations and experiments in electrophysiology, and show how eventually this became a science of its own. Electrocardiography arose as a particular phase of electrophysiology, and developed almost wholly through advances in electrophysical concepts and instrumentation.

Knowledge of electrical phenomena in ancient times was derived from four sources: the electric ray or torpedo fish, rubbed amber, the lodestone, and terrestrial lightning. For many centuries there was no awareness that any relation existed between them. It has been a special achievement of the discoverers, the "frontier" men (196), in this branch of science to have had the imagination and the experimental skill to bring together these apparently disparate phenomena. These interrelations were established over a total period of nearly two hundred years. One of the sciences created out of this conjunction was electrophysiology.

Let us briefly sketch the available knowledge of these four elements of electricity, as it existed before the age of experiment.

Torpedo mamorata, the torpedo fish or electric ray, and *Malapterurus electricus*, the electric catfish, were known to the ancients. The shock or torpor produced by the sting of the fish was said to have been used by the Greeks to treat headaches, epilepsy, and even the pains of childbirth (6).

Amber, the Greek *electron*. The property possessed by fossilized resins, such as amber, or fossilized carbon, such as jet, to attract straw, feathers, or other light objects when rubbed, was apparently known in early antiquity (*84*), though in recording this, legend may often have taken the place of fact. The property was said to have been familiar to the Chinese Emperor Hoang-Ti, 2635 B.C., to King Solomon (1033–973 B.C.), to Thales of Miletus (600 B.C.), and thence to succeeding Greek and Roman philosophers.

Lodestone. Magneta stone, stone from Magnesia in Thessaly. The attraction of the lodestone, magnetized iron, for other iron was familiar to the ancients at least as far back as 800 B.C. (*19*). It is mentioned in Homer, and was well known to philosophers during and after the Age of Pericles. Plato, in his charming dialogue on the reading of Homer (*176*), uses the lodestone in a major theme of his discourse:

> *"For as I was saying just now, this is not an art in you, whereby you speak well on Homer, but a divine power, which moves you like that in the stone which Euripides named Magnetis, but most people call Heraclea. For this stone not only attracts iron rings but also imparts to them a power whereby they in turn are able to do the very same thing as the stone, and attract other rings; so that sometimes there is formed quite a long chain of bits of iron and rings, suspended one from another; and they all depend for this power on that one stone."*

Centuries later, Lucretius (96–55 B.C.), in *De rerum natura*, carried the study further, noting that bronze particles were inert, and that sometimes iron particles would be repelled rather than attracted. He attributed the attraction to a sort of vacuum or "emptiness" in the space around the lodestone, causing iron particles to rush in to fill it.

The history of the relation of the lodestone to the magnetized needle, and thus to the mariner's compass, is more intriguing and more uncertain (*19*). The legend that the compass was invented in ancient China, and transmitted after many centuries to Europe via Arabia, is now considered doubtful (*84*). The earliest record, in a Chinese dictionary of A.D. 121, mentions only that the lodestone can attract an iron needle. The Chinese seem to have known also that a freely moving magnetized needle points to the meridian, though they probably did not use this as a compass in navigation. How or where this invention was discovered, whether it occurred in the Orient, or Arabia, or Europe, remains obscure. The earliest Italian compasses were needles lying on reeds and floating freely in water.

One of the first clear descriptions of the use of the magnetic needle in navigation is given in the writings of the English schoolman Alexander Neckam (1157–1217) (*16, 41*). This distinguished scholar was famous also for the fact that he was born on the same night as Richard the Lion-hearted, and was indeed the prince's foster brother; Neckam's mother, a healthy young matron of Saint Albans, nursed them both. Neckam wrote two books on science, *De utensilibus* and *De naturis rerum*. In these he discussed the mariner's compass as though it were a matter of common knowledge of the time. His description (*41*) was precise:

"*Mariners at sea when, through cloudy weather in the day which hides the sun, or through the darkness of the night, they lose the knowledge of the quarter of the world to which they are sailing, touch a needle with the magnet, which will turn around till, on its motion ceasing, its point will be directed toward the north.*"

Neckam apparently was writing about a needle suspended on a pivot. By the thirteenth century, the standard mariner's compass was known throughout Europe.

Terrestrial lightning, the thunderbolt of Zeus, was an object of awe and terror. Everyone knew its incredible destructive power. Not until the eighteenth century was the possibility explored of a relation between lightning and the small devices made by man.

The first scientist to study the phenomena of electricity methodically, and one of the great scientists of all time, was William Gilbert (1544–1603) (*6, 84*). He was also one of the earliest of the long succession of scientific men to come out of the University of Cambridge. He entered St. John's College in 1558 and received his medical doctorate from the University in 1569. After traveling and studying in various parts of Europe for three years, Gilbert returned to England and settled down to practice medicine in London. He rose steadily in his profession, was president of the College of Physicians in 1599, and two years later became physician to Queen Elizabeth. The Queen died in 1603, and Gilbert survived her by only a few months, dying, probably of the plague, in the last days of that same year.

The characteristic of William Gilbert's scientific achievement was his strict adherence to experiment: "Nothing has been set down in his

THE HEART

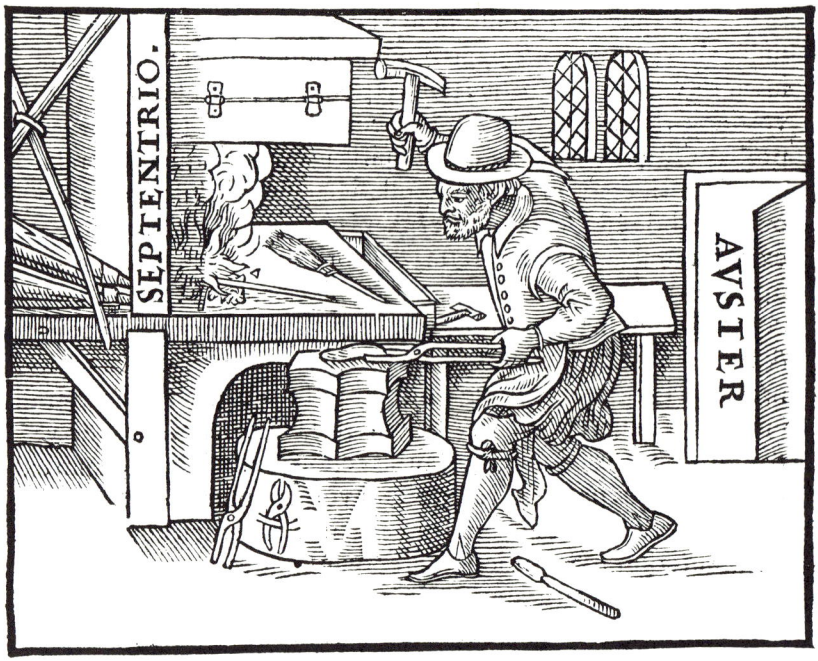

Figure 1. Gilbert's method of magnetization by repeated blows to a bar of metal held in the direction of the Earth's magnetic field.

book which hath not been explored and many times performed and repeated by himself" (*19*).

Gilbert coined the terms "electric" and "charged body." He showed that rubbed or charged amber attracted the magnetic needle, and that a rod of iron, if pointed toward the meridian, acquired a magnetic charge when heated and hammered. In terrestrial magnetism he made the broad and remarkably imaginative generalization that the Earth itself, a large rotating body, is a magnet, and so the ultimate cause of the constant deflection of the magnetic needle.

His major findings were published in 1600 in his book, *De Magnete, magneticisque corporibus, et de magno magnete tellure* (*94*).

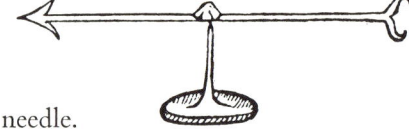

Figure 2. Gilbert's versorium or electrical needle.

William Gilbert established on a firm experimental basis the first principles of the new science of electricity. A few years the senior of William Harvey, he preceded the latter as Royal physician, and Gilbert's life ended just as Harvey's active life began.

The next hundred years, the "Century of Genius" in science (*220*), brought fundamental discoveries in electricity. The elegance and the striking character of the experiments made electricity also a highly fashionable topic of the time.

Otto von Guericke (1602–86), at the age of seventy, invented the first electric machine. This machine was a rotating globe of sulphur (later made of glass), which became highly charged when rubbed against the hand (*23*). Robert Boyle showed that the attraction between rubbed body and test object is mutual (*84*). Stephen Gray (1696–1736), in 1732, made the fundamental distinction between insulators and conductors; and at about the same time Charles Du Fay (1699–1739) discovered the mutual repulsion of similarly charged and the attraction of dissimilarly charged bodies. Du Fay also showed that "all substances could be electrified by friction, but that to electrify conductors they must be insulated or supported by non-conductors" (*84*). By successive advances the basic properties of this strange force were being established.

In the mid eighteenth century, spectacular experiments with frictional electricity were exciting popular as well as scientific interest. In 1745, Ewald von Kleist, Bishop of Pomerania, transferred the charge from an electric machine and stored it in a glass bottle. Von Kleist was one of the first to receive an electric shock from these powerful static machines (*101*). Having pushed an iron rod through the cork of a bottle full of mercury, he held the rod to the conductor of an electric machine. Accidentally he touched the conductor with his other hand and received a violent shock in his arm.

At almost the same time a group of physicists in Leiden, led by Pieter van Musschenbroek (1692–1761), were conducting similar experiments with charged bottles (*101*).

"*Cuneus, . . . a celebrated physicist . . . was one day trying to electrify some water in a wide-necked bottle. For this purpose he held the bottle in one hand after having placed in the bottle a metal rod connected to the machine.*

When he thought the water was sufficiently electrified, he tried to remove the iron rod with one hand, without loosing his hold of the bottle with the other hand. He received a shock that surprised him. [His teacher,] Musschenbroek repeated Cuneus's experiment, but the shock that he received in his arm, shoulders, and chest was so great that he lost consciousness, and he was so frightened that, in writing to Réaumur about this, then new, discovery, he wrote that for nothing in the world, not even for the crown of France, would he go through it again."

Abbé Nollet (Jean-Antoine Nollet, 1700–70) learned of Musschenbroek's experience and recognized the spectacular significance of this accident. He adopted the name, Leyden jar, in his excellent report (*101, 23*).

Soon the Leyden jar was improved, lined inside and out with metal foil, and handled with greater caution. With the development of powerful frictional machines, it was possible by 1750 to produce large sparks with the charge of a Leyden jar and discharges great enough to kill small animals or to be transmitted through long circuits of wire or water. The Leyden jar or condenser aroused considerable interest in electrical experimentation, besides providing occasional "hair raising" entertainment for the laity (*201*), such as shocking 180 soldiers of the guard of Louis XIV or 700 monks from the Convent de Paris, each joined to the next by a piece of wire clasped in the left hand of one and the right hand of his neighbor (*46*). Sir William Watson (1715–87) in England first observed the flash of light when a Leyden jar is discharged.

A number of earlier scientists, such as Francis Hawksbee and Abbé Nollet, had noted the similarity between lightning and the electric spark, and between thunder and the snap and crackle of the spark, but it remained for the great American scientist Benjamin Franklin (1706–90) to establish their identity by experiment. He was not aware at the time of European theories and experiments. Franklin had noticed the powerful action of pointed conductors in "drawing off" a charge silently, and speculated that if thunderclouds were positively charged, the fact could be shown by drawing electricity away to a high pointed conductor. In his famous kite experiment at Philadelphia in 1752, Franklin charged a Leyden jar from the key attached to the twine of the kite which he flew among the thunderclouds. From the electricity thus obtained and stored, he performed many experiments formerly made by excited "electrics" (*84, 89*).

In the latter half of the eighteenth century, electrical science became preoccupied with quantitative measurement, instrumentation, and theory (*102*). Examples include the gold leaf electroscope invented in 1786 by the Rev. Abraham Bennet, Henly's semaphore electroscope, and Coulomb's magnetic torsion balance (*102, 23*).

This was an exciting era. Elsewhere in Europe, other developments were taking place. John Canton (1718-72) discovered electrostatic induction. Pyroelectricity, the power of some minerals to become electrified when merely heated and their ability to exhibit positive and negative electricity, was characterized. Henry Cavendish (1731-1810), that strange and lonely genius, made exact measurements of electrical capacity. In 1781, he anticipated the fundamental law of electric flow, which was later rediscovered independently by G. S. Ohm in 1827, and became known as Ohm's Law. By the close of the eighteenth century, Laplace, Biot, Poisson, Priestley, Robison, and Coulomb had made their contributions to the mathematical formulation of electricity (*84, 102*).

Animal Electricity: Early Development

The strange, numbing power of the torpedo fish, familiar to the ancients, began to arouse interest of inquiring experimenters again toward the end of the seventeenth century. E. Bancroft in 1676 made the definite suggestion that the active discharge of the torpedo fish might be electrical in origin (*84*). In 1773, John Walsh reported to the Royal Society a study of "Torpedoes found on the coast of England," and "conceived of the shock as being due to the release of a compressed electric fluid" (*216*). In the same issue of the Royal Society proceedings, John Hunter confirmed Walsh's anatomical and physiological findings (*125*). Four years later Henry Cavendish reported the reverse experiment, "An account of some attempts to imitate the effects of the torpedo, by electricity," in which an artificial torpedo made of wood and leather "gave shocks when submerged in salt water, its supply of electricity being a Leyden jar" (*44*).

But this approach to electrophysiology was soon overshadowed by the effects on animal tissues of powerful electric discharges from electric

THE HEART

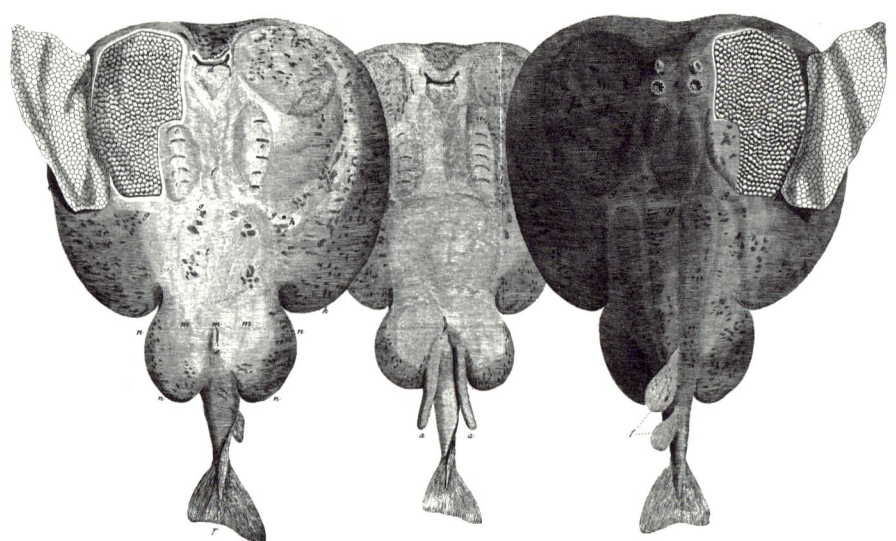

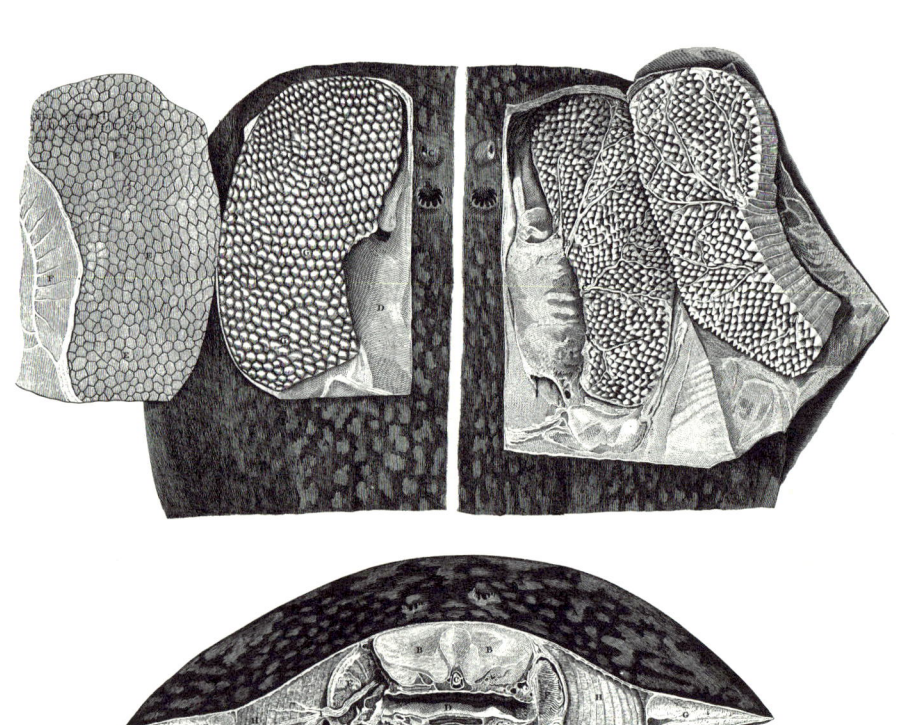

machines and Leyden jars. We have noted the violent shocks that early experimenters suffered from the discharge of these mechanical devices; their use in killing small animals; and the fashionable tricks of shocking large numbers of persons connected to one another by wire. In 1752, the year of Franklin's famous kite experiment in Philadelphia, Professor Richmann in St. Petersburg, Russia, was killed while performing a similar experiment, but with an improperly insulated rod (*102*).

In 1756, Leopoldo Caldani (1725–1813), former student of Morgagni, and then professor of medicine in Bologna, demonstrated the excitation of isolated nerve and muscle by discharge from a Leyden jar. Luigi Galvani was a student of Caldani's at the time.

Electricity had become the popular topic of the day, for hypothesis and speculation even more than for experiment. Here is a quotation from Felice Fontana, of the University of Pavia, in his "Treatise on the Venom of the Viper" (1781) (*85*):

"The considerable size of the nervous cylinders and blood-vessels, when compared with the primitive fleshy threads, leads me to suspect that these threads are not in motion, in any immediate way however, either by the blood, or by the nerves. In a word, we are not only ignorant of muscular motion, but we cannot even imagine any way to explain it, and we shall apparently be driven to have recourse to some other principle; that principle, if it be not common electricity, may be something, however, very analogous to it. The electrical gymnotus and torpedo, if they do not render the thing very probable, make it at least possible, and this principle may be believed to follow the most common laws of electricity. It may likewise be more modified in the nerves than in the torpedo or gymnotus. The nerves should be the organs destined to conduct the fluid, and perhaps also to excite it, but here everything yet remains to be done. We must first assure ourselves by certain experiments, whether there is really an electrical principle in the contracting muscles; we must determine

---

Figure 3. The torpedo fish.

A. Drawings by Walsh, who established that the numbing action of the torpedo fish is electrically comparable to that obtained from a Leyden jar.

B. Details of dissection by John Hunter. *Upper left:* the upper surface of the electric organ. *Upper right:* the right electric organ divided horizontally at the site of entry of the nerves. *Bottom:* a perpendicular section of the torpedo a little below its inspiratory openings.

the laws that this fluid observes in the human body; and after all it will yet remain to be known what it is that excites this principle, and how it is excited. How many things are left in an uncertain state, to posterity!"

THE HEART

Such was the "state of the art," when Luigi Galvani (1737–98) performed the first of his classic experiments, some time about the year 1780.

The career of this remarkable man was a mixture of triumph and frustration. His initial great discoveries were followed by years of controversy, during which he strove vainly to uphold a mistaken hypothesis. His personal life was equally tragic. Sue, a French contemporary, writing a "history of galvanism" in 1802, summarizes his life thus (*205*):

"Louis Galvani was born in Bologna, September 9, 1737. . . . After his studies, he became a doctor and soon after married the daughter of Professor Galeazzi whose works are so renowned in Italy. Galvani was still very young when he was given work as honorable as it was important. He had great success in comparative anatomy, made many dissections on birds, and published an article on the urinary apparatus of birds. . . .

"Such was his work before that which led him to the discovery of Galvanism. This great man was a victim of all the misfortunes which can afflict a sensitive and tender soul. He saw his dear Lucia (the name which he gave to his wife) die in his arms; he lost all his positions because he constantly refused to give the civic oath required by the decrees of the Cisalpine Republic. Death struck him, took away from him almost all those near to him. Finally, tormented himself for a long time by severe pain in his stomach, which medical men suspected came from an obstruction of the pylorus, he fell into a state of marasmus and languor, the progress of which the care of doctors . . . could not stop. He died on the fourteenth of Frimaire of the seventh year [of the French Republic, 1797], at the age of 60."

The course of Galvani's scientific achievement is of first importance in the history of this subject. Appointed lecturer at the University of Bologna at the age of twenty-five, and later appointed professor of anatomy, Galvani continued the experiments with the electric machine and with animal tissues which he had begun as a student under Caldani.

The key observation, identifying nerve-muscle contraction with

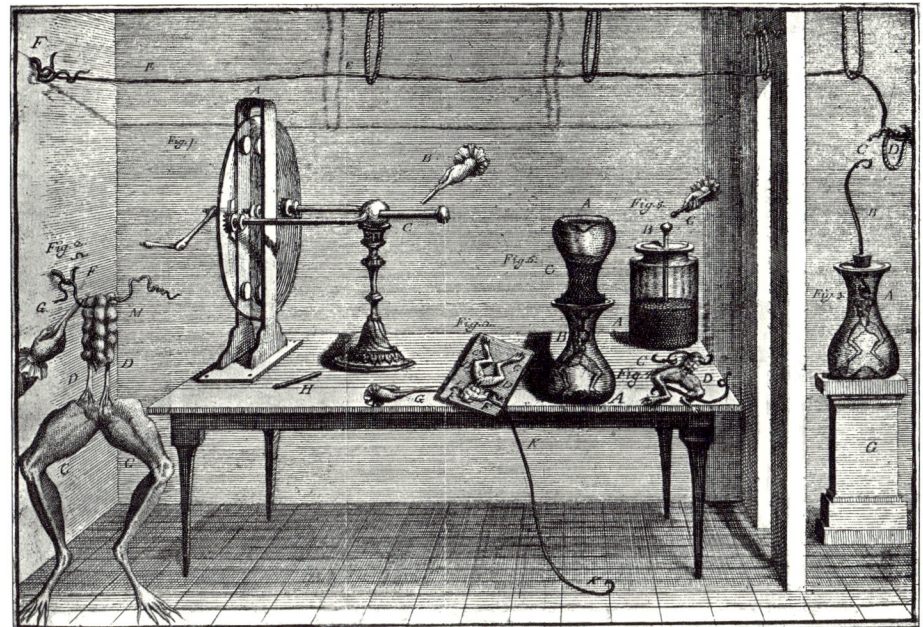

Figure 4. Galvani's drawing of his friction machine.

electrical stimulation, occurred, according to Galvani's own description, as follows (*90, 46*):

"*The course of the work has progressed in the following way. I dissected a frog and prepared it.... Having in mind other things, I placed the frog on the same table as an electrical machine ... so that the animal was completely separated from and removed at a considerable distance from the machine's conductor. When one of my assistants by chance lightly applied the point of a scalpel to the inner crural nerves ... suddenly all the muscles of the limbs were seen so to contract that they appeared to have fallen into violent tonic convulsions. Another assistant who was present when we were performing electrical experiments thought he observed that this phenomenon occurred when a spark was discharged from the conductor of the electrical machine.... Marvelling at this, he immediately brought the unusual phenomenon to my attention when I was completely engrossed and contemplating other things. Hereupon I became extremely enthusiastic and eager to repeat the experiment so as to clarify the obscure phenomenon and make it known. I myself, therefore,*

[275]

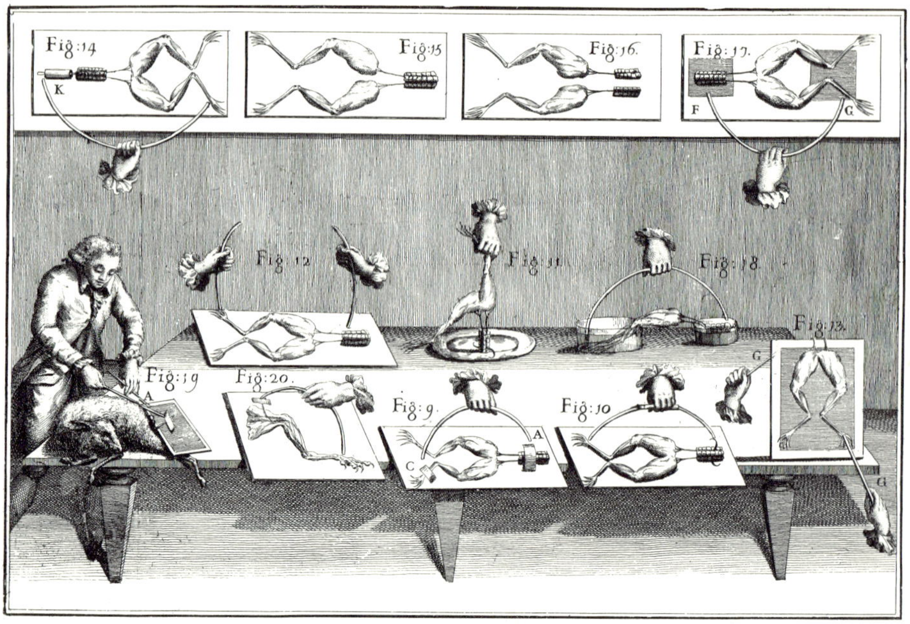

THE HEART

Figure 5. Experiments designed by Galvani to show animal electricity.

applied the point of the scalpel first to one then to the other crural nerve, while at the same time some one of the assistants produced a spark; the phenomenon repeated itself in precisely the same manner as before. Violent contractions were induced in the individual muscles of the limbs and the prepared animal reacted just as though it were seized with tetanus at the very moment when the sparks were discharged."

The next experiment, even more fundamental to the advancement of science, proved also to be the source of the great Galvani-Volta controversy. It was performed on September 20, 1786. Influenced by Franklin, Galvani tried to demonstrate that lightning flashes acted upon the limb in an identical fashion when similar electrical connections were made for it. To test the influence of atmospheric electricity on the muscles of the frog, he hung up a number of skinned frogs' legs on the balcony of his house, hooking the hind legs to the iron of the balcony by a copper wire which passed under the lumbar (crural) nerves. Galvani noted with surprise that every time their feet touched the balcony, the frog's limbs contracted, even though at that moment there were no signs of a storm cloud, and therefore no particular electric influence of the atmosphere. At first he thought this was due to the escape to earth of some atmospheric electricity accumulated in the frog. But he noticed that stimulation occurred when both metals (copper and iron) were in contact with some part of the body. Galvani pursued this new line of investigation with vigor and enthusiasm. He recreated the same conditions indoors. Placing a frog on an iron plate and pressing a brass hook against it produced similar muscular contractions. Other combinations of metals or even a circuit through his own body or a homogenous wire with which he made a conducting arc between nerve and muscle had the same effect, but insulators did not. Galvani reached the reasonable but erroneous conclusion that there was accumulated electricity inside the muscles which could be discharged by dissimilar metals, and thereby cause electrical stimulation. His account of these experiments was published in 1791, in his classic monograph, *Die viribus electricitatis in motu musculari commentarius* (*90, 182*).

Volta's alternative and correct theory, that the electric charge in Galvani's experiment was caused by the coupling of two dissimilar metals, spurred Galvani to extensive further investigations. Among these was his third great contribution, the "experiment without metal," in which he showed that if the nerve of a nerve-muscle preparation was laid along an injured point on a second muscle, the first muscle would contract. These studies were published in 1794 (*91*).

Du Bois-Reymond in a later generation summarized Galvani's theory (*59*):

"1. *Animals have an electricity peculiar to themselves, which is called Animal Electricity.*

"2. *The organs to which this animal electricity has the greatest affinity, and in which it is distributed, are the nerves, and the most important organ of its secretion is the brain.*"

At this time the German scientist Alexander von Humboldt took time off from his vast geophysical explorations to study muscle irritability, which intrigued him, and he published his findings in 1797, *Versuche über die gereizte Muskel- und Nervenfaser* (*124*). In this he essentially resolved the Galvani-Volta controversy, showing that Galvani had indeed made two great discoveries, a bimetallic and a biological source of electricity, but that the first was not a new kind of electricity but rather a new invention, a new electrical instrument. This was, of course, Volta's theory.

Alessandro Volta: Founder of Electrochemistry. Volta, professor of natural philosophy at Pavia, at first accepted Galvani's explanation of his experiments, and hailed these discoveries as being of epochal value, equivalent to those of Franklin. However, within a year he uncovered facts which forced him to differ from Galvani. With bold experiments and clever inventions, Volta was able to demonstrate that the electricity developed was of the same nature as that which an electric apparatus produced. With the most delicate electrometer of the day he could detect no electricity in animal tissues. He found that application of a stimulus confined to the nerve of his nerve-muscle preparation was sufficient to produce muscular contraction. Volta showed that the behavior of muscle described by Galvani was not caused by animal electricity, but rather by the action of physical electricity between two different metals, one of the metals being charged with positive and the other with negative "electrification." These charges combined to traverse the nerve and muscle (*101*). He asserted in a letter to the Royal Society that the frog's leg as prepared by Galvani was nothing other than a delicate electrometer, and that most of the phenomena attributed to "animal electricity" were the effects of feeble artificial electricity, generated by the simple application of two different metals (*209*).

Undaunted by the controversy which continued even after Galvani's death, Volta moved forward to create the science of electrochemistry. He found that metals whose contact caused a flow of electricity could be arranged in a definite order, that other conductors, such as carbon, had the same effect, and that any moist conductor, such as water or animal tissues, served to bridge the different metals. By 1795 he had propounded his law, that whenever two dissimilar metallic conductors were placed in contact with each other and a moist conductor, a flow of electricity took place. In 1796, Volta showed the identity of galvanic and frictional electricity by demonstrating that the mere contact of different metals produced equal and opposite charges, made visible with a condensing electroscope which he also developed. (This electroscope was approximately 120 times more sensitive than the currently available goldleaf electroscope.)

ELECTRO-
CARDIOGRAPHY

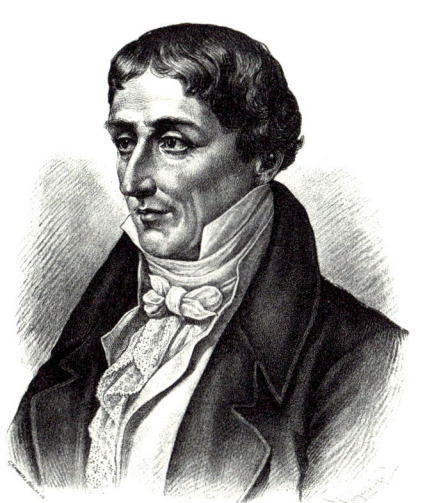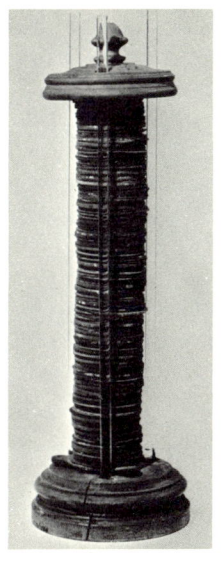

Figure 6. Alessandro Volta (1745–1827) and a voltaic pile that was probably used by Volta.

In 1799, Volta devised his famous pile (*209*). In a letter to Sir Joseph Banks in England, Volta wrote:

"*After a long silence, for which I shall offer no apology, I have the pleasure of communicating to you, and through you to the Royal Society, (of which I am a Fellow), some striking results I have obtained in pursuing my experiments on electricity excited by the mere mutual contact of different kinds of metal, and even by that of other conductors, also different from each other, either liquid or containing some liquid, to which they are properly indebted for their conducting power. The principle of these results, which comprehends nearly all the rest, is the construction of an apparatus having a resemblance in its effects (that is to say, in the shock it is capable of making the arms, &c. experience) to the Leyden flask.... The apparatus to which I allude, and which will, no doubt, astonish you, is only the assemblage of a number of good conductors of different kinds arranged in a certain manner. Thirty, forty, sixty, or more pieces of copper, or ... silver, applied each to a piece of tin, or zinc, which is much better, and as many strata of water, or any other liquid, which may be a better conductor, such as salt water, lye, &c. or pieces of pasteboard, skin, &c. well soaked in these liquids; such strata interposed between every*

[279]

pair of combination of two different metals in an alternate series, and always in the same order of these three kinds of conductors, are all that is necessary for constituting my new instrument....

"To this apparatus, much more similar fundamentally, as I shall show, and even such as I have constructed it, in its form, to the natural electric organ *of the torpedo or electric eel, &c., than to the Leyden flask and electric batteries, I would wish to give the name of the* artificial electric organ....

"*All the facts which I have related in this long paper in regard to the action which the electric fluid* [has] *excited, and when moved by my apparatus, exercises on the different parts of our body which the current attacks and passes through, — an action which is not momentary, but which lasts, and is maintained during the whole time that this current can follow the chain not interrupted in its communications; in a word, an action the effects of which vary according to the different degrees of excitability in the parts, as has been seen, — all these facts, sufficiently numerous, and others which may be still discovered by multiplying and varying the experiments of this kind, will open a very wide field for reflection, and for views, not only curious, but particularly interesting to medicine. There will be a great deal to occupy the anatomist, the physiologist, and the practitioner.*"

The origin of the electromotive force in the pile was soon disputed. Volta had erroneously maintained that mere contact of metals was sufficient to produce the electrical difference of the end plates of the pile. However, the electrochemical theory of the voltaic pile was soon correctly described and extended by Faraday, Davy, Carlisle, Nicholson, and others (*101, 201*). In modern theory the voltaic cell consists of copper, electrolyte, and zinc, and the electromotive force is considered to arise "from the summations ... of all the metal-metal, metal-liquid, and liquid-liquid junctions" (*201*).

The extensive development of voltaic batteries, and the scientific discoveries and technical applications derived from their use, are beyond the scope of this chapter.

The Galvanometer. Action Potentials. William Gilbert's observation that rubbed amber deflected the magnetic needle had first clearly demonstrated a connection between electricity and magnetism, although even before this sailors had noted disturbance in the action of the mariner's compass during electric storms. In the two centuries following, the effects of discharges from Leyden jars on magnetic needles, and later similar effects of electric currents from voltaic batteries, had been shown by many investigators.

The precise and quantitative description of the magnetic action of the electric current was announced to the scientific world in 1820 by Hans Christian Oersted (1777–1851), professor of natural philosophy in the University of Copenhagen (*6, 168*).

He showed that when a wire joining the end plates of a voltaic pile is held near a pivoted magnet or compass needle, the latter is deflected and places itself transversely to the wire, the direction depending upon whether the wire is above or below the needle, and on the manner in which the copper or zinc ends of the pile are connected to it. Oersted clearly recognized the existence of a magnetic field around the conductor. Oersted's discovery, like Volta's, stimulated further important investigations leading to the development of the galvanometer.

A. M. Ampère was the first to use Oersted's discovery to measure the intensity of currents (*101*). Johannes S. C. Schweigger (*120*) and J. C. Poggendorff (*177, 178*), working independently around 1820 (*84, 101*), conceived of the idea of multiplying the action of electricity on the magnetized needle. Schweigger's multiplicator consisted of a wooden frame on which was wound a number of turns of insulated copper wire. The frame was placed vertically on one of its sides, in the plane of the magnetic meridian, and inside the frame there was placed a magnetic needle freely suspended on a vertical pivot. Such an instrument was suitable for detecting an electric current by the deviation of the needle. The influence on the magnetic needle was multiplied by the number of turns of the wire in the coil, hence the name multiplier. In 1825, Leopoldo Nobili (1784–1834) of Florence modified this galvanometer (*120*). To gain more power by the multiplier, Nobili substituted an astatic system for the magnetic needle. This consisted of a pair of magnetized steel needles fixed to the same axis but with their magnetic poles pointing in opposite directions, thus neutralizing the force of terrestrial magnetism.

Only after Nobili constructed his astatic multiplier was it possible to measure the amount of current passing through a Galvani frog nerve-muscle preparation. He detected the frog current; muscle positive to nerve, feet positive to head (*6*). Nobili used his improved instrument to

THE HEART

demonstrate galvanic contraction without metals (*120*), thus justifying the reluctance of the followers of Galvani to dismiss his claims. Here a more sensitive galvanometer clarified a scientific controversy existing because of inadequate instrumentation.

With the development of more sensitive galvanometers, the electric phenomena of muscle, nerve, and other tissues could be both identified and measured, and Nobili's observations were confirmed and extended.

Carlo Matteucci (1811–68), professor of physics successively at Bologna, Ravenna, and Pisa, showed, in 1838, the difference of potential existing between a nerve and its damaged muscle (*158*). Four years later he demonstrated the "rheoscopic frog," i.e. that the muscle of a nerve-muscle preparation will contract if its nerve is laid across another contracting muscle. He found, in fact, an electrical current of contraction in all muscle masses, including the heart. In all cases he obtained a current which flowed from the interior of the muscle to the surface. In his report in 1843, the influence of the voltaic pile is nicely shown in the design of his experiment (*159*). He prepared a pile of frogs, putting the leg of one of the frogs on the nerve of another. The extremities of the pile were connected to the terminals of the galvanometer. The application of a potassium solution at a junction of nerve and muscle was followed by a contraction which was accompanied by an electric current. The strength of the current was found to be proportional to the number of elements, as in the voltaic pile. Not only did Matteucci make attempts to characterize the strength of the source, but he also compared the conductivity of several tissues—nerves, marrow, and brain.

The great Johannes Müller (1801–58) of Berlin became interested in Matteucci's publications, and as early as 1841 he directed his young associate Emil Du Bois-Reymond to start investigations in the field. This inquiry was to occupy Du Bois-Reymond for the next forty years. Du Bois-Reymond soon confirmed Matteucci's observations on the flow of current in cut or injured muscle. He found, in 1843, that there is also a current of rest in muscle and that this diminishes with muscular contraction. He labeled this "negative fluctuation" the "action potential," a term which has survived. Du Bois-Reymond's rather naïve theory was that these currents were produced by "electromotive molecules" of prismatic form, arranged in series end to end, unbroken circuits being maintained because the units were all moist conductors.

ELECTRO-
CARDIOGRAPHY

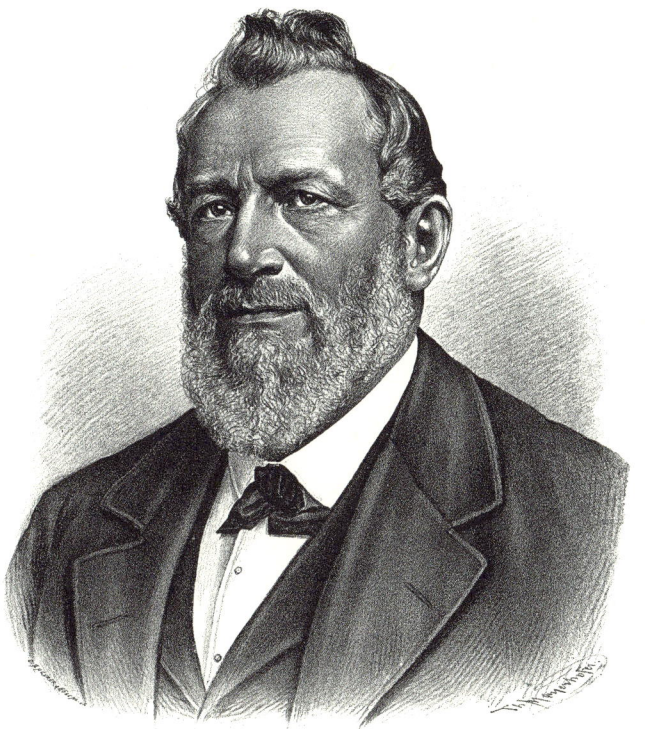

Figure 7. Emil Du Bois-Reymond (1818–96).

In 1848, he confirmed Matteucci's observations on electrical activity in the frog heart (*59*). These were, however, currents in injured and not in undamaged heart muscle. These were but a few of Du Bois-Reymond's many contributions during these years. Some others are mentioned later in this chapter.

Electrophysiology of the Heart

Fluctuation of the resting potential of spontaneously beating hearts was demonstrated in 1855, a few years after Du Bois-Reymond's presentation (*59*), by A. Kölliker and H. Müller (*139*). They placed the nerve of a nerve-muscle preparation of a frog on the surface of a beating heart, and observed that the frog leg contracted with every systole. They noted that when very sensitive nerve-muscle preparations were used, the muscles of the limb contracted just before the systole of

THE HEART

the ventricle (R wave) and, in certain cases, a second feeble twitch was observed at the beginning of the diastole (T wave). The action potential of the heart was demonstrated in this way as well as with the multiplier. It is noteworthy that Kölliker and Müller, like Galvani, used the frog nerve-muscle preparation as a sensitive galvanometer or electrometer. The action potential was crudely characterized by these investigators. They showed that the apex of the whole heart of the frog is electrically negative to any point on the anterior or posterior surface of the ventricles. The effects of injury were noted in that the cardiac apex was found to be positive compared to any cut section of the myocardium.

The next logical step was the characterization of the time and intensity curves of the negative variations of the heart beat. The deficiencies of the available instruments were obvious. Without the development of new instruments, further progress would have been impossible. As Burdon-Sanderson noted, "the phenomena observed are [limited by] ... the instruments we employ rather than [by] ... the organs we explore" (35).

Du Bois-Reymond at this juncture made his next significant contribution, the invention of the rheotome, or current interrupter. The essential feature of this instrument was that the connection between stimulus and tissue could be abruptly cut off, and the tissue then connected with a galvanometer so that the tissue's own electric currents could be recorded. Earlier workers, Saxton, Page, Lenz, Pouillet, and Morin, had already made significant contributions as a basis for this development (121). To separate the shock artefacts from the negative variation,

"... *he [Du Bois-Reymond] constructed a two-position switch operated by a rocker arm, by which in one position the connections of the nerve to the galvanometer were broken and a stimulus delivered, while in the opposite position the stimulating circuit was interrupted and the nerve reconnected to the galvanometer. Between these two extremes, both circuits were disconnected. The rocker arm was activated by a pusher-rod riding on a cam operated by clockwork, so constructed that with each revolution a cycle of stimulation and registration was carried out. By varying the shape of the cam, the duration of the stimulus and the subsequent interval of time before the galvanometer was reconnected could be varied independently ..."* (121).

This instrument made possible the first graphic analysis of the time course and amplitude of the action current in nerve and muscle. It was really the first instrument of quantitative electrophysiology.

The rheotome was used by Bernstein (*18*) and Helmholtz (*112*) to characterize the excitatory process and the negative variations in nerve, i.e., to measure the rate of conduction of the nerve impulse in frogs. The rheotome was noteworthy in that it could be used to plot accurately the time course of the action potential and to determine its rate of propagation, even though this process was complex and time-consuming. Surprisingly, the data obtained nearly match measurements made today.

The rheotome was important also in enabling R. Marchand in 1877 (*156*) and T. W. Engelmann in 1878 to chart the electrocardiogram (*74*). They showed that a stimulated spot on the heart is negative compared with a nonstimulated area. Marchand first expressed a concept, later valuable for the analysis of the electrocardiogram, of differential leads (*156*). When two spots on an uninjured heart are connected to a galvanometer, the generated negative current of each will be superimposed, but in opposite directions, to give the resultant curve.

Burdon-Sanderson and Page established the basis of present understanding of the nature of the T wave with the rheotome (*36, 37*). They also studied the order of excitation and the nature of the excitatory process in the ventricles of the heart of the frog, showed that during the excitatory state every excited part of the surface of the ventricle is negative to every unexcited part, and demonstrated that the excitatory state was propagated in all directions. They measured the duration of the excitatory state in frogs and showed that partial warming of the surface of the ventricle shortens the local duration of the excitatory state at the warmed part (*37*).

Soon the rheotome was supplanted by more versatile instruments, but it should be emphasized that it was the paramount instrument of electrophysiology for a brief time. During this period many advances were made, and the experimental basis was provided "for the hypothesis of nerve conduction and nerve and muscle bioelectricity which was to be elaborated and enunciated more clearly by Bernstein himself during the next forty years" (*121*), the first charting of the electrocardiogram, and the basic beginning of our understanding of the nature of

THE HEART

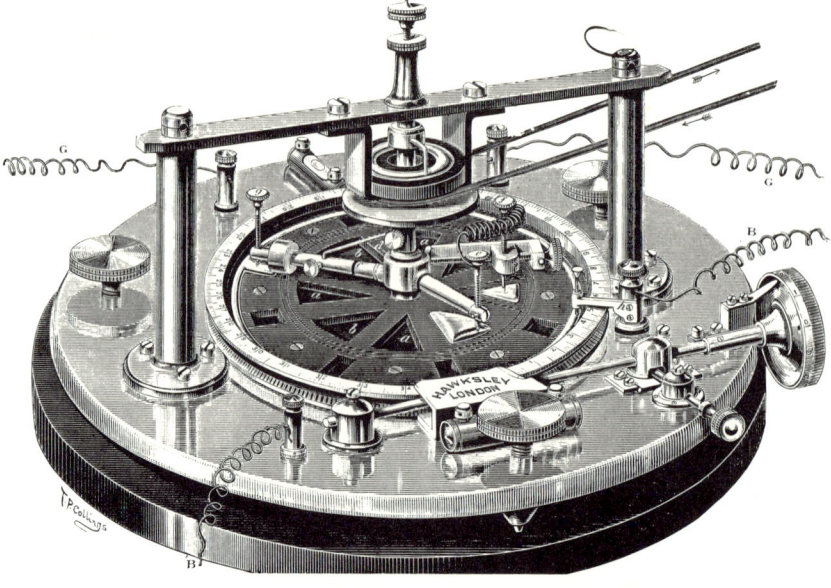

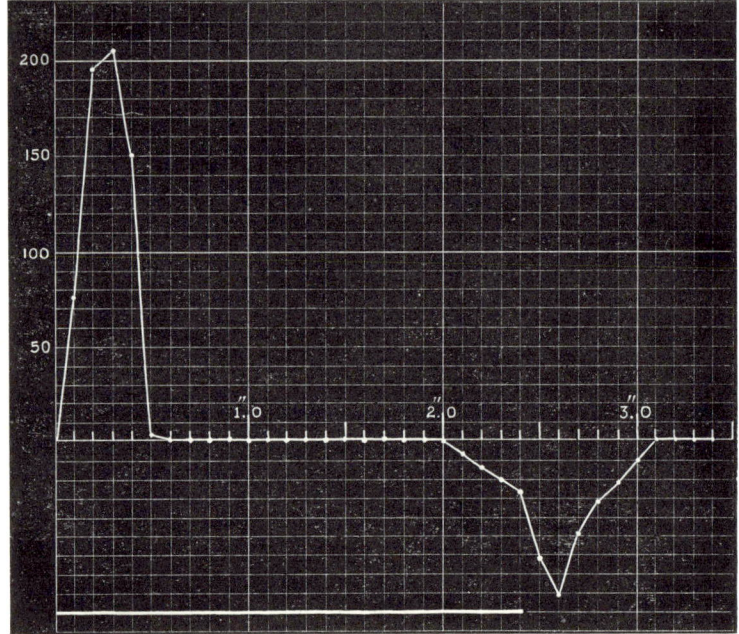

Figure 8. Top: The rheotome of J. Burdon-Sanderson and F. J. M. Page. *Bottom:* Plot of the electrocardiogram of the tortoise constructed from 35 points obtained with the rheotome.

the T wave (*35*). The rheotome has been valuable, even in the twentieth century. When "stripped of its 'scanning' function it continued to be useful in the form of a variety of stimulus-triggering devices linked with a recording system. Finally, with the advent of the cathode ray tube, similar mechanical devices triggered the stimulus and generated the sweep of the electron beam, to place a standing wave before the viewer" (*121*).

ELECTRO-
CARDIOGRAPHY

Until the 1870's, the study of the heart potentials in intact subjects had not yet been made, or if made, had not been recognized. Du Bois-Reymond had performed experiments on man relating to the electromotive action accompanying voluntary muscular tetanic contraction. In Du Bois-Reymond's experiment, "the two hands [were] led off to a galvanometer by two vessels into each of which a finger [was] dipped. The voluntary contraction of the muscles of either arm gave a deflection, which indicated the passage of a current through the galvanometer from the passive to the contracting and through the body from the contracting to the passive arm" (*59*). The action potential of the human heart was apparently not detected or registered by the galvanometer in these experiments.

In 1875, Gabriel Lippmann (1845–1921) first devised an instrument capable of recording the voltages of the heart of the intact subject (*149*). While still a student, he prepared abstracts of German papers and became acquainted with contemporary research in electricity. In 1873, he was appointed to a scientific mission and visited Germany, where he worked first at Heidelberg, under the physiologist Kühne and the physicist Kirchoff, and later at Berlin, under Helmholtz. In 1883, he was appointed professor of mathematical physics in the Faculty of Science at Paris. While at Heidelberg, Lippmann was shown an experiment presented routinely to students. A drop of mercury, covered with dilute sulphuric acid, is touched lightly with an iron nail near its upper edge; the mercury contracts, but recovers its original shape as soon as the contact with the nail is broken. These changes were ascribed to an increase in the surface tension of the mercury brought about by a change in the electrical conditions existing between the mercury and acid, the iron being in some way responsible. Lippmann made a systematic study of the phenomenon in Kirchoff's laboratory at Heidelberg which led to the publication in 1875 of his account of the capillary electrometer (*149*).

The instrument consists of a glass tube, containing mercury, with one end drawn out into a fine capillary (20 to 30mμ), and immersed in dilute sulfuric acid. The position of the mercury meniscus depends in part on surface tension existing at the boundary between mercury and acid, and movements of the meniscus occur when the potential difference between them is changed. "Permanent records are obtained by projecting a magnified image of the meniscus on sensitized paper moving uniformly at right angles to the direction in which the image is displaced" (*138*). The instrument was simple and inexpensive. It was thus described by Waller (*210*):

"... *the instrument is, in fact, an exceedingly delicate electrical manometer; a rise of electrical pressure on the mercury side or a fall of electrical pressure on the sulphuric acid side, causes the mercury to move towards the point of the capillary; a fall of electrical pressure on the mercury side or a rise on the sulphuric acid side, causes the mercury to recede from the point of the capillary.*

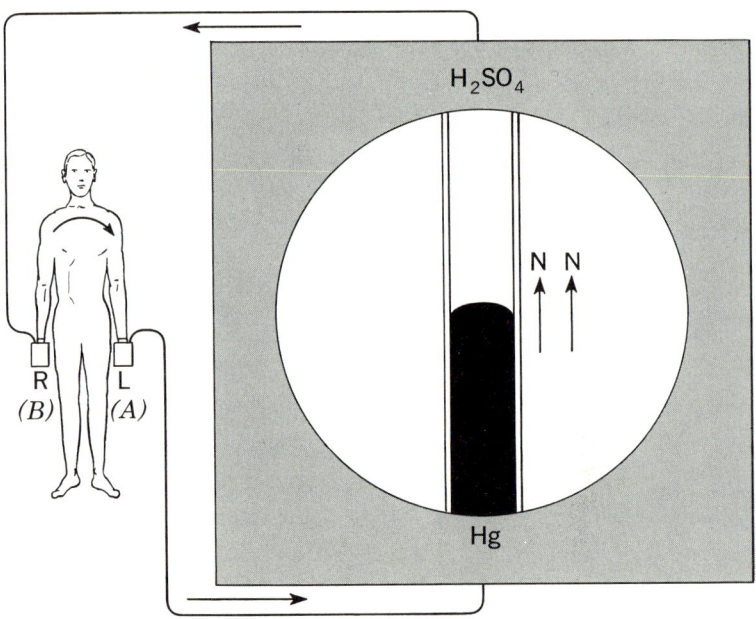

Figure 9. The mercury capillary electrometer of Lippmann.

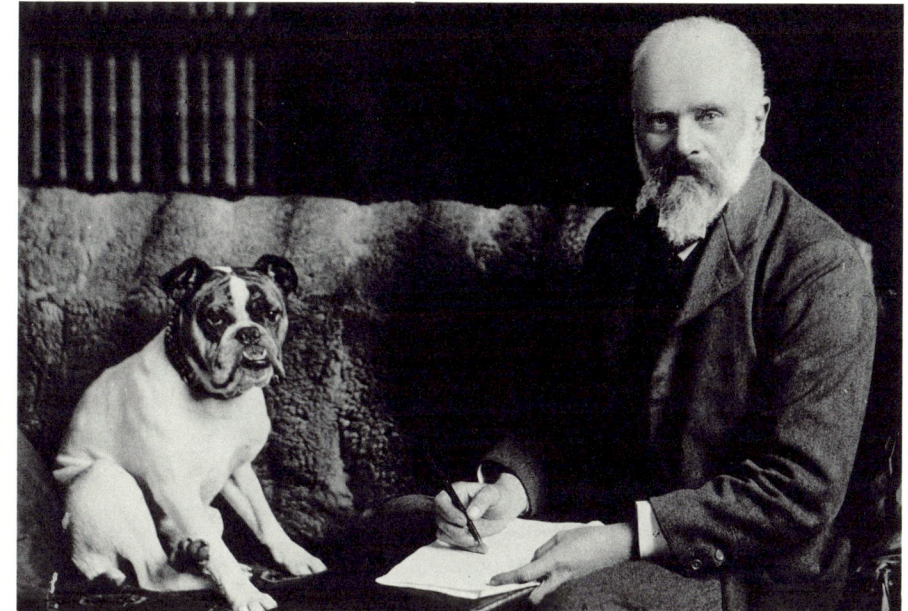

Figure 10. Augustus Waller (1856–1922) and friend.

The instrument accordingly is an indicator of "potential" or "pressure"; not of "current." Its delicacy is such that it will react to as little as 1/40,000 volt. It offers, moreover, the following advantages: the indications are practically instantaneous, free of lost time, and of after-oscillation; the resistance in circuit is immaterial; unpolarisable electrodes may for most purposes be dispensed with."

The First Electrocardiogram in Intact Animals and Man: Waller. The first records of the heart were obtained by Marey in 1876 (*157*), but the most significant advance was made by Waller. Augustus Desiré Waller, son of a distinguished father, the neurophysiologist Augustus Volney Waller, was born in Paris, studied in Geneva, then at Aberdeen, later was a student of Burdon-Sanderson's, came to London as lecturer in the School of Medicine for Women, worked at St. Mary's Hospital, and in 1902 became Director of the new Physiological Laboratory at the University of London. He was said to have been "a good talker, eager, emphatic, sometimes a little brusque, and impatient with slower witted folk" (*213*). Sir Thomas Lewis's verdict was: "Waller was the first to show that currents set up by the beating of the human heart can be recorded; he was the first to obtain a human electrocardiogram" (*213*).

THE HEART

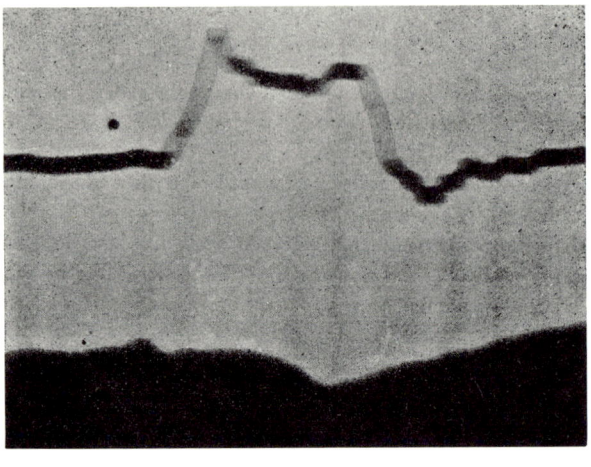

Figure 11. First electrometer record of the human heart. Time in 0.1 sec.

In his experiments both on animals and man, Waller found that currents accompanying the beat of the heart *in situ* could be recorded with the capillary electrometer when the electrodes were placed on the front and back of the chest. His classic demonstration of the electrocardiogram of the human heart took place in his laboratory at St. Mary's Hospital, London, in May 1887 (*214, 211*). A group of distinguished physiologists, including Willem Einthoven of Leiden, attended this demonstration (*116*). In addition to leads from the front and back of the chest, Waller took other combinations between the mouth and various extremities. In subsequent discussions (*211, 212*) his designation of deflections, concepts of the electrical field, of favorable and unfavorable leads (*211*), of axis of the electrical force, and of vector representations were presented in detail. In his original reports, he noted the difficulty of determining whether there were one or two movements of the mercury column, and whether each movement indicated a single variation or double variation in the same direction. He was aware of the effects of the differences of the position of the electrodes on the magnitude and form of the tracing. However, his interpretation of the original deflections was erroneous (*211*). Waller thought that the apex of the heart became negative before the base because he believed the first deflection corresponded to the negativity of the tip of the heart and the second deflection corresponded to the negativity of the base.

Improvements of the electrometer were soon made. In 1892, Bayliss and Starling, the famous brothers-in-law at University College, London, obtained the first satisfactory mammalian curves on intact man and dog with an improved electrometer (*15*). These investigators used an electric arc light in place of the limelight and obtained greater magnifying power on the projecting microscope. Their electrometer yielded a triphasic initial response, instead of the diphasic reported by Waller.

The usefulness of the capillary electrometer was of brief duration. Investigators soon realized that Waller's original satisfaction with the frequency response was not warranted. The effects of friction of the mercury, of invisible particles of dust, and of electromagnetic suppression were significant. The form of the registered curves required correction for the size of the capillary tube used, the degree of magnification, and the speed of the photosensitive plate (*64*). Nevertheless, it served as a useful tool in the study of the normal and the diseased heart. Waller, Bayliss and Starling, and Einthoven employed this electrometer between 1887 and 1900.

It is not generally known that Einthoven expended considerable effort to correct for the inertia of the capillary electrometer (*65*). In 1895, on the basis of mathematical calculations, he corrected the tracings of the capillary electrometer and increased the number of points originally found in the records of this machine from four (ABCD) to five. To avoid bias of interpretation, he introduced the PQRST designation for the several deflections, a nomenclature which has persisted to date. Interestingly, in this phase of Einthoven's research, which seems methodical and uninspiring compared to later events, emphasis was placed on the definition of component parts of the tracings, and no hint can be found in his publications of his later thoughts on vector analysis, the effect of position, etc.

New Methodology. The String Galvanometer. In 1897, events occurred which were completely unrelated to medicine and electrophysiology, but which had a momentous influence in the latter field (*84, 24*). After 1845, when a telegraph cable was laid across the English Channel, the people of Europe, Africa, and America were no longer satisfied to be separated by distance. Communication was an essential prerequisite for progress. Considerable effort had been expended in the development of the telegraph and the telephone, and Kelvin and others had developed the knowledge and instruments necessary for laying a transatlantic submarine cable. Kelvin's mirror galvanometer (1858), siphon-recorder (1867), and automatic curb sender were important practical inventions (*24*). Several submarine cables for telegraphic messages had been laid, with both failure and success, and there was an urgent need for development of improved instruments to receive submarine dispatches.

In 1897, Ader invented a new type of galvanometer now known as the string galvanometer or thread galvanometer (*3*). This galvanometer works on the principle that a current generates a magnetic field acting at right angles to its course, which varies with the strength of the current, and which may thus exert a varying attraction or repulsion upon a second magnetic field in its vicinity. Ader's string galvanometer was used on the transatlantic cable from Brest to Saint Pierre and from Marseilles to Algiers. A high frequency response of 600 to 1600 signals per minute could be obtained with it. The influence of the modes and needs of ordinary society again played an important role in the development of apparatus and thus of knowledge of electrophysiology.

Einthoven's Galvanometer: The Modern Electrocardiogram. Willem Einthoven, professor of physiology in the University of Leiden, was the founder of modern electrocardiography. His fundamental early achievement was the recognition of the potential value of Ader's new, elegant galvanometer, and his own construction of an improved and more sensitive modification of this machine (*66, 67*). In Einthoven's instrument (*69*):

"... *the string galvanometer is essentially composed of a thin silver-coated quartz filament, (about 3 μ thick): which is stretched like a string, in a strong magnetic field. When an electric current is conducted through this quartz filament, the filament reveals a movement which can be observed and photographed by means of considerable magnification; this movement is similar to the movements of the mercury contained in the capillary-electrometer. It is*

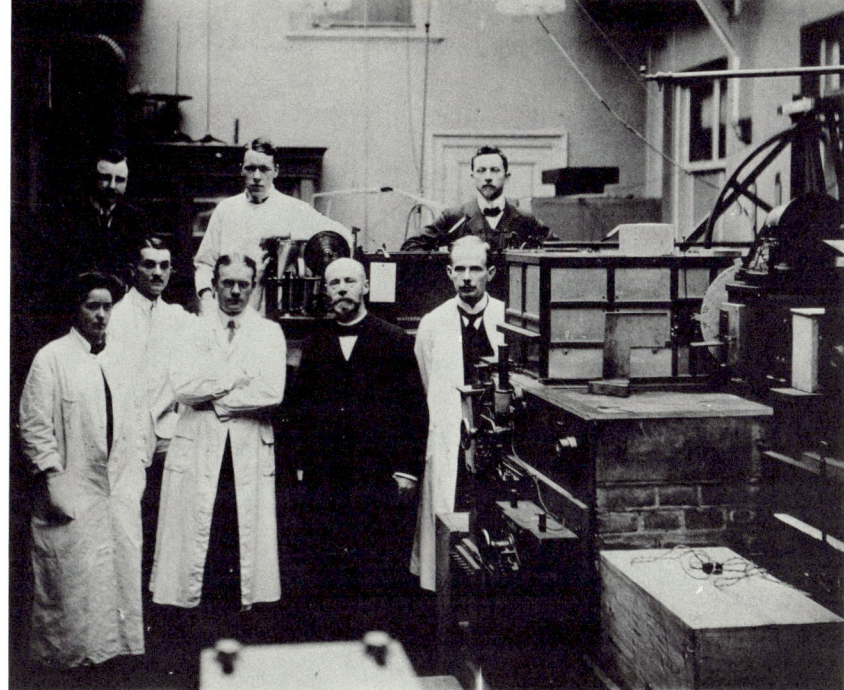

Figure 12. Willem Einthoven (1860–1927) and his co-workers.

possible to regulate the sensitivity of the galvanometer very accurately within broad limits by tightening or loosening the string."

The movements of the thread were recorded by projecting its shadow under the magnification of a high power (660-fold) microscope upon the slit of a specially devised camera about 6 feet away. The speed of movement of the photographic plate was 25 mm. per second, so that an abscissa of 1 mm. had a value of 0.04 second, while the tension of the filament was so adjusted that an ordinate of 1 mm. corresponded to 10^{-4} volt of electromotive force. By selection of these arbitrary values, Einthoven's curves met the requirements of the International Committee (*68, 69*).

Soon Einthoven's galvanometer superseded all others throughout the scientific world and provided a practical tool for electrocardiography.

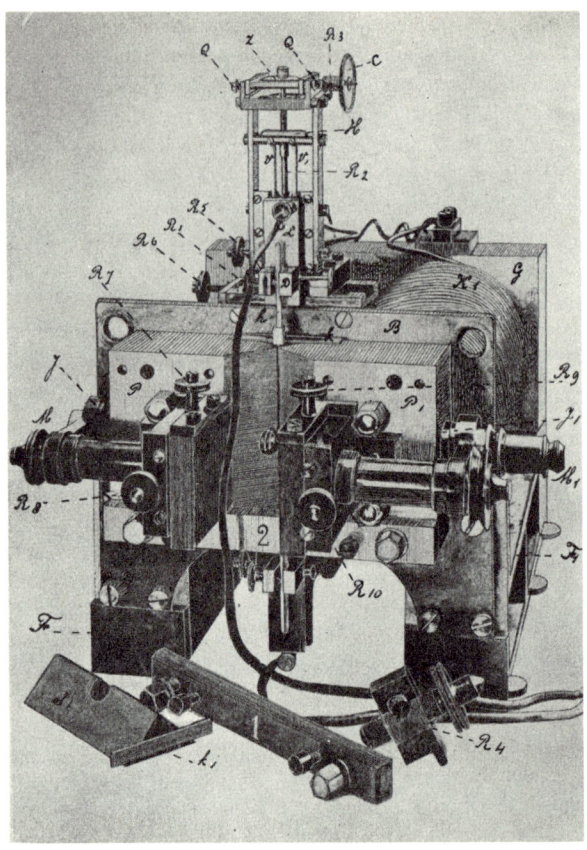

Figure 13. Einthoven's string galvanometer, Leyden model.

In his first report, Einthoven showed perfect agreement between the record obtained with his new string galvanometer and the mathematically corrected curves obtained with the capillary electrometer (*68, 69*).

Einthoven should also be credited with the recognition of the vast potential importance of the electrocardiogram as a diagnostic and investigative tool. He cooperated with the University Hospital in Leiden by laying a cable between the Institute of Physiology and the clinic; in this way he took "telecardiograms" of patients (*70*). Einthoven showed that it was by no means necessary that the patient be kept in the same room with the bulky instrument, but that the wards of the hospital could be connected by wires with the electrocardiographic laboratory and the patient thus examined without leaving his bed or even changing his position. The wiring was placed underground and was very thoroughly insulated. Einthoven's laboratory, in which his original work was done, was located 1.5 kilometers from the hospital. Although this arrangement was possible because of the character of the Dutch soil, and required a massive pillar to be sunk to keep the sensitive galvanometer free of mechanical vibration artefacts, it led to the realization that, with proper care, even greater distances were feasible. Today, for example, teleoelectrocardiography is a promising new development (*12*).

Soon the electrocardiograph superseded the clinical polygraph and the capillary electrometer. As Waller stated, "Einthoven's galvanometer

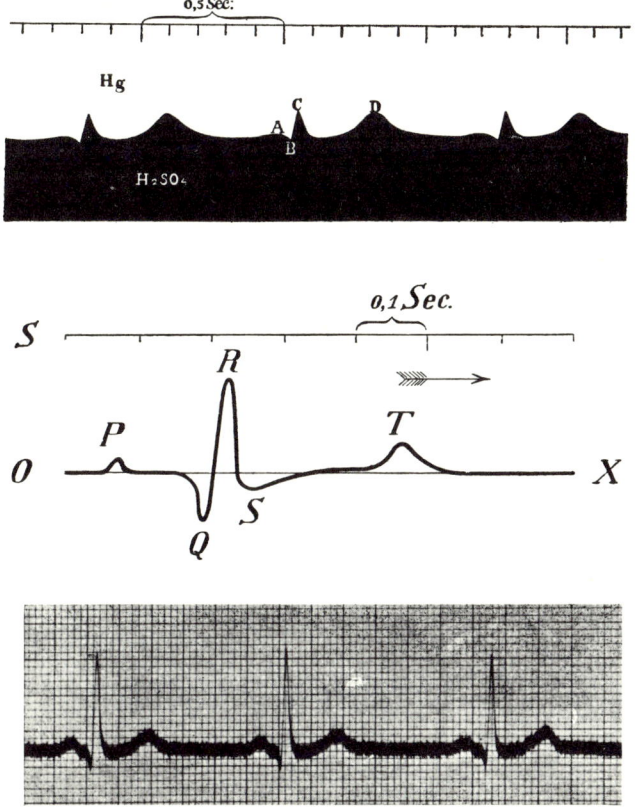

Figure 14. Evolution of the electrocardiogram from the electrometer. *Upper record*, by capillary electrometer; *middle record*, "corrected curve"; *lower record*, by Einthoven's string galvanometer.

is to the capillary electrometer as a high is to a low power of the microscope. It has opened a new chapter in the clinical study of heart disease, and played a part in medical literature that exhibits no sign of its physiological origin" (*212*).

The brilliant success of Einthoven's instrument, and the world renown which came to him on the basis of this achievement, undoubtedly pushed into the background the basic discoveries of earlier physiologists upon which his own work actually rested. This was particularly true of Augustus Waller. But Waller's own attitude was generous. He noted, that "Professor Einthoven has always acknowledged with the utmost frankness that his own work was the direct continuation of mine, and that his string-galvanometer was invented with the direct object of providing a more adequate recording of the human electrocardiogram than was afforded by the capillary electrometer" (*212*).

In 1924 (two years after Waller's death), Einthoven was awarded the Nobel prize in physiology and medicine, "for the discovery of the mechanism of the electrocardiogram."

Anatomical Structure of the Conduction System of the Heart

The characterization of the mechanism of the heart beat on an electrocardiographic basis which followed Einthoven's investigations acted as a spur to the clarification of the anatomical structures responsible for impulse initiation and conduction.

The myogenic theory of the heart beat was firmly established by the beginning of the twentieth century, when electrocardiography became a clinical tool. This theory stated "that the automatic movement of the heart muscle lies wholly in the ordinary muscular tissue and that the existing nerve centers in the heart muscle, as well as those nerve paths leading to and from the heart, only serve to mediate reflexes from the heart to the rest of the vascular system and the entire organism" (*7, 8*).

On the basis of the work of Stannius in 1852, Gaskel in 1881, and McWilliam and Engelmann in the 1880's and 1890's, the following concepts were widely accepted: first, that the heart's impulse is conducted by the cardiac muscle tissue, and second, that the impulse normally arises in the musculature of the sinus venosus and sets the heart's rhythm; it passes from here to the atria and ventricles, finally reaching the bulbus cordis (*135*).

In 1906, Tawara noted a special system of musculature within the mammalian heart which begins as a small node in or near the base (A-V junction) of the interatrial septum on the right side, and eventually spreads out in an arborescent form beneath the endocardium of both ventricles, with its final twigs becoming everywhere continuous with the ordinary musculature of the ventricles (*207*). This discovery of the A-V conduction system prodded Keith and Flack to determine if the musculature in which the heart impulse was supposed to arise and by which it was supposedly conducted differs in form and structure from that part which is mainly contractile in nature. They found that in the region of the sino-atrial junction "in the human heart the fibers are striated, fusiform, with well-marked elongated nuclei, plexiform in arrangement, and embedded in densely packed connective tissue—in fact, of closely similar structure to the Knoten (node)" (*135*). Keith and Flack's demonstration of the sino-atrial node completed the major pattern of the present concept of the anatomic structures related to impulse initiation.

The time sequence of the development of knowledge of this anatomy is interesting, in that Purkinje described his fibers in 1839 (*173*); His, in 1893 (*114*, *115*), demonstrated the atrioventricular bundle in the septal region of the A-V junction in a number of animals including man and, in 1895, reported that its section caused dissociation of the atria and ventricles (*145*); Tawara (*207*) described the A-V node in 1906 and showed the continuation of the A-V node into the common A-V bundle and Purkinje's fibers. Approximately thirty years later, Abramson showed that the Purkinje fibers penetrated deeply into the ventricular myocardium, forming a three-dimensional meshwork, rather than a subendocardial network (*42*).

Thorel, in 1909 (*208*), described an elaborate system of fibers thought to be of similar nature to Purkinje fibers, running downward toward the inferior vena cava from the superior vena cava and sino-atrial node. Other workers attributed these appearances to pathological processes (*163*). Eyster and Meek (*79*) presented physiological evidence for such preferential paths of conduction, but this was denied by others (*145*). Until the last few years it was the general view that no special path connects the sino-atrial with the atrioventricular node. However, the possibility of such a specialized tract has once again been raised recently by the demonstration of a distinct fiber bundle running from the sino-atrial to the atrioventricular node along the caval edge of the crista terminalis (*171*). Transmembrane electrical potentials from this bundle show characteristics of specialized conducting fibers (*171*). Today, as in the past, the interplay continues between anatomists and physiologists, and it has extended to electron microscopists and students of transmembrane action currents.

Current anatomic studies are influencing the understanding of the electrical events of the myocardium. The time-honored concept of the heart as a syncytium has been seriously challenged. Electron microscopic studies have indicated that the myocardium consists of cells whose ends are joined to each other by intercalated discs (*164*). Not only are there double membranes at the intercalated discs, but also double membranes enclose the nucleus, mitochondria (sarcosomes), and possibly other component subcellular structures. The intracellular milieu has been found to be much more complex than previously believed, particularly in regard to the relationship of the contractile myofibrils to the endoplasmic reticulum (*179*), the extracellular surroundings, the intercalated discs and the area of their insertion, and to the metabolic activity of the cell (*20*). Also it is now being recognized that events at the cell membrane are much more intricate than envisioned by Bernstein (*18*) and even by modern "axonologists" and cardiac physiologists. The use of these concepts for the interpretation of arrhythmias today is summarized elsewhere (*133*).

After Einthoven

With the development of a practical useful galvanometer for recording electrocardiograms, and with the advances in knowledge of the anatomy of the conduction system, a great outburst of work in electrocardiography developed which has continued to the present. Most of the workers belonged to the "interior science" (*196*) who ploddingly, by their very numbers, slowly filled in the bulk of the gaps in that knowledge which constitutes the science of electrocardiography.

Einthoven's instrument was used by many clinicians to establish cardiac diagnoses. Empirically, signs of right and left ventricular hypertrophy, of heart block, and of interruption of the right or left branch of His's bundle were defined. Following the example of Einthoven, clinicians recorded pulse curves and heart sounds simultaneously with the electrocardiogram. While the clinical gambit was pursued empirically, a new experimental era also began.

The mechanism of the heart beat was the chief concern of prominent investigators in the immediate decades after Einthoven's contribution, as it is even now (174). Foremost in characterizing various clinical arrhythmias (e.g., atrial fibrillation and the mechanism of circus rhythm) and the spread of the excitatory process through the atrial and ventricular myocardium were Lewis (145), Rothberger (186), Wenckebach and Winterberg (219), and their colleagues and students.

With the development of the string galvanometer, the exploration of new vistas of cardiac physiology began. As in the past, the invention of a new instrument or new method of investigation determined the lines along which knowledge was to advance.

"The introduction of the stethoscope by Laennec in 1819 interested physicians in heart murmurs, and focused attention on lesions of the heart valves. Thirty years later, the invention of the sphygmograph provided a graphic method of recording the pulse and opened up new possibilities of studying irregular heart action" (22).

The clinical polygraph, even prior to the innovation of the string galvanometer, had been very valuable in the study of arrhythmias in the hands of Mackenzie and others. Synchronous records of venous and arterial pulses made it possible to study the time relations of atrial and ventricular systole.

Two major divergent trends of study have marked the more recent development of cardiac electrophysiology. On the one hand, there has been a growing understanding of the relationship between the spread of the impulse (and its retreat) within the heart, and the electrical field so created within the body (and on its surface) of the animal or man. On the other, there has been a growing interest in the appearance of the action potentials at the surface membrane of each heart cell, their changes during the heart cycle, and the theories which can best account for these transmembrane electrical variations.

The Body as a Solid Conductor, the Electrical Field, the Cardiac Vector. The fact that the heart lies within the animal body, which is in essence a three-dimensional solid conductor, was known to Waller (210) and was the subject of a theoretical analysis by Einthoven (73). In such a solid conductor, an electrical field can be envisioned and the electrical currents created by the heart can be considered as a fluctuating vectorial force subject to mathematical analysis. This has occupied the energy of many investigators, physicists, mathematicians, physiologists, and clinicians, ever since its clear enunciation by Einthoven (72, 73). The

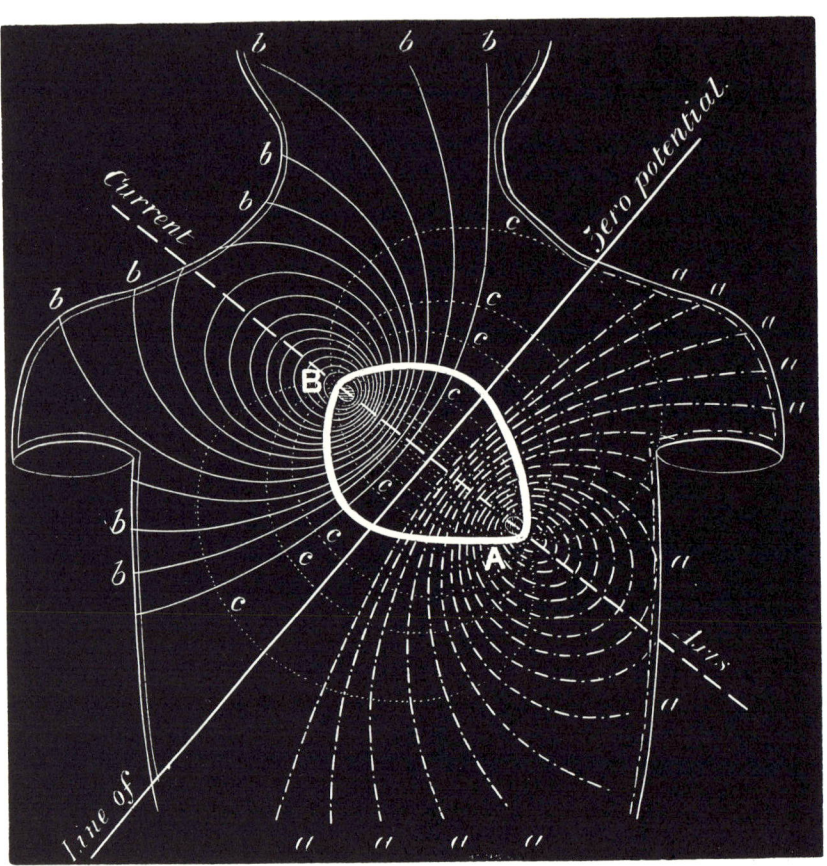

Figure 15. Distribution of potentials produced by the human heart, according to Waller.

"The contraction of the ventricles is not simultaneous throughout the mass, but traverses it as a wave.... Inequalities of potential, at different parts of the mass, are consequently established at the beginning and at the end of each systole.... The distribution of these inequalities of potential is represented diagrammatically ... [in this figure]."

laws governing the behavior of electric currents in solid conductors were established by Helmholtz as early as 1853 (*112*).

Waller evidently knew the laws governing the distribution of potential differences within solid conductors. In 1899, he presented, without explanation, a schematic drawing of the trunk with a system of electrical isopotential surfaces, seen in cross section, around the heart. He used this diagram to illustrate the "current axis of the heart" and its role in producing larger deflections in some leads than in others. Waller recognized that the position of the heart in the body influences the pattern of distribution of its potential; he illustrated this by using his observations on a human subject with situs inversus viscerum (*211*).

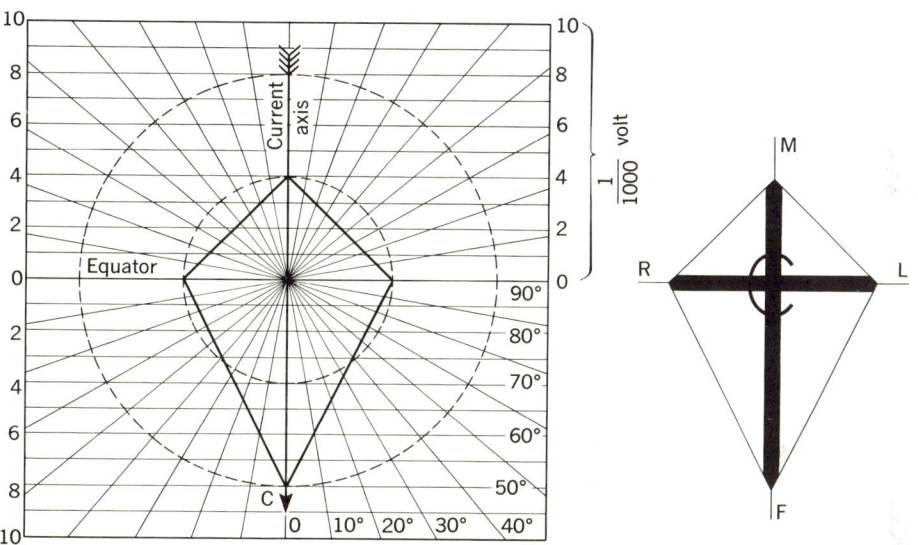

Figure 16. Axial reference system of Waller.

"Diagram serving to show how the electromotive values of the five leads, R.L., R.F., L.F., M.R., M.L., alter with altered values of the axial angle ... the current axis is vertical and the axial angle = 0°; the potential differences between, e.g., R and F and between L and F are then of course equal, i.e., the right and left hand spikes are equal.

"If [the figure on the right is] superposed upon [that on the left] centre to centre by a pin and then rotated in relation to each other so as to bring the current axis into various angular relations with M.R.L.F. the altered values of the different leads can be realized by counting the number of equipotential (parallel) lines between any two points M.R.L.F."

By means of various lead combinations, he was able to separate the vertical, horizontal, and sagittal components of the heart vector. Subsequently (212), he depicted the three-dimensional electrical field of the heart as a four-sided figure, a "tetrahedron," formed by the mouth, right arm, left arm, and left leg. From this tetrahedron he obtained five cardinal leads. He also developed an axial reference system for plotting the cardiac vector.

In 1913, Einthoven, Fahr, and de Waart described a new method for determining the direction and the "manifest value" of the potential difference produced by the heart beat at any instant in the cardiac

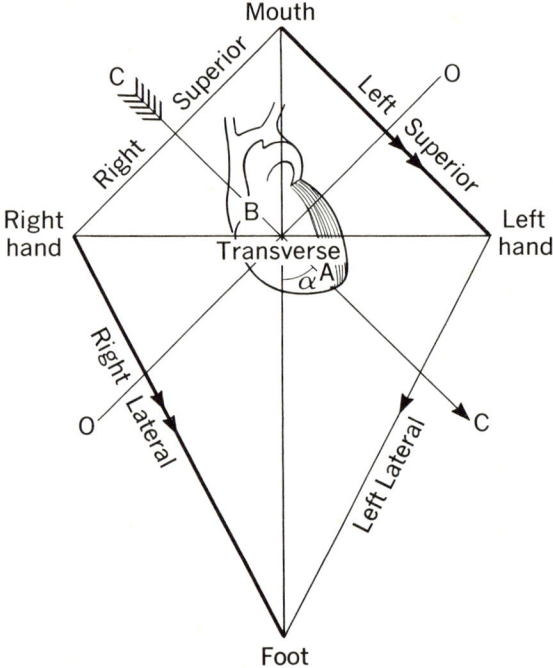

Figure 17. Schema of Waller to show current axis and equator.
"The axis of any electrical current resulting from difference of potential between base and apex is in the direction of line BA. [The arrow CC indicates the current axis]. The line of no current, or zero difference of potential, [between base and apex] is then at right angles to the current axis BA in the direction of a line OO representing the equator between potentials B and A."

Figure 18. Schema of the equilateral triangle of Einthoven.

"R corresponds to the right hand, L to the left hand, and F to both feet. The heart H is located in the center. The arrow indicates the direction of the potential difference in the heart. α = 76°."

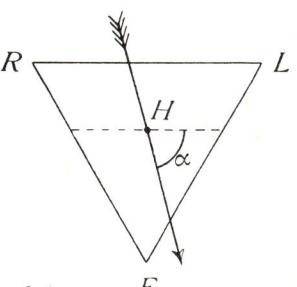

cycle (72). They were concerned with the effect of the position of the heart upon the form of the electrocardiogram; they attempted to determine the direction of the potential difference in the frontal plane of the body from the three limb leads. For this undertaking, they *assumed* that the electromotive forces of the heart in the frontal plane may be represented by a single vector in the center of an equilateral triangle (73).

Implicit in this schema are at least five subsidiary assumptions. (1) The body is a large conducting medium, (2) this medium is homogeneous and resistive, (3) the source of the potential is a single dipole, (4) the dipole is located at the center of the medium, and (5) the dipole undergoes no change in location during the cardiac cycle (132). Unfortunately, in the excitement engendered by this new approach, Einthoven's associates and students since then often mistook these assumptions for facts. Consequently, during the third of a century following the original publication of the idea of the equilateral triangle, many electrocardiographic reports appeared which either expanded electrocardiographic theory on the premise that Einthoven's postulates were absolutely valid or debated the validity of the postulates.

Considerable clarification of the issues was provided by Frank N. Wilson in the 1930's, who was the natural successor of Einthoven (and Lewis, whose pupil he was) in dominating the field of electrocardiography. His was a major contribution. With his associates at the University of Michigan, he described the laws which govern the distribution of electromotive force in solid conductors more precisely than before, assuming that the conductor is homogeneous, that its boundaries approach infinity, and that the electrical currents created by the heart are equivalent to a single fixed dipole (234). Their results were a natural extension of the deductions of Helmholtz and Einthoven (49). They transposed Craib's findings on strips of cardiac and skeletal muscle and medullated nerve fibers (50, 51) to the conditions existing in the intact body. The laws governing the flow of currents in volume conductors were shown to apply to limb leads and were considered to be relevant to the analysis of records obtained by precordial leads and by direct leads (*225*).

These theoretical outgrowths of Einthoven's postulates led, in turn, to the development of practical devices such as the central terminal, unipolar limb leads, V leads, and augmented unipolar limb leads (*230–233, 96*). By proper use of these combinations, it was believed possible to determine the potential variations produced by the heart beat at any

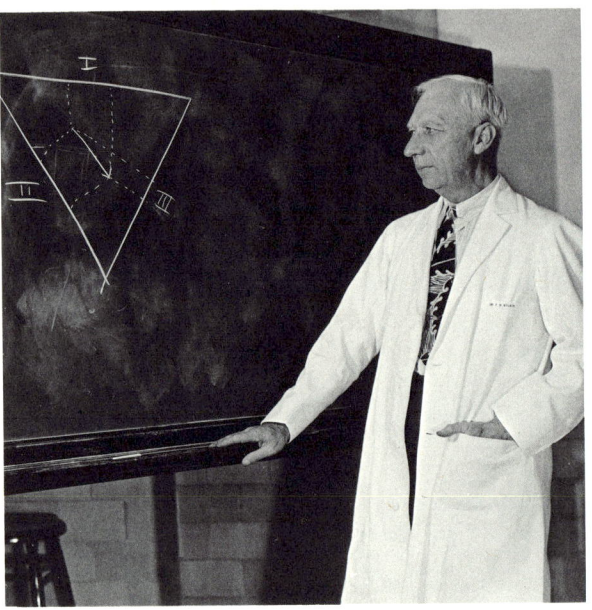

Figure 19. Frank N. Wilson (1890–1952).

point in or on the body, free from the effects of potential variations at the distant, supposedly indifferent, electrode (*231, 233*). Not only were Wilson's ideas used to practical advantage in the clinic, but they were also put to theoretical use for the analysis of the distribution of action currents and injury currents of cardiac muscle (*234*).

Over the years, these extensions of Einthoven's postulates were tested in many different ways. Particularly, the use of Wilson's central terminal as an indifferent electrode was investigated and debated (*29, 113, 55, 14*).

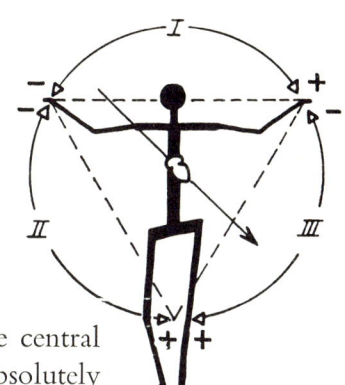

Figure 20. Diagram of the equilateral triangle, the absurdity of which stimulated Burger's interest. The extended fingers and left foot are represented as forming an equilateral triangle.

It is now well established that although the potential of the central terminal is less than that of other reference electrodes it is not absolutely at zero, and it shows fluctuations during the heart cycle. However, this inaccuracy introduced by the potential variation of the central electrode (0.2 to 0.3 mv.) (*15*) has not impaired its practical clinical usefulness (*203*).

Refutation of Einthoven's Hypothesis. By 1946, it was generally appreciated that, at best, the Einthoven triangle could only provide a rough approximation of the momentary forces which exist in the heart (*132, 237, 226*). The reasons for its inadequacies were also quite clear: the torso of the body, which constitutes the conducting medium, is not spherical; compared to the size of the heart, the torso does not comprise a large field; instead of being in the center of the body, the heart is closer to the sternum than to the back, closer to the arms than to the legs, and closer to the left arm than to the right arm; the limb leads used to obtain the vectors in the frontal plane do not form an equilateral triangle; the body is not composed of a homogeneous conducting resistive medium (*132, 237, 226*); and the blood within the heart has a short-circuiting effect.

A more realistic triangle and approach to the cardiac vector was provided by H. C. Burger and his associates. Burger, a relative newcomer to this subject, was a theoretical physicist with experience in handling problems involving boundary conditions. His interest in the problem began in 1939 when he saw a schematic representation of Einthoven's concept in a book sent to him by his brother. He was struck by the absurdity of the diagram of the man with outstretched hands whose extended fingers and left foot formed an equilateral triangle!

Recognizing that the body was electrically heterogeneous and not homogeneous, he could not imagine why the field in the frontal plane should take the shape of an equilateral triangle. It seemed to him that more could be learned about the heart vector from realistic phantoms than from equations. And, unfamiliar with either the prevailing controversy about the validity of Einthoven's assumptions or the recent

THE HEART

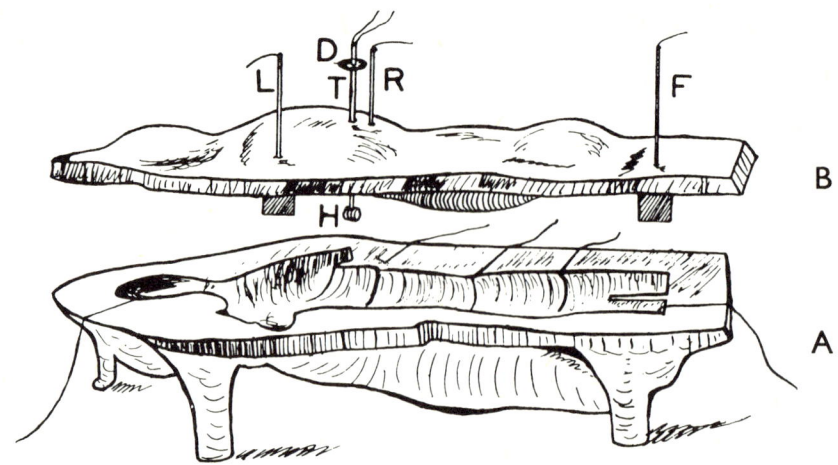

Figure 21. Phantom of Burger and van Milaan to determine the relation between heart vector and leads.

experiments in favor of these assumptions (*231*), he began his own investigations using models and making measurements. His observations on the electrical conductivity of human tissues and on the voltages obtained from a dipole contained within a glass model of the human body soon confirmed his disbelief in the accuracy of the Einthoven concept.

In 1946, Burger and van Milaan introduced the idea of using "lead vectors" to replace the geometric lead lines of Einthoven's triangle; this was followed by the concept of "image surface" to take into account the facts that the medium surrounding the heart ("dipole") is neither homogeneous nor simple in geometric design and that the "dipole" is not centered (*38, 39*). It is based on Kelvin's (1845) mathematical solution of electrical images for boundary problems in highly conductive liquids (*105*). These concepts were based on their studies of the electric fields generated by an artificial dipole in a model of the human body. By measuring the potential differences between electrodes placed according to the location of the conventional limb leads, they were able to construct a triangle of current flow. In any single lead, the deflection was regarded as "the scalar product of two vectors ('dot' product), one of which represents the lead and the other the electromotive force responsible for the field" (*226*). Instead of an equilateral triangle in the frontal plane, the triangle of Burger and van Milaan was a scalene.

The implication of this new approach was immediately recognized. Old ideas based on Einthoven's postulates were re-examined and some were found wanting. For example, "so-called unipolar and augmented unipolar leads are shown by means of lead fields to be of essentially the same genre as bipolar leads, and thus may be relegated to their proper role in the scheme of things" (*29*). Also, a new method for constructing an accurate triangle for a given subject was reported by Wilson; such a triangle was usually oblique instead of equilateral (*226*).

Under the influence of the observations and theory of Burger and van Milaan, thinking shifted from the simple projections depicted by the Einthoven triangle to more complicated pictures of "lead fields" and the patterns of current flow which they represent (*150, 30, 86, 198, 28*). A landmark in the development of the concept of lead field was the revival of the reciprocity theorem, proved by Helmholtz in 1853 (*112*) to apply for both homogeneous and heterogeneous volume conductors. According to this theorem,

"Every single element of an electromotive surface will produce a flow of the same quantity of electricity through the galvanometer as would flow through

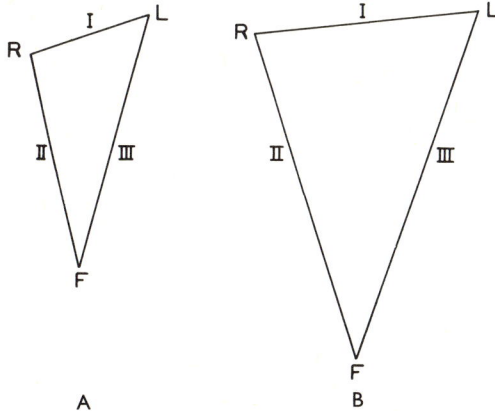

Figure 22. Triangles of Burger and van Milaan.
"(A) Triangle, representing the relation of heart vector and leads, deduced from a phantom with lungs and spine. (B) The same, without lungs and spine."

that element itself if its electromotive force were impressed on the galvanometer wire. If one adds the effects of all the electromotive surface elements, the effects of each of which are found in the manner described, he will have the value of the total current through the galvanometer" (*128*).

Thus, the theoretical knowledge which would have made so many restrictive assumptions unnecessary had already been available for fifty years at the time of Einthoven. Apparently, this information also escaped the attention of Waller, Lewis, and many subsequent investigators (*143*).

It is clear that considerable electrocardiographic and vectorcardiographic theory now hinges on the ideas of "lead vector" and "dipole" (*128*). Therefore, it would be misleading to ignore the fact that both of these ideas have their own inadequacies. For example, lead fields apply only to the particular form of the thorax and to the position, shape, size, and type of hypertrophy of the heart from which they were obtained; they make no direct provision for the real anatomy of the heart or for variations in the architecture of the thorax. Also, it is not generally accepted that a single fixed dipole may be used to represent the electromotive force generated by the heart at any instant (*88*), and many complicated attempts have been made to correct for the inaccuracies of the concept of the single fixed dipole (*87*). But even these unsettled problems have been rewarding in pointing up more precisely the questions to be asked. For example, if the interest of the observers is to gain insight into local cardiac events, the objective is the accurate registration of proximal potential by direct, precordial, or esophageal leads; but in this case, the heart cannot be considered to act as a dipole in any sense (*167, 104*). On the other hand, if interest centers around the recording of the over-all cardiac vector, proximal potentials must be minimized; in this situation the heart may be regarded as a dipole, but meaningful records can only be obtained if the lead field penetrates the heart in parallel and uniform flow lines (*191*).

The Wave of Excitation. Its Spread Through the Heart. Another aspect of electrocardiography has dealt with the manner in which the wave of excitation spreads through the various parts of the heart. The heart is relatively large compared to the body. A general idea can be obtained of this relationship by comparing the size of the subject's fist

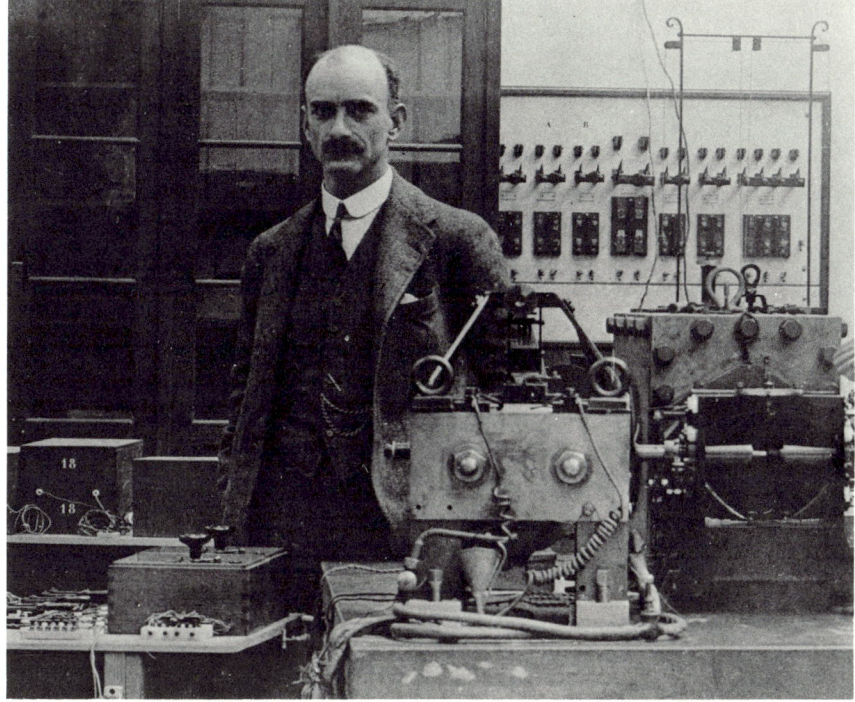

Figure 23. Thomas Lewis (1881–1945).

ELECTRO-
CARDIOGRAPHY

with the size and shape of the torso. If the heart were tiny compared to body size, a fixed dipole would readily be applicable and only the vectorial aspect of the direction of spread of excitation would be of significance in electrocardiography. However, this is not the case. It is important, therefore, to determine the order of excitation.

A fundamental prerequisite for the study of the *order* of the excitation process has been the detection of its arrival at a particular site. The earliest studies (*45, 77*), employing closely paired electrodes, led to the erroneous conclusion that the entire epicardial surface becomes negative almost simultaneously. However, the use of such electrodes has been criticized on the ground that they are unable to distinguish between the electrical activity of the subjacent region and more remote electrical activity (*152*).

Sir Thomas Lewis, one of the stalwarts of electrocardiography, a disciple of Sir James MacKenzie, Einthoven's scientific successor and

Wilson's teacher and scientific predecessor, made many important contributions during his long stay at University College in London. Lewis showed that different points on the epicardium were activated at different times when a "unipolar" lead was used. The exploring electrode that he used was a non-polarizable one, consisting of a small glass tube, plugged with salted kaolin, and half filled with a saturated copper sulfate solution into which a copper wire was immersed. This electrode, which was placed on the dog's heart, was paired with a distant electrode, providing the "unipolar" lead. The validity of this type of lead was based on the assumption that the "intrinsic deflection" is a true indicator of the time of local activation. According to Lewis (*145*),

"... *when electrodes are placed on the muscle of the auricle, they produce deflections of two kinds. ... The chief deflections are those which result from the arrival of the excitation process immediately beneath the contacts; these I term* intrinsic. *They are deflections which represent relatively large electrical potentials and they have correspondingly large amplitudes. The deflections of the second order are those yielded by the activation of muscle lying at a distance from the actual contact points. These I qualify by the adjective* extrinsic."

From records obtained at multiple epicardial points on the dog's heart, Lewis and Rothschild developed a concept of the course of the excitation wave through cardiac muscle. As may be seen in Figure 24, the

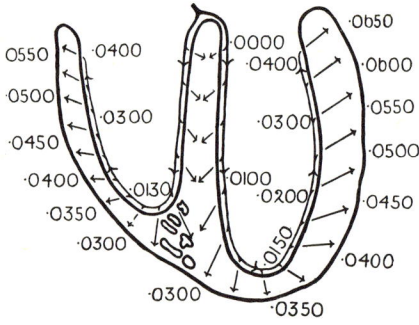

Figure 24. Lewis's diagram of the excitation process of the human ventricle.

differences between time intervals were often exceedingly small. Nonetheless, from such measurements, they estimated the rate of spread of the excitation wave to be 1000 mm./sec. in the atria, 4000 mm./sec.

in the Purkinje system, and 400 mm./sec. in the ventricular wall. Lewis emphasized the slow passage of impulses through the ventricular muscle as compared to the bundle of His and the Purkinje system, and attributed the different times of epicardial activation to regional variations in thickness of the ventricular myocardium. These studies also proved that the pattern of excitation corresponded to that of the specialized conduction system rather than to the arrangement of the cardiac muscle fibers.

Lewis and Rothschild also conducted elaborate studies on the activation of the interventricular septum. They concluded that the upper part of the septum was activated first, from left to right, by means of a special branch of the left bundle; the remainder of the septum was believed to be excited equally from both directions (*145*).

"*Since the impulse passes to the ventricle by two distinct channels, the right and left divisions of the bundle, and since no anatomical union is known to exist between the arborisations of the two sides, it might be assumed that the spread to a given ventricle is distinct and confined to that ventricle; that is to say, the wave does not normally cross the interventricular groove, but right and left waves meet somewhere in the septum . . . it seems reasonable to suppose that the normal electrocardiogram is really composite, displaying the superimposed effects of the separate ventricular activities.*"

The excitation wave was pictured as proceeding down the septum from the A-V junction to the ventricular walls. Section of one bundle branch in the dog resulted in an abnormal spread of the activation wave on the affected side, without modifying the pattern on the opposite side; the wave traversed the septum from the uninjured to the injured side of the ventricle (*145*).

Subsequent investigations confirmed that not all of the epicardium is activated simultaneously (*79, 132, 2*). Most convincing in this regard were the experiments of Harris, in which he used riding contiguous electrodes (*103*).

The Concept of the Intrinsic Deflection. According to Lewis, the intrinsic deflection represents the time of arrival of the excitation process in the myocardium beneath the exploring electrode (*145*). With the advent of precordial leads, the term "intrinsicoid" was coined to mean the same thing recorded from a "semidirect" lead (*152*). This was supported by the similarity of records obtained with the "semidirect" precordial leads (*26*) to those obtained by direct leads from either the subjacent epicardium or myocardium (*152, 230, 100*).

Refinements in the techniques of recording gradually placed the concepts of intrinsic and intrinsicoid deflections in a new perspective. The "exact time" of depolarization was shown to occur not at the beginning of the intrinsic deflection of Lewis, but just after its start; depolarization is completed at the end of this deflection. Durrer found that the differential spike occurs at the beginning of the fast portion of the intrinsic deflection; extrinsic effects are represented by initial and terminal slow portions (*61*). According to Sodi-Pallares and his associates, the moment of activation occurs during the lower part of the intrinsic deflection (*202*); in their opinion, the end of the intrinsic deflection signifies the completion under, rather than the arrival of the activation wave at, the exploring electrode.

It is evident that the time intervals under consideration are brief, a matter of a few milliseconds. The brevity of these intervals is relevant to the interpretation of the precise time of activation. As Durrer has indicated, the "moment of activation" is an abstract idea; in reality, activation involves a finite time interval (*61*). This time interval depends, in part, upon the size of the area affecting the electrode. These considerations are also relevant to the meaning of the term "intrinsic deflection." It seems that this term should be reserved for the fast component of the electrocardiogram recorded by an epicardial lead; the other components should be regarded as extrinsic. Also, unipolar leads from the surface of the body represent "the excitation processes of the whole heart, symbolized by an electrical vector as a resultant of all excitation waves at that respective moment" (*190*); in general, and with few exceptions, they should be regarded to be in the same category as extremity leads. Thus, unipolar limb leads are not truly "direct"; nor are precordial leads "semidirect." Finally, the term "intrinsicoid deflection," a pragmatic outgrowth of the use of precordial leads, seems to have more empirical than theoretical meaning.

Atrial Activation. The current concept of activation of the atria is essentially that presented by Lewis, et al. (*145, 181, 171*). The impulse that initiates the heart beat originates in the sino-atrial (sinus) node as a barrage of cascading discharges (*61*). The mechanisms involved in the generation of the impulses are unknown. The wave of excitation spreads radially from the sinus node toward the peripheral portions of the atria and the interatrial septum at an estimated rate of 360 to 1000 mm./sec. (*107*). According to current concept, based on Bernstein's membrane theory as applied to heart muscle by Craib (*50, 51*) and by Wilson, et al. (*234*), activation consists of a band of local dipoles progressing through the atrial myocardium undergoing activation.

The wave of excitation normally reaches the right atrium before the left. Activation of atrial musculature appears to be laminar since records obtained by unipolar endocardial and unipolar epicardial leads in the atria are identical. This lack of an endocardial-epicardial gradient of activation in the atria is in striking contrast to the gradients encountered in the ventricles. The intrinsic deflection in the atria varies in time depending on the position of the electrode and on the order of atrial activation; since the right atrium is normally activated before the left, the right atrial intrinsic deflection occurs during the first half of the atrial complex of the limb electrocardiogram whereas that of the left occurs during the second half. The roughly spherical shape of the atria, the laminar type of activation, the order of activation, and the relative lack of cancellation effects have encouraged efforts to identify strictly local effects in records obtained from distant leads (*187*).

Ventricular Activation. Until the 1950's, ideas about the activation of the ventricular wall were based predominantly on experiments using leads applied to the endocardial and epicardial surfaces of the ventricle (*145, 234, 33*). As indicated previously, these electrodes registered not only local but remote electrical events. Moreover, since these electrodes only registered summated electrical events, the records they provided could not be accurately analyzed in terms of the passage of the excitation wave through the successive layers of the subadjacent myocardial wall. This picture was drastically changed in the 1950's when technical advances made possible the use of penetrating electrodes in conjunction with improved cathode ray oscilloscopes and amplifiers (*193*).

It is now clear that activation of the ventricular wall does not proceed in the straightforward fashion postulated for a simple muscle strip (*50, 51*). Instead of an evenly propagated advance of dipoles from endocardium to epicardium, the inner layers are activated at a faster rate than the outer layers (*161, 63, 136*). Large areas of the subendocardium apparently undergo instantaneous excitation. And, instead of proceeding directly from endocardium to epicardium, the impulse may even reverse direction. These observed differences in the rate and direction of propagation of the excitation wave have stimulated a lively interest in an aspect of electrophysiology that had presumably been settled by the masterly experiments of Lewis and his associates.

The simultaneous excitation of the deeper layers of the myocardium is generally attributed to the presence of Purkinje fibers (*185*). This view is consistent with the earliest anatomical (*42*) and electrophysiological studies (*2*). However, the precise extent and ramifications of the Purkinje network are not entirely clear, especially in the hearts of different species. Also, recent electrophysiological observations have not settled the depth of myocardium involved in the simultaneous excitation (*136, 161, 63, 235*). As a result, many uncertainties remain about the penetration of the Purkinje fibers. These uncertainties are troublesome not only to anatomists and electrophysiologists but also to clinical electrocardiographers.

Activation of the Interventricular Septum. Direct epicardial leads in man (*100*) as well as intracavitary electrocardiograms (*195, 193*) have revealed that Lewis's ideas of activation of the septum were only partially correct. Lewis had proposed that the first portion of the ventricular myocardium to be activated was the interventricular septum, high on its left side; the wave of excitation then proceeded apically in the septum and from both endocardial aspects of the septum to the center of the septum. However, Sodi-Pallares, et al. (*161*) have found that instead of the wave of activation proceeding from above downward in the septum, it actually proceeds in the opposite direction. These observations using intracavitary electrodes have been confirmed on the isolated heart by Burchell, et al. (*34*). Lewis was apparently correct in believing that the excitation wave penetrates the muscle mass from the endocardial surfaces toward the center. However, there is controversy concerning the pattern of activation of the muscle within the septum. For example, Sodi-Pallares, et al. (*161*) have adduced evidence that the ventricular septum acts as though it were functionally two-fold, with its major portion controlled by the left bundle branch. On the other hand, Scher, et al. (*193*) could not demonstrate such a functional division of the septum and even found that a considerable portion of the septum is controlled by the right bundle.

Current View. From the experiments summarized above (primarily performed on the dog), the following sequence of ventricular activation has emerged to replace the simpler scheme of Lewis and Rothschild (146). Ventricular depolarization begins with activation of the left septal surface; the initial activity is predominantly from left to right and anteriorly in the septum. Following this initial septal activation, there is rapid conduction of the excitation wave through the Purkinje system, resulting in an invasion of the impulse from the endocardial to the central aspects of the septum and an irregular spread of excitation from the endocardial to epicardial surfaces of the free ventricular walls; the resultant forces are predominantly directed from base to apex, somewhat posteriorly, and to the left. Finally, the diaphragmatic portion of the left ventricle and the basal portions near the A-V grooves are activated; the forces are then oriented mainly from apex to base, posteriorly, and to the left (*193*).

Intraventricular Block. Further information about the spread of the impulse came from studies of block in the ventricular conduction system. Shortly after the turn of the present century, intraventricular block was produced independently by two groups of investigators: Eppinger and Rothberger produced the block by injection of silver nitrate into the myocardium of the dog (*75*); Barker and Hirschfelder sectioned the left main bundle of the heart of the dog (*10*). The characteristic electrocardiographic pattern of prolonged QRS complexes that followed interruption of the bundle to one ventricle in the dog was soon confirmed experimentally by others (*145, 229*). Within a few years, clinical counterparts were also reported (*160, 43*).

However, controversy arose when the patterns obtained in the experimental limb leads after experimental interruption of a particular bundle in the dog were held to apply to man. The view that the results in the dog were directly applicable to man was defended by Eppinger and Rothberger (*75*) and vigorously supported by Lewis (*145*). In 1930, Barker, Macleod, and Alexander showed conclusively that the QRS patterns of delayed conduction in the standard leads obtained from human subjects were diametrically opposite to those of the dog (*11*). In 1931, Wilson, et al. (*233*) explained the erroneous basis of Lewis's strong support of Eppinger and Rothberger: in part, Lewis had been misled by the histological studies of human bundle branch block reported by Eppinger and Stoerk (*76*); in addition, in his own experimental attempts to clamp the right bundle of the dog he had apparently injured conducting tracts on the left side of the septum. It appeared that much of the confusion in interpreting the limb leads had arisen from the different positions of the heart in dog and man; indeed, when precordial leads were used, they showed a delay in the activation of the free wall of the ventricle on the side of the block in both dog and man (*233, 185*).

Gaps in our knowledge of clinical heart block still persist. Conspicuously absent are detailed histologic examinations of the conduction system in both normal and abnormal hearts. The sporadic reports of the anatomical lesions in clinical bundle branch block that have appeared have been inconsistent or unconvincing (*185*). Recently, however, a surprisingly good agreement was found between the occurrence of anatomic lesions and of the patterns of complete bundle branch block in a series of 197 patients with delayed intraventricular conduction (*142*); but an adequate series of normal hearts with normal electrocardiograms were not included for comparison.

There are still other unsettled problems in relation to intraventricular block which may have important bearing on the spread of excitation. The anatomical meaning of the "arborization block" described in 1917 by Oppenheimer and Rothschild (*169*) is still unsettled. These investigators ascribed the pattern to a defect in conduction through the finer ramifications, rather than the large branches, of the conduction system; others have since offered other interpretations (*229*). Right bundle branch delay occurs, for some unknown reason, in presumably normal subjects (*32*) and in patients with exceedingly few lesions of the conduction system (*142*). Functional influences, such as fatigue of conduction tissue, may be the cause of intraventricular block (*47*) in the absence of histological lesions in the conduction system. The occasional functional prolongation of the QRS complex produced by stimulating the vagus reported by Wilson (*224*) has been attributed to the pre-excitation syndrome rather than to block.

Pre-excitation Syndrome. The foregoing described by Wilson, and similar cases subsequently described by others, were not understood properly until the report by Wolff, Parkinson, and White in 1930 (*239*).

This report originated through the study of a vigorous young athlete who had been referred in 1928 to White's laboratory;

"... *because his physician was perplexed by the occurrence of paroxysmal atrial fibrillation in a healthy individual. History, physical examination, and x-ray failed to reveal any evidence of heart disease except for episodes of rapid heart action. The electrocardiogram disclosed abnormal ventricular complexes, and the PR interval was 0.10 seconds. Since paroxysmal tachycardia had occasionally occurred during a workout in the gym, he was requested to run up and down four flights of stairs in the hope of provoking an attack. The effect of exercise was unexpected: the ventricular complex became normal, and the PR interval increased to 0.16 seconds, although the heart rate rose to levels of 120 to 140.*

"*The anomalous type of electrocardiogram was again observed on the young man's next visit to the laboratory, and this time the subcutaneous injection of atropine had the same effect as had exercise during the preceding visit.*

"... *On one occasion, the control electrocardiogram was normal and the carotid sinus massage was followed at once by prolongation of the QRS interval and abbreviation of AV conduction time.*

"*The electrocardiographic files were searched and six similar cases were found.*

"... *It so happened that White had started out on a visit of foreign medical centers at this time, and he had taken with him the electrocardiograms that were our great concern. The reaction to them in two cities is worth recording. In Vienna, the opinion was expressed that the tracings did not represent anything more unusual than bundle-branch block and AV nodal rhythm. In London, Sir John Parkinson's interest was aroused and he offered to look through his files in the hope of finding similar cases. He found three or four and graciously sent the material to us for incorporation in our paper.*"

The report of Wolff, Parkinson, and White stimulated considerable interest in this syndrome. The literature was soon filled with reports of other clinical examples of short PR intervals and prolonged QRS complexes, either freshly observed or exhumed from electrocardiographic files. With mounting experience, it also became clear that the syndrome has a graver prognosis than originally believed. Physiologically (*239*);

"... *it became a matter of considerable importance to know whether an explanation within the framework of current knowledge of cardiac physiology was adequate, or whether new concepts were needed for this purpose. It is generally agreed that premature activation of a fraction of ventricular musculature is responsible for both the short PR interval and the abnormally wide QRS complex, but there is considerable difference of opinion concerning the manner in which it is brought about."*

A number of different mechanisms have been invoked to account for the characteristic combination of short PR interval and the broad QRS (*184*). One hypothesis is that transmission of impulses from the atria to the ventricles occurs by way of an accessory bundle, either the bundle of Kent or a similar one close to or within the A-V node. Accessory atrioventricular bundles are not unique to the hearts of patients with the syndrome but may also be found in normal hearts (*184*). An alternate hypothesis is based on the concept of "accelerated" conduction. This derives from the observation that similar electrocardiographic complexes have been observed in a variety of clinical cardiac situations and in response to experimental probing and manipulation of the heart. Unfortunately, in these clinical and experimental circumstances, it is generally difficult to distinguish between the pre-excitation phenomenon on the one hand and fusion beats due to ventricular premature beats on the other. Of these two hypotheses, the bulk of the evidence favors, but does not establish, the operation of an accessory pathway (*133*).

An important by-product of these studies has been the clarification of some aspects of the function of the A-V node. The delay between atrial and ventricular activations had been postulated by Lewis to be due to the retardation of the atrial impulse in passing through the A-V node, and by Erlanger to occur at the terminal endings of the Purkinje system (*78*). Experimental stimulation of the A-V node and of the bundle of His, as well as direct electrograms, have demonstrated that the "delay in normal A-V conduction occurs at the A-V node, and not at the periphery of the conduction system" (*133*). Actually, newer evidence suggests that much of it occurs at the upper junction of the A-V node with the atrium (*172*).

Recovery From Excitation. Little work has been done on the electrocardiograph manifestations of recovery of the atria from excitation, but a considerable effort has been made to understand the T wave as a manifestation of the recovery of the ventricles from excitation (*130, 132, 141*).

That recovery from excitation in the ventricle is associated with electrical activity was first recognized by Kölliker and Müller in 1856 (*139*). The presence of this activity was confirmed in 1862 by Meissner and Cohn, who noted that a twitch of the rheoscopic frog preparation occasionally occurred at the start of diastole as well as of systole (*132*). In 1872, Donders made graphic recordings of these twitches (*133*). The contributions of Burdon-Sanderson and Page in 1878 (*36*) to the understanding of the T wave have been discussed earlier in this chapter.

Since the 1870's, considerable evidence has accumulated to indicate that the T wave occurs because the manifestations of the active state disappear asynchronously in the various parts of the heart. In addition, besides the influence of the *topography* of excitation, the *duration* of the excitatory process in different regions of the heart has been implicated in the genesis of the T wave (*130*).

Interest in distinguishing primary from secondary T wave changes led Wilson, et al. to the concept of the ventricular gradient (*235*). This was an attempt to measure the electrical effects produced by local variations in the duration of the excitatory process and particularly by local variations in the duration of the excited state. When expressed as a vector quantity, the ventricular gradient portrays the direction and magnitude of this lack of uniformity in the duration of the excitatory state. This concept was subsequently developed and applied to the frontal plane by Ashman, et al. (*9*); recently, an attempt has been made to apply it stereovectorally (*129*). However, the hope that the ventricular gradient would bring "order to a variety of electrocardiographic phenomena that are otherwise without order" (*93*) has not yet been realized. Instead, it emerges as an important conceptual tool for distinguishing primary from secondary T wave changes, with little apparent value in solving the practical, day-by-day problems of clinical electrocardiography.

That differences exist between the T waves of endocardial and epicardial leads of normal hearts is well known (*107*). Although various reasons for these differences have been considered, including the effects of heating and cooling on action potentials (*109, 52*), and much has

ELECTRO-
CARDIOGRAPHY

been learned about experimentally induced changes in T waves, it is not possible to account for the *normal* endocardial or epicardial T waves in terms of either action potentials or myocardial temperature gradients (*109*).

Recently, the pattern of recovery has been subjected to critical analysis. Not only is this pattern influenced by the chain of events set up within the fiber by depolarization and by the pattern of excitation, but it may be initiated by an external anodal current (*175*). The latter observation raises the possibility that recovery, like excitation, may be initiated as a propagated disturbance in excited tissue when resting unstimulated tissue is present (*53*). Many other questions, such as the role of propagation of repolarization in the normal electrical recovery of the heart, remain to be answered.

The T wave is often followed by a U wave. The contour of the U wave is influenced by changes in electrolyte composition of the body (*58*). Too little is known about the genesis of the U wave to warrant any further comments here (*144*).

The Influence of Myocardial Injury Upon the Electrocardiogram. Injury of the myocardium has a great influence upon the rate, order, and intensity of the processes of activation (depolarization), and of recovery (repolarization) of the cell membrane of the myocardium and of its specialized conduction tissue. Furthermore, one of the most valuable clinical uses of the electrocardiogram is to recognize, evaluate, and classify damage to the heart, particularly that produced by coronary disease, or localized or generalized myocarditis, as a result of muscle injury (*131*). Such an analysis has made the electrocardiogram indispensible in cases of ischemic heart disease of various types.

When injured, the myocardium shows changes in its electrical characteristics. This occurs in both the atria and ventricles. The effects of injury of the atrial myocardium are often obscured by overlap of the deflection of atrial electrical recovery and of ventricular excitation (*204, 106*). Injury of the ventricles, however, is much more readily detected.

Following acute injury, change in the electrocardiographic contour is only in small part due to change in the shape and position of the heart; for the most part, it occurs because certain regions of the heart become inactive and hence fail to contribute their full share to the electrical forces during the inscription of the electrocardiogram generated by the ventricles.

The late effects of injury on the ventricular activation process result in the presence of Q or (QS) waves ("electrical windows") in surface or direct leads over the destroyed muscle (236); in other words, injury removes part of the ventricular electrical activity, leaving the rest unbalanced. A completely transmural dead zone in the free ventricular wall fails to produce any action potentials and serves merely to transmit passively the negative intracavitary potential to the overlying exploring electrode.

More recently another effect of injury has been recognized—that is, an alteration of the pattern of activation. Due to alterations in the time course and order of depolarization of injured areas, acute changes in the duration, form, and magnitude of the ventricular excitation complex occur in the individual fiber and whole heart (83). The early effect of injury on activation has received far less attention than its effects on the ventricular recovery process (repolarization).

It is now generally agreed that the manifestations of injury can be explained on a cellular level, as will be discussed later in the chapter (140). The injury current of activity has been shown to occur when the resting membrane potential is normal; during systole, the injury prevents complete depolarization of the cell membrane in the area injured, and a current of injury flows to displace the S-T segment from the zero-potential line. Injury current of rest on the other hand occurs because injury causes incomplete polarization of the resting cell membrane in the area injured; a current of injury flows during diastole. This

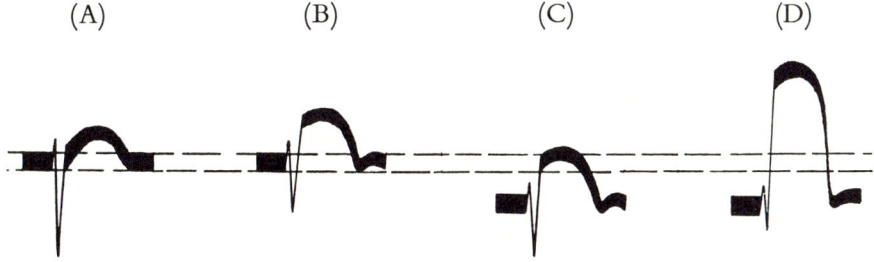

Figure 25. Effects of injury during rest and activity. A. Control record. B, C, D. Curves after injury.

produces displacement of the T-Q segment. A combination of injury during rest and activity has also been demonstrated (causing displacement of both T-Q and S-T segments). Injury currents occurring during repolarization modify the T wave (*108*).

The electrocardiographic representations of these injury currents of rest, activity, and repolarization depend on their magnitude and on their spatial location with reference to the body surface or intracavitary leads. To be represented in the external field of the heart, such injured regions must reach and occupy a portion of the endocardial or epicardial surfaces of the heart. A myocardial injury, of any given size, on the endocardial surface of a given part of the left ventricle would tend to have exactly the opposite effect of that on the corresponding epicardial surface. Also, the degree to which a myocardial injury is indicated in a given lead by displacement of the S-T segment depends on the spatial relation of the exploring electrode to the area involved (*108*).

The production of monophasic curves of injury by endocardial pressure injury in the atria and ventricles has demonstrated that these areas, as well as others, are capable of producing electrocardiographic changes. But for some time there has been disagreement about the contributions of the deeper layers of the heart to the electrocardiogram (*165, 180*). There is no doubt that an injury that does not surface upon the endocardium or epicardium is electrically silent. Injured subendocardial myocardium is not electrically silent, but produces displacement of the S-T segment in a predictable fashion depending upon how far it surfaces upon the endocardium (*108*). Unreconciled differences of various experimenters (*183*) may be due in part to differences in experimental technique (*140*).

Despite the knowledge currently available and its practical utility in clinical medicine, much still needs to be learned about the important fundamental processes of injury which follow upon ischemia and injury to parts of the heart.

The Vectorcardiogram. Most of clinical electrocardiography has been based on the recording of scalar tracings (magnitude of deflections written over time) of a number of heart cycles, employing many different lead combinations. The recording of the vectorial fluctuations of the electrocardiogram during a single cycle has been less fully developed and employed. The vector approach to electrocardiography, however, has been in use ever since Waller; recently time signals on the vector record have been added.

In the first description of the direction and magnitude of the potential variations in the frontal plane, by Einthoven, Fahr, and de Waart in 1913, vector analysis was essentially confined to the peak of the R wave (*72*). With the development of multichannel simultaneous recording, it soon became evident that the apexes of the R wave in the standard leads were not simultaneous. Williams, in 1914, attributed this discrepancy to the vectoral nature of the changing potential during the heart cycle (*223*). Accordingly, vector analysis was recognized to be inaccurate unless the two reference leads were taken simultaneously and homologous points were used. Within the next year (*82*), vectors were plotted at short intervals in the cycle, instantaneous electrical axes thereby showing changes in the direction of the electrical axis from moment to moment. Lewis and his associates used this method to study bundle branch block and hypertrophy, and to plot the course of atrial activation in experimental flutter and other arrhythmias (*145*).

The first known attempt to plot the electrocardiogram as a vector-time trace was made by Mann in 1920 (*153*). He constructed a monocardiogram for the frontal plane, a fusion of the three leads of the electrocardiogram into a single curve. He used lead I as the horizontal (X axis), and the average of leads II and III for the vertical component (Y axis). This method consisted of plotting the instantaneous axes of two leads, preferably recorded simultaneously, in a rectangular coordinate system. The terminals of the instantaneous axes were then joined to form a loop, the "monocardiogram." Mann was cognizant of the need to portray the monocardiogram in three dimensions and suggested that three leads be taken in the horizontal plane to obtain a transverse monocardiogram. This suggestion bore fruit nine years later when Savjoloff reported a method for obtaining stereomonocardiograms (*188*). Mann calculated the monocardiogram of right and left bundle branch block (*154*). He suggested that the Lewis designation for bundle branch block, then in common use, was in error; the same conclusion had previously been reached by Fahr in 1920 using vector analysis (*81*).

Unfortunately, instrumental methods were not yet available in 1920 for deriving the monocardiogram. Mann attempted to use a cathode ray oscilloscope with a pair of three stage amplifiers for this purpose,

ELECTRO-CARDIOGRAPHY

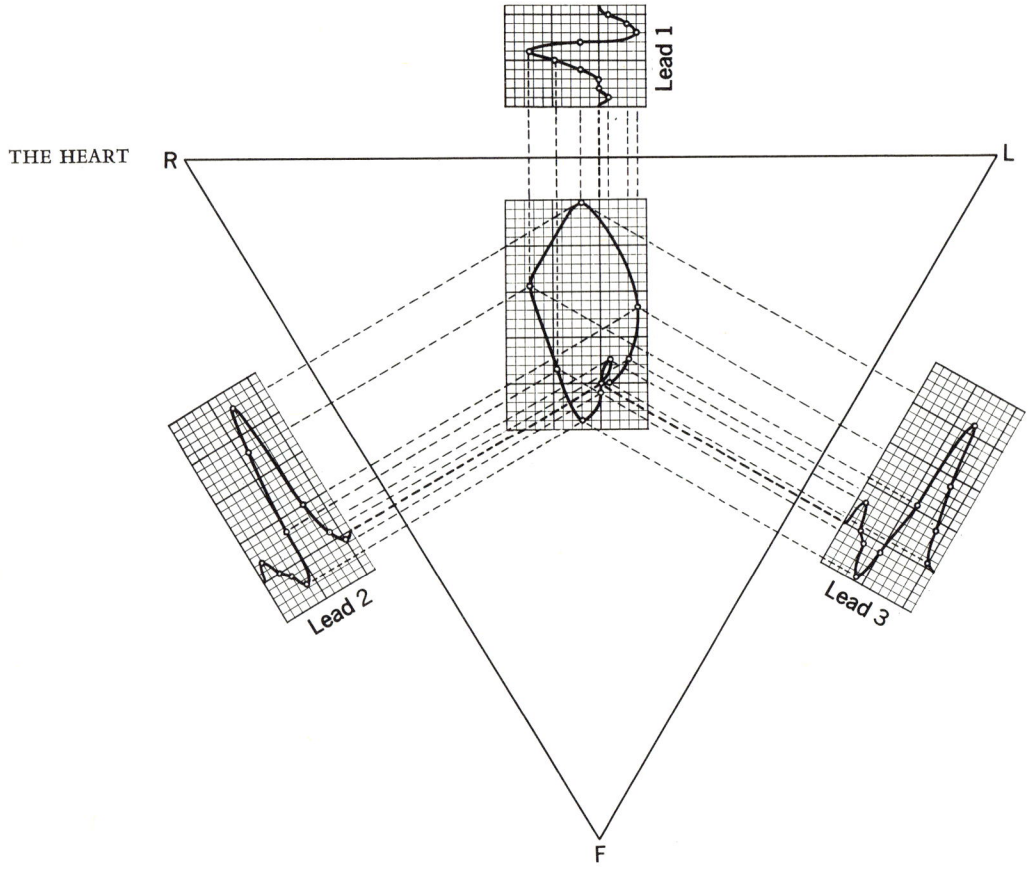

Figure 26. First vectorcardiogram, the monocardiogram of Mann.

but because of serious technical difficulties he abandoned the attempt. The cathode ray tube was still inadequate in 1931, when Mann developed a special galvanometer with three movable coils which caused a mirror to oscillate. At this time he reported a vector analysis of ventricular premature systoles, of hypertrophy, and of bundle branch block (*154*). In 1938, he presented a detailed report of the results with his special galvanometer (*155*), already obsolete because of contemporary improvements in the cathode ray oscilloscope and thermionic tube.

By the late 1930's the cathode ray oscilloscope and amplifiers were sufficiently developed to be used for the registration of vectorcardiograms. In 1936, Sulzer of Geneva, unaware of Mann's investigations, used the cathode ray oscilloscope to study the isolated rabbit heart. He presented frontal plane loops, "electrocardiograms in two dimensions," of the normal heart beat and of ventricular fibrillation (*206*). In the same year, Schelong presented his method for obtaining vectorcardiograms in man using the Braun tube (*192*). In this country, Wilson, Johnston, and Barker, unaware of the European efforts, constructed a similar apparatus to obtain satisfactory vectorcardiograms (*228*).

In 1937 and 1938, a great deal was published on vectorcardiography. Particularly noteworthy were the monocardiograms or vectorcardiograms obtained by H. E. Hollmann and W. Hollmann, who fed the output from three leads (VR, VL, and VF), taken simultaneously, through a special cathode ray tube; in this tube three sets of plates, placed at an angle of 120 degrees to each other, replaced the usual two sets placed perpendicular to each other (*123*). Interest in vectorcardiography lagged during World War II but revived, particularly in Europe, immediately after the war (*60, 40*). The American phase began somewhat later (*1, 98*).

It has been pointed out previously that many practical advances in electrocardiography were made even though the theoretical bases were not completely understood. The question arises why vectorcardiography has not flourished in a similar fashion. There are several reasons.

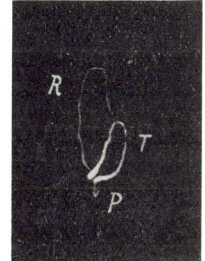

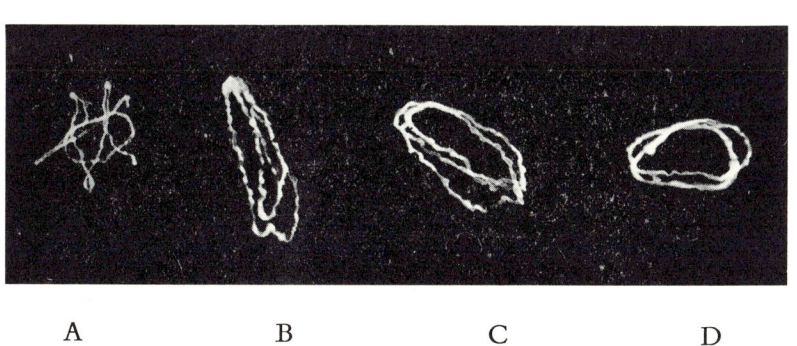

A   B   C   D

Figure 27. First vectorcardiograms recorded with cathode ray oscilloscope. *Upper right:* "Electrogram in two dimensions of the activity of the normal heart of a rabbit." *Lower left:* "Electrogram in two dimensions of the heart of a rabbit in ventricular fibrillation. A, B, C, D: four successive stages."

Paramount among these is the strangeness of the configuration of the vectorcardiogram. Also, there have been, and still remain, technical problems in developing and using suitable instrumentation. One major difficulty has been superimposition of P, QRS, and ST-T components on the screen of the cathode ray oscilloscope; not only the components of single loops, but also entire successive loops, may superimpose when the heart rate is rapid. Many different attempts have been made to solve the problem of superposition; these include stereoscopic viewing (*192*), moving the film during a portion of the loop (method of Milovanovich) (*56*), and gaiting techniques to record each of the three component parts of the vectorcardiogram separately (*27, 97, 111*) or in various combinations. Improvements in amplifiers, apparatus to calculate correction coefficients, stereoscopic or panoramic viewing, light registration of images without photography by ultraviolet or other methods, and simplification of design of equipment, all promise to make suitable apparatus widely available soon (*17, 197, 162, 189, 25*).

In addition to these intrinsic problems, the evolution of vectorcardiography has shared other growing pains with electrocardiography. The question of uniformity in recording and in terminology has been particularly troublesome. At the moment, although all concerned with vectorcardiography appreciate the need for standardization, there is no immediate solution in prospect.

Transmembrane Potentials

Fundamental to the understanding of the electrophysiology of the heart is the understanding of the electrical activity of the individual muscle cells in particular, and of bioelectric phenomena in general. As indicated earlier, the first insights into the electrical activity of muscle were gained in the frog by Galvani and his successors. These observations indicated that unless muscle (or nerve) were injured, there would be no potential difference between any two points on their surfaces. On the other hand, injury would make the injured area negative with respect to the rest of the tissue; the injury or "demarcation" potential was not only present at rest but decreased with each contraction of the muscle (*159, 151*).

Collateral information gradually accumulated from other sources.

The action potential was described in 1872 by Du Bois-Reymond. He pointed out that the electrical sign of the changes produced by the excitatory process originates in the membrane of muscle (59). In 1871, Bowditch described the all-or-none response, indicating that suprathreshold stimuli failed to augment the amplitude of cardiac muscular contraction (21). The magnitude of the injury potentials was measured in frog ventricles by Engelmann and his associates in 1873. According to their results the injury potentials were of the order of 100 mv. and the electrical potential reversed its sign during excitation (74). However, their findings could not be duplicated by everyone (36); indeed, sixty years were to elapse before the reversal phase (or overshoot) was established beyond cavil by Eyster, Meek, and their associates, who used surface electrodes for recording (80). Unfortunately, this technique is uncertain with respect to the "zero" reference potential so that acc-

ELECTRO-
CARDIOGRAPHY

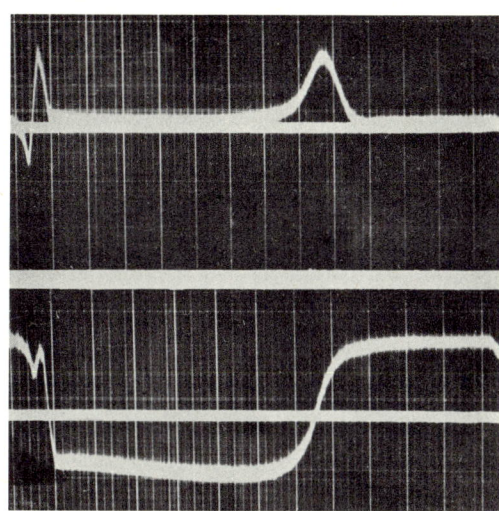

Figure 28. Reversal of polarization following injury of heart muscle according to Eyster and Meek.
"Potential time curves from a tortoise heart *in situ*, one electrode on the mid-anterior ventricle, the other on the muscles of the left hind leg. The upper curve is recorded before, the lower curve after the region under the electrode was burned with a hot iron. The deviations above the horizontal line represent negativity; the deviations below the horizontal line represent positivity."

urate delineation of the magnitude and time course of the action potentials was not possible. This last step had to await the advent of transmembrane recording (*148*), and was accomplished in the squid giant axon by Hodgkin and Huxley (*117*), and by Curtis and Cole (*54*).

The Classical Theory of Bernstein. In 1910, Julius Bernstein, one of Du Bois-Reymond's best students, presented the famous theory which accounted for bioelectric phenomena on the premise that nerve conduction was a surface phenomenon (*18*). This was an important advance. The cell surface (or membrane) was considered to be impermeable to all cations but potassium; the resting potential, in turn, was pictured as originating in the marked difference between the intra- and extra-cellular potassium, K_i^+, K_o^+. According to this scheme, the selectively permeable membrane of the nerve fiber is polarized when the nerve is at rest; a layer of cations on the outside is separated by the membrane from a layer of anions on its inside. When a stimulus is applied locally to the membrane it loses its selective permeability; the point of stimulation becomes negative with respect to the immediately adjacent section of nerve. A potential difference is set up and a current flows between the active and inactive portions. The flow of current initiated in this way initiates, in turn, similar changes in nearby regions, thereby causing the propagated electrical pulse, the "spike." In support of his theory, Bernstein was able to show a fairly good correlation between the resting membrane potential and $\log K_i^+/K_o^+$.

Bernstein's theory did not wear well. As electrochemistry developed, the reactions at the cell surface were shown to be more complicated than originally imagined (*4*). Moreover, the assumption that potential differences between an injured spot and an uninjured area were derived exclusively from the uninjured area was shown to be untenable (*234, 221, 80*). Also, by no reasonable extension of concept or analogy could Bernstein's theory account for either the rapid rate of propagation of the impulse or for the rapid recovery (*199*). Finally, experimental measurements by more refined techniques failed to find the close correspondence between the magnitude of the resting potential and the concentration gradient for potassium across the cell membrane (*4, 199*). Nonetheless, despite the inadequacies of Bernstein's hypothesis in explaining either excitation or contraction, it served admirably to promote serious consideration of excitation, conduction, electrical manifestations, and contraction as parts of a unified process rather than independent phenomena.

The Upset of the Classical Theory. In proposing his theory of bioelectric phenomena, Bernstein had disregarded Engelmann's observations on the overshoot (*74*). The most telling blow against his theory came from observations on the overshoot in the giant axon of the squid and the demonstration that selective permeability was not lost but merely altered.

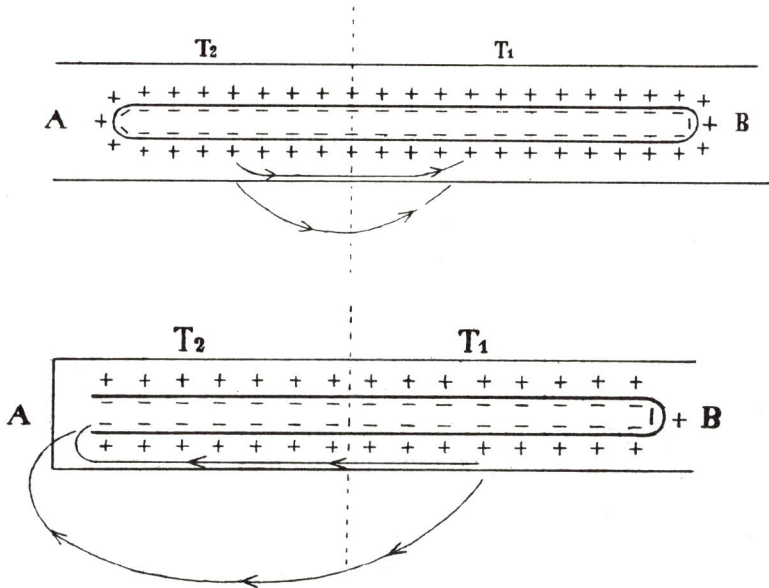

Figure 29. Bernstein's membrane theory.
Upper: Normal fiber in fluid. The potential difference between the inside and outside of the fiber (AB) is everywhere the same; the fiber appears to be without current. *Lower:* Injured fiber in fluid. At the cut end (A) the membrane is removed so that a current arises.

In the 1930's, the English biologist, J. Z. Young, rediscovered the giant nerve system in the squid and introduced the fibers of this system into neurophysiology (*242*). The squid is jet-propelled. Its squirting is controlled by nerves of enormous size. A single squid fiber is a half millimeter in diameter, approximately twenty times larger than a nerve fiber in the leg of a rabbit (*48*). The use of these huge fibers has made pos-

THE HEART

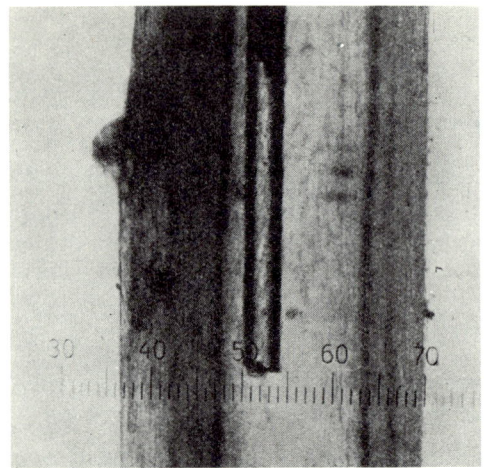 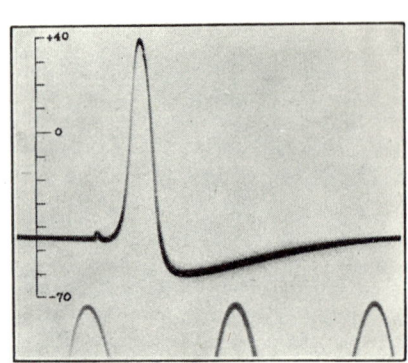

Figure 30. First demonstration of overshoot during the action potential showing reversal of polarization with electrode placed inside a nerve fiber. *Left:* "Photomicrograph of electrode inside giant axon. One scale division equals 33μ." *Right:* "Action potential recorded between inside and outside of axon."

sible investigations that could never have been attempted otherwise. Axoplasm can be sampled and analyzed for its content of ions, proteins, etc. The squid fiber or axon can be isolated and kept alive and functioning for hours (54). A fairly large electrode (from 1 to 100μ) can be placed within it, and electrical properties, such as conductance, potential, resistance, and capacitance, can be studied (117).

By using this preparation, it was confirmed that ions cross a membrane with greater ease during the passage of an impulse than at rest and that the potential recorded by the inside electrode is about 60 mv. at rest. However, instead of merely declining after the application of a stimulus—as would be expected if only loss of selective permeability were involved—the potential rapidly overshoots the reference ("zero") potential so that the transmembrane potential in the region of the applied stimulus actually reverses its polarity and the inside of the fiber becomes positive with respect to the outer surface. The rising phase of the spike overshoots the "zero" level by as much as 20 to 50 mv. After the peak of the reversal, the transmembrane potential returns to its resting level at a much slower rate than occurs during the rising phase.

This overshoot has since been found in a wide variety of bioelectric tissues (52).

The Ionic Hypothesis. At the turn of the present century, Overton had sought to explain the excitation of muscle in terms of an exchange of sodium and potassium ions (*170*). However, he could conceive of no physical process by which the natural distribution of potassium between the inside and outside of the cell could be restored. Fifty years later, following the demonstration of the overshoot, ionic flux and membrane pumps were used to explain excitation and conduction in a striking and convincing way.

Again at the root of the explanation were observations on the giant nerve fiber of the squid, particularly those by Hodgkin, A. F. Huxley, B. Katz, and their associates (*118, 119*). According to these members of the "Cambridge School," the propagation of the nerve impulse depends on the exchange of sodium and potassium across the membrane at the surface of the fiber under the control of the potential difference across the membrane. Also, the rising phase of the action potential is effected by an increase in permeability to sodium ions so that positive charges enter the fiber at a rapid rate; the declining phase of the action potential arises from the combination of a reduced permeability of the membrane to sodium and an increased permeability to potassium, resulting in a net efflux of positive charges (potassium ions) (*118, 52*). The observations on the squid giant axon did not determine whether the membrane potential is the cause or effect of the ionic shifts.

Resting and Action Potentials of Cardiac Muscle. The exploration of heart muscle through the same technique as was used in studying the squid giant axon had to await improvements in methodology. In 1950, Nastuk and Hodgkin (*166*) improved the microelectrode technique which Ling and Gerard had introduced the previous year (*148*); in 1951 the microelectrode was successfully applied to the ventricle of the frog heart by Woodbury, Hecht, and Christopherson (*241*) and to the isolated Purkinje fiber of the dog and kid heart by Draper and Weidmann (*57*). Improvements in technique have continued. Outstanding among the more recent modifications of the Ling-Gerard electrode is the "riding" tungsten-wire glass capillary which leads off from inside a single fiber of the moving heart (*240*). At rest, the potential difference

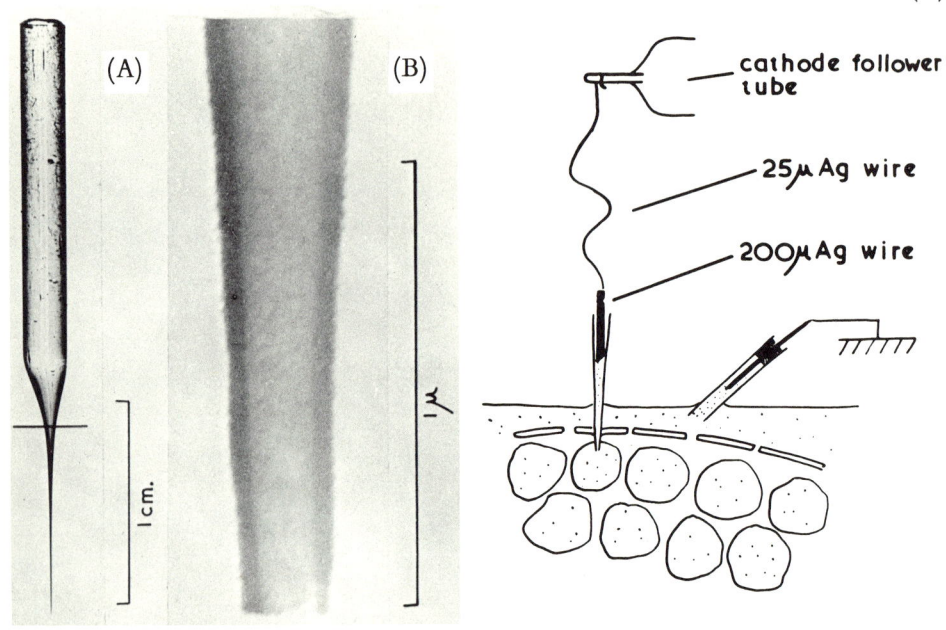

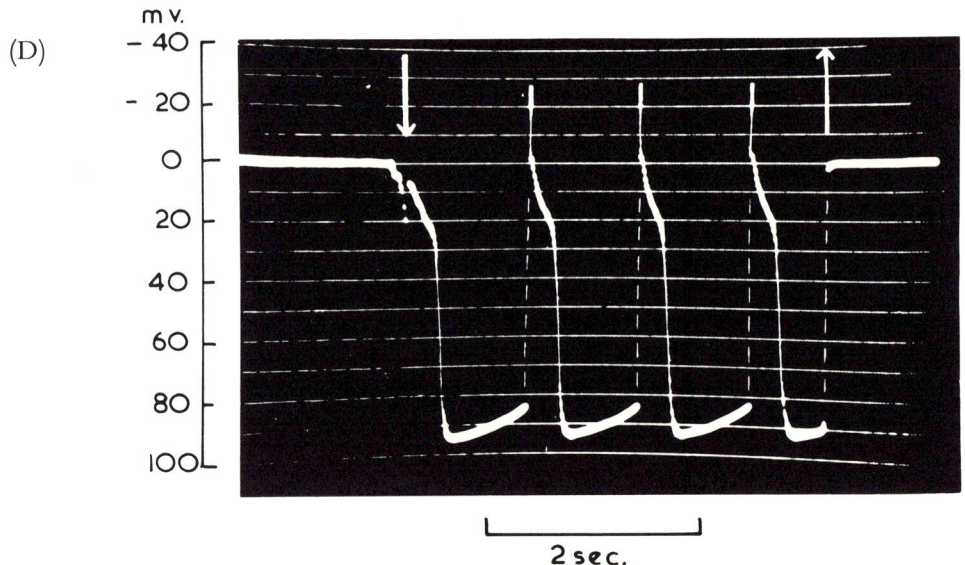

[332]

across the membrane varies from 50 to 90 mv., the outside being electrically positive to the inside. During activity, the membrane voltage reverses temporarily, the outside becoming negative to the inside.

Five periods of voltage change can be identified in a cardiac action potential (52): rapid depolarization, rapid repolarization (spike), slow repolarization (plateau), terminal repolarization, and diastole. During the spike, sodium moves into the fiber; during and after the plateau, potassium moves out.

Distribution of Ions in Cardiac Muscle. In the resting muscle fiber, K_i^+/K_o^+ is of the order of 40:1, while the corresponding ratio for sodium ion is of the order of 1:10 (217, 52). Many hypotheses exist to account for the maintenance of such concentration gradients across any biological membrane which is permeable to these ions. For the heart muscle fiber in particular, the hypothesis must also account for the extrusion of sodium ions from the interior of the fiber during activity, against both a concentration gradient and an electrical gradient. The most popular concept is that of the "sodium pump" according to which sodium is actively moved and potassium is distributed passively (31). The energetics involved in driving this hypothetical pump, as well as the details of its operation, are entirely speculative.

The Movement of Ions During the Cardiac Action Potential. In general, the movement of ions in cardiac muscle corresponds to that in the giant nerve of the squid. The influx of sodium ions seems to be responsible for depolarization (119), the efflux of potassium for repolarization (222). Following activity, sodium ions are ejected and potassium ions are accumulated to restore the resting ionic strength before the onset of the next action potential.

Figure 31. Use of microelectrode for recording action potentials of cardiac muscle.

A. Ling-Gerard electrode, 2.5x natural size. B. Electron micrograph of tip of the microelectrode, 55,000x natural size. C. "Riding" microelectrode leading off from inside single fiber of moving heart. D. Potential changes recorded when the tip of the Ling-Gerard electrode is introduced into a single Purkinje fiber of the dog heart and then withdrawn.

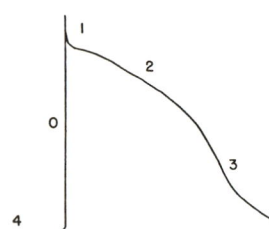

Figure 32. Schematic representation of a cardiac membrane action potential showing the various phases.

Pacemaker and Non-Pacemaker Action Potentials. Draper and Weidmann also described a fundamental difference between pacemaker and non-pacemaker tissues, namely, the presence of a slow depolarization or prepotential in pacemaker tissues (*57*). In non-pacemaker tissues, where the prepotential rise does not occur, the resting membrane potential remains at constant value until the area is abruptly depolarized by a propagated action potential. On the other hand, in pacemaker tissues there is a gradual "upward" convex part of the curve, a "prepotential" suggestive of a gradual transition from rest to activity (*217*). Similar types of pacemaker activity have been observed in the S-A and A-V nodes of the hearts of various mammals, fowl, and amphibia, and in mammalian Purkinje fibers.

Once the prepotential had been characterized by Draper and Weidmann in 1951, a considerable effort was made to relate it to the excitability of pacemaker and non-pacemaker tissues, to determine the factors that influence the prepotential, and to establish the effects on the prepotential of agents that were known to alter rhythmicity (*122*). This effort has been most rewarding with respect to excitability. A propagated action potential is initiated when the prepotential reaches a critical level; when this "threshold potential" has been attained, a regenerative process is automatically stimulated to effect further depolarization and a reversal of potential (*31*).

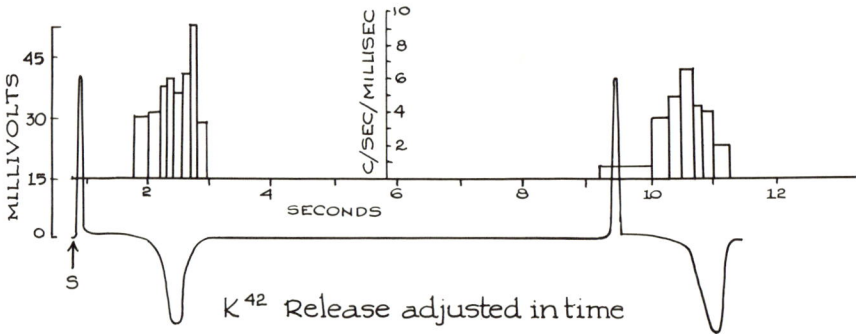

Figure 33. Potassium efflux during action potential according to Wilde.

Spontaneous rhythmicity appears to originate in the instability of the membrane of pacemaker tissues. Moreover, changes in the rate of spontaneous depolarization after repolarization, as well as the height of the threshold potential, influence the rate at which a pacemaker fires. These insights have led to a new characterization of agents that are known to alter cardiac frequency. These agents include autonomic mediators, changes in temperature, ions, hypoxia, and cardiac drugs such as procaine, quinidine, and digitalis. Vagal stimulation decreases the slope of the prepotential so that more time is required to reach the threshold potential. The opposite effect occurs during sympathetic stimulation; the slope of the prepotential is increased. Prolonged vagal stimulation not only decreases the slope of the prepotential but also effects hyperpolarization which prevents the pacemaker from firing (the "Gaskell Effect," 1887) (*122*).

Changes in ionic concentrations also modify the prepotential significantly. For example, a decrease in the concentration of extracellular sodium ions decreases the rate of depolarization. Conversely, a decrease in extracellular potassium ions increases the slope of the prepotential and lowers the threshold potential. An increase in extracellular calcium slows the heart rate by lowering the threshold potential; the slope of the prepotential is not altered (*52, 31*).

Other Lessons from the Recording of Transmembrane Potentials. The few examples cited above comprise only a small fraction of the gains in the understanding of cardiac electrophysiology that have followed the introduction of precise techniques for recording transmembrane potentials (*194, 126*). Even at this time, enough has been learned to indicate that not only will old concepts be clarified and extended but that new areas for investigation will be disclosed.

Epicrisis

It is plain that we are at the beginning of what may be called a "biophysical" revolution—a period during which we may expect many new discoveries about the cell, its membrane, microsomes, mitochondria, and cytoplasm. The particular causes of this current development are obvious. It is easy to point to several new techniques whose use within the last few years make it possible to mount revealing and significant experiments. The electron microscope, the newer

THE HEART

characterization of proteins chemically, and spatial orientation of their amino acids and their genetic coding, tracer isotopes, etc., have made the study of the cell's interior possible, and indeed the whole region of the cell between its interior and its surface can now be investigated in a depth of detail which would have been beyond the most extravagant hopes of electrophysiologists even a few decades ago. The development of new techniques is not the only factor in current investigations. The great periods of discovery in science are marked by a sudden synthesis of knowledge from different fields. The creative achievements of Du Bois-Reymond, Helmholtz, Kelvin, Lippmann, Waller, Hodgkin, A. F. Huxley, B. Katz, Ader, Einthoven, Lewis, Wilson, Burger, etc., were derived from experience in fields as apparently dissimilar as electricity, atomic theory, field theory, and chemistry. The recognition of the unity of scientific enquiry is largely due to patient research in diverse disciplines. The fertilization of one field by another makes new and important problems apparent; it also makes simpler solutions of old problems possible.

Out of current diversified and exploitive research we can reasonably expect to know a great deal more about the basic nature of the electric current source, the nature of the spread of the impulse in the heart, of cardiac recovery, and of distribution of electrical potentials within the body and upon the body surface. This understanding will probably be clear and coherent, since we are now applying more accurate data from many fields, as well as using finer instrumentation. Instruments and techniques naturally determine in great part what observations will be made.

A man was seen in the street one night, looking for something on the ground by the light of the street lamp.
"What are you looking for?"
"My door key."
"Have you lost it?"
"Yes."
"Is this where you lost it?"
"I don't know."
"Then why are you looking here?"
"Because here I can see" (218).

BIBLIOGRAPHY

1. ABILDSKOV, J. A., G. E. BURCH, and J. A. CRONVICH. The validity of the equilateral tetrahedron as a spatial reference system. Circulation, 2:122, 1950.
2. ABRAMSON, D. I., and K. JOCHIM. The pathway taken by the impulse in the mammalian ventricles. Amer. J. Physiol., 119:257, 1937.
3. ADER, C. Sur un nouvel appareil enregistreur pour câbles sous-marins. C.R. Acad. Sci. (Paris), 124:1440, 1897.
4. ADRIAN, R. H. The effects of membrane potential and external potassium concentration on the potassium permeability of muscle fibres. J. Physiol. (Lond.), 143:59P, 1958.
5. ALEXANDER, J. T., and W. L. NASTUK. An instrument for the production of microelectrodes used in electrophysiological studies. Rev. sci. Instrm., 24:528, 1953.
6. AMBERSON, W. R. The influence of fashion in the development of knowledge concerning electricity and magnetism. Amer. Sci., 46:33, 1958.
7. ASCHOFF, L. Zur Myocarditisfrage. Verh. dtsch. path. Ges., 8:46, 1904.
8. ASCHOFF, L. Concerning the question of myocarditis. Tr. by F. A. Willius. In Cardiac Classics. F. A. Willius and T. E. Keys, Eds. St. Louis, Mosby, 1941.
9. ASHMAN, R., E. BYER, and R. H. BAYLEY. The normal human ventricular gradient. I. Factors which affect its direction and its relation to the mean QRS axis. Amer. Heart J., 25:16, 1943.
10. BARKER, L. F., and A. D. HIRSCHFELDER. The effects of cutting the branch of the His bundle going to the left ventricle. Arch. intern. Med., 4:193, 1909.
11. BARKER, P. S., A. G. MACLEOD, and J. ALEXANDER. The excitatory process observed in the exposed human heart. Amer. Heart J., 5:720, 1930.
12. BARR, N. L. The radio transmission of physiological information. Milit. Surg., 114:79, 1954.
13. BAYLEY, R. H. Exploratory lead systems and "zero potentials." Ann. N.Y. Acad. Sci., 65:1110, 1957.
14. BAYLEY, R. H., E. W. REYNOLDS, JR., C. L. KINARD, and J. F. HEAD. The zero of potential of the electric field produced by the heart beat. The problem with reference to homogeneous volume conductors. Circulat. Res., 2:4, 1954.
15. BAYLISS, W. M., and E. H. STARLING. On the electromotive phenomena of the mammalian heart. Proc. roy. Soc. B, 50:211, 1891.

16. BEASLEY, C. R. Alexander Neckam. Encyclopedia Britannica (11th ed.), 19:336, 1910.
17. BECKING, A. G. TH., H. C. BURGER, and J. B. VAN MILAAN. A universal vectorcardiograph. Brit. Heart J., 12:339, 1950.
18. BERNSTEIN, J. Die Thermoströme des Muskels und die "Membrantheorie" der biolektrischen Ströme. Pflügers Arch. ges. Physiol., 131:589, 1910.
19. BIDWELL, S. Magnetism. Encyclopedia Britannica (11th ed.), 17:321, 1910.
20. BOURNE, G. H. Enzymes of the intercalated disks of heart muscle fibres. Nature, 172:588, 1953.
21. BOWDITCH, H. P. Ueber die Eigenthümlichkeit der Reizbarkeit, welche die Muskelfasern des Herzens Zeigen. Arbeit. physiol. Anst. Leipzig, 6:139, 1871.
22. BRAMWELL, C. The Approach to Cardiology. London, Oxford University Press, 1951.
23. BRAZIER, M. A. B. The Evolution of Concepts Relating to the Electrical Activity of the Nervous System, 1600 to 1800. In The Brain and its Functions. Springfield, Ill., Thomas, 1958.
24. BRIGHT, C. The Story of the Atlantic Cable. New York, Appleton, 1903.
25. BRILLER, S. A. The integrated electrocardiogram. Ann. N.Y. Acad. Sci., 65:894, 1957.
26. BRILLER, S. A. Dipole theory in the analysis of the electrocardiogram and the vectorcardiogram. In C. E. Kossmann, Ed. Advances in Electrocardiography. New York, Grune and Stratton, 1958.
27. BRILLER, S. A., N. MARCHAND, and C. E. KOSSMANN. A differential vectorcardiograph. Rev. sci. Instrm., 21:805, 1950.
28. BRODY, D. A. The meaning of lead vectors and the Burger triangle. Amer. Heart J., 48:730, 1954.
29. BRODY, D. A. Discussion: Part IV (Distribution of electrical potentials in volume conductors). Ann. N.Y. Acad. Sci., 65:1051, 1957.
30. BRODY, D. A., and W. E. ROMANS. A model which demonstrates the quantitative relationship between the electromotive forces of the heart and the extremity leads. Amer. Heart J., 45:263, 1953.
31. BROOKS, C. McC., B. F. HOFFMAN, E. E. SUCKLING, and O. ORIAS. Excitability of the Heart. New York, Grune & Stratton, 1955.
32. BRYANT, J. M. Intraventricular Conduction. In C. E. Kossmann, Ed. Advances in Electrocardiography. New York, Grune & Stratton, 1958.
33. BURCHELL, H. B. Current problems of excitation. Ann. N.Y. Acad. Sci., 65:741, 1957.

34. BURCHELL, H. B., R. D. PRUITT, and H. E. ESSEX. Excitation of the isolated ventricular septum of the heart. Proc. Soc. exp. Biol. Med., 77:117, 1951.
35. BURDON-SANDERSON, J. The mechanical, thermal, and electrical properties of striped muscle. In E. A. Schäfer, Ed. Text-Book of Physiology, vol. 2. Edinburgh, Pentland, 1900.
36. BURDON-SANDERSON, J., and F. J. M. PAGE. Experimental results relating to the rhythmical and excitatory motions of the ventricle of the heart of the frog, and of the electrical phenomena which accompany them. Proc. roy. Soc. B, 27:410, 1878.
37. BURDON-SANDERSON, J., and F. J. M. PAGE. On the time-relations of the excitatory process in the ventricles of the heart of the frog. J. Physiol. (Lond.), 2:384, 1879–80.
38. BURGER, H. C., and J. B. VAN MILAAN. Heart-vector and leads. Brit. Heart J., 8:157, 1946.
39. BURGER, H. C., and J. B. VAN MILAAN. Heart-vector and leads. Part II. Brit. Heart J., 9:154, 1947.
40. BURGER, H. C., J. B. VAN MILAAN, and W. DEN BOER. Comparison of different systems of vectorcardiography. Brit. Heart J., 14:401, 1952.
41. BUTLER, F. H. Compass. Encyclopedia Britannica (11th ed.), 6:808, 1910.
42. CARDWELL, J. C., and D. I. ABRAMSON. The atrio-ventricular conduction system of the beef heart. Amer. J. Anat., 49:167, 1931.
43. CARTER, E. P. Clinical observations on defective conduction in the branches of the auriculo-ventricular bundle. Arch. intern. Med., 13:803, 1914.
44. CAVENDISH, H. An account of some attempts to imitate the effects of the torpedo by electricity. Phil. Trans., 66:196, 1776.
45. CLEMENT, E. Über eine neue Methode zur Untersuchung der Fortleitung des Erregungsvorganges im Herzen. Z. Biol., 58:110, 1912.
46. COHEN, I. B. Introduction. In L. Galvani. Commentary on the Effects of Electricity on Muscular Motion. Tr. by M. G. Foley. Norwalk, Conn., Burndy Library, 1954.
47. COHN, A. E., and T. LEWIS. The pathology of bundle branch lesions of the heart. Proc. N.Y. Path. Soc., 14:207, 1914.
48. COLE, K. S. Ions, potentials, and the nerve impulse. In T. Shedlovsky, Ed. Electrochemistry in Biology and Medicine. New York, Wiley, 1955.
49. COLE, K. S. Introduction to Part I (Cellular events during the cardiac cycle). Ann. N.Y. Acad. Sci., 65:657, 1957.
50. CRAIB, W. H. A study of the electrical field surrounding active heart muscle. Heart, 14:71, 1927.

51. CRAIB, W. H. A study of the electrical field surrounding skeletal muscle. J. Physiol. (Lond.), 66:49, 1928.
52. CRANEFIELD, P. F., and B. F. HOFFMAN. Electrophysiology of single cardiac cells. Physiol. Rev., 38:41, 1958.
53. CRANEFIELD, P. F., and B. F. HOFFMAN. Propagated repolarization in heart muscle. J. gen. Physiol., 41:633, 1958.
54. CURTIS, H. J., and K. S. COLE. Membrane action potentials from the squid giant axon. J. cell. comp. Physiol., 15:147, 1940.
55. DOLGIN, M., S. GRAU, and L. N. KATZ. Experimental studies on the validity of the central terminal of Wilson as an indifferent reference point. Amer. Heart J., 37:868, 1949.
56. DONZELOT, E., J. B. MILOVANOVICH, and H. KAUFMANN. Études pratiques de vectographie. Paris, L'Expansion scientifique française, 1950.
57. DRAPER, M. H., and S. WEIDMANN. Cardiac resting and action potentials recorded with an intracellular electrode. J. Physiol. (Lond.), 115:74, 1951.
58. DREIFUS, L. S., and A. PICK. A clinical correlative study of the electrocardiogram in electrolyte imbalance. Circulation, 14:815, 1956.
59. DU BOIS-REYMOND, E. Untersuchungen über thierische Elektricität, vols. I & II. Berlin, Reimer, 1848–60.
60. DUCHOSAL, P. W. and R. SULZER. La vectocardiographie. Méthode d'exploration du champ électrique créé dans le corps humain par les courants d'action du coeur dans les conditions normales et pathologiques. Bibl. cardiol., Fasc. 3, 1949.
61. DURRER, D. Electric activity of the sinus node, atrial myocardium and atrioventricular node. Circulation, 12:697, 1955.
62. DURRER, D., and L. H. VAN DER TWEEL. Spread of activation in the left ventricular wall of the dog. II. Activation conditions at the epicardial surface. Amer. Heart J., 47:192, 1954.
63. DURRER, D., L. H. VAN DER TWEEL, and J. R. BLICKMAN. Spread of activation in the left ventricular wall of the dog. III. Transmural and intramural analysis. Amer. Heart J., 48:13, 1954.
64. EINTHOVEN, W. Ueber den Einfluss des Leitungswiderstandes auf die Geschwindigkeit der Quecksilberbewegung in Lippmann's Capillarelectrometer. Pflügers Arch. ges. Physiol., 60:91, 1895.
65. EINTHOVEN, W. Ueber die Form des menschlichen Electrocardiogramms. Pflügers Arch. ges. Physiol., 60:101, 1895.
66. EINTHOVEN, W. Un nouveau galvanomètre. Arch. néerl. Sci., Ser. II, 6:625, 1901.
67. EINTHOVEN, W. Ein neues Galvanometer. Annal. d. Physik Folge IV, 12:1059, 1903.

68. EINTHOVEN, W. Die galvanometrische Registrirung des menschlichen Elektrokardiogramms, zugleich eine Beurtheilung der Anwendung des Capillar-Elektrometers in der Physiologie. Pflügers Arch. ges. Physiol., 99:472, 1903.
69. EINTHOVEN, W. The galvanometric registration of the human electrocardiogram, likewise a review of the use of the capillary-electrometer in physiology. In Cardiac Classics. Tr. by F. W. Willius. F. A. Willius and E. Keys, Eds. St. Louis, Mosby, 1941.
70. EINTHOVEN, W. Le télécardiogramme. Arch. int. Physiol., 4:132, 1906.
71. EINTHOVEN, W. Die Konstruktion des Saitengalvanometers. Pflügers Arch. ges. Physiol., 130:287, 1909.
72. EINTHOVEN, W., G. FAHR, and A. DE WAART. Über die Richtung und die manifeste Grösse der Potentialschwankungen im menschlichen Herzen und über den Einfluss der Herzlage auf die Form des Elektrokardiogramms. Pflügers Arch. ges. Physiol., 150:275, 1913.
73. EINTHOVEN, W., G. FAHR, and A. DE WAART. On the direction and manifest size of the variations of potential in the human heart and on the influence of the position of the heart on the form of the electrocardiogram. Tr. by H. E. Hoff and P. Sekelj. Amer. Heart J., 40:163, 1950.
74. ENGELMANN, T. W. Ueber das Verhalten des thätigen Herzens. Pflügers Arch. ges. Physiol., 17:68, 1878.
75. EPPINGER, H., and C. J. ROTHBERGER. Ueber die Folgen der Durchschneidung der Tawaraschen Schenkel des Reizleitungssystems. Z. klin. Med., 70:1, 1910.
76. EPPINGER, H., and O. STOERK. Zur Klinik des Elektrokardiogramms. Z. klin. Med., 71:157, 1910.
77. ERFMANN, W. Ein Beitrag zur Kenntnis der Fortleitung des Erregungsvorganges im Warmblüterherzen. Z. Biol., 61:155, 1913.
78. ERLANGER, J. Observations on the physiology of Purkinje tissue. Amer. J. Physiol., 30:395, 1912.
79. EYSTER, J. A. E., and W. J. MEEK. Experiments on the origin and propagation of the impulse in the heart. The point of primary negativity in the mammalian heart and the spread of negativity to other regions. Heart, 5:119, 1914.
80. EYSTER, J. A. E., W. J. MEEK, H. GOLDBERG, and W. E. GILSON. Potential changes in an injured region of cardiac muscle. Amer. J. Physiol., 124:717, 1938.
81. FAHR, G. An analysis of the spread of the excitation wave in the human ventricle. Arch. intern. Med., 25:146, 1920.
82. FAHR, G., and A. WEBER. Über die Ortsbestimmung der Erregung im menschlichen Herzen mit Hilfe der Elektrokardiographie. Dtsch. Arch. klin. Med., 117:361, 1915.

83. First, S. R., R. H. Bayley, and D. R. Bedford. Peri-infarction block; electrocardiographic abnormality occasionally resembling bundle branch block and local ventricular block of other types. Circulation, 2:31, 1950.
84. Fleming, J. A. Electricity. Encyclopedia Britannica (11th ed.), 9:179, 1910.
85. Fontana, F. Traité sur le vénin de la vipère, sur les poisons américains, sur le laurier-cerise, et sur quelques autres poisons végétaux. Florence, 1781. Cited by H. E. Hoff. Galvani and the pre-Galvanian electrophysiologists. Ann. Sci., 1:157, 1936.
86. Frank, E. The image surface of a homogeneous torso. Amer. Heart J., 47:757, 1954.
87. Frank, E. Measurement and significance of cancellation potentials on the human subject. Circulation, 11:937, 1955.
88. Frank, E. Spread of current in volume conductors of finite extent. Ann. N.Y. Acad. Sci., 65:980, 1957.
89. Franklin, B. Experiments and Observations on Electricity, made at Philadelphia, 1751-1754. London, 1769.
90. Galvani, L. De viribus electricitatis in motu musculari commentarius. De Bononiensi Scientarium et Artium Instituto atque Academia Commentarii, 7:363-418, 1791.
91. Galvani, L. Dell'uso e dell'attività dell'Arco conduttóre nelle contrazioni dei muscoli. Bologna, Tommaso d'Aquino, 1794.
92. Galvani, L. Il "Taccuino" di Luigi Galvani. Riproduzione in facsimile dell'autografo conservato nella biblioteca dell'Archiginnasio di Bologna.... Bologna, Zanichelli, 1937.
93. Gardberg, M., and I. L. Rosen. The ventricular gradient of Wilson. Ann. N.Y. Acad. Sci., 65:873, 1957.
94. Gilbert, W. De Magnete, magneticisque corporibus, et de magno magnete tellure; physiologia nova, plurimis & argumentis & experimentis demonstrata. London, Short, 1600.
95. Gilbert, W. On the Magnet, Magnetick Bodies also on the Great Magnet, the Earth. Tr. by S. P. Thompson. London, Cheswick, 1900.
96. Goldberger, E. A simple, indifferent, electrocardiographic electrode of zero potential and a technique of obtaining augmented, unipolar, extremity leads. Amer. Heart J., 23:483, 1942.
97. Grant, R. P., and E. H. Estes, Jr. Spatial Vector Electrocardiography. Philadelphia, Blakiston, 1951.
98. Grishman, A., and L. Scherlis. Spatial Vectorcardiography. Philadelphia, Saunders, 1952.
99. Groedel, F. M. Das Extremitäten-, Thorax- und Partial-Elektrokardiogramm des Menschen, eine vergleichende Studie. Dresden, Steinkopff, 1934.

100. GROEDEL, F. M., and P. R. BORCHARDT. Direct Electrocardiography of the Human Heart and Intrathoracic Electrocardiography. New York, Brooklyn Medical Press, 1948.
101. GUILLEMIN, A. V. Electricity and Magnetism. Tr. by S. P. Thompson. London, Macmillan, 1891.
102. HALL, A. R. The Scientific Revolution, 1500–1800; the Formation of the Modern Scientific Attitude. New York, Longmans, Green, 1954.
103. HARRIS, A. S. The spread of excitation in turtle, dog, cat, and monkey ventricles. Amer. J. Physiol., 134:319, 1941.
104. HARTMANN, I., R. VEYRAT, O. A. M. WYSS, and P. W. DUCHOSAL. Vectorcardiography as studied on the isolated mammalian heart suspended in a homogeneous volume conductor. Cardiologia, 27:129, 1955.
105. HECHT, H. H. Research in electrocardiography. Editorial. Circulat. Res., 3:231, 1955.
106. HELLERSTEIN, H. K. Atrial infarction with diagnostic electrocardiographic findings. Amer. Heart J., 36:422, 1948.
107. HELLERSTEIN, H. K. Contributions of cardiac catheterization to electrocardiography. In H. A. Zimmerman, Ed. Intravascular Catheterization. Springfield, Ill., Thomas, 1959.
108. HELLERSTEIN, H. K., and L. N. KATZ. The electrical effects of injury at various myocardial locations. Amer. Heart J., 36:184, 1948.
109. HELLERSTEIN, H. K., and I. M. LIEBOW. Electrical alternation in experimental coronary artery occlusion. Amer. J. Physiol., 160:366, 1950.
110. HELLERSTEIN, H. K., and I. M. LIEBOW. Factors influencing the T wave of the electrocardiogram. An experimental study employing intracavitary and extraventricular (epicardial) leads. I. Effect of heating and cooling the endocardium and the epicardium. Amer. Heart J., 39:35, 1950.
111. HELLERSTEIN, H. K., D. SHAW, and T. SANO. Dissection of the vectorcardiogram: differential vectorcardiography. Amer. Heart J., 47:887, 1954.
112. HELMHOLTZ, H. Über einige Gesetze der Verteilung elektrischer Ströme in körperlichen Leitern, mit Anwendung auf die tierisch-elektrischen Versuche. Poggendorff's Annalen, 1853.
113. HILL, A. The genesis of the normal electrocardiogram. Brit. Heart J., 8:147, 1946.
114. HIS, W., JR. Die Thätigkeit des embryonalen Herzens und deren Bedeutung für die Lehre von der Herzbewegung beim Erwachsenen. Arb. med. klin. Lpz., 14, 1893.
115. HIS, W., JR. The function of the embryonic heart and its significance in the interpretation of the heart action in the adult. In Cardiac

Classics. Tr. by F. A. Willius. F. A. Willius and T. E. Keys, Eds. St. Louis, Mosby, 1941.
116. HISTORICAL NOTES. Augustus Désiré Waller (1856–1922): Pioneer in electrocardiography. Med. Press, 236:80, 1956.
117. HODGKIN, A. L., and A. F. HUXLEY. Action potentials recorded from inside a nerve fibre. Nature, 144:710, 1933.
118. HODGKIN, A. L., A. F. HUXLEY, and B. KATZ. Measurement of current-voltage relations in the membrane of the giant axon of Loligo. J. Physiol., 116:424, 1952.
119. HODGKIN, A. L., and B. KATZ. The effect of sodium ions on the electrical activity of the giant axon of the squid. J. Physiol. (Lond.), 108:37, 1949.
120. HOFF, H. E., and L. A. GEDDES. The rheotome and its pre-history: A study in the historical interrelation of electrophysiology and electromechanics. Bull. Hist. Med., 31:212, 1957.
121. HOFF, H. E., and L. A. GEDDES. The rheotome and its pre-history: A study in the historical interrelation of electrophysiology and electromechanics. Bull. Hist. Med., 31:327, 1957.
122. HOFFMAN, B. F., A. P. DE CARVALHO, W. C. MELLO, and P. F. CRANEFIELD. Electrical activity of single fibers of the atrioventricular node. Circulat. Res., 7:11, 1959.
123. HOLLMANN, H. E., and W. HOLLMANN. Das Einthovensche Dreiecksschema als Grundlage neuer elektrokardiographischer Registriermethoden. Z. klin. Med., 134:732, 1938.
124. VON HUMBOLDT, F. W. H. A. Versuche über die gereizte Muskel- und Nervenfaser nebst Vermuthungen über den chemischen Process des Lebens in der Thier- und Pflanzenwelt. Vol. I. Posen, Decker, 1797.
125. HUNTER, J. Anatomical observations on the torpedo. Phil. Trans., 63:481, 1773.
126. HUXLEY, A. F., and R. E. TAYLOR. Activation of a single sarcomere. J. Physiol., 130:49P, 1955.
127. JOHNSTON, F. D. Electrocardiography, p. 352. In O. Glasser, Ed. Medical Physics. Chicago, Year Book Publishers, Inc., 1944.
128. JOHNSTON, F. D. The spread of currents and distribution of potentials in homogeneous volume conductors. Ann. N.Y. Acad. Sci., 65:963, 1957.
129. KARNI, H. S. TsE loop in left ventricular hypertrophy. Amer. Heart J., 56:518, 1958.
130. KATZ, L. N. The significance of the T wave in the electrogram and electrocardiogram. Physiol. Rev., 8:447, 1928.
131. KATZ, L. N. Electrocardiography. 2nd ed. Philadelphia, Lea & Febiger, 1946.

132. KATZ, L. N. The genesis of the electrocardiogram. Physiol. Rev., 27:398, 1947.
133. KATZ, L. N., and A. PICK. Clinical Electrocardiography, Part I, The Arrhythmias. Philadelphia, Lea & Febiger, 1956.
134. KATZ, L. N., E. SIGMAN, I. GUTMAN, and F. H. OCKO. The effect of good electrical conductors introduced near the heart on the electrocardiogram. Amer. J. Physiol., 116:343, 1936.
135. KEITH, A., and M. FLACK. The form and nature of the muscular connections between the primary divisions of the vertebrate heart. J. Anat. (Lond.), 41:172, 1907.
136. KENNAMER, R., J. L. BERNSTEIN, M. H. MAXWELL, M. PRINZMETAL, and C. M. SHAW. Studies on the mechanism of ventricular activity. V. Intramural depolarization potentials in the normal heart with a consideration of currents of injury in coronary artery disease. Amer. Heart J., 46:379, 1953.
137. KLEINFELD, M., E. STEIN, and J. MAGIN. Electrical alternans in single ventricular fibers of the frog heart. Amer. J. Physiol., 187:139, 1956.
138. KOCH, E. Allgemeine Elektrokardiographie. 8th ed. Dresden, Steinkopff, 1945.
139. KÖLLIKER, A., and H. MÜLLER. Zweiter Bericht über die im Jahr 1854/55 in der physiologischen Anstalt der Universität Würzburg angestellten Versuche. VII. Nachweis der negativen Schwankung des Muskelstroms am natürlich sich contrahirenden Muskel. Verh. phys.-med. Ges. Würzb,. 6:528, 1856.
140. KOSSMANN, C. E., Ed. Advances in Electrocardiography. New York, Grune & Stratton, 1958.
141. KOSSMANN, C. E. Recovery of cardiac muscle, a particular problem. Ann. N.Y. Acad. Sci., 65:869, 1957.
142. LENÈGRE, J. Contribution a l'étude des blocs de branche, comportant notamment les confrontations électriques et histologiques. Paris, Baillière, 1958.
143. LEPESCHKIN, E. Modern Electrocardiography. Vol. I. Baltimore, Williams & Wilkins, 1951.
144. LEPESCHKIN, E., L. N. KATZ, H. SCHAEFER, A. M. SHANES, and S. WEIDMANN. The U wave and afterpotentials in cardiac muscle: Panel Discussion. Ann. N.Y. Acad. Sci., 65:942, 1957.
145. LEWIS, T. The Mechanism and Graphic Registration of the Heart Beat. 3rd ed. London, Shaw, 1925.
146. LEWIS, T., and M. A. ROTHSCHILD. The excitatory process in the dog's heart. Part II. The ventricles. Phil. Trans. B, 206:181, 1915.
147. LINDNER, E., and L. N. KATZ. The relative conductivity of the tissues in contact with the heart. Observations on animals with closed chests. Amer. J. Physiol., 125:625, 1939.

148. LING, G., and R. W. GERARD. The normal membrane potential of frog sartorius fibers. J. cell. comp. Physiol., 34:383, 1949.
149. LIPPMANN, G. Rélations entre les phénomènes électriques et capillaires. Ann. Chim. (Phys.), ser. 5, 5:494, 1875.
150. McFEE, R., R. M. STOW, and F. D. JOHNSTON. Graphic representation of electrocardiographic leads by means of fluid mappers. Circulation, 6:21, 1952.
151. MACINNES, D. A. The Principles of Electrochemistry. New York, Reinhold, 1939.
152. MACLEOD, A. G. In F. D. Johnston and E. Lepeschkin, Eds. Selected Papers, F. N. Wilson, Note, p. 275. Ann Arbor, Edwards, 1954.
153. MANN, H. A method of analyzing the electrocardiogram. Arch. intern. Med., 25:283, 1920.
154. MANN, H. Interpretation of bundle-branch block by means of the monocardiogram. Amer. Heart J., 6:447, 1931.
155. MANN, H. The monocardiograph. Amer. Heart J., 15:681, 1938.
156. MARCHAND, R. Beiträge zur Kenntniss der Reizwelle und Contractionswelle des Herzmuskels. Pflügers Arch. ges. Physiol., 15:511, 1877.
157. MAREY, E. J. Des variations électriques des muscles et du coeur en particulier, étudiées au moyen de l'électromètre de M. Lippmann. C.R. Acad. Sci. (Paris), 82:975, 1876.
158. MATTEUCCI, C. (Extrait d'une lettre) Nouvelles éxperiences relatives à l'électricité animale. C.R. Acad. Sci. (Paris), 15:797, 1842.
159. MATTEUCCI, C. Sur le courant électrique des muscles des animaux vivants ou récemment tués. C.R. Acad. Sci. (Paris), 16:197, 1843.
160. MATHEWSON, G. D. Lesions of the branches of the auriculo-ventricular bundle. Heart, 4:385, 1912.
161. MEDRANO, G. A., A. BISTENI, R. W. BRANCATO, F. PILEGGI, and D. SODI-PALLARES. The activation of the interventricular septum in the dog's heart under normal conditions and in bundle-branch block. Ann. N.Y. Acad. Sci., 65:804, 1957.
162. MILNOR, W. R., S. A. TALBOT, and E. V. NEWMAN. A study of the relationship between unipolar leads and spatial vectorcardiograms, using the panoramic vectorcardiograph. Circulation, 7:545, 1953.
163. MÖNCKEBERG, J. G. Zur Frage der besonderen muskulären Verbindung zwischen Sinus- und Atrioventrikularknoten im Herzen. Zbl. Herz. u. Gefasskr., v. 2:1, 1910.
164. MUIR, A. R. An electron microscope study of the embryology of the intercalated disc in the heart of the rabbit. J. biophys. biochem. Cytol., 3:193, 1957.
165. NAHUM, L. H., and H. E. HOFF. The configuration of epicardial and

endocardial extrasystoles in the chest leads. Amer. J. Physiol., 145: 615, 1946.
166. NASTUK, W. L., and A. L. HODGKIN. The electrical activity of single muscle fibers. J. cell. comp. Physiol., 35:39, 1950.
167. NELSON, C. V. Human thorax potentials. Ann. N.Y. Acad. Sci., 65:1014, 1957.
168. OERSTED, H. C. Galvanic magnetism. Phil. Mag., 56:394, 1820.
169. OPPENHEIMER, B. S., and M. A. ROTHSCHILD. Abnormalities in the QRS group of the electrocardiogram associated with myocardial involvement. Proc. Soc. exp. Biol. Med., 14:57, 1916.
170. OVERTON, E. Beiträge zur allgemeinen Muskel- und Nervenphysiologie. Pflügers Arch. ges. Physiol., 92:346, 1902.
171. PAES DE CARVALHO, A., and B. F. HOFFMAN. Evidence for specialized intra-atrial conducting paths. Fed. Proc., 17:120, 1958.
172. PAES DE CARVALHO, A., W. C. DeMELLO, and B. F. HOFFMAN, Eds. The Specialized Tissues of the Heart. Proceedings of the Symposium on the Specialized Tissues of the Heart, August 1960, Rio de Janeiro. Amsterdam, Holland, Elsevier, 1961.
173. PALICKI, B. De musculari cordis structura. Dissertation. Breslau, 1839.
174. PICK, A., R. LANGENDORF, and L. N. KATZ. Advances in the electrocardiographic diagnosis of cardiac arrhythmias. Med. Clin. N. Amer., p. 269, 1957.
175. PIPBERGER, H., L. SCHWARTZ, R. A. MASSUMI, and M. PRINZMETAL. Studies on the nature of the repolarization process. Ann. N.Y. Acad. Sci., 65:924, 1957.
176. PLATO. ION. Tr. by W. R. M. Lamb. (Loeb Classical Library). London, Heinemann, 1925.
177. POGGENDORFF, J. C. Ueber den Gebrauch der Galvanometer als Messwerkzeuge. Ann. Phys. Lpz., 56:324, 1842.
178. POGGENDORFF, J. C. On the use of the galvanometer as a measuring instrument. Tr. by J. D. Easter. A. R. Smithson. Inst., p. 396, 1860.
179. PORTER, K. R., and G. E. PALADE. Studies on the endoplasmic reticulum. III. Its form and distribution in striated muscle cells. J. biophys. biochem. Cytol., 3:269, 1957.
180. PRUITT, R. D., A. R. BARNES, and H. E. ESSEX. Electrocardiographic changes associated with lesions in the deeper layers of the myocardium. An experimental study. Amer. J. med. Sci., 210:100, 1945.
181. PUECH, P. L'activité électrique auriculaire normal et pathologique. Paris, Masson, 1956.
182. PUPILLI, G. C. In L. Galvani. Commentary on the effect of electricity on muscular motion. Introduction. Tr. by R. M. Green. Cambridge, Mass., Licht, 1953.

183. RAKITA, L., J. L. BORDUAS, S. ROTHMAN, and M. PRINZMETAL. Studies on the mechanism of ventricular activity. XII. Early changes in the RS-T segment and QRS complex following acute coronary artery occlusion. Experimental study and clinical applications. Amer. Heart J., 48:351, 1954.

184. ROSENBAUM, F. F., H. H. HECHT, F. N. WILSON, and F. D. JOHNSTON. The potential variations of the thorax and the esophagus in anomalous atrioventricular excitation (Wolff-Parkinson-White Syndrome). Amer. Heart J., 29:281, 1945.

185. ROSENMAN, R. H., A. PICK, and L. N. KATZ. Intraventricular block. Arch. intern. Med., 86:196, 1950.

186. ROTHBERGER, C. J. Allgemeine Physiologie des Herzens. In Handbuch der normalen und pathologischen Physiologie, 7:523. Berlin, Springer, 1926.

187. SANO, T., H. K. HELLERSTEIN, and E. VAYDA. P vector loop in health and disease as studied by the technique of electrical dissection of the vectorcardiogram (Differential vectorcardiography). Amer. Heart J., 53:854, 1957.

188. SAVJOLOFF, V. V. Methode der stereometrischen Elektrokardiographie. Z. Kreisl.-Forsch., 21:705, 1929.

189. SCHAEFER, H. Zur Vektortheorie des EKG, zur Funktionselektrokardiographie Kienles und zum elektrischen Herzbild. Dtsch. med. Wschr., 80:11, 1955.

190. SCHAEFER, H. The general order of excitation and of recovery. Ann. N.Y. Acad. Sci., 65:743, 1957.

191. SCHAEFFER, H., and H. G. HAAS. Electrocardiography. Chapter 13. In W. F. Hamilton and P. Dow, Eds. Handbook of Physiology. Section 2: Circulation. Washington, D.C., American Physiological Society, 1962, p. 323.

192. SCHELLONG, F., S. HELLER, and E. SCHWINGEL. Das Vektordiagramm; eine Untersuchungsmethode des Herzens. I. Mitteilung. Z. Kreisl.-Forsch., 29:497, 1937.

193. SCHER, A. M. Excitation of the heart. Chapter 12. In W. F. Hamilton and P. Dow, Eds. Handbook of Physiology. Section 2: Circulation. Washington, D.C., American Physiological Society, 1962, p. 287.

194. SCHER, A. M., M. I. RODRIGUEZ, J. LÜKANE, and A. C. YOUNG. The mechanism of atrioventricular conduction. Circulat. Res., 7:54, 1959.

195. SCHER, A. M., and A. C. YOUNG. Ventricular depolarization and the genesis of QRS. Ann. N.Y. Acad. Sci., 65:768, 1957.

196. SCHILLING, H. K. A human enterprise. Science, 127:1324, 1958.

197. SCHMITT, O. H. Cathode-ray presentation of three-dimensional data. J. appl. Physiol., 18:819, 1947.

198. SCHMITT, O. H. Lead vectors and transfer impedance. Ann. N.Y. Acad. Sci., 65:1092, 1957.
199. SCHÜTZ, E. Elektrophysiologie des Herzens bei einphasischer Ableitung. Ergebn. Physiol., 38:493, 1936.
200. SCHWAN, H. P., and C. F. KAY. The conductivity of living tissues. Ann. N.Y. Acad. Sci., 65:1007, 1957.
201. SHEDLOVSKY, T. Introduction. In his Electrochemistry in Biology and Medicine. New York, Wiley, 1955.
202. SODI-PALLARES, D., E. BARBATO, and A. DELMAR. Relationship between the intrinsic deflection and subepicardial activation, an experimental study. Amer. Heart J., 39:387, 1950.
203. SODI-PALLARES, D., and R. M. CALDER. New Bases of Electrocardiography. St. Louis, Mosby, 1956.
204. SÖDERSTRÖM, N. Myocardial infarction and mural thrombosis in the atria of the heart. Acta med. scand., suppl. 217, 1948.
205. SUE, P. Histoire du galvanisme; et analyse des différents ouvrages publiés sur cette découverte depuis son origine jusqu'à ce jour. Paris, Bernard, 1802.
206. SULZER, R. L'électrogramme à deux dimensions du battement et de la fibrillation ventriculaire du coeur de lapin. Arch. int. Physiol., 43:82, 1936.
207. TAWARA, S. Das Reizleitungssystem des Säugetierherzens. Jena, Fischer, 1906.
208. THOREL, C. Vorläufige Mitteilung über eine besondere Muskelverbindung zwischen der Cava superior und dem Hisschen Bündel. Münch. med. Wschr., 56:2159, 1909.
209. VOLTA, A. On the electricity excited by the mere contact of conducting substances of different kinds. In a letter . . . to Sir Joseph Banks, March 20, 1800. Phil. Trans., Pt. 2, p. 405, 1800.
210. WALLER, A. D. An Introduction to Human Physiology. 2nd ed. New York, Longmans, Green, 1893.
211. WALLER, A. D. On the electromotive changes connected with the beat of the mammalian heart, and of the human heart in particular. Phil. Trans. B, 180:169, 1889.
212. WALLER, A. D. The Electrical Action of the Human Heart. London, University of London Press, 1922.
213. WALLER, A. D. Obituary notice. Brit. Med. J., 1:458, 1922.
214. WALLER, A. D., and E. W. REID. On the action of the excised mammalian heart. Phil. Trans. B, 178:215, 1887.
215. WALSH, J. Of the electrical property of the torpedo. Phil. Trans., 63:461, 1773 (Table 19).
216. WALSH, J. Of torpedos found on the coast of England. Phil. Trans., 64:464, 1773-75.

217. WEIDMANN, S. Resting and action potentials of cardiac muscle. Ann. N.Y. Acad. Sci., 65:663, 1957.
218. WEIZSACKER, C. F. Some fundamental problems of natural science. Presented at Geigy Bicentenary Scientific Day Report, June 3, 1958, Basle. (Unpublished).
219. WENCKEBACH, K. F., and H. WINTERBERG. Die unregelmässige Herztätigkeit. Leipzig, Engelmann, 1927.
220. WHITEHEAD, A. N., Science and the Modern World. New York, MacMillan, 1925.
221. WIGGERS, H. C., and C. J. WIGGERS. The interpretation of monophasic action potentials from the mammalian ventricle indicated by changes following coronary occlusion. Amer. J. Physiol., 113:683, 1935.
222. WILDE, W. S. The pulsatile nature of the release of potassium from heart muscle during the systole. Ann. N.Y. Acad. Sci., 65:693, 1957.
223. WILLIAMS, H. B. On the cause of the phase difference frequently observed between homonymous peaks of the electrocardiogram. Amer. J. Physiol., 35:292, 1914.
224. WILSON, F. N. A case in which the vagus influenced the form of the ventricular complex of the electrocardiogram. Arch. intern. Med., 16:1008, 1915.
225. WILSON, F. N. The distribution of the potential differences produced by the heart beat within the body and at its surface. Amer. Heart J., 5:599, 1930.
226. WILSON, F. N., J. M. BRYANT, and F. D. JOHNSTON. On the possibility of constructing an Einthoven triangle for a given subject. Amer. Heart J., 37:493, 1949.
227. WILSON, F. N., and F. D. JOHNSTON. The vectorcardiogram. Amer. Heart J., 16:14, 1938.
228. WILSON, F. N., F. D. JOHNSTON, and P. S. BARKER. The use of cathode-ray oscillograph in the study of the monocardiogram. J. clin. Invest., 16:664, 1937.
229. WILSON, F. N., and G. R. HERRMANN. Bundle branch block and arborization block. Arch. intern. Med., 26:153, 1920.
230. WILSON, F. N., F. D. JOHNSTON, and I. G. W. HILL. The interpretation of the galvanometric curves obtained when one electrode is distant from the heart and the other near or in contact with the ventricular surface. Part II. Observations on the mammalian heart. Amer. Heart J., 10:176, 1934.
231. WILSON, F. N., F. D. JOHNSTON, F. F. ROSENBAUM, and P. S. BARKER. On Einthoven's triangle, the theory of unipolar electrocardiographic leads, and the interpretation of the precordial electrocardiogram. Amer. Heart J., 32:277, 1946.

232. WILSON, F. N., A. G. MACLEOD, and P. S. BARKER. The interpretation of the initial deflection of the ventricular complex of the electrocardiogram. Amer. Heart J., 6:637, 1931.
233. WILSON, F. N., A. G. MACLEOD, and P. S. BARKER. The potential variations produced by the heart at the apices of Einthoven's triangle. Amer. Heart J., 7:207, 1931.
234. WILSON, F. N., A. G. MACLEOD, and P. S. BARKER. The distribution of the currents of action and of injury displayed by heart muscle and other excitable tissues. Ann Arbor, University of Michigan Press, 1933.
235. WILSON, F. N., A. G. MACLEOD, P. S. BARKER, and F. D. JOHNSTON. The determination and the significance of the areas of the ventricular deflections of the electrocardiogram. Amer. Heart J., 10:46, 1934.
236. WILSON, F. N., A. G. MACLEOD, P. S. BARKER, F. D. JOHNSTON, and L. L. KLOSTERMEYER. The electrocardiogram in myocardial infarction with particular reference to the initial deflections of the ventricular complex. In F. D. Johnston and E. Lepeschkin, Eds. Selected Papers, F. N. Wilson. Ann Arbor, Edwards, 1954.
237. WOLFERTH, C. C., M. M. LIVEZEY, and F. C. WOOD. The relationships of Lead I, chest leads from the C_3, C_4, and C_5 positions, and certain leads made from each shoulder region: The bearing of these observations upon the Einthoven equilateral triangle hypothesis and upon the formation of Lead I. Amer. Heart J., 21:215, 1941.
238. WOLFF, L. The clinical entity of the syndrome. (Anomalous atrioventricular excitation: Panel discussion). Ann. N.Y. Acad. Sci., 65:828, 1957.
239. WOLFF, L., J. PARKINSON, and P. D. WHITE. Bundle-branch block with short P-R interval in healthy young people prone to paroxysmal tachycardia. Amer. Heart J., 5:685, 1930.
240. WOODBURY, J. W., and A. J. BRADY. Intracellular recording from moving tissues with a flexibly mounted ultramicroelectrode. Science, 123:100, 1956.
241. WOODBURY, L. A., H. H. HECHT, and A. R. CHRISTOPHERSON. Membrane resting and action potentials of single cardiac muscle fibers of the frog ventricle. Amer. J. Physiol., 164:307, 1951.
242. YOUNG, J. Z. Structure of nerve fibres and synapses in some invertebrates. Cold Spr. Harb. Symp., quant. Biol., 4:1, 1936.

Part Two

BLOOD VESSELS

VI

The Capillary Circulation

THE modern understanding of the capillary circulation represents a fusion of information about structure and function accumulated over the last three hundred years. The clear definition of structure depended upon the development of increasingly powerful light microscopes and, more recently, upon the great resolving capacity of the electron microscope; the comprehension of function involved the knowledge and techniques of physiology, physics, chemistry, and pathology. Therefore, it is not surprising that the growth of ideas about the capillary circulation has been uneven; often progress was completely arrested because essential information from other fields was not yet available.

Since a simple chronological account would be both fragmented and repetitious, the evolution of concepts will be considered in the present chapter as a series of lineages beginning with the first identification of the capillaries and progressing to their functional anatomy and quantitative histology, the variability of capillary blood flow and the question of independent contractility, the capillary blood pressure, the passage of substances through capillary walls and, finally, the nature of the capillary wall as a membrane.

Identification of the Capillaries

The idea of an invisible and capillary portion of the circulation preceded actual discovery of the blood capillaries themselves by almost fifty years. William Harvey's experiments and conclusions made it a reasoned necessity that there be pathways for the flow of blood from the smallest visible arteries to the smallest visible veins. These terminal, minute portions of the circulatory system were quite beyond the power of Harvey's unaided vision, but they were not beyond the power of his logic.

BLOOD VESSELS

The first references to this peripheral part of the circulation are therefore particularly noteworthy because they consist of speculative, yet cautious, phrases such as *porositates carnis* (porosities of the flesh), *per caecas porositates* (through invisible porosities), and even the word capillary itself, in terms of *e venis capillaribus* (from capillary veins). The predictive connotations of these terms become clearer when they are read in context as, for example, in the following from Chapter 14 of *De motu cordis* (24, 25):

"Since calculations and visual demonstrations have confirmed all my suppositions, to wit, that the blood is passed through the lungs and the heart by the pulsation of the ventricles, is forcibly ejected to all parts of the body, therein steals into the veins and the porosities of the flesh, flows back everywhere through those very veins from the circumference to the centre, from small veins into larger ones, and thence comes at last into the vena cava and to the auricle of the heart...."

In the final section of Chapter 15 the term *capillary veins* appears in connection with a quite recognizable reference to the *muscle pump* mechanism for venous return.

"... the blood is expressed by the movements of the limbs and the compression exerted by the muscles, from capillary veins into venules and thence into comparatively large veins, and is thus more disposed and prone to move centrally than the opposite (even supposing the valves offered no obstacle)...."

But this vague idea of peripheral communications between arteries and veins was not enough for either the proponents or the critics of Harvey's theory. Some proponents denied the existence of porosities and believed that the blood passed by a sort of seepage through the parenchyma of the organs. Some critics held that the volume flow described by Harvey required vascular continuity in the periphery and declared that the theory as a whole must remain doubtful until some form of direct communication between arteries and veins was clearly demonstrated. This demonstration had to await the development of lenses to extend human vision into smaller dimensions.

This was accomplished by Marcello Malpighi, professor of medicine in Bologna, thirty-three years after the appearance of Harvey's book. A double convex lens, and later probably a pair of them, allowed Malpighi

[356]

to see blood passing from arteries to veins and so to make Harvey's *circuitum sanguinis* demonstrable. In 1661, Malpighi was studying various internal organs, among them the lungs of frogs. At first, he could not

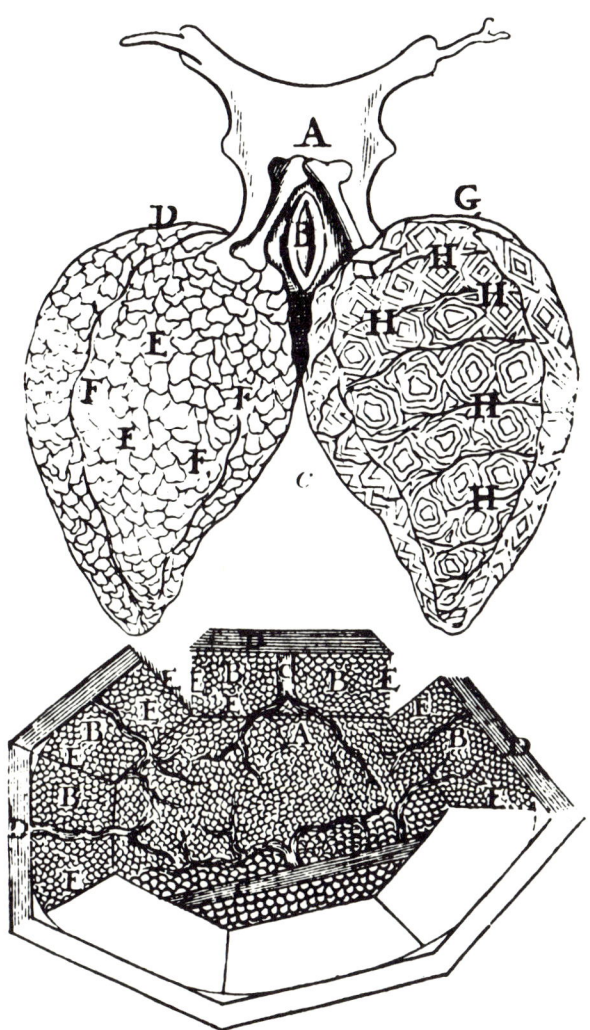

Figure 1. Drawings by Malpighi (1681).
Above: Frog lungs with attached trachea. *Below:* Enlarged view of complete "unit chamber" with adjacent walls showing (A) interior of chamber, (B) walls avulsed and spread out, (C) pulmonary artery and branches, (D) pulmonary vein with confluent vessels, and (E) ramifying network.

decide whether the finest vessels anastomose or "gape into the substance of the lung" (*63*). But, with the use of a more perfect lens, he resolved the difficulty.

BLOOD VESSELS

"... *And so great is the divarication of these vessels, here from a vein, there from an artery, that order is no longer preserved, but a network appears made up of prolongations of both vessels. This network occupies not only the whole floor, but extends also to the walls, and is attached to the outgoing vessel, as I could see with greater difficulty but more abundantly in the oblong lung of a tortoise, which is similarly membranous and transparent. Here it was clear to sense that the blood flows away through the tortuous vessels, that it is not poured into spaces but always works through tubules, and is dispersed by the multiplex winding of the vessels.*"

Malpighi's lenses were still not powerful enough to do more than characterize blood as a liquid consisting "of an almost infinite number of particles" (*63*).

Red blood corpuscles had been seen and described by Jan Swammerdam of Amsterdam as early as 1658, but it remained for Antony van Leeuwenhoek, in 1674, using his own beautifully ground lenses, to see the cells and plasma flowing in the capillary stream. His instrument was a small glass sphere supported between two perforated silver plates. Even with a pinhole aperture this instrument offered only imperfect definition and was not at all achromatic; but it did offer higher magnifying power. Leeuwenhoek, in turning his attention to the *tail of frog-worms* (tadpoles), and then to fish, devised an aquatic microscope which permitted more prolonged study than was possible by lens alone. He could distinguish single *globules* following each other, compressed and in single file, through the narrowest channels. Sometimes the *corpuscles* changed into long ovals as the vessel narrowed. Both the narrowness and number of these parallel pathways arrested his attention. Whereas Aristotle had surmised that "As the blood vessels advance, they become gradually smaller and smaller, until at last their tubes are too fine to admit the blood," Leeuwenhoek realized that "arteries and veins are one and the same continued blood vessels" (*40*).

Leeuwenhoek illustrated the continuity of the arteries and veins by a simple figure which he described in the following way (*40*):

THE CAPILLARY
CIRCULATION

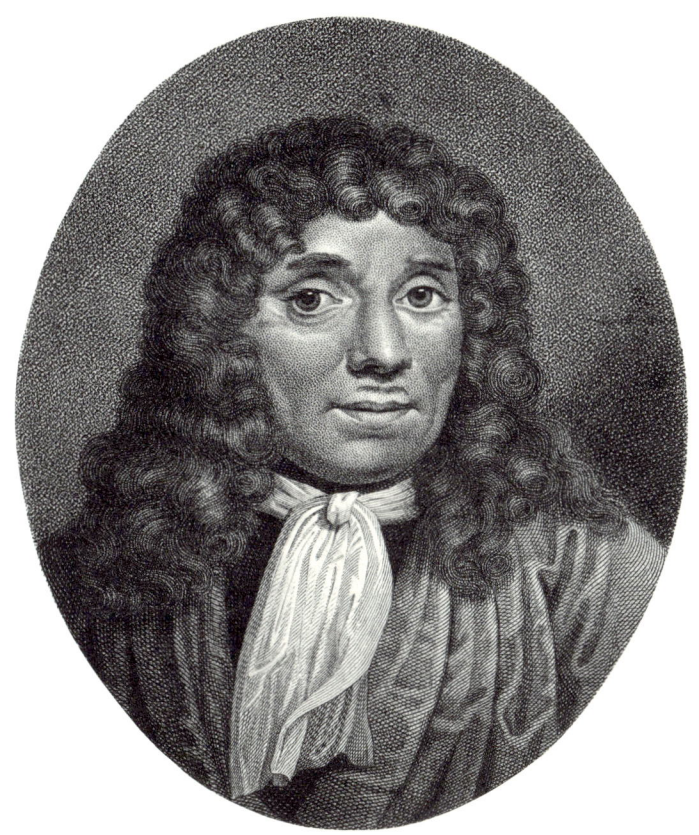

Figure 2. Antony van Leeuwenhoek (1632–1723).

". . . *I saw that the Fig. 6A [of Fig. 4] artery DE. divided into two branches as in E. and that each of these branches continued in a curve as is indicated by EF. and EG. If now we assume DEF. and DEG. to be arteries, because they carry the blood away from the heart, it follows that FH. and GIK. are veins, because both of them carry the blood back to the heart. . . .*"

"*If now in the tail-fin of such a small fish . . . we see thirty-four separate circulations of the blood, how immense must not then be the number of circulations in our own body. This being so, we need not wonder any longer that blood appears when we prick ourselves with a needle or other small instrument.*

"*Nay, after my observations described, I feel sure that in a space the size of a nail, there are on our forefinger, or I may say all over our skin, generally more than a thousand separate circulations of the blood. . . .*"

BLOOD VESSELS

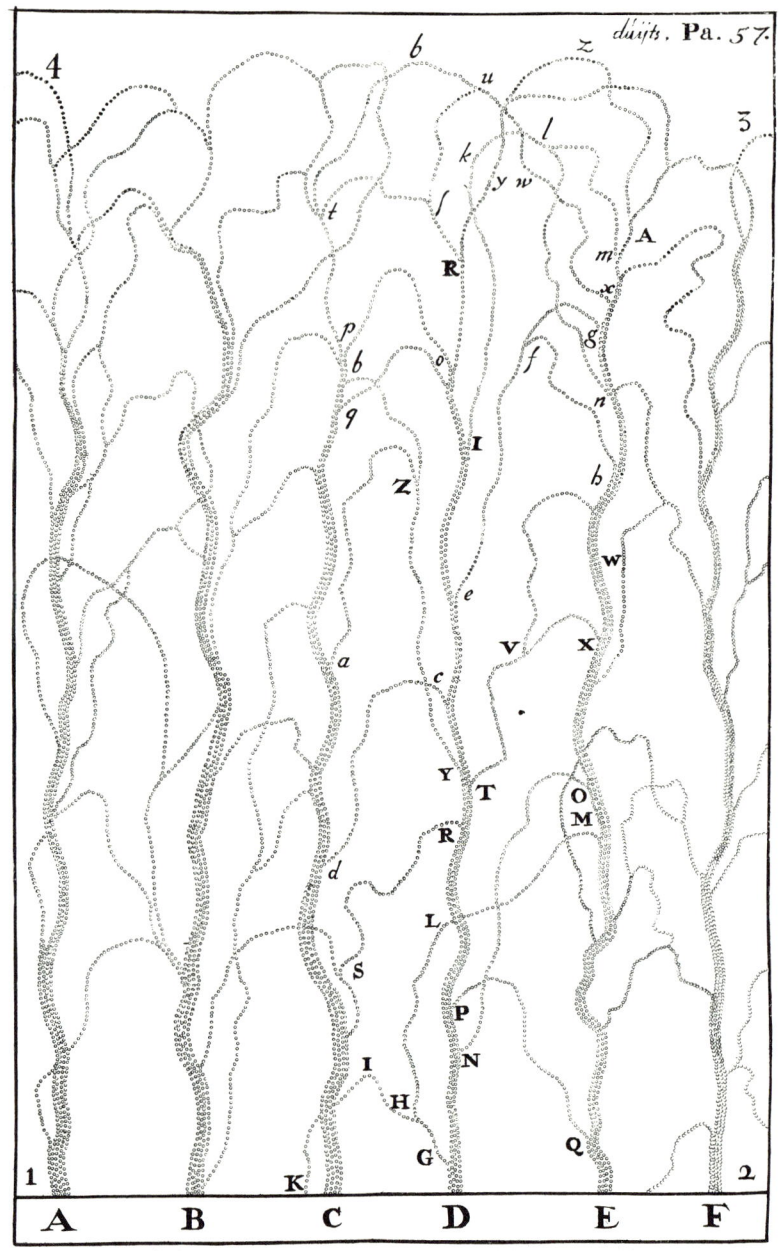

Figure 3. Sketch by Leeuwenhoek (1686) of the blood vessels in the tail of the eel.

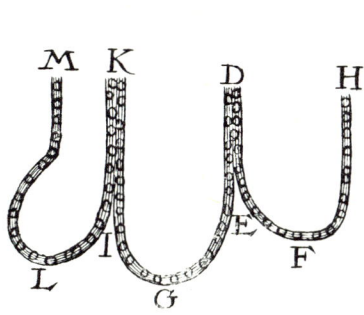 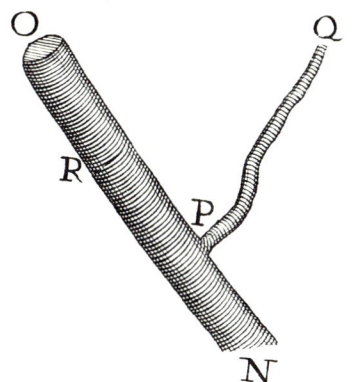

THE CAPILLARY CIRCULATION

Figure 4. Drawing by Leeuwenhoek (1688) to show capillary connections between artery and vein (left) and larger vessels (right).

Thus was completed, in terms of multiple capillary channels, Harvey's necessarily partial description of the circulation. The blood vessels and their contents emerged as a system around which anatomists and early physiologists could begin to arrange their thoughts concerning the mysteries of nutrition and the provisioning of the body as a whole. But, despite the small size of the capillaries and the thinness of their walls, their functions proved to be multiple, confusingly simultaneous, and highly variable from unit to unit. In subsequent decades, methods of investigation, both physiologic and histologic, were repeatedly strained to their very limits and often beyond, leaving much to interpretation and speculation. All this remains true today, although at a different level. For these reasons, the knowledge of capillary function at any stage in its development has usually seemed to be a matter of differences of opinion, and even controversies, grouped around specific issues.

Functional Anatomy and Quantitative Histology of the Capillary System

In later sections of this chapter it will become evident repeatedly that many discrepancies in observation and interpretation arose from lack of any clear definition of the term *capillary*. Much of the writing done in the eighteenth century is difficult to evaluate because the finest arterioles, the capillaries, and the finest venules were not differentiated. Therefore, we will leap a full century and a half, to find the first real effort in this direction. This was made in 1831 by Marshall Hall, in *A Critical and Experimental Essay on the Circulation of the Blood, Especially as Observed in the Minute and Capillary Vessels of the Batrachia and of Fishes*.

Marshall Hall of Nottingham, England, studied in Edinburgh and was appointed resident physician in the Royal Infirmary in 1811. He resigned after two years to take a walking tour and to visit the medical schools in Paris, Berlin, and Göttingen. He returned after some years to Nottingham, where he became a practicing physician of great renown. He wrote extensively on clinical subjects. In physiology, his outstanding achievements are represented by the essay on the circulation of the blood, mentioned above, and a paper read before the Royal Society in the following year (1832), *On the Reflex Function of the Medulla Oblongata and the Medulla Spinalis*.

Marshall Hall's account (22) was the first to distinguish capillaries from arterioles and venules clearly on anatomical grounds. After describing his use of Dollond's microscope and giving reasons for using tissues that could be transilluminated, he defined the vessels as follows:

"The minute vessels may be considered as arterial, as long as they continue to divide and subdivide into smaller and smaller branches. The minute veins are those vessels which gradually enlarge from the successive addition of smaller roots. The true capillary vessels are obviously distinct from each of these. They do not become smaller by subdivision, nor larger by conjunction; but they are characterized by continual and successive union and division, or anastomoses, whilst they retain a nearly uniform diameter."

Observing conspicuous anatomic differences in the arrangements of capillaries in the several tissues studied, he emphasized their functional significance. The following conclusions were based on comparisons of the capillary networks in the fin and tail of the stickleback, the mesentery of the toad, and the lungs of the salamander, frog, and toad.

"The number and distribution of the minute and capillary vessels, is accurately proportioned and adapted to the object of the circulation. When the structure of the part is simple, and the object of the circulation is its nutrition merely, the vessels are few in number; when the part is more complicated, or other objects besides its nutrition are to be fulfilled, the number, character, and mode of distribution of the vessels, are appropriately modified."

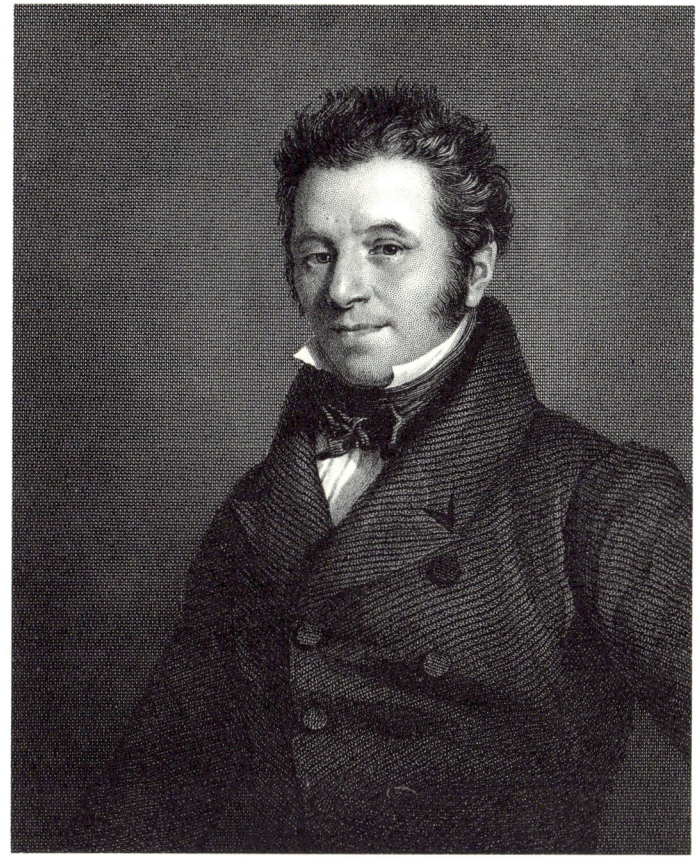

Figure 5. Marshall Hall (1790–1857).

Some observers before him had described frequent large connections between arteries and veins. Hall described in great detail that when he focused his microscope very carefully he could identify vessels at two depths and what seemed to be a connection between artery and vein was merely a crossing of the two vessels at different levels without any confluence or fusion of their lumina. On the other hand he described for the first time the finer arteriolo-venular communications known in modern terminology as *direct channels* or *thoroughfare channels*. In the mesenteric circulation, arteries were seen to give off a minute branch, "and this early to turn around and pursue a venous course." In explaining the distribution of the vessels in the tail of the stickleback he wrote:

BLOOD VESSELS

"The arteries run immediately along the ray, giving off a few capillary vessels in its course; where the ray divides, the artery gives off a branch to supply the new space formed by this division; at the extremity of the ray, the artery turns and assumes the character of a vein."

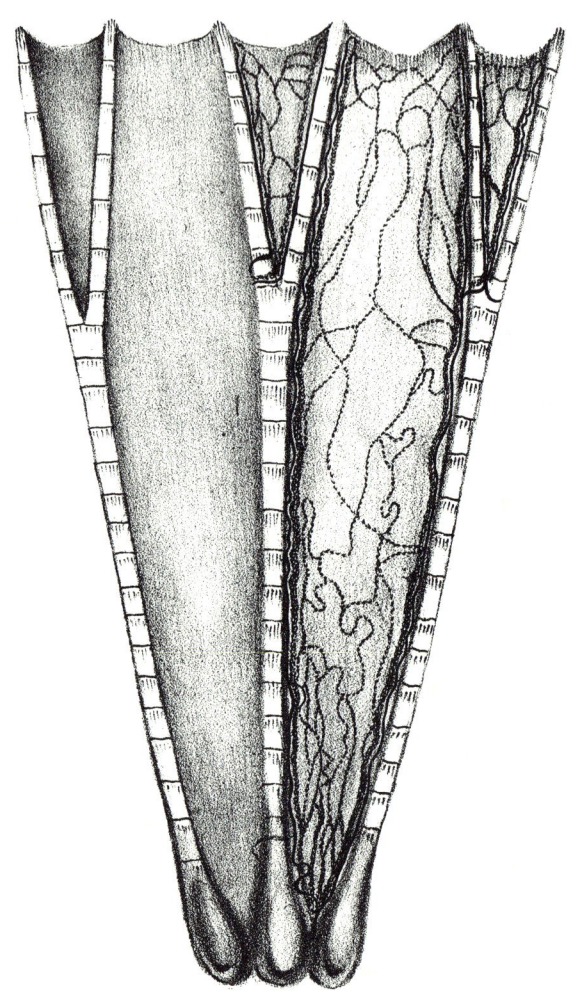

Figure 6. Marshall Hall's drawing (1831) of capillaries in the tail of the stickleback with first definition of capillaries and a description of an "artery that turns and assumes the character of a vein."

Hall also recognized occasional anastomoses of small and large veins, and described the to and fro flow through them, with formation of eddies and with periods of stagnation, despite rapid flow in the connected veins.

In 1838, the study of the capillary circulation received impetus from a new source. Johannes Müller, professor of anatomy and physiology in the University of Berlin, published a review of existing ideas and questions on this subject (*44, 45*). This commanding genius, eminent in almost all medical sciences, has been called the founder of scientific medicine in Germany. His interests included human and comparative anatomy, pathology, psychology, physiology, and physiological chemistry. Among his students were Virchow, Schwann, Henle, Du Bois-Reymond, and Helmholtz.

Müller accepted Marshall Hall's general definition of the capillaries but found it difficult to define exactly the point at which the arteries terminate and the minute veins commence. He agreed that the transition from artery to vein is a gradual one, but noted that the small vessels which comprise the intermediate network are uniquely uniform in diameter, neither tapering like arteries in one direction nor enlarging like veins in the opposite direction.

Müller gave diameters of capillaries for many regions of the body; he found that they ranged from 1/4700 inch in the brain to 1/1149 inch in the skin. He described the form of the capillary network as, "in general, very uniform," varying "merely in the size of the meshes, or in being elongated or not." On the other hand, he also cited many examples of special configuration. For example, Müller quoted Soemmering as follows:

> "... *that the mode of ramification in the small intestines resembles a tree which is not in leaf, in the placenta a tuft, in the spleen an asperge or sprinkling-brush, in the muscles a branch of twigs, and in the choroid plexus of the brain a lock of hair, in the Schneiderian membrane a trellis-work. These meshes are smallest in the lung, liver and kidneys; largest and most sparse in ligaments and tendons.*"

Müller also remarked on the absence of capillaries in the cornea and their ingrowth during ulceration, as described by Henle.

The rest of the review consisted of questions and balancing of evidence. The first of these was one that had troubled Malpighi. "Have the minute arteries open mouths?"

"*Microscopic observations and minute injections have shown that the capillary vessels are merely the fine tubes which form the medium of transition from arteries to veins, and that no other kind of vessel arises from them; that the minute arteries have no other mode of termination than the communication with the veins by means of the capillaries; in a word, that there are no vessels terminating by open extremities. It is the more necessary to demonstrate this fact, which minute anatomy has clearly shown, since Haller unfortunately adopted, and thus contributed to confirm, the crude notions of his predecessors regarding the open terminations of arteries. He admitted that arteries terminate in five ways: 1st, by openings on the surface of membranes; 2nd, in lymphatics; 3rd, in secreting canals; 4th, in fat; and, lastly, in veins.*"

Müller described a whole series of experiments, including some injections of his own, to negate all but the last of these possibilities.

He invoked "invisible pores" to explain the passage of fluid through the capillary wall.

"*An exhaling membrane, such as the peritoneum, has merely reticulated capillary vessels spread out over a great superficies, and the fluids are exhaled into the cavities by permeating the substance of the organ itself; all animal textures being permeable to fluid by virtue of the pores which, though not visible, must necessarily exist even in the smallest molecules of the animal substance which are capable of being softened by fluids. It is owing to this porosity that when arteries are injected with a solution of size coloured with cinnabar, a colourless fluid exudes on the surface of the membranes, as was pointed out by Mascagni, the colouring particles not being able to pass through the pores.*"

He weighed the evidence for the existence of *serous* vessels. These vessels had long been regarded as "branches of the blood vessels which are too minute to allow the passage of the *red particles*," and which are traversed therefore merely by the "lymph of the blood." Müller admitted that they might exist but felt that they had not been demonstrated.

Müller also considered the question of the existence of a continuous capillary wall, a problem which had been debated vigorously for decades, but could still not be answered definitely. His own studies were clearly in favor of a continuous capillary wall, but he conscientiously

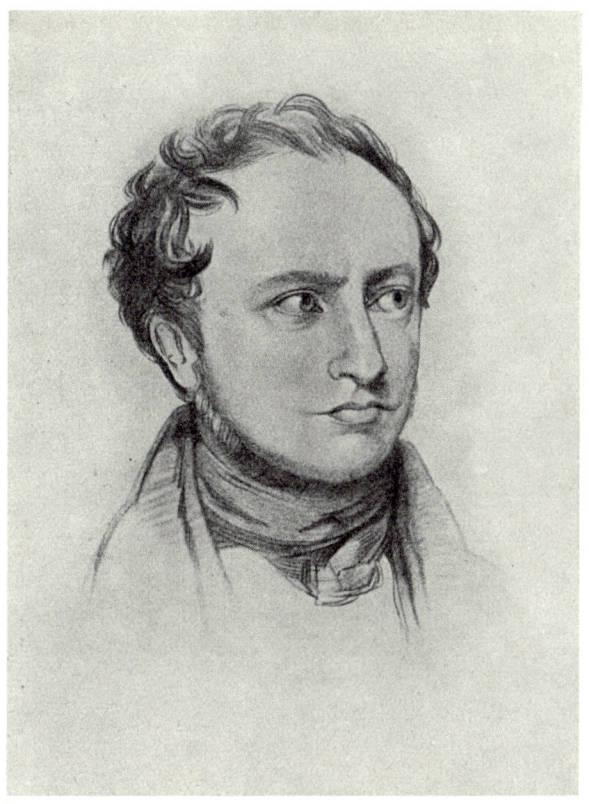

THE CAPILLARY CIRCULATION

Figure 7. Johannes Müller (1801–58).

described the claims on both sides of the question. Malpighi and John Hunter were among the famous who had denied, at one time or another, the existence of such a wall; Leeuwenhoek, Haller, Spallanzani, and Bichat were among those who had preceded Müller in affirming that some form of separate wall existed, with rare exceptions in some tissues.

The methods of the new science, histology, which developed gradually after 1840, eventually confirmed the views of the latter group. This occurred not by any single large discovery but by a long series of small contributions. One of the earliest of these, the silver staining method, deserves special mention. In 1844, C. Krause (*26*) immersed fragments of skin in a dilute solution of silver nitrate, exposed the tissue to light, and noticed dark granular deposits where cells touched each other. In 1862,

BLOOD VESSELS

F. von Recklinghausen (50) studied this silver staining in many tissues and found in lymphatic vessels and veins that best differentiation of their *epithelium* occurred if only the *Kittsubstanz* or cement substance was stained; his results with capillaries were equivocal. Finally, in 1865, three brief papers appeared in one volume of the *Centralblatt für die medizinische Wissenschaften*, and all three described clearly the cellular nature of the capillary wall. Auerbach and Eberth separately confirmed von Recklinghausen's observations in the lymphatics and extended them to the blood capillaries, though with considerable difficulty. Finally, having carefully washed out all blood and injected 1 or 2 per cent silver nitrate solution, Auerbach (2) identified dark streaks outlining in the true capillaries very long "spindle shaped elements arranged parallel to the long axis of the capillary." In each cross section of the frog's capillary there were generally three to four cells, in mammalian capillaries generally two. In adjacent larger vessels the cells were shorter, broader, and more varied in shape. Auerbach concluded:

"The wall of the blood capillary is multicellular, its lumen an intercellular space. This brings a certain similarity to the structure of all portions of the vascular system and many uncertainties, e.g. transition to larger vessels, are clarified, and this will certainly be consequential in physiology and pathology."

In a footnote, the editor called attention to receipt of a paper from Eberth with similar conclusions which would appear in the issue of the next week. Using aniline red to stain nuclei, Eberth (17) identified more securely still the spindle-shaped cells of the capillary wall in many tissues and several species. Again the editor added a footnote acknowledging receipt of still a third paper (1) with similar conclusions which would appear in the following issue. This note, presented by Aeby, read in part:

"Few conclusions in histology have been so firmly established as the view that the wall of the capillaries is structureless. Embryologic research and observations on fully grown forms seem to have supported this view. Therefore I was no little astonished by a recent observation which established the opposite. While investigating the lung of a frog injected with one per cent silver solution I discovered at first glance a delicate network of black, occasionally broadened, lines which previously had been found only on the inner surface of larger blood vessels. Further study revealed this pattern in its most beautiful form in the

capillaries of muscle and intestine. In many places it was possible to follow these lines into the very finest tubes. No less clear was the picture in various organs of the rabbit. There is no doubt that this is a general rule. . . . The entire science of blood capillaries is hereby transformed. . . . The capillaries are simply epithelial tubes."

THE CAPILLARY CIRCULATION

A period of descriptive histology, based upon improved injection masses and special stains of thin sections and reconstructions, expanded and extended this cellular concept of the capillary wall to all parts of the body. In terms of functional histology, however, the next large ideological step was made by August Krogh in the opening paragraphs of his Silliman lectures delivered at Yale University in 1922 (*31*).

"The circulatory system of man and the vertebrate animals can be considered as made up of a small number of organs or subordinate systems, which are easy to recognize anatomically, and the functions of which are on the whole quite distinct. We have a propulsive organ: the heart; a distributing organ: the system of arteries; an organ for interchange of substances between the blood and the tissues: the capillaries; and an organ for collecting the blood and carrying it back to the heart: the venous system. It is evident that the organs of propulsion, distribution and carrying back are all subservient to the functions of exchange carried out in the capillaries, and though, of course, each of the great organs is absolutely necessary for the functioning of the whole, it will be difficult to challenge the proposition that the capillaries constitute the most essential part of the whole circulatory system. It is a little strange, therefore, to find that, far from being a favourite subject for anatomical and physiological research, the capillaries have been neglected in an extraordinary degree. Though about two hundred years have passed since the capillaries were discovered you can find them dealt with in a few lines in quite modern textbooks on physiology, and the references to their structure, given in text-books of histology, are likewise of the most summary character.

"In the last few years, however, the capillaries have been, so to speak, 'rediscovered' as a subject worthy of study and experimental research. Interest in them must have been 'in the air' for the study was taken up independently and almost simultaneously in different countries about seven years ago and has been developed at a rapid rate by quite a number of new workers."

In this paragraph Krogh probably refers to conclusions concerning variations in capillary volume and flow arrived at independently and

BLOOD VESSELS

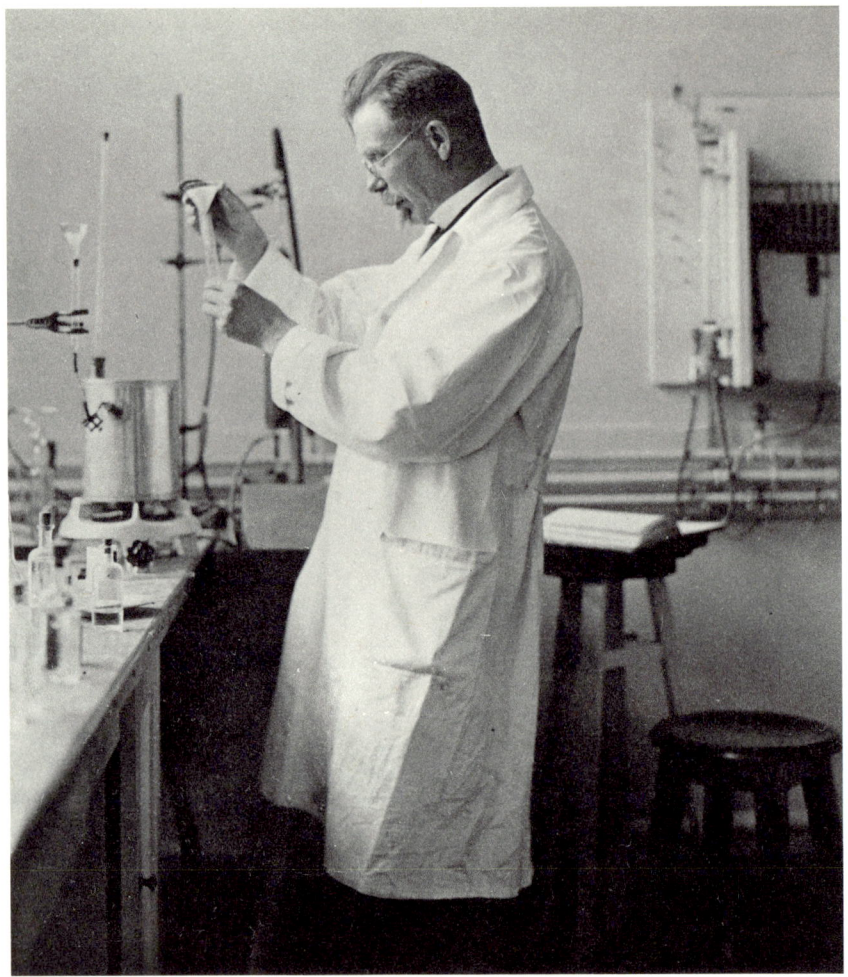

Figure 8. August Krogh (1874–1949).

with quite different methods by H. H. Dale and A. N. Richards, by Thomas Lewis, by Ebbecke, and by himself. These will be considered in the next section; for the present we can return to Krogh's discussion of quantitative histology.

"*By way of introduction I think I can do nothing better than to state briefly the problem with which I was confronted seven years ago, when I began seriously to study the physiology of the capillaries. My problem was the supply of* oxygen to the fibres of striped muscle, the mechanism by which it was brought about and, especially, how it could be regulated. . . .

"In order to solve this general problem or the more modest part of it, which had forced itself upon my mind in 1915, information of a very varied nature must be brought together; but as I have said just now, the first thing to do must be to find out about the number, distribution and surface of capillaries in those tissues in which we are interested.

"For information of this kind we naturally turn to the anatomical literature, but I regret to have to say that in the main we are disappointed. We cannot find there that quantitative information which we require. We will find a certain number of papers in which the distribution of capillaries in different organs is described, and we will find numerous figures illustrating the distribution, but the capillaries have practically never been counted, and the illustrations, from which at least approximate countings could in many cases be made, are as a rule deficient in that one respect which is for our purpose the most essential: the magnification is not given at all, or is given in such an ambiguous way that it is impossible to be sure whether it is the actual magnification of the figure as published, the magnification of the original drawing (which is usually arbitrarily reduced in reproduction) or merely the magnification of the microscope employed, which is meant."

THE CAPILLARY CIRCULATION

Krogh then described his own results in the quantitative histology of the capillary system, which transformed Leeuwenhoek's "a thousand circulations" to square meters and revealed the collective magnitude, as a membrane, of what had previously been considered as microscopic structures.

"On the same assumptions the volume of blood in the muscle capillaries works out as between 3.3 per cent (horse) and 10.6 per cent (dog) of the muscle volume, and the surface of 1 cc. blood contained in capillaries as 2700 cm.^{2} (frog) to 7300 cm.^{2} (horse). It is evident that very large exchanges of substances can take place in a short time through such enormous surfaces. Supposing a man's muscles to weigh 50 kg. and his capillaries to number 2000 per sq. mm., the total length of all these tubes put together must be something like 100,000 kilometers or $2\frac{1}{2}$ times round the globe and their total surface 6300 sq. meters. . . . It is evident that much more work could be done, and ought to be done, on what I should like to term the quantitative anatomy of muscle capillaries."

Much more work has been done since, but not nearly as much, one can be sure, as Krogh felt necessary. His approximate figures have been revised downward to some extent in a few detailed calculations, but even when thus reduced their magnitude still remains astonishing. The lowest of them still expresses better than many descriptive paragraphs the collective significance of the capillary circulation and the importance of the mechanisms by which flow through single capillaries can be adjusted to meet the needs of the immediately adjacent tissue cells.

The Pattern of Capillary Blood Flow

Pulsatile variations in the flow of blood cells through capillaries were described by their discoverer, Leeuwenhoek, in the following terms (*40*):

"This circulation was not regular in its movement, but at very short intervals it was continually brought about anew with sudden impulses, and before there was another sudden impulse we might (in case we had not observed a continual increase in the rapidity) have thought that a stoppage in the circulation would follow. But scarcely had the blood begun to move more slowly, when there was again a sudden impulse of the blood, so that there was an uninterrupted current; and trying accurately to measure the very short time in which each impulse took place, I found that in the time wanted to count rapidly to a hundred, there were as many as a hundred sudden impulses. From this I concluded that as often as these sudden impulses occurred, the blood was driven from the heart.

"But it is remarkable that in the very small vessels mentioned above and placed furthest from the heart, as here at the end of the tail, the impulse was not by far so sudden and strong as in the vessels nearest to the heart. And though the uninterrupted current could be clearly observed, it could be distinctly seen that at each impulse from the heart the current was a little quicker."

Ascribing the "sudden impulses" in capillary blood flow simply to blood "driven from the heart" has not passed uncontested. A considerable number of writers during the eighteenth century fancied the existence of peristalsis-like waves of muscular contraction that swept along the larger arteries and even into the capillaries. Robert Whytt, better known for his work on reflexes, summarized these papers up to 1755 and criticized them drastically (*62*). After considering the factors "which promote the circulation of fluids in the very small vessels of animals," he concluded "the principal cause which propels the blood through the body is, without doubt, the contraction of the heart." He also mentioned that pulsation of arteries is greatest near the heart and becomes less vigorous, though still detectable by variations in flow, as "capillaries of the first order" are approached. This thesis that capillary blood flow depends in part on arterial peristalsis has appeared many times, and most recently in a series of papers published between 1910 and 1922. It was then even more specifically related to the capillaries themselves, which were referred to as a "peripheral heart." Refutation again followed in a review by A. Fleisch (*18*) in 1923. Quantitatively, by calculations of times, pressures, and flows it was shown that, even if present, any such mechanism could have only the most trifling effect compared to cardiac systole.

The Measurement of Blood Flow and the Concept of Resistance

The period from Harvey to Leeuwenhoek, from 1616 to 1700, was essentially one of speculation followed by qualitative description. In 1733 Stephen Hales added quantification. The extraordinary variety of careful measurements which this remarkable man performed in both the vegetable and animal kingdoms included a series of ingenious perfusions of the peripheral vessels of animals. In these experiments he imposed known pressures and measured outflows under a variety of conditions. In describing his results he used many now familiar terms in quite modern contexts (*21*).

EXPERIMENT IX. *1. I slit open with a Pair of Scissors, from end to end, the Guts of a Dog, on that side which was opposite to the insertion of the mesenteric Arteries and Veins; and having fixed a Tube 4 + 1/2 Feet high to the descending Aorta a little below the Heart, I poured blood warm Water thro' a Funnel into the Tube, which descended thence into the Aorta, with a Force equal to that, with which the Blood is there impelled by the Heart: This Water passed off thro' the Orifices of innumerable small capillary Vessels which were cut asunder thro' the whole length of the slit Gut. But notwithstanding it was impelled with a Force equal to that of the arterial Blood in a live Dog, yet it did not spout out in little distinct Streams, but only seemed to ouze out at the very fine Orifices of the Arteries, in the same manner as the Blood does from the capillary Arteries of a Muscle cut transversely.*

2. Having provided a Pendulum which beat Seconds, and pouring in thro' the Tube known Quantities of warm Water, I found that 342 cubic Inches of Water passed off in 400 Seconds or 6.6 Minutes.

3. Then cutting all the mesenteric Arteries asunder close to the Guts, and taking away the Guts, I found that a like Quantity of Water passed thro' these larger Ramifications of the Arteries in 140 Seconds, or 2.3 Minutes, that is in one third of the Time.

4. Then cutting asunder the crural Arteries, which were before tyed, and cutting off the mesenteric and emulgent Arteries close to the Aorta, a like Quantity of Water passed thro' this thus cut Aorta in .308 Minute, that is in 1/21.4th part of the Time, in which it passed thro' the capillary Arteries of the slit Guts."

But Hales found that these rates of flow when calculated for the whole body were greater than his earlier calculations of cardiac output. He ascribed this discrepancy to a series of factors. These include "the much greater fluidity of Water than of viscid Blood," "the more relaxed state" of the arteries in the dead animal, the small size of the "capillary Arteries," and the "Resistance of the venal Blood, which rising six Inches in the Tube fixed to the jugular Vein is = 1/13.33 part of the Force of the arterial Blood, and must therefore proportionably retard its Motion." He found that the "finest arteries" had a diameter of 1/3240th of an inch, "that is so fine that only single Blood globules can pass them into the Veins; here Therefore so viscid a Fluid as the Blood must needs meet with a very great Resistance." Hales also compared the cross-sectional area of the aorta with areas of its branches and found "the Sum of the Areas of their transverse Section is considerably greater than that of the Aorta." But he returned again to a consideration of the "extream capillary arteries."

"19. And to this Resistance which the Blood meets with in passing the capillary Arteries, is owing the great Difference of the Force of the Blood in the Arteries to that in the Veins, viz. as 10 or 12 to 1.

"20. For tho' the Velocity of the Blood at its first Entrance into the Aorta, depends on the Proportion the Area of its Orifice bears to the Quantity thrown into it at each Systole, and also on the Number of those Systoles in a given time: Yet the real Force of the Blood in the Arteries, depends on the Proportion, which the Quantity of Blood thrown out of the left Ventricle in a given time, bears to the Quantity which can pass thro' the capillary Arteries into the Veins, in that time.

"21. But the Resistance which the Blood meets with in those capillary Passages, may be greatly varied, either by different Degrees of the Viscosity or Fluidity of the Blood, or by the several Degrees of Constriction or Relaxation of those fine Vessels; Instances of which may be seen in Experiments XV, XVI, XVII, XVIII.

"22. And as the State of the Blood or Blood vessels are in these Respects continually varying from diverse Causes, as Motion, Rest, Food, Evacuations, Heat, Cold, etc. so as probably never to be exactly the same, any two Minutes, during the whole life of an Animal; so nature has wisely provided, that a considerable Variation in these, shall not greatly disturb the healthy State of the Animal."

The Experiments XV to XVIII mentioned above have been cited by some as the first mention of independent contractility of capillaries, but this interpretation seems unjustified, because Hales's "capillary Arteries" probably included arterioles. As already mentioned, Marshall Hall, in 1833, was the first to differentiate clearly by microscopic examination and by anatomic criteria between the finest terminal arterioles and the true capillaries. Hales habitually used the term capillary as an adjective, viz. "capillary Arteries" and "capillary Veins." With this limitation the many ingenious perfusions made by Hales "according to hydraulic and hydrostatic method" nevertheless established clearly both dilatation and constriction of the minute vessels, though without exact localization.

By the thoroughly modern method of alternating experimental and control periods, plus quantitative measurements of perfused volumes, Hales described constriction by cold, by "strong Decoction of Peruvian Bark," and by "strong Decoction of Oak Bark." Dilatation was produced by mildly warm perfusions of water, but a "scalding hot Decoction" reduced the rate of outflow. Most interesting of all, however, is the caution with which Hales extrapolated from experimental conditions to the living animal.

"4. We see in this and the three foregoing Experiments, how the Vessels of the Body are manifestly contracted or relaxed, by different Degrees of Warmth, Heat or Cold, or from the different Qualities of the Fluids which pass thro' them, as to Restringency or relaxing: And such Qualities of the Fluids must have very considerable Effects on the finer capillary Vessels, whose Coats bear a much greater Proportion to the contained small cylindrical

Fluid, than in larger Vessels. Tho' it is not to be imagined that the Effects are so sudden and great in a live Animal, as in these Experiments; because in a live Animal, the several Fluids which are taken in, are more gradually and in smaller Proportion blended with the Blood. . . ."

BLOOD VESSELS

In a later section still, Hales observed the abnormal filtration of fluid, and its effects on perfusion.

"4. If we could be so happy as to find a Liquor of such a due Consistence, as to pass freely thro' from the Arteries to the Veins, as the Blood does in its natural State, then many curious and useful Experiments might in this manner be tried on several Parts of the Body.

"5. It was with this View that I made Columns of warm Water flow into the Arteries of dying Dogs . . . to try if by this means I could wash all the glutinous Blood out of the finer capillary Arteries and Veins . . . but I was soon disappointed in my Expectations; for the Water tho' a much more dilute Fluid than the Blood, had no free Passage from the Arteries to the Veins."

The reason for this is referred to in an earlier experiment in which perfusion was quite prolonged:

"3. . . . for I always found that by a long Continuance to pour in Water, the Vessels did gradually let less and less pass; the capillary Vessels being compressed by the Water that insinuated into all Parts of the Coats of the Guts, so as to make them much thicker than they were at first. . . ."

Another century elapsed before "insinuated" was replaced by "filtered," and another half a century still until Starling's "absorption" explained why the change from "glutinous blood" to "warm water" made perfusion studies so difficult.

Patterns of Blood Flow in Individual Capillaries and Capillary Contractility

That blood flow through a single capillary may vary from moment to moment, or even reverse direction, has never been doubted. Moreover, careful comparisons have shown that in two adjacent capillaries, originating close together from one arteriole and ending close together in one venule, flow may be slow in one and rapid in the immediately adjacent one. Conversely, no one has ever claimed that rates of flow in all the capillaries from a given arteriole are identical, nor that flows in groups of capillaries increase and decrease together. Hence, independent variability of flow from capillary to capillary has been generally accepted and even emphasized as a striking finding. But the history of ideas concerning the mechanism or mechanisms which produce these variations has been quite different. Indeed, views concerning the independent contractility of capillaries have continued to be affirmed and denied up to recent times.

Controversies prior to 1833 can be passed over quite briefly, because until that date neither anatomic nor physiologic descriptions of the minute vessel system differentiated clearly between capillary arteries, capillaries per se, and capillary veins. Stephen Hales, in 1733, described "different Degrees of Constriction or Relaxation," but this finding was based on results obtained from perfusion and referred simply to "capillary Passages," which we would now consider to include fine arterioles. Albrecht von Haller, in 1756, denied contractility (*23*), and the weight of his authority lasted for a long time. James Black (*3*) described constriction and dilatation of vessels in 1825, but again in terms of capillary arteries and veins with most emphasis on the arteries. Marshall Hall (*22*), in 1831, confirmed observations of others on contractility of arteries but could never observe any "irritability in the true capillaries" or any "automatic power in them."

A number of investigators had studied the effects of applying to the minute vessels a variety of substances, including ammonia, alcohol, ice, opium, tartaric acid, and dilute muriatic acid. The results were uncertain, conflicting, and confusing, as indicated by Müller's summary:

"*Action of different substances on the capillaries. Direct experiments to determine the action of different substances on the capillary vessels, by watching the changes produced by the application of these substances to the vessels of transparent parts, promised at first to increase considerably our knowledge of the action of the capillaries. But these experiments have left our knowledge of the subject in the greatest confusion.*"

Shortly after this was written the cell theory and improved microscopy encouraged renewed attacks on the problem. In 1858, Lister (*41*) produced inflammation in the web of the frog and described great widening of the capillaries. This he ascribed simply to increased pres-

BLOOD VESSELS

sure within them produced by dilatation of the arteries. Stricker (*60*), in 1865, observed irregular and spontaneous contractions and relaxations of capillaries in the nictitating membrane of the frog. This tissue was excised so that changes in blood pressure were excluded. Conditions were, however, far from physiological, and consequently the findings were not widely accepted. Rouget in 1873 (*52*) and 1879 (*53*) studied the recently formed blood vessels of the developing larvae of amphibians and concluded that the endothelium per se was not contractile. Contractility, he suggested, resided in amoeboid cells which, as the vessels developed, applied themselves to the endothelial tube and partially encircled the vessel by branching protoplasmic extensions. After extending his studies to the nictitating membrane of newly born or embryonic mammals, he concluded that a contractile tunic surrounds the "whole system of blood vessels from heart to capillaries inclusive." It should be noted that the tissues studied were chiefly from larvae of amphibians (tadpoles) or from embryonic or newborn mammals, so that active growth, including rapid formation of new blood vessels, was still present. Cohnheim (*11*) in 1880 once more discounted the importance of capillary contractility and denied the existence of muscular elements in the capillary wall. More than twenty years elapsed before Steinach and Kahn (*59*) repeated Stricker's studies and stimulated the excised nictitating membranes of the frog and the omentum of young cats. They reaffirmed contractility of capillaries, but the subject received little attention until 1917–18, when investigators in four independent laboratories studied the subject in order to explain a series of new observations, all involving the peripheral vessels.

Ebbecke (*16*), from observations on the frog's web during drying, and in human skin during application of heat and cold, concluded that to explain his results it was necessary to postulate (a) dilated arterioles without dilated capillaries and (b) contracted arterioles with dilated capillaries (and venules). Independently, from their studies of dermographism, Cotton, Slade, and Lewis (*12*) came to a similar tentative conclusion. Later, however, Sir Thomas Lewis habitually used the term "minute vessels" to include collectively the smallest arterioles, the capillaries, and the subpapillary venous plexus. He found that it was this plexus, rather than the capillaries, that gives human skin its color. One year later Dale and Richards (*13*) published a detailed and closely

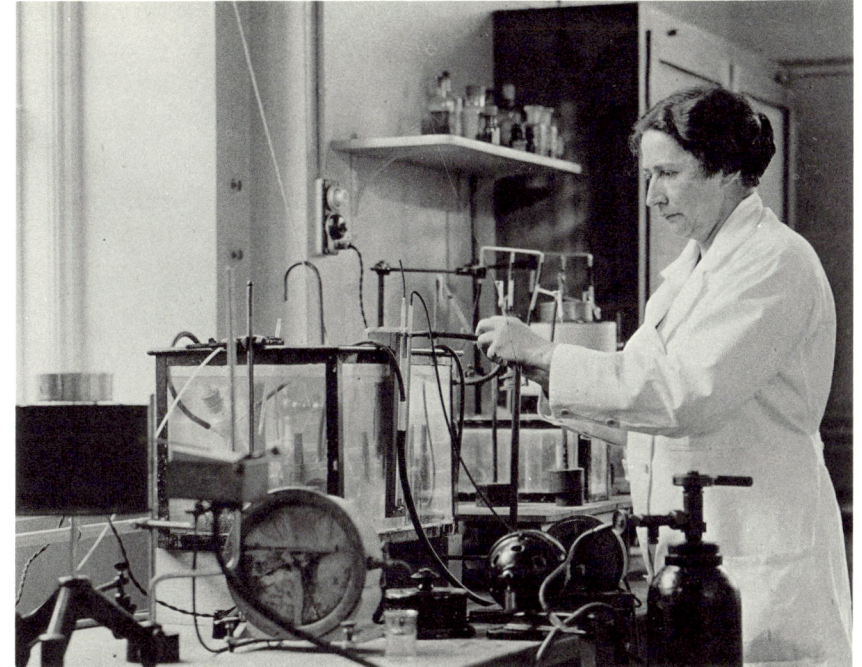

Figure 9. Marie Krogh (1874–1943).

reasoned comparison of the actions of histamine, epinephrine, and acetylcholine which led to the suggestion that independent responses of arterioles and capillaries were probable. They pointed out, however, that their evidence did not warrant any sharp distinction between the capillaries proper and the smallest arteries.

In 1918, August Krogh's attention was directed to the problem in order to explain the mechanics of tissue respiration (*28, 29, 30*). The following excerpts from his own account indicate the reasoning which underlay his thesis of independent contractility of capillaries. However, it applies equally well to the less controversial independent variability of flow through capillaries.

In a fascinating lecture (*32*), *Reminiscences of Work on Capillary Circulation*, given in 1946 at the Harvard Medical School, Krogh traced the development of his idea to three basic questions. (1) Having first doubted, and then, by experiment, disproved Christian Bohr's theory that oxygen was secreted in the lungs, Krogh and his wife Marie, his

BLOOD VESSELS

co-investigator, had, by 1910, formed "a personal, but rather strong, belief that diffusion would be found almost everywhere to be the mechanism for gas transport in organisms." (2) In 1910, studies of oxygen consumption and cardiac output in man indicated that exercise produced enormous increases in both. "It also became clear at a fairly early stage that the increase in oxygen consumption must take place mainly in the working muscles (including the heart)...." (3) In the course of writing a monograph, *Respiratory Exchange of Animals and Man*, he concluded "that the oxygen tension in tissues, and particularly in muscles, was probably very low and that the tension might be the limiting factor for the rate of oxidations."

Krogh described the problem and its solution as follows:

"The final arterioles in muscles are more or less at right angles to the muscle fibres; they branch out into a comparatively large number of capillaries which run parallel to the fibres and finally—that is after about 1/2 mm.—unite into small veins which are again at right angles to the fibres. On a cross-section vertical to the fibres, the injected capillaries show as stained dots between the fibre cross-sections, and sometimes even running inside a fibre [Fig. 10].

"You will understand that, while I had undertaken to write only on the metabolism of organisms and their parts at rest, I could not, with the background I have sketched to you, well avoid speculating on the function of this mechanism during work; and such speculations could not, with the premises enumerated, avoid bringing me into considerable difficulties. I felt pretty certain that the supply of oxygen to the fibres must take place by diffusion from the capillaries. Every capillary could be conceived as a tube with walls permeable to oxygen and surrounded by a cylinder of tissue through which oxygen would diffuse toward the periphery, being reduced all the way by the metabolic processes. Now if the supply was just right during rest, so that the oxygen pressure at the surface of the cylinder would be negligibly small, no increase in the rate of flow through the same capillaries could make it sufficient during work, when oxygen was used up, say at a tenfold rate. If, on the other hand, the density of the capillary network was sufficient to provide by diffusion all the oxygen necessary during heavy work, the arrangement would be very wasteful during rest and would result in an oxygen pressure in the tissue practically identical with that of the venous blood.

"One day while pondering over this problem in the University library, the idea suddenly struck me that the anatomical arrangement would work beautifully if it could be assumed that during rest, only a certain small fraction of the capillaries, suitably distributed, are open to the passage of blood while all the rest are closed; and that increasing numbers are opened with increase in work. This mechanism would become ideal if local lack of oxygen forced the opening-up of the nearest capillary, while a certain higher concentration of the dissolved gas allowed the capillary to close, so that, in the resting muscle, or during moderate work, capillaries would open and close in certain alternation. While discussing this idea the same evening with my wife, who was always my nearest colleague, I illustrated it with a diagram something like that in . . . [Fig. 11], and the outcome was that it seemed worth while to make an experimental test.

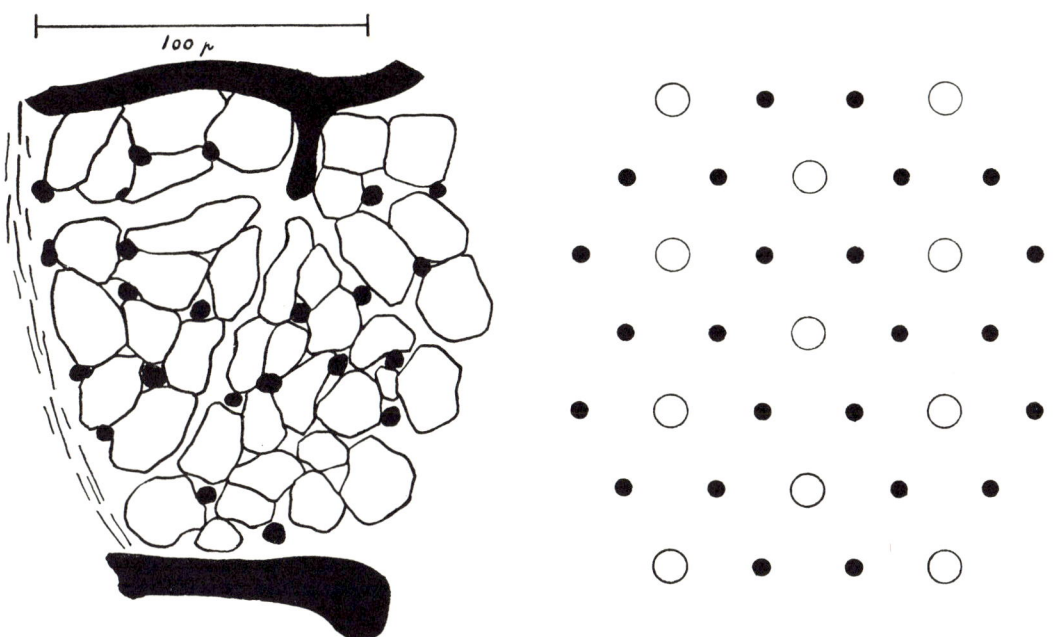

Figure 10. Cross section of skeletal muscle of frog showing capillaries after perfusion with carbon.

Figure 11. Diagram by Krogh to illustrate his idea that capillaries might "open and close in certain alternation."

BLOOD VESSELS

The experimental test consisted of several steps. (1) It was necessary to measure the rate of diffusion of oxygen and carbon dioxide through masses of tissue in vitro. (2) By direct observation or by injecting dialyzed India ink the number of perfused capillaries per sq. mm. of muscle was determined at rest in four species and during exercise in two. (3) Combining the results of 1 and 2 permitted the calculation of conditions existing during rest and exercise as summarized in Tables I and II, in which R is the cross-sectional area of the diffusion cylinder supplied by each capillary.

TABLE I

Calculated Maximum Oxygen Tension Difference $(T_o - T_r)$ Between Blood and Muscular Tissues of Four Species[1]

	Weight (kg.)	Metabolism (cal./kg./hour)	Number of capillaries per mm.^{2} cross-section of muscle	R (μ)	Diameter of red corpuscles ($2r$) (μ)	$T_o - T_r$ (mm. Hg)
Frog	0.04	0.4	400	28	15	0.25
Horse	500	0.5	1400	15	5.5	0.1
Dog	5	3	2500	11.3	7.2	0.2
Guinea pig	0.5	6	3000	10.3	7.2	0.3

[1]From A. Krogh (29).

TABLE II

Numbers of Capillaries and Oxygen Tension Differences $(T_o - T_r)$ Between Blood and Muscular Tissues of Frog and Guinea Pig during Rest and Exercise[2]

	O_2 consumed per minute in vol. per cent. of tissue	Number of capillaries per mm.^{2} cross-section	R (μ)	$2r$ (μ)	$T_o - T_r$ (mm. Hg)	Capacity of capillaries per vol. per cent. of tissue
FROG MUSCLE						
Minimum, Rest	0.03	10	180	4.4	10	0.015
Work	0.3	325	31	6.8	1.2	1.2
GUINEA PIG MUSCLE						
Rest	0.5	31	100	3	45	0.02
Work	5	2500	11	5	1.4	5.5
Maximum	10	3000	10	8	1.2	15

[2]From A. Krogh (30).

"*In the resting muscles of the frog with ten open capillaries per mm.^{2} there must be lack of oxygen in considerable portions of the muscle, but during work, with 325 open capillaries per mm.^{2} the oxygen pressure in the muscular tissue becomes practically equal to that of blood. Similar relations hold in the muscles of the guinea pig. The last column of Table II shows the total volume of capillaries in per cent. of tissue or, what amounts to the same, the percentage of capillary blood present in the muscles during rest and work.*

"*These results make good the contention that the distances between open capillaries are closely related to the metabolic requirements, but of the shifting of open capillaries from one position to another in the resting muscle I was never able to obtain convincing proof.*"

Krogh, who was always interested in new techniques and their usefulness in biological research, used motion picture photomicrography with great effectiveness to illustrate regional differences in capillary structure and variations in capillary blood flow (*31*).

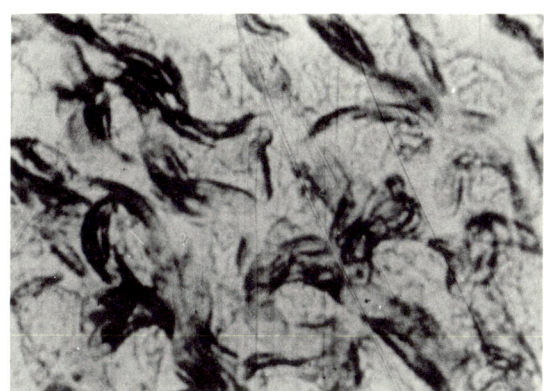

Figure 12. Pulmonary circulation in the frog from film prepared by Krogh.

Location of Contractile Elements Controlling Capillary Blood Flow

Comparisons of the many papers and reviews that have argued for and against independent contractility of capillaries make it clear that knowledge of structure and function is still too incomplete to permit final conclusions. Four mechanisms have been explored, viz. in-bulging of the endothelial cell itself (*60*), intrinsic tone or natural elasticity of the endothelial wall (*9, 10*), the Rouget cells already mentioned (*53*), and the Capillarpförtnerzelle (capillary gate-keeper cells) described most clearly by Tannenberg (*61*) and photographed in action as arteriocapillary sphincters by Fulton and Lutz (*19*) as shown in Fig. 13. The arteriocapillary sphincter mechanism is certainly the most widely distributed, as well as the most generally accepted. A recent reclassification of the minute vessel system by Chambers and Zweifach (*7*) excludes from the category of true capillaries any vessels which have contractile elements along their length. Figure 14 shows this classification for comparison

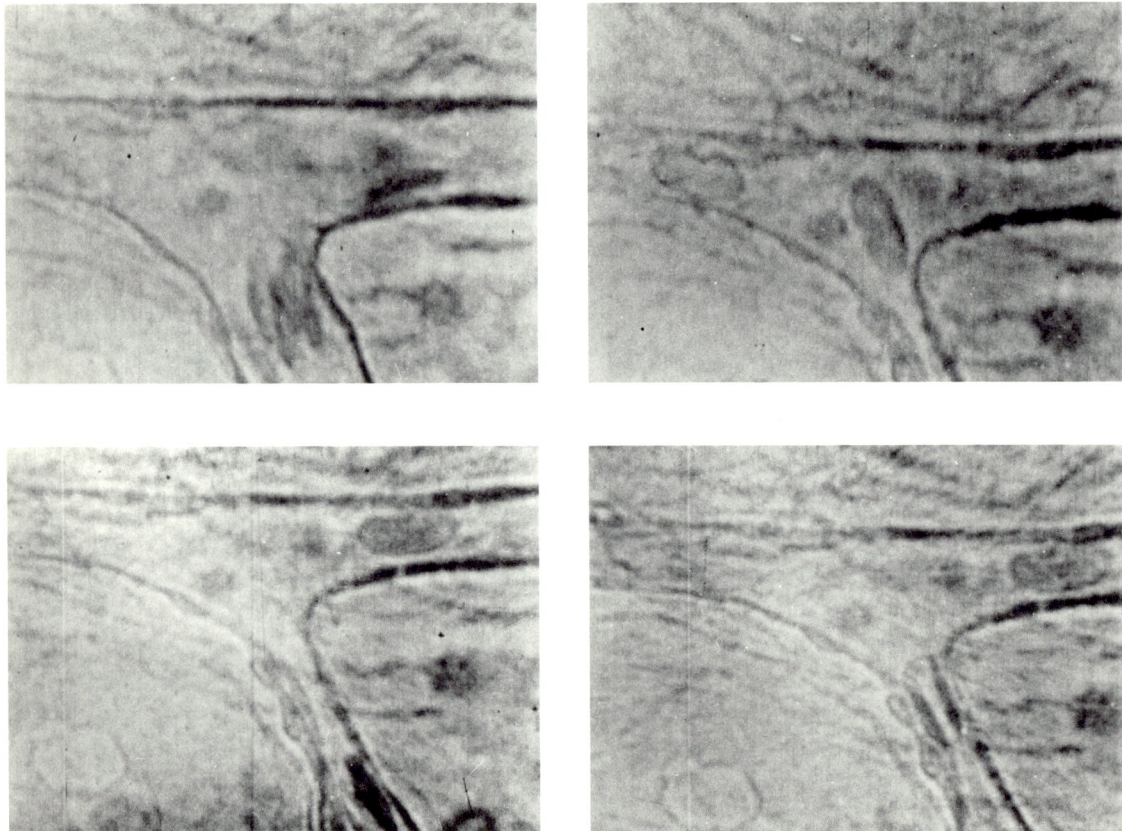

Figure 13. Four stages in constriction of arteriocapillary sphincter from film by Fulton and Lutz.

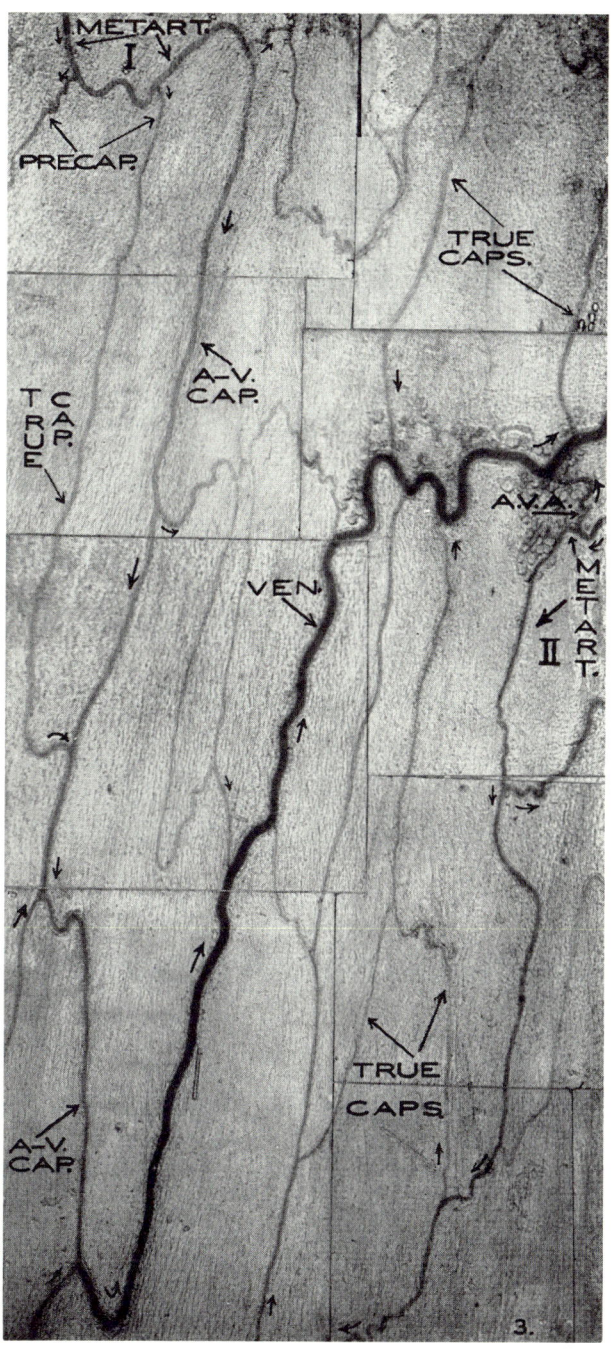

THE CAPILLARY
CIRCULATION

Figure 14. Mosaic of photomicrographs of the mesoappendix of the rat by Chambers and Zweifach (1944), to show metarterioles, "true capillaries," and "arterio-venous capillaries" or "direct channels" or "thoroughfare channels."

with Marshall Hall's far simpler drawing of 1831 (Fig. 6). Differences of opinion have arisen in part from the tendency to extrapolate from capillaries in embryonal forms (tadpoles) or growing tissues to adult forms and tissues. In part also it has been assumed that observations in one tissue or one species can be extended to all tissues and species. It seems clear that in this area the fusion of knowledge concerning structure and function is still quite incomplete. Electron microscopy is revealing regional differences in the capillary wall but has not yet approached the question of determining whether the gate-keeper cells are simply the usual vascular type of smooth muscle in a special location or whether they are differentiated elements with encircling extensions of a Rouget type.

Physiologically, however, the important point is that independent variability of blood flow from capillary to capillary, and in any one capillary from moment to moment, is a fact agreed to by all investigators from Leeuwenhoek to Krogh and beyond.

Capillary Blood Pressure

Knowledge concerning blood pressure within the capillaries, as was the case with their structure, began with the grossly visible and, through two centuries, penetrated stepwise to the microscopic unit. In 1733, about a century after Harvey, Stephen Hales's direct measurements (21) revealed the mean blood pressure at two sites in the circulatory system. The intubated carotid artery of the horse supported a column of blood eight to nine feet high; the intubated jugular vein, a column less than a foot high. This difference led Hales to his calculations of the force of the blood in the minute vessels.

The next hundred years produced little more than some rough calculations based on questionable assumptions. In 1817, Poiseuille (49) tested the then current view that arterial pressure began to fall as soon as blood passed the aortic valve, and declined by a steady gradient through the larger arteries to the veins. He devised the first U-tube mercury manometer and established the validity of the pressures indicated by it. He also used an anticoagulant to prevent clotting. With cannulae of decreasing size he measured arterial blood pressure in smaller and smaller vessels to the then existing limits of cannula size (about 2 mm.), and concluded:

"A molecule of blood moved with the same pressure during its entire course through the arterial system, a conclusion that a priori *with all physiologists we were far from thinking."*

But he was not able to penetrate to the minute vessels and hence could not determine, except by exclusion, where, and how rapidly, arterial pressure fell to reach venous pressure. Thwarted in this direction, he turned his attention to glass capillary tubes and from them derived the relation which flow per unit time bears to pressure, tube radius, viscosity, and length. Thus Poiseuille's equation, which in its modern modifications is now an important part of hydrodynamics, emerged from attempts to measure blood pressure in the smaller blood vessels.

THE CAPILLARY CIRCULATION

Direct cannulation in animals being technically beyond existing methods, von Kries (27), in 1875, approached the problem indirectly in man by using a *blanching* method. Five years later Roy and Brown (55) improved the indirect methods somewhat by using a capsule with a distensible transparent membrane to determine under the microscope the pressures required to modify or to obstruct flows through single arterioles, capillaries, and venules in the transparent tissues of animals. They showed that, in the frog, with aortic pressures of 23 to 30 cm. water, pressures in large arterioles could be as high as 19 to 25 cm. water whereas a pressure of as little as 2 cm. water was enough to modify, and 2.5 to 4 cm. water enough to stop flow through the veins. They found, too, that capillary blood pressure could be quite different from moment to moment and quite different in capillaries arising from the same arteriole. Again a series of modifications followed, with emphasis on observations in the skin of man and with reported capillary blood pressures ranging from 1 to 45 mm. Hg. For example, Sir Thomas Lewis and August Krogh, each using his own indirect method and criterion of balance between imposed pressure and capillary blood pressure, came to different conclusions. Lewis found higher pressures, and Krogh found lower pressures. By 1925 it was clear to most observers that indirect methods were quite inaccurate, and that their criteria were based on assumptions of doubtful validity. The effectiveness of transmission of pressure from the plate or capsule through the skin to the vessels within the tissues beneath remained a basic uncertainty.

The first attempts to cannulate capillaries directly, with minute glass tubes, were made by Carrier and Rehberg in Krogh's laboratory in 1923 (*4*). Inserting a saline-filled pipette, connected to a manometer, into the larger venous capillary loops at the base of the finger nail of human subjects, they found that blood entered these pipettes at manometer pressures of 3.3 to 5.5 mm. Hg when the subject's finger was at heart level. But these pipettes were held in the hand of the observer so that observations were necessarily brief and fleeting in nature. Continuity between the lumen of the capillary and the lumen of the pipette could not be maintained for any long period of time. Moreover, not enough account was taken of the pressure drop required to produce entry of plasma and corpuscles into a tube through an orifice approaching corpuscular size. Hence their values proved to be much too low.

At about the same time Prof. Merkel H. Jacobs at the University of Pennsylvania suggested that the relatively new micromanipulators and microinjection methods of Robert Chambers (*5*) might be helpful in studying the permeability of the capillary wall. This was tried on single capillaries of the frog's mesentery and was shown to be a promising approach (*34*). However, the results of the first few successful injections of dye solution into the single capillaries were exceedingly variable and emphasized that, to be meaningful, this type of study required measuring the blood pressure in the capillary or capillary net during the injection.

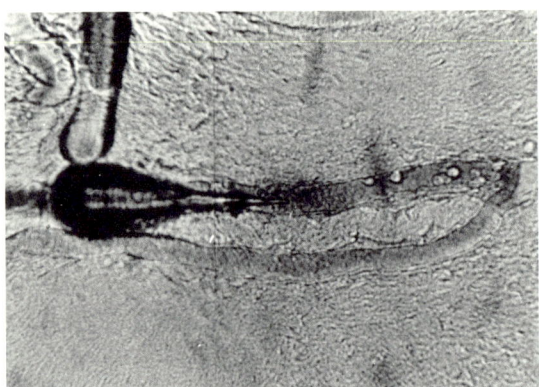

Figure 15. Micropipette in mesenteric capillary of the frog with glass rod to hold the mesentery and capillary stationary. Dilute dye being washed through capillary (i.e., pressure in manometer slightly greater than capillary pressure) preparatory to measurement of capillary pressure by exact balance.

The performance of such measurements required that micropipettes be held in position within the capillary lumen for periods of time long enough to adjust the pressure within the manometer-pipette system until it exactly balanced the existing capillary blood pressure without net flow of liquid in either direction through the 5 to 10μ orifice of the micropipette. From these studies of pressures in single arteries, arterioles, capillaries, venous capillaries, and veins, it was concluded (34):

"*At the average rate of flow the fall of pressure in the peripheral vessels of the mesentery does not cease abruptly at the junction of the arterioles and capillaries, but continues to the venous capillary before flattening, though pulse pressure is sharply diminished at the junction of arteriole and capillary. The gradient varies markedly under different conditions of arteriolar resistance, capillary pressure, and flow.*

"*Pressure and velocity of flow in the capillary vary in the same direction and with rather close relationship....*

"*Pressure differs not only in different capillaries coming from the same arteriole, but also in the same capillary from moment to moment. Pressure may be above or below the reported osmotic pressure of plasma colloids throughout the whole length of any capillary in successive moments....*"

At this point quantitative information concerning capillary blood pressure began finally to contribute to another line of ideas, namely, the movements of fluid, by filtration and absorption, through the capillary wall.

Passage of Substances Through Capillary Walls: Diffusion, Filtration, and Absorption

The idea that the capillaries are directly concerned in the nutrition of the tissues appeared quite late and, in a sense, secondarily. Even in 1828, Marshall Hall wrote, "When the structure of the part is simple, and the object of the circulation is its nutrition merely, the vessels are few in number." In contrast, the lymphatics had been much discussed as the vessels of nutrition ever since Aselli, in 1622, had discovered the lacteal vessels and thought that they carried foodstuffs from the intestines direct to the liver, to be elaborated there into blood. The "suction theory" of lymph production, the postulation of special "exhalant" blood vessels, together with hypothetical secretory activities of lymphatic vessels or tissue cells, all served to continue the idea that nutrition was chiefly a lymphatic function.

Concurrently, however, an irrigation theory of tissue nutrition was considered in several forms but failed to find general acceptance. As early as 1653, Bartholin proposed that water and solids might well be transuded from the blood vessels, that the tissues could then take up the solids, and that the pure water which was left over could return via the lymphatics to the blood. Nevertheless, throughout the eighteenth century the "suction theory" remained dominant.

In 1850, Noll's studies (46) in Ludwig's laboratory began a new era in the history of knowledge concerning lymphatics and blood capillaries. Aided by Poiseuille's mercury manometer and by Ludwig's kymograph and smoked paper for continuous recording, Noll concluded that the chief factor in forming lymph was the pressure of blood in the capillaries. Ludwig summarized the filtration theory thus in 1861 (42):

"The blood which is contained in the vessels must always tend to equalize its pressure and its chemical constitution with those of the extravascular fluids, which are separated from it only by the porous bloodvessel walls. If, for example, the quantity of blood in the vessels has increased, the mean blood pressure is also increased and at once a portion of blood is driven out into the tissues by a mere process of filtration. A similar result is brought about when the constitution of the blood is altered by the absorption of food or by increased excretion by the kidneys, blood, or skin, or when the composition of the tissue fluids is altered in consequence of increased metabolic changes taking place in the tissues. In the latter case, the changes brought about in the lymph are produced by processes of diffusion."

In view of present-day attempts to clarify the still uncertain semantics, and interlocking roles, of diffusion and filtration in capillary physiology, the definitions of a century ago have more than usual interest. Ludwig's two-volume textbook of physiology (42), published in 1858 and 1861, provided the following:

"Filtration. This term refers to the driving of a stream of liquid through capillary pores of a membrane by a hydrostatic pressure.... In this filtering stream one must consider the chemical composition of the liquid before and after its passage through the membrane and also the mass of liquid that has passed through the membrane in unit time."

Diffusion required a more lengthy description. In 1809 Magendie (43) questioned the view that the lymphatics were the sole pathway by which substances entered the blood stream from the tissue spaces. He had found that when crude extracts containing strychnine were introduced into the peritoneal cavity, or into the tissues of a leg, they produced characteristic effects in spinal cord function in seconds or minutes. This seemed too brief a time for transport through a circuitous lymphatic route only. His experiments with the isolated leg of a dog established passage from interstitial fluid to blood directly through the capillary wall.

THE CAPILLARY CIRCULATION

"In a dog, previously made sleepy with opium (to avoid the pain of a difficult experiment) we separated a leg from the body; this separation was so made that the leg was connected to the trunk only by the crural artery and vein.... We carefully isolated them for a distance of four centimeters and we removed their tunics to destroy lymphatic connections.... We then placed two grains of poison in the paw and we awaited the production of symptoms. These appeared with promptness and intensity as if the leg had not been separated from the body; thus the first signs of action appeared during the fourth minute, and the animal was dead before the tenth."

In 1855, Adolph Fick published two papers on diffusion in physical systems, and, in 1858, Ludwig (42) devoted a chapter of twenty-five pages to the subject of *aggregation states and diffusion*. He described the latter, beginning with its simplest case and then proceeding to the more complex examples that might be found in the animal body.

"Two fluids, liquid or gaseous, penetrate through each other, provided that they exhibit no interfering capillarity with each other when they are directly mixed, and also provided that finally the space originally occupied by each can be occupied by the other without intervention of chemical affinities and of mechanical shaking....

"In connection with the presumption of impenetrability of bodily structures and their being composed of minute particles (molecules) this occurrence is explicable only if the molecules do not fill the entire volume but leave spaces (molecular pores) between them."

For the more specific case of "blood flowing through a series of tubes which are themselves immersed in a liquid," Ludwig considered the

BLOOD VESSELS

barrier which the walls of the blood vessels must present to the movements of molecules to and from the blood, and concluded:

"In view of the great importance of hydrodiffusion it is all the more regrettable that no studies are available for the diffusion properties of those very liquids and membranes which are most important for life. . . ."

In spite of these uncertainties, the importance of diffusion in the molecular transport of nutrients and wastes through the capillary wall was generally appreciated after 1850, and was gradually amplified. Both theory and qualitative evidence held diffusion primarily responsible for maintaining constancy of solute concentrations. Many studies showed that when dyes, salts, and sugars were injected into blood they were quite soon afterward found in the lymph. Conversely when such substances were introduced into the tissue spaces or into the pleural or peritoneal cavities they could be found very promptly in the general blood stream. In general, the smaller the molecule the more rapid was the development of equality of solute concentrations inside and outside the capillary wall.

On the other hand, attempts to explain the control of the volume of lymph flow and the regulation of the constancy of blood volume remained unsuccessful. Many of Ludwig's earlier experiments supported his belief that this was accomplished by a direct relationship between blood pressure, filtration, and lymph formation, followed by return of this lymph to the blood stream. Elevating arterial pressure in perfused tissues increased lymph flow, as did elevating venous pressure in portions of the circulation in the entire animal. But others showed very soon that elevations of blood pressure produced by vasomotor changes did not always produce the predicted increase of filtration. From the resting limb little lymph could be obtained, whereas Ludwig's filtration hypothesis required that even resting capillary blood pressure should have produced some filtration and some lymph flow.

The problem became still more obscure after 1880, when Heidenhain began studying the abundant flow of lymph from the thoracic duct, which continued even during rest. The actions of his two classes of "lymphagogues," coupled with slight but definite inequalities of solute concentrations in plasma and lymph, led him to postulate active secretion by the cells of the capillary walls and possibly by the lympha-

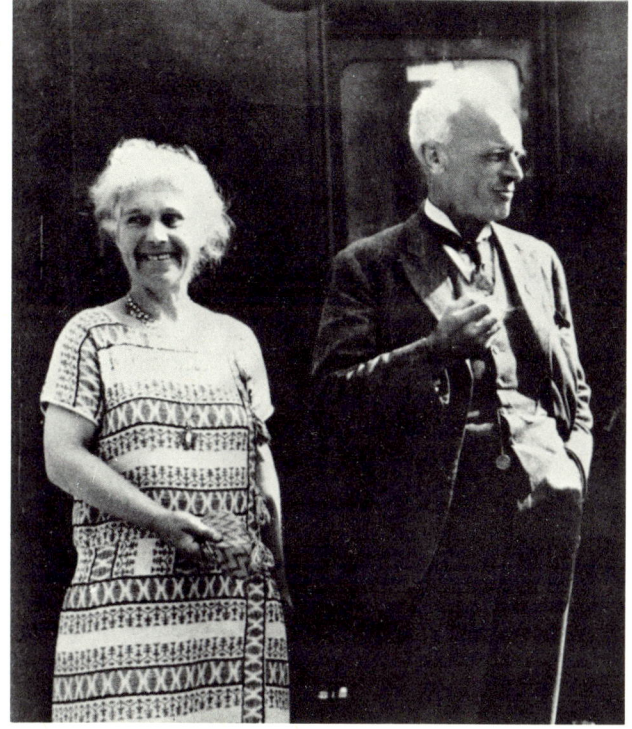

Figure 16. Ernest H. Starling (1866–1927) and Mrs. Starling.

tics. Heidenhain found Ludwig's simple filtration hypothesis adequate for some conditions and quite unable to explain many others. On the other hand, Heidenhain's secretion hypothesis was supported by no direct proof. All these studies were the background for Starling's measurement of the osmotic pressure of the plasma proteins and his addition of absorption to Ludwig's filtration. In 1896, Starling wrote

On the absorption of fluids from the connective tissue spaces (57):

"*Until within the last few years, all workers who investigated the question of absorption by the blood vessels, confined their experiments to cases in which some substance, not occurring normally in the blood, was introduced into some connective tissue space. That, under these conditions, absorption by the blood vessels does take place, was shown by Magendie, and confirmed in recent years by Ascher as well as by Tubby and myself. Although the ease, with which this interchange by a process of diffusion between blood and extravascular fluids*

BLOOD VESSELS

takes place, must be of great importance for the normal metabolism of the tissues (as, e.g. the much discussed supply of CaO to the mammary gland cells), yet such processes will not serve to explain the absorption by the blood vessels of fluids having the same tonicity and the same approximate constitution as the circulating plasma. The fluids contained in the tissue-spaces have the same tonicity and the same composition in salts as blood-plasma. We have to inquire first whether the blood vessels do absorb such isotonic fluids, and secondly the manner in which this absorption takes place."

Having provided evidence that isotonic fluid could be absorbed by capillaries (a) after hemorrhage and (b) after artificial edema, Starling proceeded with the mechanism of absorption by the blood vessels.

"We have now to consider how this absorption is effected. Are the capillary walls so constituted as to react to a lowering of the capillary pressure with an active absorption of extravascular fluid, i.e. is the absorption due to vital activity of the cells? or can we find mechanical conditions that will account for this absorption? . . .

"I believe the explanation is to be found in a property on which much stress was laid by the older physiologists, and which they termed the high endosmotic equivalent of albumen. It must be remembered that the earlier workers used animal membranes in their experiments on osmotic interchanges. These membranes permit the passage of water and salts, but hinder the passage of coagulable proteid. The application of semi-permeable membranes by Pfeffer to the measurement of osmotic pressures, showed that the osmotic pressures of salts and other crystalloids are enormously higher than those of such substances as albumen, and it has therefore been supposed that the osmotic pressure of the proteids in serum being so insignificant must be of no account in physiological processes. The reverse is however the case. Whereas the enormous pressures of the salts and crystalloids in the various fluids of the body are of very little importance for the function of absorption by the blood vessels, the comparatively insignificant osmotic pressure of the albumens is I believe of great importance. . . .

"To decide these points I have attempted to measure the osmotic pressure of the proteids in the serum directly. The osmometer consists of a small glass bell provided near the top with two vertical tubulures. Over the mouth of the bell is tied a peritoneal membrane similar to that used by Dr. Lazarus Barlow.

This was however rendered absolutely watertight by soaking it for some minutes, after it had been tied on, in a 10% solution of gelatin. The membrane is prevented from bulging by fixing over it a perforated silver or copper plate. The wider of the two tubulures is used for filling the bell with serum. The other one is connected either with a long narrow tube, or with a small mercurial manometer. Three or four of these osmometers are fixed in a wooden disc and arranged to revolve in alternating directions by means of a kitchen jack with their lower ends immersed in salt solution. The salt solution was in most cases 1.03% NaCl and was therefore slightly hypertonic to the serum.

"In all my experiments the fluid in the osmometer began to rise in the tube within two or three hours after the commencement of the experiment, and rose steadily for 3 or 4 days, the final height varying from 30 to 41 mm. Hg.

"The importance of these measurements lies in the fact that, although the osmotic pressure of the proteids of the plasma is so insignificant, it is of an order of magnitude comparable to that of the capillary pressures; and whereas capillary pressure determines transudation, the osmotic pressure of the proteids of the serum determines absorption. Moreover, if we leave the frictional resistance of the capillary wall to the passage of fluid through it out of account, the osmotic attraction of the serum for the extravascular fluid will be proportional to the force expended in the production of this latter, so that, at any given time, there must be a balance between the hydrostatic pressure of the blood in the capillaries and the osmotic attraction of the blood for the surrounding fluids. With increased capillary pressure there must be increased transudation, until equilibrium is established at a somewhat higher point, when there is a more dilute fluid in the tissue-spaces and therefore a higher absorbing force to balance the increased capillary pressure. With diminished capillary pressure there will be an osmotic absorption of salt solution from the extravascular fluid, until this becomes richer in proteids; and the difference between its (proteid) osmotic pressure and that of the intravascular plasma is equal to the diminished capillary pressure.

"Here then we have the balance of forces necessary to explain the accurate and speedy regulation of the quantity of circulating fluid."

This elegant concept did not find easy acceptance. First, much difficulty was encountered in measuring the osmotic pressure of the plasma proteins accurately. It was not until the 1920's that osmometers were developed in sufficiently dependable form to permit reproducible

BLOOD VESSELS

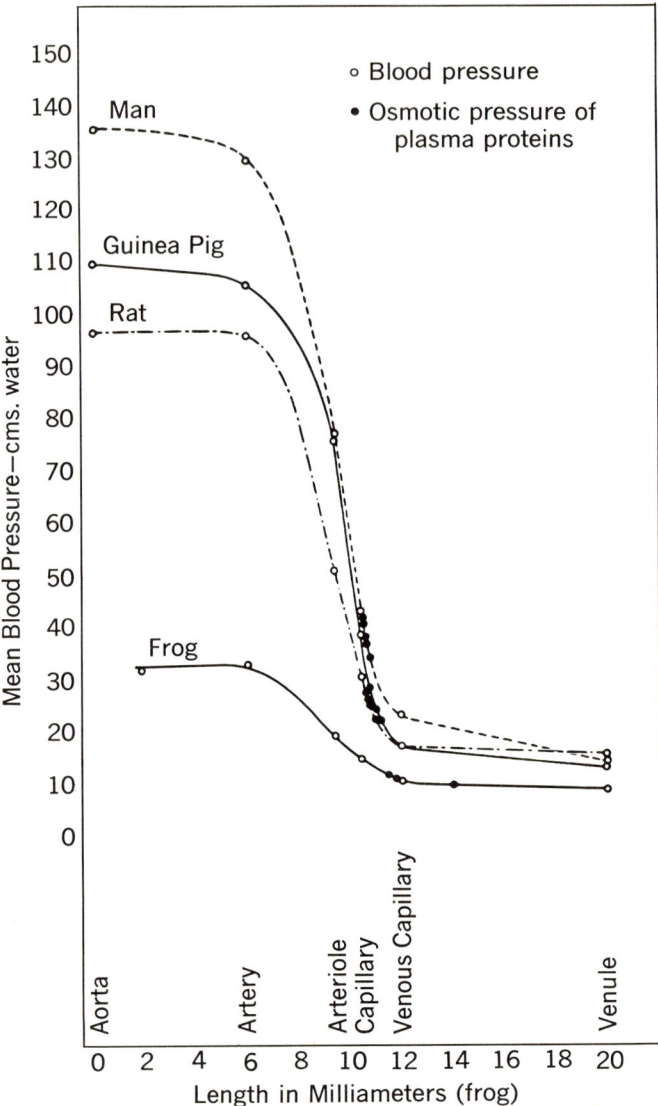

Figure 17. Chart showing relation between the average blood pressure gradient, capillary blood pressure, and the osmotic pressure of the plasma proteins in four species.

measurements in experimental animals and in patients with various types of edema. Even then skeptics could still point to the discrepancies between the measured osmotic pressures and the total concentration of the plasma proteins. As increasingly pure solutions of separated plasma proteins were studied, however, their molecular weights were established. The relative contributions of the albumins and globulins to the total osmotic pressure of the plasma proteins then became clear.

Equally uncertain for some decades was the validity of Starling's assumption that a balance existed between capillary blood pressure and the osmotic pressure of the plasma proteins. By 1931 this point was clarified by direct measurements of capillary blood pressure in several species—frog, rat, guinea pig, and man. On the average, and for each species, arteriolar capillary pressure was greater than, and venous capillary pressure less than, the osmotic pressure of the plasma proteins. With respect to absolute levels of pressure, the balance was found to be maintained at a lower level in the frog (about 11 cm. water) and at a higher level in man (about 34 cm. water or 25 mm. Hg). Moreover, in each species, pressures in single capillaries could be temporarily above or temporarily below this average balance (34, 37), depending on arteriolar dilatation, venous pressure, position relative to the heart, temperature, injury, etc.

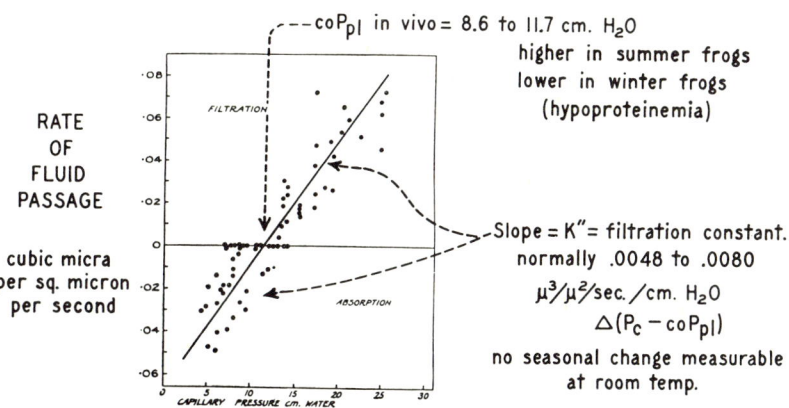

Figure 18. Chart showing, for single capillaries of frog's mesentery, the relation between filtration, absorption, and capillary blood pressure measured directly by micro-injection methods.

More direct quantitative proof of filtration and absorption was found in 1927 by micromanipulation and micro-injection of single capillaries in the frog's mesentery (*35*), in 1932 by studies with the pressure plethysmograph in the forearm of man (*33*), and in 1951 by Pappenheimer's elegant studies of the perfused limb of the cat (*47*). These are only a few of the many studies of normal and injured capillaries which verified Ludwig's filtration hypothesis and Starling's absorption hypothesis. More significantly still, they provided quantitative measures of fluid movement through normal and injured (*36*) capillary walls which

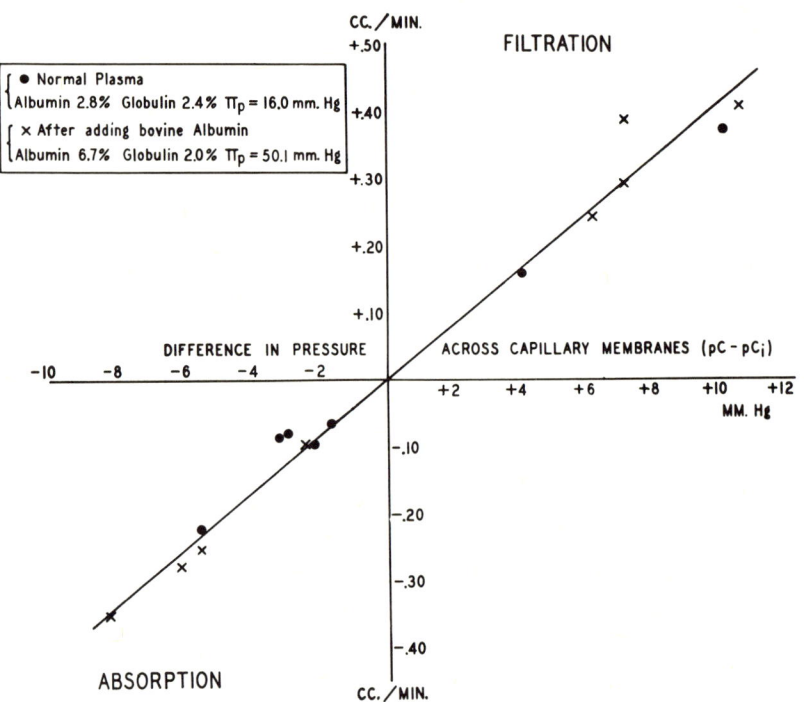

FLUID EXCHANGE IN HINDLIMB OF CAT
Exp. C - 25 Limb Weight 302 grams
Filtration Constant = Slope ÷ 3.02 = .014 cc./min./mm. Hg per 100 g. Tissue

Figure 19. Chart showing relation between net filtration, net absorption, and the average pressure difference across the capillary walls in the perfused hind limb of the cat.

made it feasible to consider, as a next step, the size, nature, and distribution of the interstices in the capillary wall through which these interchanges might conceivably take place.

The Capillary Wall as a Membrane

In 1858, Ludwig discussed the nature of the capillary membrane chiefly to express regret that so little was known about it. His linking of filtration and capillary blood pressure implied, however, that the capillary wall was passive. As mentioned previously, Heidenhain felt that secretory activity must be added to Ludwig's filtration in order to explain the action of his "lymphagogues," and also to explain differences between chloride concentrations in blood plasma and in lymph. In the 1890's the experiments of Starling and others negated secretory activity and provided much convincing, though still indirect, evidence in favor of inertness or passivity of the capillary wall. But regional and functional differences in the capillary wall were also already evident to Starling in 1898 when he wrote in Schäfer's Textbook of Physiology (*58*) as follows:

"The permeability of the capillary wall itself. The dependence of lymph formation on capillary pressure is not the only important relationship brought to light by these experiments. The amount and composition of the transudation through a membrane depend not only on the pressure at which the transudation is effected, but also on the nature of the membrane. According to the permeability of the membrane, so the amount and composition in proteids of the transuding fluid will vary. . . . We can therefore arrange the capillaries of the body in a descending order of permeability, the liver capillaries being the most permeable and the limb capillaries the least permeable. . . ."

Still unexplained, however, were the slight but definite differences in concentrations of ions on blood plasma and in the extravascular fluids. In the early 1920's it was demonstrated that these differences were qualitatively in the direction predicted by the Gibbs-Donnan equilibrium, though not quite in quantitative agreement with theory. A number of studies agreed in showing that dialysis and ultrafiltration of plasma in vitro produced the same exceptions and indicated that the discrepancies in vivo could be attributed to complex physico-chemical properties of plasma and extravascular fluids, which the simplifying assumptions of the Gibbs-Donnan theory did not include. The essential conclusion that emerged was that the electrolyte pattern observed when the capillary wall separated plasma and extravascular fluid was identical with the pattern observed when a collodion membrane of similar permeability separated the two fluids. This substantiated on chemical grounds the abundant physiological evidence concerning the inertness of the endothelial membrane.

Simultaneously, Drinker (*15*) and his students were exploring the passage of plasma proteins and particulate matter through the capillary wall into the interstitial fluid and lymph. At the same time, from observations on dyes of graded molecular size, Rous and his co-workers (*54*) postulated a gradient of capillary permeability with diffusion occurring more rapidly in the venous end of the capillary network. By 1934, a review (*38*) of physiological and chemical studies justified a few semiquantitative conclusions of which the first and most basic was that the capillary wall is a living, but inert, ultrafiltering membrane; no valid evidence of secretory activity had been found. Measured by fluid movement, the permeability of the capillary wall in the frog's mesentery ranged from 100- to 3000-fold greater than that of typical cell membranes studied up to that time. Filtration and absorption could be described quantitatively as relatively slow processes which ensured constancy of solvent volumes in plasma, interstitial fluids, and lymph. Diffusion, on the other hand, was much more rapid over short distances and ensured the equally important constancies of solute concentrations and cell nutrition.

In the twenty-five years since then, theory, experiment, and speculation have pressed onward to considerations of the area, size, number, location, and nature of the interstices or pores in the capillary wall. Three centuries ago the first lenses were being pushed to the limit of their resolving power to describe the blood capillaries and the passage of erythrocytes along their lumina. Now the methods of physiology, physical chemistry, isotopic tracer techniques, and electron microscopy are, in their turn, being pushed to their respective limits to describe the ultramicroscopic channels in the capillary wall itself, through which solvent and solute molecules must pass. As described by Pappenheimer in 1953 (*47*), in the introduction to his review, *Passage of molecules through capillary walls:*

"Only occasionally are discontinuities in the capillary wall made evident by the diapedesis of one of the formed elements of the blood and even in such cases it is hard to be certain that a microscopically visible channel of egress is present. . . . There are good reasons for supposing, however, that the capillary blood is in intimate contact with extravascular fluid and that the visible flow of blood through the capillaries is, in fact, very small in comparison with the invisible flow of water and dissolved materials through the capillary walls. . . . Indeed it is by means of this ultramicroscopic circulation through the capillary wall that the circulatory system as a whole fulfills its ultimate function in the transport of materials to and from the cells of the body."

THE CAPILLARY CIRCULATION

It is much too early to draw final conclusions concerning the location and nature of the actual channels through which this ultramicroscopic circulation takes place. As with the capillaries themselves three centuries ago, so now with the pores of those capillaries, views and objections seem balanced. Chambers and Zweifach (7) proposed that the intercellular cement substance must be the site for exchanges by filtration, absorption, and diffusion. Pappenheimer's (47) estimate that the collective pore area equals 0.2 per cent of the capillary wall is compatible with this view. However, electron microscopy has not so far identified this postulated intercellular substance and in some areas the capillary endothelium seems to resemble an interrupted syncytium rather than a mosaic of cells.

As to pore size, as soon as physical chemists established the equatorial dimensions of the plasma proteins it seemed clear that some pores at least must have diameters well in excess of 35 Angstrom units (39). Pappenheimer and his co-workers (47), by combining diffusion and filtration data from their perfusion experiments, concluded for limb capillaries:

"Uniform cylindrical pores of radius 30 to 45 Angstrom units and a population density of 1 to 2 $\times$ 10^9 per cm.^{2} of capillary wall would account for the observed rates of passage of water and lipid-insoluble molecules of various sizes. However, there are no reasons for supposing that the channels are actually cylindrical and we may regard this value of effective pore radius as analogous to the Einstein-Stokes molecular radius which, by itself, tells nothing of the actual shape of the molecule."

An abundance of questions and problems remains. Adsorption of protein, blockage by platelet fragments (*14*), sieving (*47*), and lipid solubility (*51*) can modify the passage of molecules through the capillary wall. Chinard (*8*) has criticized the filtration hypothesis and pore concept on physicochemical and thermodynamic grounds. Pappenheimer, on the other hand, has postulated graded restriction of diffusion related to molecular radius together with a changing ratio between hydrodynamic flow and diffusion depending upon pore radius. Grotte (*20*), after measuring the passage of dextrans through the capillary wall, has postulated in addition to smaller *pores* a series of *leaks*, 250 Angstrom units in diameter and numbering from 30,000 to 60,000 per cm.² of limb capillary wall. The possibility of increased *pore* size whenever the capillary wall is stretched proposed by Krogh in 1922 (*31*) has been raised again (*56*). Meanwhile, electron microscopy has revealed, in some capillary endothelial cells, minute clear spaces near the inner and

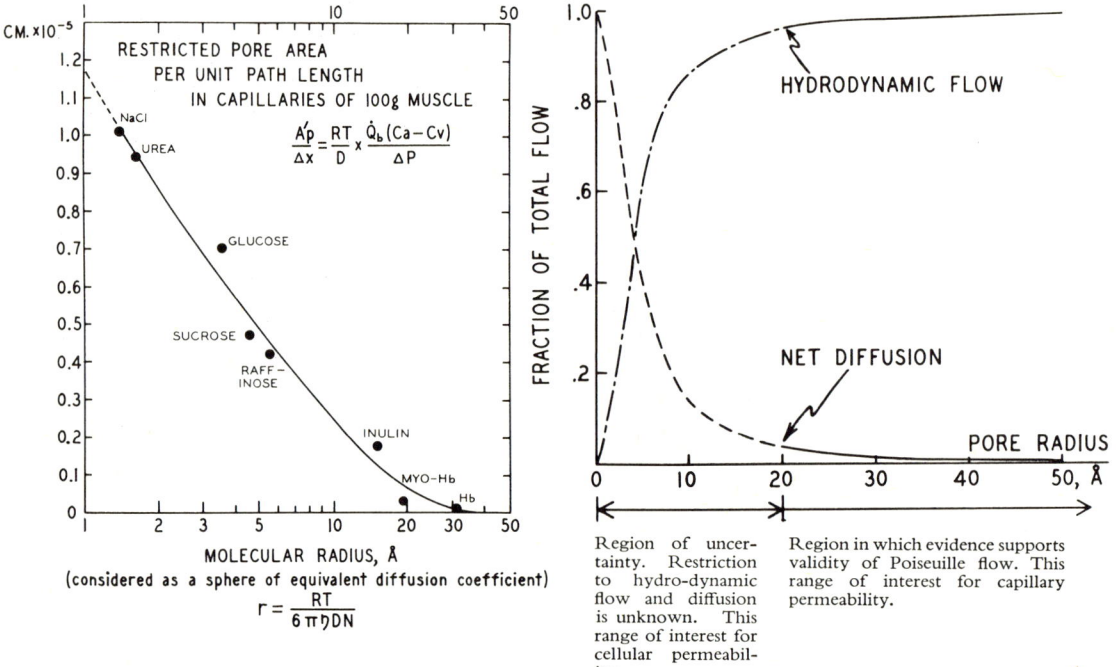

Figure 20. Charts showing (left) postulated relation of restricted diffusion to molecular radius and (right) a possible relation of hydrodynamic flow and diffusion to pore radius.

outer cell membranes as well as in the cytoplasm. It has been suggested that these may indicate transport by pinocytosis. In other capillaries, e.g. renal and hepatic, electron micrographs are showing large interstices or even gaps in the endothelial membrane sometimes with a more continuous, and, to current resolving powers, amorphous, basement membrane just outside. It has been suggested that the properties of this basement membrane may well be more significant than those of the endothelial wall.

Three centuries ago, when the science of physiology was just beginning, theory and experiment dealt with the *porositates carnis* of Harvey and the *divarications* of Malpighi, measurable in micra. Now attention is focused on *porositates capillorum* measured in Angstrom units. Physiologists, looking into the unknown, have made a full turn of the spiral. At this writing, the *porosities of the capillary wall* present as great a challenge to ingenuity, theory, and experiment as did the *porosities of the flesh* postulated by William Harvey in 1628.

BIBLIOGRAPHY

1. AEBY, C. T. A.   Ueber den feineren Bau der Blutcapillaren. Zbl. med. Wiss., 3:209, 1865.
2. AUERBACH, L.   Ueber den Bau der Lymph- und Blut-Capillaren. Zbl. med. Wiss., 3:177, 1865.
3. BLACK, J.   A Short Inquiry into the Capillary Circulation of the Blood; with a Comparative View of the More Intimate Nature of Inflammation, and an Introductory Lecture. London, Longman, 1825.
4. CARRIER, E. B., and P. B. REHBERG.   Capillary and venous pressure in man. Skand. Arch. Physiol., 44:20, 1923.
5. CHAMBERS, R.   The microvivisection method. Biol. Bull., 34:121, 1918.
6. CHAMBERS, R., and B. W. ZWEIFACH.   Topography and function of the mesenteric capillary circulation. Amer. J. Anat., 75:173, 1944.
7. CHAMBERS, R., and B. W. ZWEIFACH. Intercellular cement and capillary permeability. Physiol. Rev., 27:436, 1947.
8. CHINARD, F. P., G. J. VOSBURGH, and T. ENNS.   Transcapillary exchange of water and of other substances in certain organs of the dog. Amer. J. Physiol., 183:221, 1955.
9. CLARK, E. R., and E. L. CLARK.   B. The relation of "Rouget" cells to capillary contractility. Amer. J. Anat., 35:265, 1925.

10. CLARK, E. R., and E. L. CLARK. Caliber changes in minute bloodvessels observed in the living mammal. Amer. J. Anat., 73:215, 1943.
11. COHNHEIM, J. Vorlesungen über allgemeine Pathologie. Berlin, A. Hirschwald, 1877-80.
12. COTTON, T. F., J. G. SLADE, and T. LEWIS. Observations upon dermatographism with special reference to the contractile power of capillaries. Heart, 6:227, 1917.
13. DALE, H. H., and A. N. RICHARDS. The vasodilator action of histamine and of some other substances. J. Physiol. (Lond.), 52:110, 1918.
14. DANIELLI, J. F. Capillary permeability and oedema in the perfused frog. J. Physiol. (Lond.), 98:109, 1940.
15. DRINKER, C. K., and M. E. FIELD. Lymphatics, Lymph and Tissue Fluid. Baltimore, Williams and Wilkins, 1933.
16. EBBECKE, U. Die locale vasomotorische Reaktion (L.V.R.) der Haut und der inneren Organe. Pflügers Arch. ges. Physiol., 169:1, 1917.
17. EBERTH, C. J. Ueber den feineren Bau der Blutcapillaren bei den Wirbelthieren. Zbl. med. Wiss., 3:196, 1865.
18. FLEISCH, A. Die aktive Förderung der Capillaren. In Handbuch der normalen und pathologischen Physiologie. Berlin, Springer, 1927, 7:1083.
19. FULTON, G. P., and B. R. LUTZ. The control of small blood vessels. Amer. J. Physiol., 133:P284, 1941.
20. GROTTE, G. Passage of dextran molecules across the blood-lymph barrier. Acta chir. scand. Suppl. 211:1, 1956.
21. HALES, S. Statical Essays: Vol. 2 Containing Haemastaticks; or, an Account of Some Hydraulick and Hydrostatical Experiments made on the Blood and Blood-vessels of Animals. London, W. Innys and R. Manby, 1733.
22. HALL, M. A Critical and Experimental Essay on the Circulation of the Blood; Especially as Observed in the Minute and Capillary Vessels of the *Batrachia* and of Fishes. London, Seeley and Burnside, 1831.
23. HALLER, A. VON. Deux mémoires sur le mouvement du sang, et sur les effets de la saignée; fondés sur des experiences faites sur des animaux. Lausanne, M.M. Bousquet, 1756.
24. HARVEY, W. Exercitatio anatomica de motu cordis et sanguinis in animalibus. Frankfurt, W. Fitzer, 1628.
25. HARVEY, W. Movement of the Heart and Blood in Animals. Tr. by K. J. Franklin. Springfield, Ill., Thomas, 1957.
26. KRAUSE, C. Haut. In R. Wagner. Handwörterbuch der Physiologie. Braunschweig, F. Vieweg, 1844, 2:108.
27. KRIES, N. VON. Ueber den Druck in den Blutcapillaren der menschlichen Haut. Ber. Akad. Wiss., Leipzig, 27:149, 1875.
28. KROGH, A. Vaevenes Frosyning med Ilt og Kappillaerkredslöbets Regulering. Biol. Medd., Kbh., 1:No. 6, 1918.

29. KROGH, A. The number and distribution of capillaries in muscles with calculations of the oxygen pressure head necessary for supplying the tissue. J. Physiol. (Lond.), 52:409, 1919.
30. KROGH, A. The supply of oxygen to the tissues and the regulation of the capillary circulation. J. Physiol. (Lond.), 52:457, 1919.
31. KROGH, A. The Anatomy and Physiology of Capillaries. New Haven, Yale University Press, 1922.
32. KROGH, A. Reminiscences of work on capillary circulation. Isis, 41:14, 1950.
33. KROGH, A., E. M. LANDIS, and A. H. TURNER. The movement of fluid through the human capillary wall in relation to venous pressure and to the colloid osmotic pressure of the blood. J. clin. Invest., 11:63, 1932.
34. LANDIS, E. M. The capillary pressure in frog mesentery as determined by micro-injection methods. Amer. J. Physiol., 75:548, 1926.
35. LANDIS, E. M. Micro-injection studies of capillary permeability. II. The relation between capillary pressure and the rate at which fluid passes through the walls of single capillaries. Amer. J. Physiol., 82:217, 1927.
36. LANDIS, E. M. Micro-injection studies of capillary permeability. III. The effect of lack of oxygen on the permeability of the capillary wall to fluid and to the plasma proteins. Amer. J. Physiol., 83:528, 1928.
37. LANDIS, E. M. Factors controlling the movement of fluid through the human capillary wall. Yale J. Biol. Med., 5:201, 1933.
38. LANDIS, E. M. Capillary pressure and capillary permeability. Physiol. Rev., 14:404, 1934.
39. LANDIS, E. M. Capillary permeability and the factors affecting the composition of the capillary filtrate. Ann. N.Y. Acad. Sci., 46:713, 1946.
40. LEEUWENHOEK, A. VAN. Den Waaragtigen Omloop des Bloeds, als mede dat de Arterien en Venae gecontinueerde Bloed-Vaten zijn, klaar voor de Oogen gestelt. Verhandelt in een Brief, geschreven aan de Koninglijke. Societeit tot London. 65th Missive, Sept. 7, 1688. Opuscula selecta Neerlandicorum de Arte medica. Fasc. 1:45, 1907.
41. LISTER, J. L. On the early stages of inflammation. Philos. Trans., 148:645, 1858.
42. LUDWIG, C. Lehrbuch der Physiologie des Menschen. Leipzig, C. F. Winter, 1858-61.
43. MAGENDIE, F. Mémoire sur les organes de l'absorption chez les mammifères. Paris, 1809.
44. MÜLLER, J. Handbuch der Physiologie des Menschen für Vorlesungen. Coblenz, J. Hölscher, 1834-40.
45. MÜLLER, J. Elements of Physiology. Tr. by W. Baly. London, Taylor and Walton, 1838-42.

46. NOLL, F. Ueber den Lymphstrom in den Lymphgefässen und die wesentlichsten anatomischen Bestandtheile der Lymphdrüsen. Z. rat. Med., 9:52, 1850.
47. PAPPENHEIMER, J. R. Passage of molecules through capillary walls. Physiol. Rev., 33:387, 1953.
48. PAPPENHEIMER, J. R., and A. SOTO-RIVERA. Effective osmotic pressure of the plasma proteins and other quantities associated with the capillary circulation in the hindlimbs of cats and dogs. Amer. J. Physiol., 152:471, 1948.
49. POISEUILLE, J.-L.-M. Recherches sur la force du cœur aortique. Thèse. Paris (No. 166), 1828.
50. RECKLINGHAUSEN, F. VON. Die Lymphgefässe und ihre Beziehung zum Bindegewebe. Berlin, A. Hirschwald, 1862.
51. RENKIN, E. M. Capillary permeability to lipid-soluble molecules. Amer. J. Physiol., 168:538, 1952.
52. ROUGET, CH. Note sur le développement de la tunique contractile des vaisseaux. C.R. Acad. Sci. (Paris), 79:559, 1873.
53. ROUGET, CH. Sur la contractilité des capillaires sanguins. C.R. Acad. Sci. (Paris), 88:916, 1879.
54. ROUS, P., H. P. GILDING, and F. SMITH. The gradient of vascular permeability. J. exp. Med., 51:807, 1930.
55. ROY, C. S., and J. G. BROWN. The blood pressure and its variations in the arterioles, capillaries and veins. J. Physiol. (Lond.), 2:323, 1880.
56. SHIRLEY, H. H., JR., C. G. WOLFRAM, K. WASSERMANN, and H. S. MAYERSON. Capillary permeability to macromolecules: stretched pore phenomenon. Amer. J. Physiol., 190:189, 1957.
57. STARLING, E. H. On the absorption of fluids from the connective tissue spaces. J. Physiol. (Lond.), 19:312, 1896.
58. STARLING, E. H. The production and absorption of lymph. In E. A. Schäfer. Text-Book of Physiology. Edinburgh, Pentland, 1898, 1:285.
59. STEINACH, E., and R. H. KAHN. Echte Contractilität und motorische Innervation der Blutcapillaren. Pflügers Arch. ges. Physiol., 97:105, 1903.
60. STRICKER, S. Studien über den Bau und das Leben der capillären Blutgefässe. S. B. Akad. Wiss. Wien. Math. Nat. Kl. 2. Abt., 52:379, 1865.
61. TANNENBERG, J. Über die Kapillartätigkeit. Verh. dtsch. path. Ges., 20:374, 1925.
62. WHYTT, R. Physiological Essays. Edinburgh, Hamilton, Balfour and Neill, 1755.
63. YOUNG, J. Malpighi's "De Pulmonibus." Proc. roy. Soc. Med., 23:1, 1929.

VII

Vasomotor Control and the Regulation of Blood Pressure

THE vascular system is the great transport mechanism of the body. It serves as the link between the tissue fluid bathing the cells and the external environment. For the vascular system to fulfill its purpose, the blood supply to the tissues must be adapted to their metabolic needs. This flexibility is accomplished by changes in vascular caliber and in the output of the heart.

VASOMOTOR CONTROL

It is generally accepted that the peripheral circulation of the blood is determined by the arteriovenous pressure gradient across the vascular bed and by the vascular resistance to blood flow. The resistance to flow depends on both the viscous properties of the blood and on the calibers of the resistance blood vessels. By far the most potent variable affecting resistance is the tone of the vascular smooth muscle cells. Although, basically, this tone appears to be an inherent and automatic characteristic of muscle, it may be strongly modified, and even dominated, by extrinsic influences such as nervous stimuli and chemical agents. These influences constitute the most powerful tools for the control of the vascular bed; this chapter will deal with the development of our concepts concerning their role in the regulation of the circulation.

Vasomotor Control: The First Insights

The term "tone" was apparently first used in reference to veins. In his *De corde*, which appeared in 1669, Lower employed the phrase "*relaxatio venorum tono*" in considering the effect of venous dilatation on the heart beat (*144*). Lower also noted that veins which have long been over-dilated cannot easily recover their tone and contract; "*non ita facile in pristinum tonum resistui possunt aut coarcti.*" About two hundred years

BLOOD VESSELS

were to elapse before anything fundamental was added to Lower's statements about veins; not until 1864 was the idea of a nervous control of veins introduced (*88, 76*).

The first insights into the vasomotor control of the arterial part of the peripheral circulation came in the early part of the eighteenth century. Credit for the discovery of the vasomotor nerves is probably due to Pourfois du Petit, who reported in 1727 that dilatation of the conjunctival vessels occurred after section of the cervical sympathetic nerves (*168*).

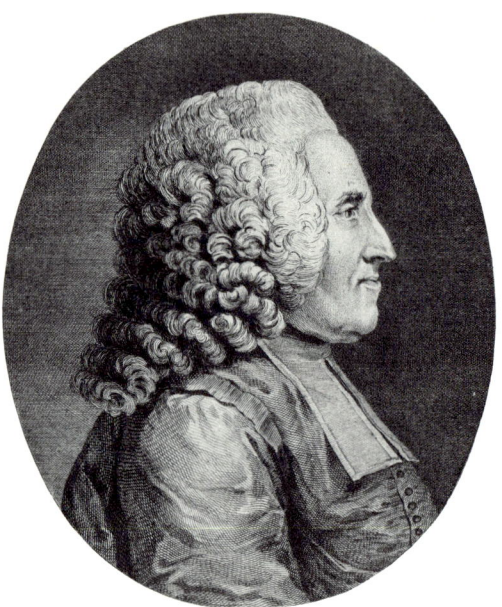

Figure 1. Jean-Baptiste de Sénac (1705–70).

However, the first clear statement of the control of the caliber of the arteries was provided by the French physician, Sénac, who wrote in 1777 (*180*):

"*The arteries which are so active are true hearts in another guise; they have the same functions, the same movements.* . . . *These movements are alternate dilatations and contractions which succeed each other without pause.* . . . *The force inherent in the tissue of the arteries depends on the muscular fibers the very existence of which has been doubted.* . . ."

By the early nineteenth century, histologists were well aware that nerves extended into and around the walls of blood vessels (*199*). Also, information was accumulating about the structure of the blood vessels and the functions of the vasomotor nerves. For example, in 1831, Weber reported that blood vessels change their dimensions not only as a result of their elasticity but also due to the influence of nerves on their muscular coat (*195*). In 1840, Henle presented the first clear description of smooth muscles in the walls of the smallest blood vessels (*94*), and shortly thereafter, Kölliker isolated individual muscle cells for the first time (*172*). Finally, in 1840, Stelling (*187*) concluded from his studies that the vasomotor fibers emerge from the central nervous system by way of the sympathetic nerves, regulating "die Bewegungen, der Tonus, die lebendige Zusammenziehung der Kapillargefässe und der Gefässe überhaupt, arterieller wie venöser." Indeed, we owe to him the term "vasomotor," a term which came into common use in the form of "nerfs vasomoteurs" after the important papers of Claude Bernard, Brown-Séquard, and Waller were published some ten years later.

VASOMOTOR CONTROL

When considering these early contributions one should remember that even though scientists had begun to realize 150 to 200 years ago that the blood vessels were contractile and controlled by nerves, they had little understanding—in either quantitative terms or in terms of the dynamics of the cardiovascular system as a whole—of what this control actually meant for the blood supply to the tissues. Poiseuille's law concerning flow through narrow tubes was yet to be published, and there was little knowledge of hemodynamic principles. These early views of what happens within the vascular bed have, therefore, little resemblance to current knowledge.

From Bernard to Bayliss

A giant step towards a more analytic and systematic study of the nervous vascular control was taken at the middle of the nineteenth century. This period is generally regarded as the starting point in the discovery of the mechanisms involved in the nervous control of the blood vessels. Within a period of only a few months, three separate papers of approximately equal content were presented by three men: Charles-Édouard Brown-Séquard on November 1, 1852, in Philadelphia, Claude Bernard a few days later in Paris, and Augustus Volney Waller

BLOOD VESSELS

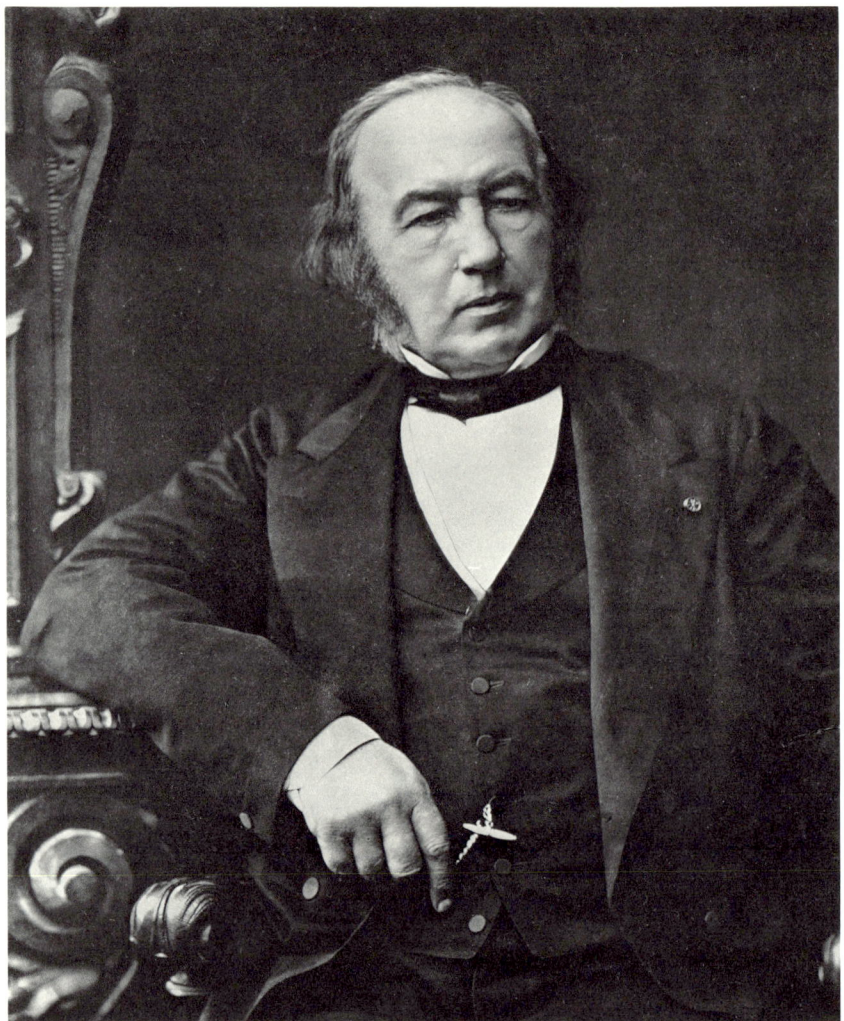

Figure 2. Claude Bernard (1813–78).

in February 1853, also in Paris. These had been anticipated in the previous year (December 1851) in a preliminary report by Claude Bernard (*14*):

"*I have seen that immediately following the section of the sympathetic nerve which connects the cervical ganglia, there occurs an increase in the temperature all over the ipselateral side of the face. This increase in temperature can be felt very easily with the hand. When one inserts the thermometer either into the ears or the nares of an animal, one finds that the temperature is higher by four to six degrees centigrade on the side where the sympathetic chain had been cut.... When one excises the superior sympathetic ganglion, one reproduces exactly the same effects and, sometimes, with greater intensity.... Along with the increase in the temperature of the parts, the circulation becomes more active, a phenomenon which is very apparent on the ears of the rabbits as I have shown to you in the course of reproducing my experiences before the Society. Later, I will explain about this modification of the circulation from the point of view of its mechanism and of the question of knowing if it is the cause or the effect of the increase in animal heat...."*

Claude Bernard was the greatest of the French physiologists. His discovery of the function of the vasomotor nerves was one of many important contributions to physiology (15, 16). This was not the product

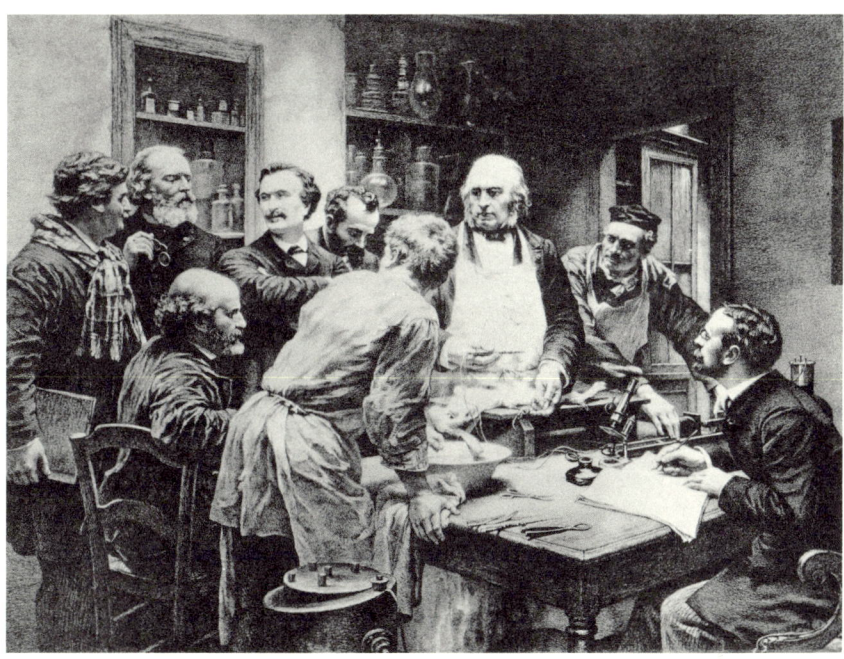

Figure 3. Claude Bernard demonstrating an experiment, presumably the effect of section of the sympathetic nerve on the rabbit's ear. Paul Bert, one of his most famous students, stands, with arms crossed, third from the left.

[411]

BLOOD VESSELS

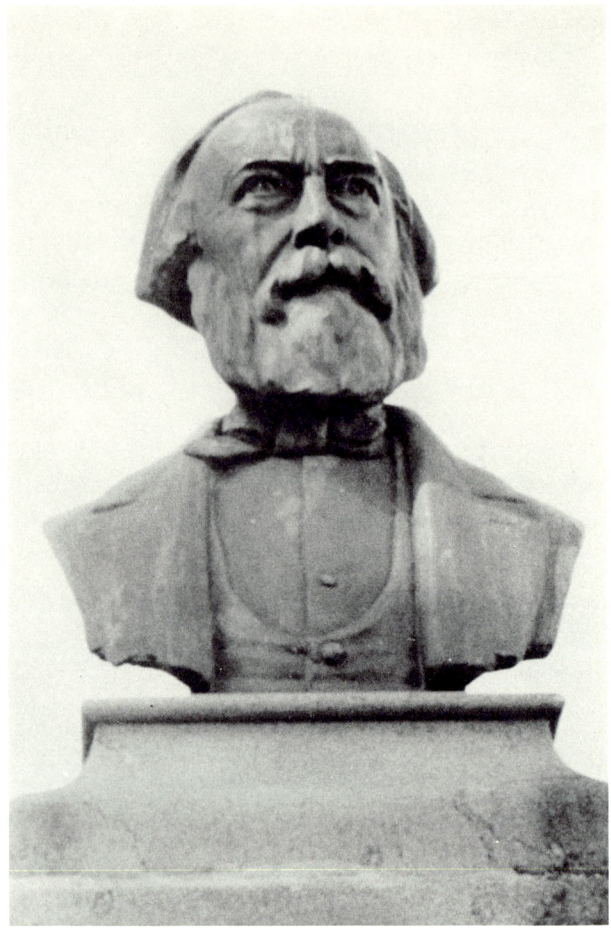

Figure 4. Bust of Charles E. Brown-Séquard (1817–94) in Port-Louis, Mauritius.

of an isolated piece of research; instead, it was a natural outgrowth of Bernard's interest in the role of the sympathetic nerves in metabolism and in the regulation of body temperature. Indeed, his preoccupation with the regulation of temperature delayed for several years his full appreciation of the role of the vasomotor nerves in the regulation of vascular dimensions. According to his student, Paul Bert, Bernard "discovered as others breathed." His was an unusual combination of scientific imagination, manual dexterity, skill in anatomy and chemistry, and scientific discipline. He devoted these talents to physiologic experimentation, on the premise that the laws which govern biological phenomena are as immutable as those of physics and chemistry and that the forces of vitalism play no part in biological phenomena. It is of interest that Bernard's prodigous scientific accomplishments were made in the face of marital difficulties, financial problems, and physical ailments, and at a time when the rewards for animal experimentation were apt to be scientific skepticism and police action (*162*).

Charles Brown-Séquard was one of the most interesting personalities of modern medicine. He was born in Mauritius, in the Indian Ocean, of American and French parentage, and studied medicine in Paris. His career was an unsettled one, beset by political and financial difficulties. In pursuing his physiological researches he crossed the Atlantic many times, and he taught and practiced medicine in Paris, Harvard, London, and New York. For a good part of his scientific life he was overshadowed by Claude Bernard. Although they were good friends, Brown-Séquard and Bernard were totally different in character. Brown-Séquard's research was motivated not so much by logic as by his brilliant intuition, where Bernard's was the product of a precise mind and a disciplined imagination.

Both of these men received their training under François Magendie (1783-1855). The leading physician of his day, Magendie was chief clinician at the Hôtel-Dieu, and professor at the Collège de France, where he conducted his experiments in physiology and pharmacology. His most notable contribution to science was his long fight in behalf of mechanism and against the vitalistic theories of his day. His philosophy was espoused with equal conviction by his two most illustrious students.

While in Paris, Brown-Séquard attended weekly meetings of the Société de Biologie, where he, Bernard, and François Magendie exchanged ideas on their current research. These discussions undoubtedly helped to shape Brown-Séquard's experiments on the vasomotor nerves (*161*). His observations on their function were published in the Philadelphia Medical Observer (*26*); however it is probable that the actual experiments were completed in Paris the year before.

In investigating the vasomotor nerves, he noted, as did Bernard, that section of the cervical sympathetic trunk evoked vasodilatation. He also made the novel observation that stimulation of the peripheral end of the

BLOOD VESSELS

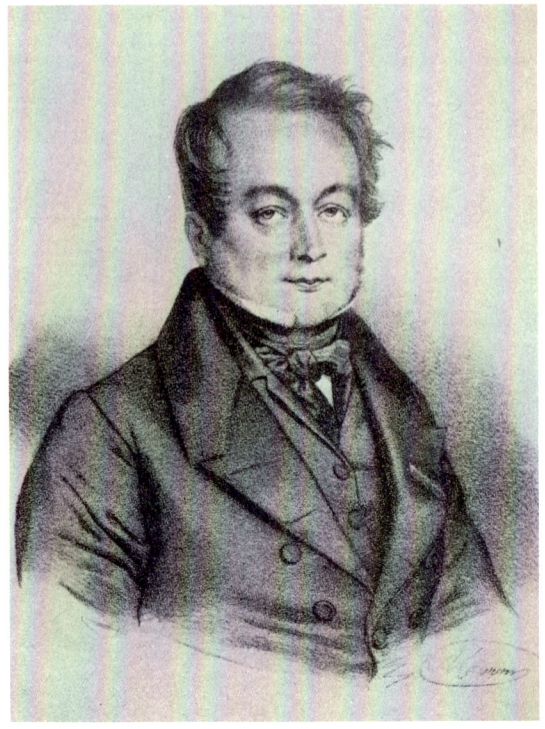

Figure 5. François Magendie (1783–1855).

same trunk induced vascular constriction. In 1854, he extended and confirmed his observations (*27*):

"(*1*) *Cutting a nerve, just like stimulating it, excites it.*
"(*2*) *When a nerve is excited, it is activated and to a variable degree, effects of its action are obtained.*
"(*3*) *The effects which are observed, some time after the section of a nerve, are the consequences of the paralysis or cessation of its activity.*"

The third contribution to the understanding of the vasomotor nerves, by the English physiologist Augustus Volney Waller (1816–70) (*194*), was the outgrowth of his continued interest in the neuron theory and the relationship between nerve fibers and nerve cells. In 1850, he had discovered that if a nerve is cut the parts of the fibers that are separated from their cells rapidly degenerate ("Wallerian degeneration") while the proximal parts remain relatively intact. By this type of experiment, which indicated that the nerve cells nourish the fibers, he established the physiologic autonomy of the nerve cell and its branches. His experiments in 1853 gave results identical with those of Brown-Séquard and Bernard: using cessation of blood flow from the cut surface of the ear as the end point, he showed that stimulation of the cervical sympathetic nerve elicited vasoconstriction.

These studies of Brown-Séquard, Bernard, and Waller established that the blood vessels are controlled by nerve fibers and that these nerve fibers are tonically active. In effect, they opened the door to the investigation of vasomotor tone and of blood pressure regulation. However, they shed no light on where or how this vasomotor tone is established and how it is controlled.

A few observations on the central control of the cardiovascular system had been made earlier. Spallanzani, as early as 1773 (*186*), had observed that damage to the brain of the frog could induce a closure of mesenteric and pulmonary vessels, and, in 1817, Nasse (*156*) had shown that high section of the spinal cord caused an increased temperature of the hind limbs. But Bernard (*17*) and Schiff (*176*) were the first systematic investigators of the centers for the vasoconstrictor fibers. On the basis of experiments that involved sectioning of the brain stem and spinal cord at different levels, they, and subsequently others (*164*), suggested the existence of special centers in the brain for the control of blood vessels. Goltz, who also studied the central control of the vascular bed, reported in 1864 that venous tone is dependent on the presence of the spinal cord and the medulla oblongata (*88*). He assumed that the centers exerted their control of the venous vessels by way of the sympathetic nerves.

Little was understood as to how the newly explored vasoconstrictor centers operated, but much insight was gained when information about reflex influences began to accumulate and when it was shown that high carbon dioxide tensions stimulated the vasomotor center (*190*), whereas abnormally low carbon dioxide tensions depressed its activity. The effects of carbon dioxide which were first shown clearly by Yandell Henderson in 1907 (*93*), made it obvious that the local chemical environment is highly important in "setting" the excitability level of the vasomotor center and thereby exerting considerable influence on the activity rate of the vasoconstrictor fibers.

BLOOD VESSELS

The concept of specific vasodilator fibers also developed in the middle of the nineteenth century. In 1853, Moritz Schiff, a German student of Magendie and Longet, who was to become professor of physiology at Florence and renowned for the first studies of the ductless glands, reported that section of the lingual and hypoglossal nerves caused a dilatation of the vessels of the tongue (*176*). A few years later, Bernard confirmed Schiff's suggestion about the function of the vasodilator nerves by demonstrating that stimulation of the chorda tympani induced an increase of blood flow through the submaxillary gland.

Bernard published the account of his study of the vasodilator nerves in a paper presented at the Académie des Sciences on August 9, 1858 (*16*) in which he stated:

"In the last analysis, we see that the two nerves which change the color of the venous blood to red and to black, are two motor nerves which act primarily by contracting or dilating the blood vessels. The sympathetic nerve is the constrictor nerve of the blood vessels; the tympanicolingual nerve is their dilator."

It is now known that this statement concerning the "tympanicolingual" nerve may be in error; but this misinterpretation hardly detracts from Bernard's contribution to the concept of vasodilator fibers.

In this paper he also provided the first demonstration of a reflex vasodilatation:

"In effect, if immediately after the exposure of the glandular vein and of the nerve in question (chorda tympani), a taste sensation is evoked in the tongue by instilling a little vinegar in the mouth, blood rapidly becomes ruddy in the vein because the taste sensation produced in the tongue is conducted to the nervous center and transmitted by reflex action, through the chorda tympani."

During the next few years, the other types of vasodilator nerve fibers were explored. In 1863, Eckhard showed that the sacral parasympathetic outflow also carries vasodilator fibers, e.g., to the penis (*54*). The first experiments demonstrating that the sympathetic nervous system also contains vasodilator fibers were performed by Dastre and Morat in 1880 (*46*), but nothing was then known about either the functional significance of these fibers or their distribution within the vascular bed. In 1876, Stricker showed clearly that the dorsal roots also carry vasodilator fibers (*188*), although the conditions under which these fibers were

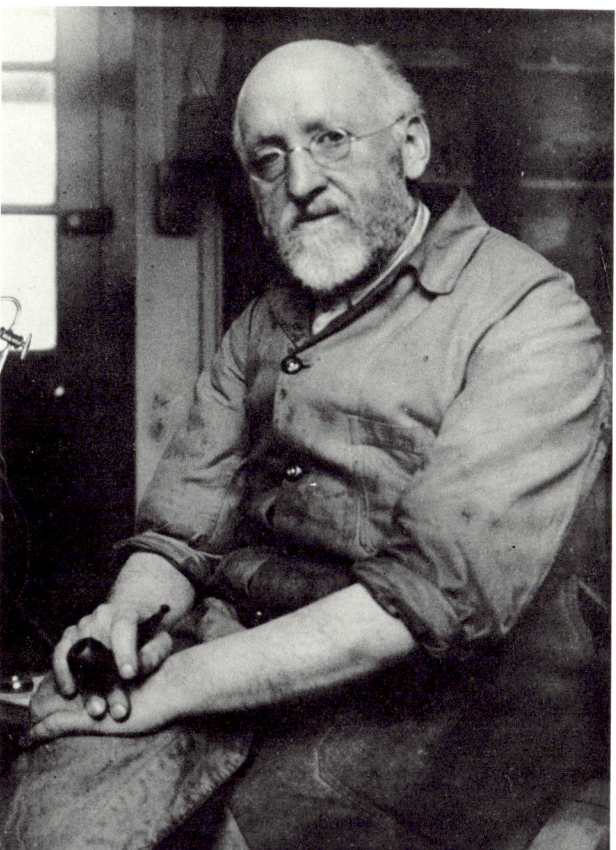

Figure 6. William Maddock Bayliss (1860–1924).

normally activated remained obscure. Evidence for the existence of a separate center for vasodilator fibers was provided by Laffont in 1880 *(134)*. He reported that destruction of the floor of the fourth ventricle or removal of parts of the medulla interfered with the reflex vasodilatation obtained when the depressor nerve was stimulated. The fact that inhibition of constrictor fiber tone is the most common type of neurogenic vasodilatation was not appreciated at that time.

At the beginning of the present century, Bayliss tried to introduce some order into the confused ideas concerning the function of the vasodilator fibers *(12, 13)*. Basing his theory on beautifully designed experiments, he proposed that all the vasodilator fibers were governed by a specific vasodilator center, in reciprocal balance with the vasoconstrictor center. Since this view was in harmony with what was already known about the nervous control of the heart, it was widely accepted, and for many decades it was standard teaching in practically all textbooks of physiology. It brought clarity and order to concepts of cardiovascular nervous control; its only drawback was that it was wrong. Indeed, it took almost fifty years to prove that the functional significance of the vasodilator fibers was far more complicated than Bayliss had conceived. Bayliss's hypothesis stands as a good example of how scientific concepts can become "canonized."

Bayliss's "error" should, by no means, detract from his stature; he was certainly one of the most erudite and disciplined physiologists of his time. Early in his academic career he had become associated with Burdon-Sanderson, disciple of Ludwig, and this association presumably directed his first researches to electrophysiology. From the electrophysiology of the salivary glands, his research progressed to the electrophysiology of the heart, and thence to the study of the circulation. His independent research was supplemented by a collaboration with Starling, which produced the discovery of "secretin" and fresh insight into the innervation of the heart and of the intestine. His classical book, *Principles of General Physiology*, illustrates his far-sighted dedication to tracing biological phenomena to their physicochemical origins.

An interesting side light on the character of William Bayliss was the episode, famous in its day, of the "Brown Dog Case." An ardent antivivisectionist had publicly accused Bayliss and Starling of cruelty in their treatment of dogs in their experiments. Bayliss, quick to defend himself, brought suit for defamation of character, and the trial became a *cause célèbre* through 1903–4. In Figure 7 is shown one of the posed photographs which was presented as evidence in court. Bayliss won his case.

As early as 1860, Brown-Séquard was on the verge of finding the hormonal link of the sympatho-adrenal system: he had observed vascular reactions which obviously depended on the discharge of catechol hormones from the adrenal medulla (*28*). However, his observations appear to have passed largely unnoticed, presumably because the time was not yet ripe for a concept which involved hormonal participation in vasomotor control. After this study, little interest seems to have been paid to the adrenal glands until Oliver, about forty years later, made some extracts of the glands and studied their remarkable cardiovascular effects on his own child; these effects were subsequently confirmed by experiments with Schäfer in 1894 on dogs (*160*). Since that time, the notions concerning the functional role of the hormonal components in cardiovascular control have undergone considerable modification, and until very recently, their importance has been exaggerated out of all proportion to the evidence presented.

VASOMOTOR CONTROL

This brief survey gives some idea of the state of our knowledge at the start of the modern era of physiological research. On superficial examination, we may gain the impression that most of our current concepts about cardiovascular control had already been fully established. On closer view, however, it is obvious that this was by no means the case. It

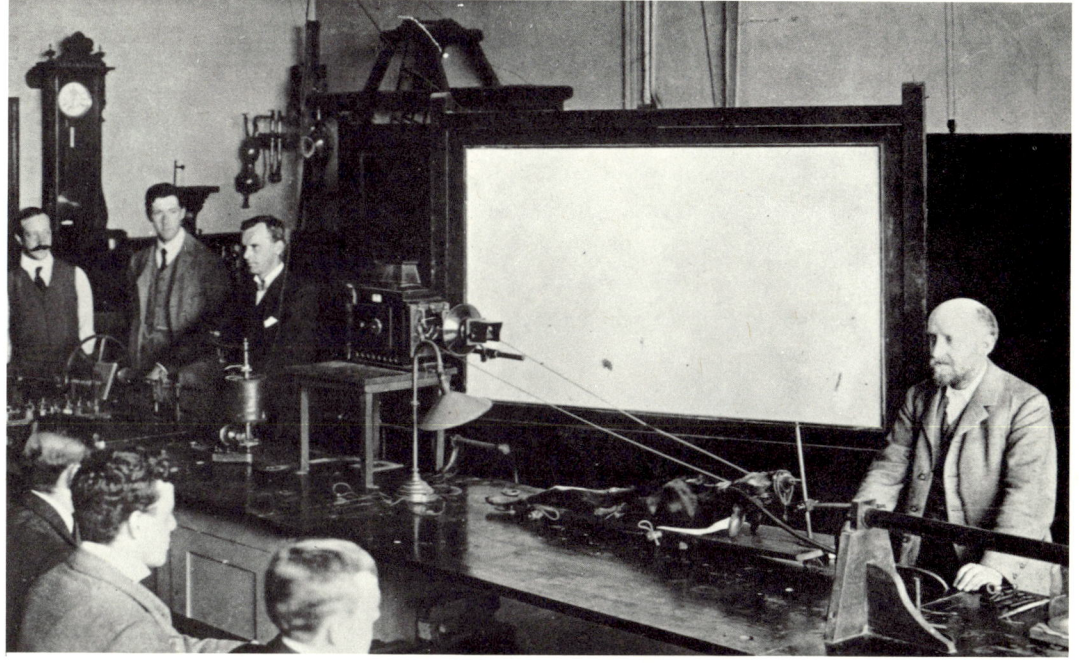

Figure 7. The "Brown Dog Case." Here the individuals concerned are of interest. On the right, "experimenting," is Bayliss. To his right, beyond the screen, is Starling, and beside him H. H. Dale, who had just arrived as a young student in Starling's laboratory. The "audience" were student volunteers, to enliven the picture.

is true that the existence of all the different links engaged in cardiovascular control was in great part known to the pioneers, but nothing, or nearly nothing, was known about their functional significance: how and when they were involved in different reaction patterns, their range of action, and their quantitative interrelationships. The cortical and diencephalic centers for circulatory control were still unknown, and so was practically every type of important cardiovascular receptor. Indeed, the innumerable contributions of later years have been built over the pioneer contributions to such an extent that our modern concepts bear but little resemblance to those of some eighty to a hundred years ago.

Functional Classification of Vascular Segments

Without knowledge of the general principles that govern the operation of vascular smooth muscle, an outline of the development of current concepts of cardiovascular control would be meaningless. Unfortunately, it has been extremely difficult to investigate the characteristics of smooth muscle in general, and vascular smooth muscle in particular. Part of the difficulty may be traced to the fact that practically no methods exist which allow a detailed, in vivo study of individual muscle cells of the smallest vessels without introducing a variety of interfering mechanisms and artefacts. Consequently, interest has focused on the behavior of the smooth muscle of isolated, large vessels. As long as it was generally accepted that vascular smooth muscle, independent of location, was fairly uniform in its behavior, this approach appeared to be valid. However, there is now considerable evidence to indicate that in some respects, the muscle cells of the smallest vessels—which are the seat of a large number of important regulatory mechanisms—behave in a strikingly different manner than the muscle cells of larger arteries or veins.

A common oversight in earlier years was the fact that not only do larger vessels react differently from the smaller ones, but also that the vascular beds of different tissues are far from uniform in their behavior. For example, erroneous generalizations concerning the principal elements responsible for vascular tone have been drawn from studies confined to the cutaneous vessels. At the other extreme, many investigators have been so impressed with the dissimilarities among various vascular beds that they have assumed that no generalizations whatsoever can be drawn concerning the contractile elements and their control mechanisms. Gradually, however, the view has emerged that the truth lies somewhere between these extremes. There certainly are considerable differences between various vascular beds and even between various consecutive sections or elements of one and the same vascular bed; but the same principal elements can be identified everywhere—the differences are more quantitative than qualitative in nature.

It now seems clear that the vascular bed should be regarded neither as a functionally uniform system of tubes nor as a network of fundamentally different tube-sections of confusing complexity, but instead as a highly differentiated system, with each part subserving important specialized functions. For this reason, the vascular bed may be considered as consisting of two categories of vessels which may be analyzed in two distinct ways: (1) *"Parallel-coupled" circuits*, i.e. of the vascular beds in different tissues. During recent years considerable information has been gained about differences and similarities among such circulations as the cerebral, myocardial, cutaneous, and muscular. (2) *"Series-coupled" sections* of the vascular bed. Little information is available as yet because only recently have reliable methods been developed to measure accurately the influence of the vasoconstrictor nerves on different portions of the vascular tree, e.g. veins as compared with arterioles.

The increased insight of recent years into hemodynamics has gradually established the advantages inherent in distinguishing between the following, functionally defined, vascular segments:

"Windkessel" vessels, which convert a rhythmic input to a fairly smooth outflow.

Resistance vessels, each with a precapillary, a capillary, and a postcapillary section, the sum of which make up the total resistance to flow, and the interrelation of which is one of the main determinants of the rate of filtration across the capillary walls.

Exchange vessels, in which blood comes into contact with the tissue across an enormous capillary surface, thus fulfilling the main purpose of cardiovascular function, the other sections serving mainly as adjustors of this contact between the internal and external environments.

Sphincter vessels, limited sections of the smallest resistance vessels, where smooth muscle "sphincters" can induce intermittent occlusion of the lumens, thus affecting the capillary surface available for perfusion, and hence exchange with the tissue, at any given moment.

Capacitance vessels, where shifts in average bore, though so moderate that they hardly affect the flow resistance, can dramatically affect the filling of the pump and thus the volume flow.

Shunt vessels, found only in certain tissues in which they serve special needs such as heat exchange; these vessels allow a by-pass of the exchange vessels.

These segments of the vascular tree show considerable overlap in function and lack morphologically distinct boundaries. However, it is important to deal with the vascular bed from a functional approach, because only from such a treatment can the peripheral circulation and its control be analyzed with due regard for all of its functional aspects. Unfortunately, adequate methods for continuous, quantitative, and simultaneous measurements of many events in these different vascular sections are still lacking.

Vascular Tone

Before examining the determinants of vascular tone, we should consider how it may be reasonably quantified. As a baseline for assessing any given degree of tone, the resistance to blood flow may be compared to the resistance which exists when the vascular bed is maximally dilated since, at a constant pressure head, only the structural characteristics of the fully dilated bed determine its resistance to blood flow. Obviously this maximally dilated state rarely occurs under natural conditions. Instead, the smooth muscle cells of the vascular bed adjust the resistance to blood flow according to the tissue requirements for blood. In practice, maximal dilatation of a vascular bed may be accomplished by a close arterial injection of a supramaximal amount of a dilator drug.

The first step in distinguishing the relative importance of each of the various factors involved in the establishment of vascular tone is determining the effect on the vascular tone of cutting the vasomotor nerves. The second and more difficult step is that of identifying the relative roles of the other factors which contribute to the "residual" or the "basal" tone. In some vascular beds, such as those of the brain, the intestine, the "metabolic" vessels of the skin, and especially the skeletal and the cardiac muscles, the basal tone is quite pronounced. In other beds, such as the arteriovenous anastomoses of the skin, there is considerably less basal tone and almost maximal dilation can be accomplished by sectioning the vasomotor nerves.

It was once widely held that the basal tone is primarily a consequence of blood-borne vasoconstrictor agents. Such a view is, however, hardly compatible with the fact that vessels with a high basal tone, like those of the skeletal muscles, are, in fact, *less* sensitive to all of the known vasoconstrictor agents than are some vessels which exhibit little or no basal tone, e.g. the anastomoses of the skin (*69*). This observation indicates that in the "resting" intact organism the blood concentration of vasoconstrictor substances is functionally insignificant and, as a corollary, that the marked basal tone which exists in some vascular areas must be due to a purely local mechanism. The question then arises, what is the nature of this local mechanism?

Myogenic Versus Extrinsic Determinants of Vascular Tone

By the end of the last century, hints were being made that the smooth muscles of the vessels, like those of the gastrointestinal tract, possess "spontaneous" activity or automaticity. Although these hints also implied that the inherent activity of smooth muscle might be a basic component of vascular tone, they were not taken very seriously, and for the next decades only nervous and humoral influences received serious attention. A fresh point of view was introduced by Bayliss in 1902, when he suggested that distension of the vessel by the blood pressure could act as a mechanical stimulus to the muscle cells, thereby contributing to their tone (*10*). However, conclusive experimental support for this concept was only forthcoming in recent years.

There is now ample reason to believe that vascular smooth muscle cells do exhibit myogenic activity, an activity which is a phylogenetically primitive characteristic of cardiac muscle and of other types of smooth muscle (*21*). Myogenic activity is manifested in isolated larger vessels as slow, spontaneous changes in tone, and in small vessels as an unsynchronized "vasomotion"; the latter phenomenon is especially pronounced in the venules of the bat's wings (*80*) and is also a striking feature of the behavior of precapillary sphincters in general. Indeed, the activity of these sphincters often induces complete, intermittent closure of their lumens, which explains why only a few of the capillaries in resting muscle are perfused at any given moment.

It has sometimes been suggested that, as in the case of the heart, this inherent activity is ultimately initiated by the local nerve plexuses. This suggestion, which merely shifts the responsibility for automaticity from muscle to nerve, solves no problems. Instead, it creates new ones. Spontaneous activity of smooth muscle is present in completely nerve-free strips, after application of local anesthesia, and in embryonic tissues before the development of nerve cells. Also, there is no clear evidence of any plexuses of nerve cells in the vascular walls. On the whole, it seems reasonable to implicate nerve elements only when their presence is necessary to account for a rapid and widespread propagation of excitation or inhibition. The available evidence indicates that while the rhythmic, unsynchronized contractions of vascular smooth muscle are, like all other manifestations of cellular function, dependent on a fairly normal environment, they are myogenic in the sense that their existence can hardly be ascribed to specific extrinsic influences; it is apparent, however, that such influences, whether nervous or humoral, can markedly affect the inherent activity.

It now seems clear that myogenic automaticity is most marked in the small resistance vessels, while the influence of nerve fibers predominates in the larger resistance vessels. Moreover, as indicated previously, contractions of the precapillary sphincters and venules may be sufficiently intense to effect closure of their lumens. It seems logical to conclude that this inherent activity of the contractile elements of the smaller muscular vessels can affect the resistance to flow, the number of capillaries perfused, and, to some extent, the blood content of the tissues at any given moment.

Granting that myogenic activity constitutes the basic element in vascular tone, there remains to be considered the balance between this basal, myogenically induced vascular tone and the superimposed extrinsic nervous influence. In general, there is an inverse relationship between the extent of the basal tone in a given vascular bed and the range of the nervous control; the vessels with little inherent activity are dominated by a rich nervous supply, and vice versa. For example, the arteriovenous anastomoses of the skin, which, under the control of the heat-loss center, are involved in the temperature control of the entire organism, have little inherent activity and are richly innervated. On the other hand, the vessels concerned with the nutrition of vital organs, such as the heart or brain, have a relatively meager extrinsic nerve supply. In these vital organs, a predominant system of external controls could not be tolerated, whereas a pronounced basal tone creates a locally controlled "blood flow reserve"; this tone relaxes promptly in response to vasodilator substances produced by the active tissue itself, the limit of the relaxation being maximal dilatation. The tonic regulation of the other vascular regions is found between these extremes.

It should be emphasized that, under normal conditions, blood-borne constrictor agents seem to exert a significant influence only episodically, i.e. during strong reflex activation of the suprarenal medulla; even then, the effect of these vasoconstrictor substances from the adrenal glands is weak compared to the effects of the vasomotor fibers. There is also no convincing evidence that there are any other specific vasoconstrictor substances in the circulating blood which play a physiological role in adjusting vascular tone.

With these aspects in mind, Bayliss's proposition, that vascular distension by the blood pressure may affect vascular smooth muscle tone, can be examined. If his suggestion were substantiated, a mechanical factor should be added to our concept about how vascular tone is built up. In 1934, and in 1939, Fog (*67, 68*) provided strong evidence that the degree of vascular distension did appear to be a factor of importance in determining cerebral vascular tone. More recently, other experimental observations have been added which are difficult to explain in any other terms. For example, in vascular regions of high basal tone, e.g. the vessels of the skeletal muscles, the reactive hyperemia after a partial obstruction of flow proves to be somewhat greater at low levels of transmural pressure than at high levels, i.e. the vessels relax somewhat more when they are less distended. The logical interpretation of such an observation is that the *continuous* distending effect of the blood pressure does noticeably enhance basal vascular tone, at least in some of the consecutive sections of some vascular beds. On *sudden* distension, undulating rhythmic changes in tone can sometimes be seen, suggesting a synchronization of normally unsynchronized myogenic activity. It should be stressed that these responses to continuous or sudden distension are not seen in regions lacking basal tone. All in all, these observations indicate that the reaction to distension caused by blood pressure is intimately connected to the existence of a myogenic activity.

However, as Gaskell and Burton pointed out (*81*), a paradox is involved in the proposition that a continuous stimulus to distension should be able to keep the vascular smooth muscles so contracted that they *remain* shorter than their initial length: in such a sequence the stretch stimulus should eliminate itself. This consideration led Gaskell and Burton to suggest the existence of local-distension reflex arcs as an alternative explanation, even though the histologists were unable to find any nervous structures which might be involved in such local reflexes.

By taking into account the behavior of other types of smooth muscle, the objection of Gaskell and Burton may be easily resolved. For example, continuous distension of intestinal smooth muscle increases the rate of myogenically induced spike potentials and thus also the rate of rhythmic contractions of these cells (*30*). It is highly probable that a continuous vascular distension, effected by a raised transmural pressure, also acts as a facilatory influence on the rate of myogenic activity so that, per unit time, a greater number of muscle contractions is obtained. This phenomenon has actually been observed in the venules of the bat's wing (*197*).

These observations raise the possibility that in regions of high myogenic activity, as in the smallest precapillary vessels, the resistance to blood flow may increase in response to an increase in transmural pressure. Also, as long as any single portion of the vascular bed exhibits significant myogenic activity, its response to distension will not only tend to nullify the effect of an increased transmural pressure on the calculated resistance to flow of the entire vascular bed, but could conceivably increase the over-all calculated resistance. Such a view does not involve any paradox; on the contrary, it is in full harmony with observed characteristics of other types of myogenically active smooth muscles and with direct observations of the behavior of the contractile elements of some small vessels. Therefore, in principle, the suggestion made by Bayliss in 1902 seems to be correct even though his original view has undergone considerable modification.

Our present concept of the manner in which vascular tone is established implies an underlying variable element of myogenic activity, somewhat enhanced by the distension imposed by the blood pressure. This latter factor should not be overemphasized; its influence is probably not marked from the quantitative point of view. Superimposed upon this myogenic activity is an extrinsic nervous influence, roughly reciprocal in extent to the automaticity. Under some circumstances, blood-borne, specific vasoexcitor agents may contribute to vascular tone, although these are apt to become prepotent only during episodes of stress or in pathological states. The blood flow reserve, created by vascular tone, is easily mobilized to the needed extent by locally produced vasodilator agents. These will be considered subsequently.

It is apparent that the vasomotor fibers should not be regarded as the initiators of vascular tone, but instead as one of several tools for adjusting it. Moreover, as mentioned previously, the extrinsic vasomotor control in different tissues and organs is far from uniform. Indeed, the outstanding feature of the nervous control is its role in ensuring prompt, and often regional, regulation of the blood flow. Not only is it superior in this respect to hormonal mechanisms, but also in the intensity of its excitatory influence (33). These characteristics of the sympathetic vascular control are not surprising since major circulatory adjustments, e.g. to sudden changes in body position, would be miserably slow and inadequate if they depended mainly on hormonal factors.

Functional Organization of Vasomotor Fibers

It was long taken for granted that the two main sets of vasomotor fibers were functionally organized in a fashion similar to that which exists for the nervous control of the heart. According to this view the vasomotor center was made up of two tonically active, reciprocal centers, one governing both the vasoconstrictor fibers and the adrenal medulla, the other the different types of vasodilator fibers. Though Bayliss himself was rather cautious in the conclusions which he drew from his experimental evidence, the concept of reciprocal interaction became so firmly established that it proved difficult to convince people that it was all wrong. The situation was one in which the burden of proof fell to the opponents rather than to the supporters of the hypothesis, even though close inspection revealed that the supporters had no convincing experimental evidence to fall back on.

The experimental work of the last two decades has gradually provided a considerably modified concept of the functional organization of the nervous control of the vessels, which may be summarized as follows:

BLOOD VESSELS

Centrally Controlled Vasomotor Fiber Systems

Sympathetic adrenergic vasoconstrictor fibers: These are the only vasomotor fibers that are tonically active; they participate in practically all types of neurogenic cardiovascular adjustments. They form the sole efferent vasomotor pathway for the control of the level of the blood pressure and for the maintenance of the temperature equilibrium, thereby serving as the most important vasomotor link of the organism as a whole. They also constitute the basis for the most common type of neurogenic vasodilatation, i.e. that simply induced by inhibition of their tonic activity.

Sympathetic cholinergic vasodilator fibers: These are distributed to the skeletal muscles and possibly also to the myocardium. They possess no tonic activity, but do engage in a specific somatomotor-visceromotor reaction pattern—probably elicited in emergency situations—whereby the cardiovascular system is rapidly adjusted to increase the blood flow to the muscles.

Adrenal medulla: The hormones from this gland lend support to the nervous pathways mentioned above. Their excitatory effects are, however, far inferior to those of the vasoconstrictor fibers. With regard to inhibitory effects even small concentrations of epinephrine may exert a vasodilator effect in some tissues, especially in skeletal muscles.

Parasympathetic cholinergic vasodilator fibers: These are distributed only to a few hemodynamically insignificant areas, in which they increase the blood flow upon activation of the tissue. In many areas vasodilatation is due to release of a specific vasodilator substance rather than to the activity of these vasodilator fibers.

Peripherally Controlled Vasomotor Fiber Systems

Dorsal root vasodilator fibers: These fibers are present in skin and superficial mucous membranes, where they create a local increase of blood flow in response to harmful stimuli; they possess no efferent function whatever. They are identical with unmyelinated C fibers, are primarily concerned with pain, and are involved in the axon reflex mechanism.

Possible local nerve cell plexuses in the vascular walls: These constitute a hypothetical system for local integration. The reactions ascribed to it may simply represent a spread of excitation and hyperpolarization along purely muscular interconnections.

Thus, the tonic vascular control in circulatory homeostasis is executed only by the constrictor fibers, while the different types of dilator fibers, which do not form a homogeneous group, are reserved for a few, highly specialized purposes.

VASOMOTOR CONTROL

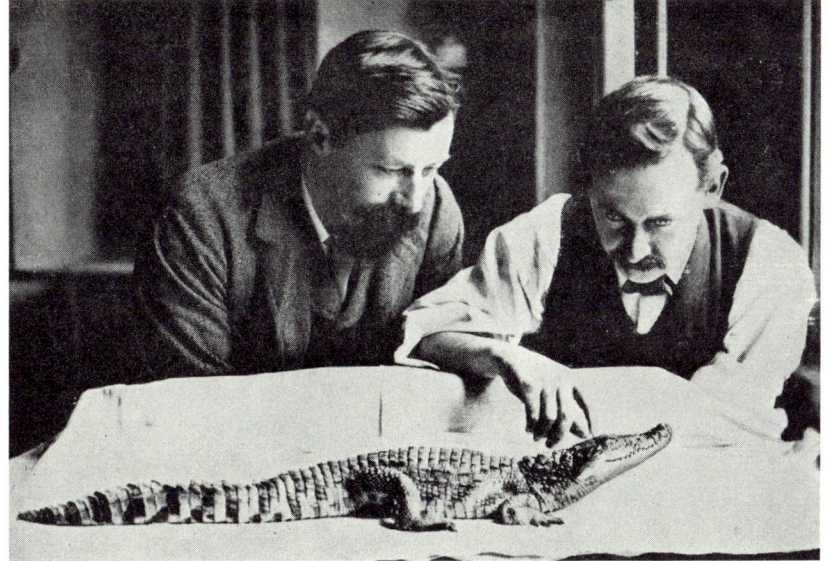

Figure 8. W. H. Gaskell (1847–1914) with his "lab-boy," Thomas Metcalfe, on his left.
In the foreground is one of the crocodiles on which Gaskell worked out the separation of the vagus and sympathetic nerve supplies to the heart.

Autonomic Pathways: Gaskell and Langley

For the first understanding of the organization of the autonomic pathways and their relay stations, physiology is indebted to W. H. Gaskell and J. N. Langley. The two men were closely associated. Both were students of Michael Foster's at Cambridge. Gaskell, who also studied with Carl Ludwig, was the first to treat the innervation of the blood vessels and of the viscera in a systematic and comprehensive manner. He is known for two major discoveries: the myogenic nature of the heart beat and the nature of the sympathetic nervous system. The first discovery upset the prevalent notion that the nerve cell is the sole cause of muscular movement and proved that the muscle cell, per se, is endowed with the property of rhythmic contraction; the second outlined the broad scheme of the autonomic nervous system (*84*).

Langley was Foster's chief disciple at Trinity College and ultimately

[429]

BLOOD VESSELS

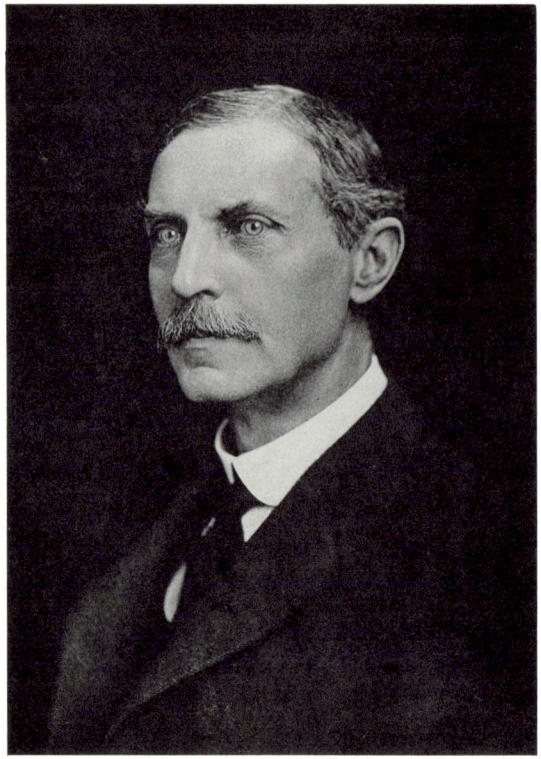

Figure 9. John Newport Langley (1853–1925).

succeeded him both as professor of physiology and as editor of the Journal of Physiology. He investigated the mechanisms of secretion and established the main anatomical and functional organization of the autonomic nervous system. Whereas Gaskell was the great generalizer, Langley was more concerned with the accurate definition of the structure and function of each part. It is interesting that Langley's research may be traced predominantly to two pharmacological agents, pilocarpine and nicotine, which he used to study glandular secretion and autonomic nervous control, respectively (*139*).

After Gaskell, Langley, and their co-workers had outlined the organization of the autonomic system, the anatomical separation of the two systems of vasomotor nerves appeared to be distinct. It was therefore somewhat puzzling to find that some vasoconstrictor reflexes could still be elicited in animals from which the sympathetic chains had been completely removed (*7*). It was, however, subsequently shown that a small fraction of vasoconstrictor fibers pass directly to the vessels via the ventral roots after traversing synapses in "intermediate" ganglia in their neighborhood. Though small, this fraction of "aberrant" vasomotor nerves may not be insignificant: due to sensitization of the effectors which follows partial denervation (*32*), the vascular effects of the few remaining fibers may be considerably potentiated after a conventional sympathectomy, conceivably even to the point of occasionally nullifying the effects of such an operation.

Discharge Rate and Vascular Response: Cannon

Before considering the control of different sections of the vascular bed by the vasomotor fibers, we shall pause to review our present views of the relationship between fiber discharge and vascular response, and of the normal discharge of the vasomotor fibers. It is somewhat surprising to note that almost a century of study of the autonomic nervous system elapsed before investigators tackled these problems, even though one encounters them whenever one deals with nerve fibers and their function. Moreover, decades elapsed before autonomic regulation began to be studied by the quantitative approach which had already contributed so much to the knowledge of the action of somatic nerve fibers.

Among the most important studies of the relationship between the discharge rate of vasomotor fibers and the vascular response were those of Cannon, Rosenblueth, and their collaborators, on the frequency-response characteristics of a number of autonomic neuroeffectors. In general, their results indicated that the curve showing this relationship is a hyperbola, slowly reaching its maximum at around 20 impulses per second (*32*). This curve also applies to the various neuroeffectors of the vascular bed. Almost invariably, the response is near-maximal at a rate of stimulation of approximately ten impulses per second. These findings suggest that the normal rate is rarely more than ten impulses per second; more direct estimations of the sympathetic discharge rates confirm this idea. Indeed, there is now good evidence that normal constrictor "tone" is maintained with a discharge rate of not more than one to two impulses per second and that the impulse flow rarely exceeds the order of ten impulses per second even during severe stress. These values, derived largely

BLOOD VESSELS

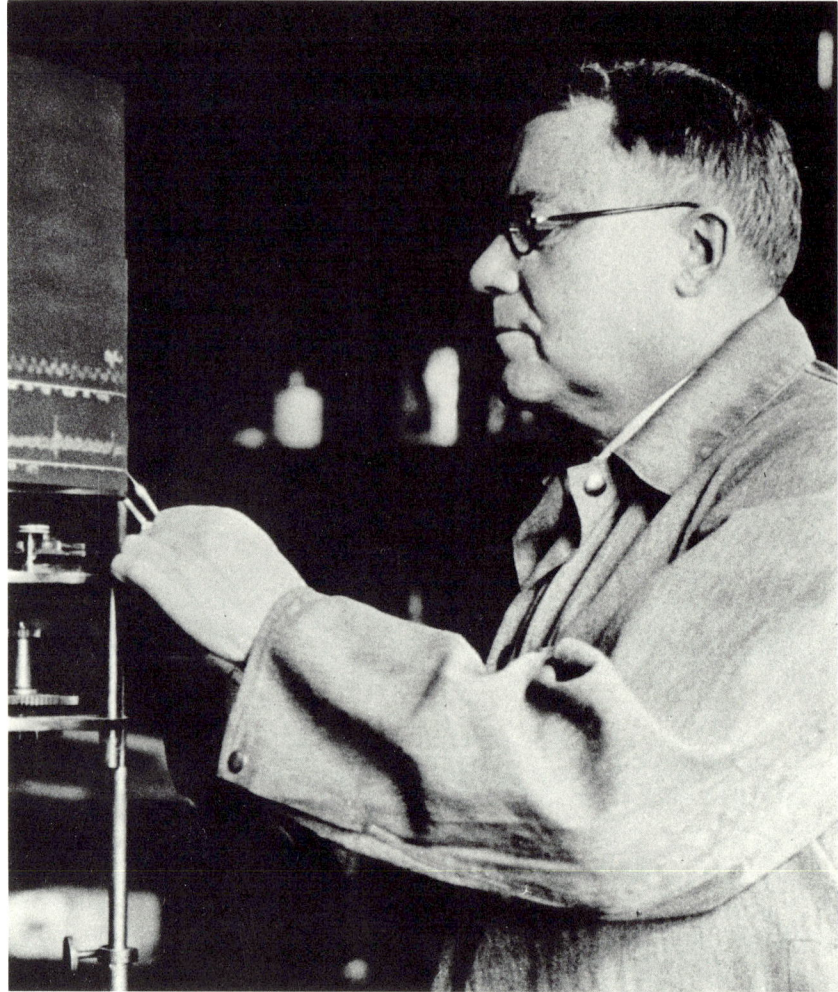

Figure 10. Walter Bradford Cannon (1871–1945).

from the cat and dog, also seem to apply to man (69). At first sight the low discharge rate may seem surprising; but in general it is quite adequate to elicit the full range of responses that can be obtained from the effector cells, and it does correspond well to the neurophysiological and structural characteristics of the autonomic nerve fibers. It is pertinent to note that there is a fairly good one-to-ten relationship between these autonomic neuroeffectors and an average motor unit within the somatic nervous system, with respect to the diameter of the fibers, their maximal discharge capacity, the rates of stimulation needed to evoke maximal contractions, and the physiological range of discharge (69, 70).

Chemical Transmitters of the Nervous Impulse: Elliott, Loewi, Dale

Research on the problem of how the autonomic nerve fibers make contact with, and influence, the effector cells was begun by T. R. Elliott, a student in the Department of Physiology at Cambridge (42, 57). His recognition of the similarity between the actions of epinephrine and of the sympathetic nerves led him to propose that epinephrine, or a related substance, might be released at the sympathetic nerve endings. It took another sixteen years and a series of important contributions, notably by Otto Loewi and Sir Henry Dale, before the existence of a humoral transmission mechanism could be proved.

Otto Loewi, a pupil of Naunyn, Schmiedeberg, Hofmeister, H. H. Meyer, and Starling, was professor of pharmacology at Graz when, in 1921, he experimentally proved the theory of the chemical transmission of the nervous impulse (142). As Loewi recalls in his autobiography:

"The hearts of two frogs were isolated, the first with its nerves, the second without. Both hearts were attached to Straub cannulas filled with a little Ringer solution. The vagus nerve of the first heart was stimulated for a few minutes. Then the Ringer solution that had been in the first heart during the stimulation of the vagus was transferred to the second heart. It slowed and its beats diminished just as if its vagus had been stimulated. Similarly, when the accelerator nerve was stimulated and the Ringer from this period transferred, the second heart speeded up and its beats increased. These results unequivocally proved that the nerves do not influence the heart directly but liberate from their terminals specific chemical substances which, in their turn, cause the well-known modifications of the function of the heart characteristic of the stimulation of its nerves" (143).

Henry Hallett Dale began his research at Cambridge, under Gaskell, Langley, and H. K. Anderson, and studied for a brief period in London in association with Starling and Bayliss. His original research on ergot led him by a serendipitous path to his major contributions in physiology and pharmacology: (1) the elucidation of the role of epine-

BLOOD VESSELS

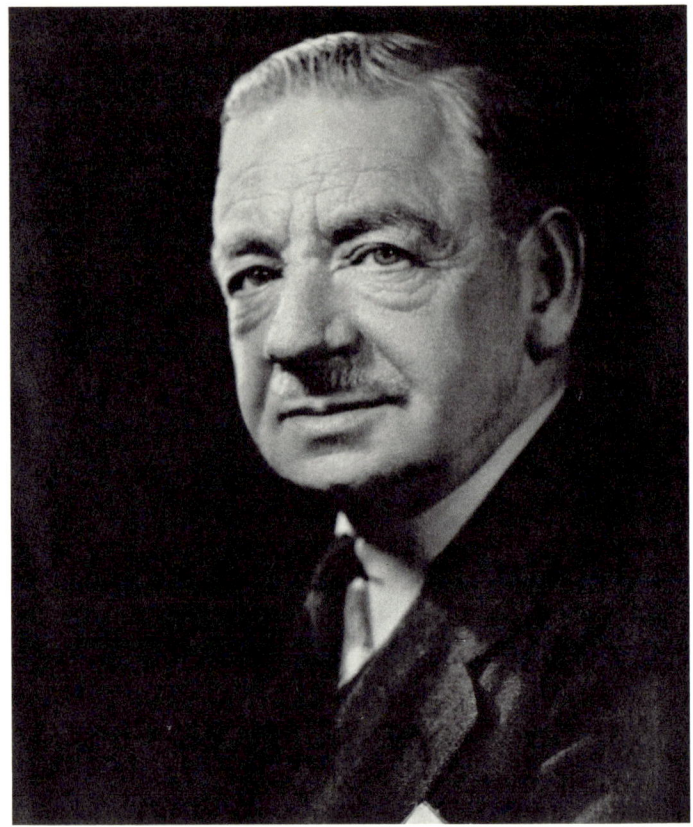

Figure 11. Otto Loewi (1875–1962).

phrine and of acetylcholine in the body economy and the concept of a chemical phase in the transmission of excitation from nerve endings to responsive cells, and (2) the use of histamine to uncover the way in which the organism and its tissues respond to a wide variety of insults to living cells. As Dale recalls:

"*Elliott had there (in the Journal of Physiology, 1905 and 1907) set out arguments in favour of regarding the motor end-plates of striated muscle fibres as homologous with autonomic ganglion cells, not only on morphological grounds, but also on that of a kinship revealed by a common sensitiveness to nicotine and curare. I must have read this discussion, introduced by Elliott towards the end of a very big paper on the innervation of the bladder; but I cannot have had it in conscious memory when I wrote this one on the choline esters, though it may well have been subconsciously effective on my line of thought. Even more curious, however, is the fact that, by this time, both Elliott and I seem to have become shy of any open allusion to the 'chemical transmission' theory, which he had originated ten years earlier. I am sure that both of us had it still in the backs of our minds; and this paper, in fact, added points of real importance for its later detailed development. As I have elsewhere suggested, the stage was now set for it, and only a piece of direct evidence was needed to ring up the curtain; and, after a further gap of years due to the first World War, direct evidence of a very convincing kind was produced, in 1921 and the following years, by another friend of ours, Otto Loewi, in Graz"* (*42*).

The history of this whole series of remarkable discoveries is recounted in detail in Dale's recent volume of selected papers, "Adventures in Physiology" (*42*). Acetylcholine, discovered by Hunt and Taveau in 1906, was studied by Dale in 1914, and its powerful parasympathetic action, as well as its rapid destruction in the body, described. Engelhart in Loewi's laboratory in 1930 found that eserine (physostigmine) blocked the action in the body of cholinesterase. In 1929 Dale and Dudley identified acetylcholine in a mammalian tissue (horse's spleen). From this point, by a succession of brilliant experiments, using particularly the technique of nerve stimulation, with the liberated acetylcholine protected by eserine administration, Dale and his colleagues demonstrated acetylcholine as the effector substance liberated by parasympathetic nerve stimulation. When he gave his Linacre Lecture in 1934, the full picture was essentially established: acetylcholine as the effector substance is liberated at all preganglionic synapses and at postganglionic parasympathetic nerve endings, whereas an "adrenaline-like" substance is liberated on stimulation of postganglionic sympathetic nerves.

A few years before Loewi's work, Cannon had noted the release of an epinephrine-like substance from the liver when its sympathetic nerves were stimulated, but he did not interpret this observation as evidence of the humoral transmission of nerve effects. Cannon and his group, especially Bacq, subsequently developed their concept of sympathin E and sympathin I. They were of the opinion that the sympathetic

BLOOD VESSELS

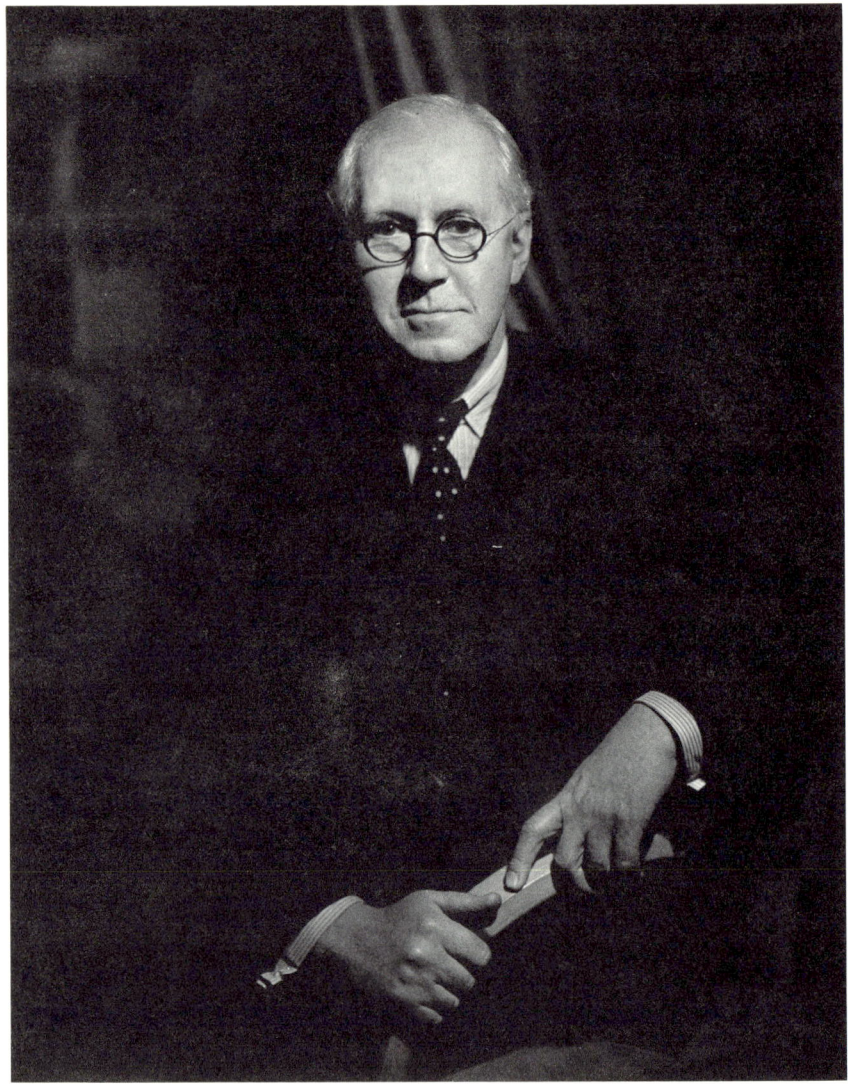

Figure 12. Henry H. Dale (1875-   ).

nerve endings made contact with a few "key cells" among the effectors, from which the adrenergic transmitter substance reached the surrounding effectors by way of diffusion. The transmitter substance was also pictured as diffusing away to the blood stream and thereby potentiating, by a combination of its remote effects on other sympathetically innervated effectors and by the release of hormone from the adrenal medulla, the direct effects of the constrictor fibers. This idea about the elimination of the transmitter substance by diffusion, in marked contrast to the immediate, local destruction of the transmitter of the cholinergic nerves, was consistent with the prevalent notion of the time that sympathetic cardiovascular control was characterized by its diffuse nature rather than by any highly developed specificity. This hypothesis was supported by the histologic evidence of the period (*173*) which indicated that the vasomotor nerve endings made contact with a fairly continuous nervous syncytium around the effector cells, an arrangement also consistent with the idea of a diffuse and undifferentiated type of neuroeffector function. Finally, the ease with which the adrenergic transmitter could be shown to appear in the blood stream during sympathetic stimulation—which never occurs with the cholinergic transmitter during parasympathetic stimulation—seemed to support these ideas.

However, it is now clear that in all of these experiments supraphysiological stimulation rates were used. In fact, an "overflow" of the adrenergic transmitter in amounts of functional significance for the control of the cardiovascular effector cells does not occur if the discharge rate of the fibers is kept within physiological limits, since the local mechanism for elimination, whatever its nature, is then able to cope promptly with the greater fraction of the released transmitter (*33, 25*). Indeed, the present evidence indicates that, with respect to the motor control of autonomic effector cells under truly physiological circumstances, the adrenergic transmitter is almost as effectively destroyed at the site of release as is the acetylcholine released at cholinergic autonomic nerve endings. Furthermore, according to modern histological views, the autonomic neuroeffector junctions appear to be well adapted morphologically for highly differentiated patterns of activity, i.e. despite considerable overlap, they appear to be arranged in the form of distinct "motor units" (*173*). Therefore, modern concepts concerning the morphological and functional characteristics of the sympathetic neuroeffector junctions have much in common with those concerning the somatomotor system. These concepts also agree with the recent evidence for a highly differentiated and swiftly operating control of the vasomotor nerves, a control which is anything but slow and diffuse in its action.

There is now little doubt that norepinephrine is liberated at the vasoconstrictor nerve endings (*117, 113*), while acetylcholine is the transmitter of both the sympathetic and the parasympathetic vasodilator nerve fibers (*59*). It is not yet established which substance is released at the vascular axon ramifications of the afferent dorsal root C fibers.

Vasomotor Innervation of the Resistance Vessels

At the present time, a comparison of the differences in the distribution of vasomotor fibers to the various "parallel circuits" has to be confined largely to their resistance vessels, simply because the control of this vascular segment is the only one we understand clearly. It has been known for many decades that all vascular beds, with the exception of the placental vessels, are provided with vasoconstrictor fibers. However, as previously outlined, these fibers are by no means evenly distributed. This uneven distribution of fibers will cause great differences in the effector responses of the various parallel-coupled circuits, even when the increase in the discharge rate of the vasoconstrictor fibers remains fairly uniform. Also, uneven distribution, together with the possibility of regional variations both in the discharge rate required to elicit certain patterns of activation and in the sensitivity of the effector to the transmitter substance, implies a potential for a wide range of vascular control by the constrictor fibers.

Theoretically, vasodilator fibers would be of little use unless distributed to vascular beds with considerable basal tone. Actually, they are found, almost without exception, in vascular beds which do possess a great deal of basal tone, e.g. the sympathetic vasodilator fibers of skeletal muscle. Stimulation of these dilator fibers has been shown to evoke intense vasodilation with increments in blood flow to near-maximal levels (*69*). Clearly, if such a response were to occur as an isolated phenomenon in the intact organism, it would elicit a profound decrease in blood pressure; instead, the activation of the sympathetic dilator fibers is part of a general reaction pattern in which there is a simultaneous and intense activation of the accelerans fibers and of the constrictor fibers to the other vascular beds. This interplay illustrates the synergistic effects of the sympathetic vasodilator and vasoconstrictor fibers, a picture which contrasts sharply with the earlier notion that reciprocal interaction of vasomotor centers dominates the nervous control of blood vessels (*193, 70*).

Far less is known about the interrelationships that govern the nervous control of the "series-coupled" vascular sections than of the "parallel-coupled" ones. Clearly, the nervous control of the resistance to blood flow is only one of several important aspects, perhaps not even the most important one, for cardiovascular homeostasis. For example, it is apparent that the relation between the influence of the vasomotor fibers on the pre- and post-capillary sections of the resistance vessels is of great importance for the level of capillary blood pressure, raising the prospect of an intimate, though indirect, nervous control of the rate of fluid exchange between blood and interstitial fluid (72). Most investigators agree that the capillary endothelium is neither contractile nor subject to other types of direct control by vasomotor fibers; but this type of control is hardly needed, since both the blood flow through the capillaries and the filtration exchange across their walls can be controlled just as effectively by the effects of the vasomotor fibers on the smooth muscles of the vascular sections that lie immediately proximal and distal to the true capillaries.

The number of capillaries that are perfused at any given moment can also be reduced drastically by the vasoconstrictor fibers if they exert some control over the sphincter sections. This implies that an obstruction to blood flow at the level of the sphincter sections would not only decrease the surface area available for nutritional exchange but also increase the average diffusion distance between cells and capillaries. Indeed, an extensive closure at the sphincter level of a vascular bed could deprive considerable parts of the tissue of the flow of blood through their exchange vessels; and, if the larger resistance vessels were less involved than the sphincters in the vasoconstrictor response, so that the total volume flow of blood to the tissue would not be reduced proportionally, those parts of the tissue in which the capillaries were still open would receive a relative excess of flow. This would give the impression that the blood had passed through "shunts," because the *average* oxygen tension within the tissue would be far less than that of the venous blood which leaves it. This theoretical, though far from unrealistic, example indicates how exceedingly important for the tissues may be the balance of control exerted by the vasomotor fibers on the pre- and post-capillary resistance vessels and on the sphincter sections.

Vasomotor Innervation of the Capacitance Vessels

Up to this point, we have been concerned almost exclusively with the control of the resistance vessels. The control of the capacitance sections is also of the greatest importance. These are vessels in which changes in dimensions, which are too slight to affect the resistance to blood flow significantly, can dramatically affect the filling of the heart. These sections—mainly the veins—constitute, therefore, a mobile blood reserve, the control of which is one of the main determinants of the venous return to the pump, and hence of the cardiac output. For many decades it has been known that the veins are under the influence of constrictor fibers; also that reflex changes in the tone of the resistance and the capacitance sections generally appear to parallel each other. Quite recently methods have been developed which allow the simultaneous and continuous recording of the quantitative interrelationship between the vasomotor fiber control of the pre- and post-capillary sections of the resistance vessels and of the capacitance vessels (153). These have shown that the constrictor fiber control of the capacitance vessels is, in some respects, even more sensitive than that of the resistance vessels. Thus, slight to moderate sympathetic stimulation may elicit more intense contraction of the capacitance vessels than of the resistance vessels; by contrast, sympathetic dilator fibers do not appear to be distributed to the venous side of the circulation.

The predominant constrictor control of the capacitance vessels means that the blood depots are mobilized more readily than the resistance to blood flow is increased; the operation of this arrangement during hemorrhage allows the cardiac output to be sustained at near-normal levels so that the tissue supply of blood is relatively little decreased. If the blood loss is severe, the cardiac output falls and the constrictor fibers increase flow resistance markedly, thereby maintaining the systemic arterial blood pressure. However, because of the uneven distribution of constrictor fibers to the various parallel circuits, the low cardiac output is preferentially distributed so that the blood supply of more important tissues is preserved at the expense of the others.

Once the resistance vessels undergo strong constriction, opportunities are created for the shift of extravascular fluid to the circulatory system: the precapillary sections of the resistance vessels appear to be affected more strongly by the constrictor fibers than are the postcapillary sections, so that increased activity of the constrictor fibers in the face of unchanged arterial and venous pressures results in a lowered mean pressure in the capillaries. As a result of this lowering of the capillary blood pressure, the Starling equilibrium across the capillary walls will be so modified that the tissue fluid will pass into the vascular bed. This "extravascular fluid mobilization," consequent to the nervous control of the resistance vessels, will thus supplement the more promptly evoked "intravascular fluid mobilization," inherent in the reflex contraction of the capacitance vessels.

Some idea has also been gained about what happens to the exchange vessels upon activation of the vasoconstrictor fibers. For example, recent evidence indicates that sympathetic stimulation causes a decrease of the capillary surface area that is perfused (29). Under special circumstances the decrease of capillary surface area can be semiquantitatively deduced from the changes in fluid exchange across the capillary surface (125).

There is little doubt that extended and more detailed studies of the control of the different consecutive sections of the various parallel circuits—concerned with the quantitative aspects of their interrelationships—will form a fascinating field for future research. It is perhaps less likely that these new studies will make fundamental changes in our present concepts of the control of the blood vessels. They promise, instead, to make our concepts broader and more richly faceted.

Central Control of Vasomotor Fibers

In this section, we will deal mainly with the centers that control the sympathetic vasomotor fibers since, for practical purposes, the sympathetic portion of the autonomic nervous system dominates the extrinsic nervous regulation of vascular tone.

The most peripheral link in the chain of sympathetic vasomotor centers consists of the preganglionic neurons in the lateral horns of the spinal medulla; these form the final common path for a variety of converging influences. Although, in general, these neurons serve only as conveyors of impulse patterns from higher levels, the old expression "spinal centers" is justified since there is little doubt that truly spinal vasomotor reflexes occur normally, and that these reflexes are sometimes confined to only a few segments.

BLOOD VESSELS

By far the most important influences on the spinal sympathetic neurons descend from the higher levels of the central nervous system. In particular, the spinal neurons are continually exposed to the effects of the medullary center for the vasoconstrictor fibers, generally called the "vasomotor center." This center is tonically active and is the point of convergence of impulses from the more important cardiovascular proprioceptors. Although it exerts no control over the vasodilator fibers, it is capable of eliciting both vasoconstriction and vasodilatation simply because its tonic activity can be changed in both directions.

Many aspects of the organization of the reflex vasomotor control are uncertain. For example, it is not clear whether the neuron pools of the vasomotor center, which control the individual "parallel circuits" and their various consecutive sections, have different "thresholds" for participation in reflexes initiated by the cardiovascular proprioceptors; for example, it is conceivable that the receptors situated on the venous side of the circulation may influence the discharge of the efferent nervous links to the capacitance vessels more than those to the resistance vessels. Furthermore, there is some evidence to indicate that anatomical peculiarities in the connections of the chemo- and baro-receptors with the neurons of the different "parallel circuits" may serve to influence the constrictor fiber discharge to some of the circuits more than to others; in this way, even slight differences in discharge rate could accomplish marked differences in effector response. Unfortunately, the appropriate techniques for resolving these problems are not yet at hand.

There is no doubt that the vasomotor center is deeply involved in reflex integration. But during recent decades it has been shown that this center also requires an additional fine regulation from higher control stations (123) in order to accomplish the complex cardiovascular adjustments involved in the control of temperature, shifts in emotional balance, or centrally induced patterns of somatomotor activity. Particularly striking has been the change in ideas about the cardiovascular responses to muscular work. Not too long ago, the view prevailed that the cardiovascular adjustments to muscular work began in peripheral cardiovascular proprioceptors as a phenomenon secondary to muscular activity. It is now generally agreed that at the start of activity, the cortical and diencephalic centers initiate the cardiovascular adjustments and that these are part of the general pattern of autonomic activation which accompanies the somatomotor one. This arrangement affords considerable advantage to the organism since the efferent connections between the higher autonomic centers and the lower ones allow adjustment of the circulation to satisfy immediately, or even to anticipate, the changing nutritional demands of the active tissues. By contrast, the peripheral cardiovascular receptors serve primarily as powerful, smoothly operating regulators which adapt the centrally triggered activation patterns to actual peripheral needs and, at the same time, protect the cardiovascular system against undue loads, e.g. inordinate increments in blood pressure. The net result of this organization is a very close coordination of central and reflex influences. This pattern of adjustment is not physiologically unique; it is reminiscent of the interplay of peripheral receptors and central influences in the regulation of respiration during muscular work; a similar parallel can be drawn for the control of the skeletal muscles in

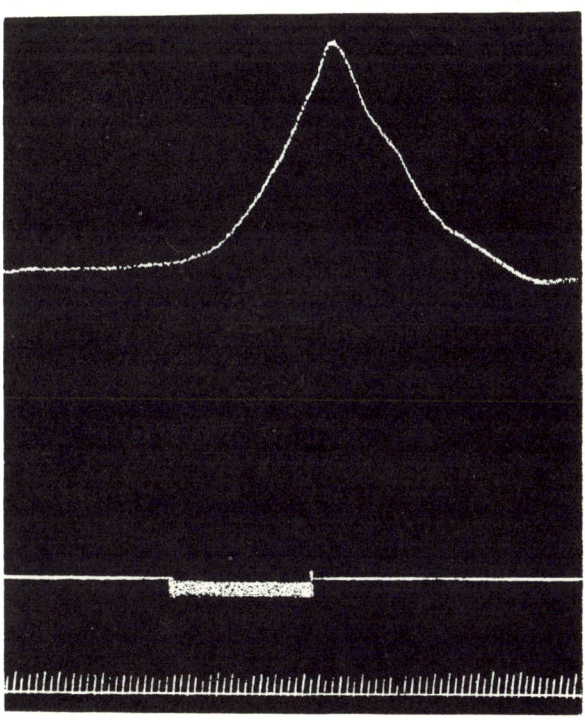

Figure 13. Increase in blood pressure following stimulation of the hypothalamic centers after extirpation of the hypophysis. Upper curve is blood pressure; middle curve shows the stimulation; beneath is the time.

BLOOD VESSELS

general. It should be noted that this view does not detract from the importance of the cardiovascular proprioceptors; it merely changes somewhat the time sequence of their involvement.

The present level of understanding of cortical autonomic control is comparable to what was known about central somatomotor control at the turn of this century. To a great extent, our lack of knowledge is a consequence of the great experimental difficulties that are involved. For example, the techniques of electrophysiology are difficult to apply to this problem because of the extremely thin diameters of the fibers; moreover, clearly distinct fiber tracts can seldom be identified for study. Indeed, even if the electrical activity of the fibers were to be recorded, troublesome questions would remain: to which vascular section do the recorded impulses run; are other vascular regions also affected by these impulses, and if so to what extent; further, will the vessels respond by constricting or by dilating? Action potentials do not settle this last question since they look about the same whether derived from vasodilator or vasoconstrictor fibers! Obviously, the functional analysis of the sympathetic nervous control of vasomotor activity requires elaborate electrophysiological and cardiovascular techniques. Unfortunately, up to the present, most of the studies dealing with the influence of higher centers on nervous cardiovascular control have dealt solely with the analysis of changes in blood pressure and heart rate. These gross circulatory responses can disclose very few details of an integrated cardiovascular response; it is well known that extensive, and highly interesting, reaction patterns can take place behind the curtain of a fairly constant arterial blood pressure.

There is no doubt that the centers at the different levels operate as a complex functional unit. Just because evolution has provided higher control stations does not mean that they are concerned only with the more complex patterns and that the reflex control mechanisms are left entirely to the phylogenetically older centers of the lower parts of the brain stem. For example, recent observations suggest that the *afferent* pathways of a number of important cardiovascular proprioceptors make reflex connections with most of the levels that are involved in vasomotor control, even though the basic reflex arcs relay via the vasomotor center (*155*, *86*). Much less is understood about the arrangement of the *efferent* connections between the highest centers and the "final common path," the preganglionic neurons in the spinal medulla. Nonetheless, it does seem that all cortical efferents need not relay in the hypothalamus: in fact, many fibers appear to bypass not only the diencephalon but possibly the medullary center as well. A priori, it is quite probable that the principles of the arrangement of the efferent autonomic pathways will prove to be very similar to those that are known to apply to the somatomotor system. Even though the vasomotor center, like the somatic "antigravity center," relays a number of highly important reflex patterns, its efferent connections may be only one of several important pathways converging on the "final common path."

VASOMOTOR CONTROL

A few additional points concerning hypothalamic and cortical influences on the circulation may illustrate our current concepts of the nature of this higher control. The hypothalamic neuron pools of the autonomic nervous system do not form histologically distinct centers as do the neurons involved in pituitary control. Functionally, nevertheless, they prove to be highly differentiated. Thus, the hypothalamic center for heat loss selectively controls the cutaneous blood vessels, especially the shunts; the discharge of the constrictor fibers to these vessels is regulated both by the temperature within the hypothalamus and by incoming messages from temperature receptors (97).

Topical stimulation in an adjacent section of the anterior hypothalamus elicits a pattern which seems to be highly suited to adjust cardiovascular function to sudden mobilization of the skeletal muscles, for example, as for defense and flight; this hypothalamic station is, in its turn, controlled by a cortical area adjacent to the motor cortex (56). The pattern, which was mentioned briefly in our discussion of the sympathetic dilator fibers, consists of the effects of exciting these dilator fibers to the muscles, of activating the constrictor fibers to the skin, intestines, and spleen, and of activating the suprarenal medulla; the heart also accelerates promptly as the result of activation of the sympathetic accelerans fibers. It is perhaps worth repeating that this pattern of vascular reactions is so precisely balanced and the change in arterial blood pressure is often so slight that the entire reaction could escape detection if only blood pressures were recorded.

A somewhat opposite pattern of reaction can be produced by stimulating a nearby restricted hypothalamic area; presumably this station is also under cortical influence. Topical stimulation in this area induces a

BLOOD VESSELS

dramatic, over-all inhibition of tonic sympathetic activity, which apparently affects the heart and both the resistance and the capacitance vessels in all vascular circuits; in this case, of course, the fall in systemic blood pressure is profound (71). So far, it is not definitely known whether respiration and the tone of the skeletal muscles are also inhibited by stimulation of this area, but preliminary observations seem to suggest that inhibition does occur. We can still only speculate whether this area forms the pathway which is concerned with the peculiar, possibly protective, pattern of reaction which we call emotional fainting or with the "playing dead" reactions of some animal species. According to studies which are still in progress, the earlier view that the sympathetic vasodilator fibers are engaged in fainting does not appear to be correct; it appears instead that a pure inhibition of vasoconstrictor fibers, together with activation of vagal fibers to the heart, are involved in producing this striking circulatory effect.

For some time the hypothalamus was regarded as the very center of autonomic adjustments to psycho-physiological activities. Now we suspect that it might be more realistically regarded as a highly developed relay station for the cortical autonomic centers. It is true that it is highly differentiated and that certain autonomic reactions can be induced by topical stimulation, but this evidence constitutes no proof that the hypothalamus ordinarily functions as an independent level of the highest order in mediating this type of response. Indeed, the evolution of the cerebral cortex implies, for psycho-physiological as well as for other fields of nervous control, a step toward further centralization; from the cortex the other autonomic stations are exposed to still more complex, and often dominating, influences.

Specific cortical areas are involved in vasomotor regulation: the motor and premotor cortex, the anterior parts of the cingulate gyrus, certain parts of the orbital cortex, the temporal lobes, and some sections of the insula, especially the "limbic" system. Indeed, the mere existence of these different areas suggests that the vasomotor fibers may participate in a number of different cortical activities and different patterns of efferent impulses.

We do not know whether the centrally induced cardiovascular adjustments that occur at the start of muscular work utilize essentially the same, or separate but similar, autonomic pathway systems as those that serve the emergency functions of the sympathetic nervous system. All we do know is that the stimuli seem to emerge from the motor-premotor area, and that there occurs a prompt increase of the cardiac output which is directed mainly to the skeletal muscles at the expense of other areas. There is also no doubt that this efferent pattern is closely correlated with reflex adjustments and with the local release of vasodilator agents from the activated muscle groups; there seems to be little purpose in debating which of these factors is most important.

Another activity of the cortical autonomic centers appears to be a more or less continuous inhibitory action on lower centers, for example, on the hypothalamus. This inhibition is reflected in the general phenomena of sympathetic release which occur after cortical lesions. Also, the cingulate gyrus—considered to be an important center for emotional expression and behavior—is characterized by the marked sympathoinhibitory effects that can often be evoked by topical stimulation of this area. Indeed, recent findings suggest that the sympatho-inhibitory pattern that can be elicited by topical stimulation of the hypothalamic inhibitory region, e.g. the "playing dead" type of reaction, may originate in these cortical autonomic centers.

Finally, both pressor and depressor responses can be elicited from many of these cortical areas. Sometimes these different responses are obtained from the same electrode position simply by changing the rate of stimulation or the depth of anesthesia. The most reasonable explanation of such findings is that there is generally a considerable morphologic overlap with regard to excitatory and inhibitory neuron pools.

The experimental analysis of the vasomotor effects that can be elicited from cortical structures is certainly a promising field for research. Particularly rewarding will be restricted cortical extirpations and topical stimulation in unanesthetized animals, with studies of behavior and expressions, as in Hess's beautiful exploration of the diencephalon (99). Then will we be able to judge under what circumstances the different autonomic cortical areas that influence cardiovascular control are normally involved.

Chemical Vasodilator Factors

When the concept of specific vasodilator fibers was established in the 1850's it was generally assumed that these centrally controlled fibers were responsible solely, or predominantly, for any improvement in the blood supply of a given tissue. We now know, however, that this is not at all the case; first, the vasodilator fibers are distributed only to a few tissues, second, they are activated only as part of specific cardiovascular adjustments, and, third, they are far from ideally suited for the continuous adjustment of the blood flow to the local needs of the tissues.

Several decades after the demonstration of the vasodilator nerves it was realized that a purely locally controlled vasodilatation occurs whenever the nutrient supply of a tissue is disproportionately low for its actual metabolic needs. In principle, such an imbalance can be caused either by some restriction of the blood flow, by an increase in the tissue metabolism, or, alternatively, by such a change in the composition of the blood that its nutritional capacity is impaired.

Cohnheim, in 1872, seems to have been the first to demonstrate that a reactive hyperemia, independent of any central influences, follows the interruption of the blood flow to a tissue (37). He ascribed the reaction to tissue metabolites. A few years later, Gaskell (83) suggested that locally produced acids might be involved, and Severini (181) was able to show that carbon dioxide has a vasodilator action. In 1879, when writing about their experiences with reactive hyperemia, Roy and Brown considered the possibility that similar mechanisms might operate normally during activation of tissues:

"It is not difficult to imagine that an increase in the chemico-vital changes of the tissue elements will have the same influence on the degree of dilatation of the vessels as temporary anemia. In both cases there will be a relative diminution of some of the constituents of the blood and a relative accumulation of the products of tissue change, one or both of which would probably, as in our experiment, stimulate the vessels to dilate" (174).

In 1877, Gaskell observed a huge increase of muscle blood flow during stimulation of the motor nerves, but, at least initially, he believed that the increase in flow was due to the stimulation of vasodilator fibers (82). A little later Chauveau and Kaufmann (35) found that the blood flow through the lip muscles of a horse increased dramatically on activation of the muscles; this study and the earlier one of Gaskell appear to be the first clear demonstrations of work hyperemia.

By the end of the nineteenth century it was realized that the vasodilatation which occurred following arterial obstruction and during work was essentially a local affair, evidently arising from chemical agents produced by the tissue itself, although, of course, extrinsic mechanisms, such as dilator fibers, could occasionally contribute.

The main question was: what is the nature of the vasodilator substance or substances; is it a single, vasodilator agent, common to all tissues, or do many factors contribute, including some which are specific only for certain tissues? Is it a normal intermediate or end-product of metabolism? Investigators realized that the nature of the chemical substances might vary to some extent with the tissues and with the type of imbalance between the nutritional need and the nutritional supply. For example, some tissues might release certain vasodilators only during activity, as their cell membranes were depolarized, in addition to those ordinarily released while the tissue was at rest.

Much of the present understanding of the vasodilator substance or substances began with Thomas Lewis, and his technically simple but brilliantly conceived experiments on man. Although Lewis realized that many factors contribute, he became convinced that one of them played a dominant role. This factor, which he designated the "H substance," was pictured as a single substance which resembled histamine in action but was possibly of a different chemical nature. Its properties included a relative stability and a slow diffusivity. Subsequent experiments (*141*) have substantiated Lewis's picture of a specific vasodilator substance, but they have left unsettled the physiological role played by other factors in producing vasodilatation (*198*).

It is easy to see why this uncertainty about nonspecific dilators should persist. The seat of the difficulty is the natural occurrence of many chemical substances that are capable of producing vasodilatation. It is, however, not enough to show that a given metabolite *can* induce vasodilatation; practically all metabolic substances may dilate blood vessels if present in sufficient concentration. It must therefore also be determined, and this is not a simple undertaking, whether this metabolite also exerts an appreciable dilator effect when applied in the concentrations which actually occur in the perivascular tissue spaces. Despite these reservations, physiological roles have been established for an increase in carbon dioxide tension or a decrease in oxygen tension as vasodilators of the systemic vessels; the coronary and cerebral vessels in particular seem to be very sensitive to shifts in the tensions of these gases (126). On the other hand, the pulmonary vascular bed seems to respond to hypoxia by vasoconstricting (60, 63). The mechanisms by which these respiratory gases exert their vasomotor effects are not entirely clear. For example, it is difficult to distinguish between a direct effect of the gas tension on the vessels and an indirect effect of a vasodilator metabolite which increases in concentration as the oxygen tension decreases.

It has often been suggested that lactic acid may be the main metabolic vasodilator, but actually this view has never been substantiated. A popular argument against this notion is the fact that there is often no correlation between the vasodilator response to muscular work and the lactic acid content of the venous blood. However, this is not a telling argument for two reasons: the diffusion of lactic acid from the cells into the blood stream may be so restricted that its local concentration in the tissues is only poorly reflected in the draining venous blood; or, if it exerts its dilator action mainly by increasing the *local* carbon dioxide tension (146), it may be that the venous blood, with its own buffer capacity, does not reflect the local tension of carbon dioxide in the tissue spaces surrounding the vascular smooth muscles. In general, it seems unlikely that the role of any local vasodilator can be accurately appraised from its concentration in blood draining the tissue, as long as the possibility exists that it may *not* diffuse readily from the cells into the passing blood stream.

When evidence began to accumulate that energy-rich phosphate bonds were responsible for the initial delivery of energy to activated cells, their possible role in producing work hyperemia was considered. Although creatine phosphate appeared to lack vasodilator properties, adenosine triphosphate and several of its derivatives proved to have an intense vasodilator action. It was therefore proposed that the energy-rich phosphate bonds, which apparently initiated metabolic activity within activated cells, might also be involved in the regional vasodilatation which occurs during tissue activation (65). If only about a few millionths of the adenosine content of a muscle, which amounts to some 3 to 4 grams per kilogram, were to diffuse into the extracellular fluid during, say, 10 seconds of activity, it would be enough to explain the observed vasodilatation. Unfortunately, it is exceedingly difficult to estimate such minute amounts of these adenosine compounds reliably.

Another type of mechanism was proposed by Dawes in 1941 (*47*). He suggested that potassium ions, known to dilate blood vessels, might be involved. This hypothesis is attractive because of its fundamental simplicity: the inevitable ionic shifts, occurring whenever cells are activated, would also initiate the needed vascular dilatation. In fact, it may also be the common denominator for the dilatation obtained during ischemia, as tissue anoxia is known to cause leakage of cell potassium out into the extracellular space.

Other, more specific vasodilator agents, like acetylcholine and histamine, have been considered and found wanting. For example it has been suggested that some of the acetylcholine released at the motor end plates might diffuse to reach and affect adjacent vessels. However, in most of the species which have been studied, large doses of atropine, sufficient to block the action of high concentrations of acetylcholine completely, have no effect on either the post-contraction hyperemia or the vasodilatation which occurs after arterial occlusion. Nor, as judged from the lack of effect of huge concentrations of antihistaminic agents, does histamine seem to be of any importance in this connection.

The recent demonstration that a specific vasodilator agent, unrelated per se to the normal metabolites, is released upon activation of tissues like the salivary and the sweat glands (*116*, *74*) is of particular interest. On activation of these gland cells a proteolytic enzyme is liberated into the tissue spaces; there, from a globulin normally present in blood and tissue fluid, it splits off a vasodilator polypeptide, identical with, or similar to, bradykinin. This mechanism, which is activated whenever the glands are stimulated, is thought to be responsible for the vasodilatation which occurs within different parts of the gastrointestinal tract whenever its parasympathetic nerves are stimulated (*78*, *116*). The discovery of this mechanism has, in turn, cast serious doubt on the view that the tissues in which it operates are supplied with parasympathetic vasodilator fibers. It is indeed curious that the original concept of vasodilator fibers was based on studies of a tissue, the salivary gland, which probably contains no vasodilator fibers.

An inevitable question raised by this work is whether all types of tissues split off a specific vasodilator agent from the local depots of normal proteins; if so, this agent might be the very principle involved in the establishment of work hyperemia. So far, however, there is no evidence that this agent is involved in work hyperemia of the muscles (*115*). It may be that this specific vasodilator agent is released only in tissues that not only depend on the blood flow for their nutrition but also use it to elaborate a secretion; in this case, the dilator agent could conceivably help to ensure a sufficient blood flow to meet both needs. However, it seems pertinent to emphasize that even if this specific vasodilator agent were shown to operate in non-glandular tissues, conventional metabolites would still seem to be involved in the vasodilatation which occurs in tissues like the muscles. It is both challenging and depressing to note that even after eighty to ninety years of study, not very much more is known about the nature of the key substances involved in hyperemia than was known by the first investigators of the problem.

Another question, raised during more recent years, is how the substances, whatever they may be, induce the prompt and fairly widespread dilatation within the activated tissue. For instance, some investigators have doubted that the released substances can reach the arterioles, since these are located up-stream from the capillaries. This doubt obviously presupposes that the substances exert their vasodilator action from the blood side of the vascular wall and has led to the suggestion that a local nervous interlink exists in the vascular wall. On theoretical grounds, there is no reason why the released chemical agents should not affect the precapillary resistance vessels from their outsides, which are bathed in tissue fluid into which substances diffuse from the cells. But the notion of a local nervous connection has been reinforced by the observation that the larger arteries, not immediately adjacent to the activated tissue, also show evidence of vasodilatation. This observation indicates clearly that there is a spread of vasodilatation along the vascular walls.

However, the intimate mechanisms involved in this spread remain uncertain. To a limited extent, there is pharmacological evidence in favor of the idea of a nervous connection. Opposing this notion is the lack of histological support for the existence of independent, local nerve plexuses in the vascular walls (*114*). Moreover, there is some experimental basis for the idea that excitation may spread along purely muscular lines. Indeed, it is not entirely impossible that a considerable spread, not only of excitation but also of inhibition, might occur along purely muscular links in the form of a hyperpolarization of the cell membranes.

If so, no local nervous links need be invoked and the vascular smooth muscles per se could form the propagation pathways.

It is obvious that our concepts of the substances mainly responsible for work hyperemia, and of their mechanisms of action, are still vague and uncertain (53). It is clear, however, that these mechanisms do have a great capacity to adapt blood flow closely to tissue needs, operating with special sensitivity in tissues like the brain, in which extrinsic neurogenic influences are not of paramount influence. For example, any change in blood pressure, and consequently in flow, shifts the local chemical environment of the brain so that vascular tone decreases as blood pressure drops, and increases as blood pressure is raised. Simultaneous changes in the mechanical stimulus of the blood pressure, facilitating myogenic automaticity, adds to the effects of the changes in the chemical environment on vascular tone. Variations in blood pressure therefore have surprisingly little effect on the blood supply to the brain, whereas an increase in cerebral metabolism immediately increases it. This interplay comprises a sort of "autoregulation," a phenomenon more or less obvious in most vascular beds endowed with a good basal tone, and in the last analysis, dependent on myogenic automaticity.

VASOMOTOR CONTROL

Baroreceptor Reflexes from the Aortic Arch

The first idea of a reflex regulation of the cardiovascular system exercised via afferent nerve endings situated within the cardiovascular system itself came from the discovery of the depressor nerve by Cyon and Ludwig in 1866 (41). They found that the stimulation of the central end of the nerve which lies adjacent to but separate from vagosympathetic trunks in the neck of the rabbit caused marked bradycardia and systemic hypotension. It was later shown that the reflex hypotension still occurred when reflex bradycardia was abolished by the administration of atropine. Cyon and Ludwig erroneously believed, however, that the depressor (aortic) nerve arose from endings in the heart itself and that these sensory endings were normally responsive to changes in intracardiac pressure: if the heart beat too strongly the reflex bradycardia and systemic hypotension would reduce the work of the heart. We now know that the aortic depressor nerve endings are located in the aortic arch and the roots of the great vessels instead of within the heart. However, the belief of Ludwig and Cyon in intracardiac receptors was to be substantiated in a curious and roundabout manner: within two years of the discovery of the depressor nerve reflexes, von Bezold and Hirt (*20*) described the reflex bradycardia and systemic hypotension caused by the injection of veratrine, and, about ninety years later, Paintal (*167*) showed that veratrine excites cardiac receptors which appear to serve a function such as that suggested by Cyon and Ludwig.

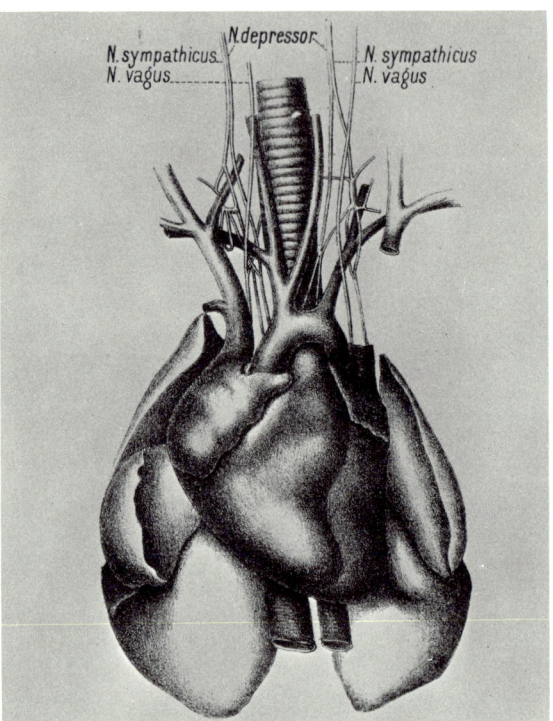

Figure 14. The depressor nerve in the rabbit.

The original observations of Cyon and Ludwig on the depressor nerve were amply confirmed in subsequent years in many different mammalian and nonmammalian species (*187, 18, 75*). It is interesting to note that Cyon and Ludwig did not believe that the aortic depressor nerves were tonically active, since bilateral section of these nerves in their experiments did not alter the level of the systemic blood pressure. In 1885, Sewall and Steiner (*182*) contested this (although very respectfully!). They claimed that the systemic blood pressure did rise by 1 to

3 cm. Hg after cutting both nerves. They also confirmed the earlier observations of others (*40, 147, 157*) that clamping the common carotid arteries caused a rise in the systemic blood pressure. They found that the increase in blood pressure was apt to be much greater if the depressor nerves were cut previously. Sewall and Steiner were puzzled by these results, and, in accord with the opinion of the time, they ascribed the effects of carotid occlusion on the blood pressure to asphyxial stimulation of the vasomotor center. But even though they did not understand the mechanism of the carotid sinus reflex, they fully appreciated the mode of action of the depressor nerves:

". . . *supposing the normal irritant of the depressor nerve to be the mechanical strain of the contracting heart muscle, this irritation would be intensified with every increase of arterial pressure, which itself is under the control of the vasomotor center. One of the principal physiological excitants of the center is a diminution of blood pressure in the brain. When, therefore, the carotids are clamped, the vasomotor center is stimulated, and this of itself would cause general vascular constriction and elevation of blood pressure; but the heart feels this increased resistance to its action in its first beginnings, and by means of afferent impulses proceeding along the depressor nerves the action of the vasomotor center is inhibited.*"

In 1902, Köster and Tschermak (*132*) proved by degeneration experiments that the aortic nerve arose mainly from the aortic arch and the roots of the great vessels, and that its cell bodies were located in the jugular vagal ganglion. They demonstrated that action potentials were aroused in the nerve by distension of the isolated aorta with saline (*133*). A few years later, Einthoven showed that electric activity in the aortic nerve occurred with every heart beat (*55*), and Eyster and Hooker (*61, 62*) elicited bradycardia in animals by distending an isolated innervated segment of the aortic arch. Similar reflex responses were subsequently reported by others (*44, 189*).

In 1924 and 1925, C. Heymans and Ladon (*111, 112*) used a donor dog (A) to perfuse the head of a recipient dog (B) (Fig. 15). The cephalic ends of the common carotid arteries of dog (B) were joined to the cardiac ends of the common carotid arteries of dog (A). The jugular veins of the two dogs were similarly joined. The head of dog (B) was completely separated from its trunk except for the vagi. When a rise of aortic

BLOOD VESSELS

pressure was induced in the trunk of (B) by any suitable means (e.g., by an injection of epinephrine) there ensued a bradycardia. This response,

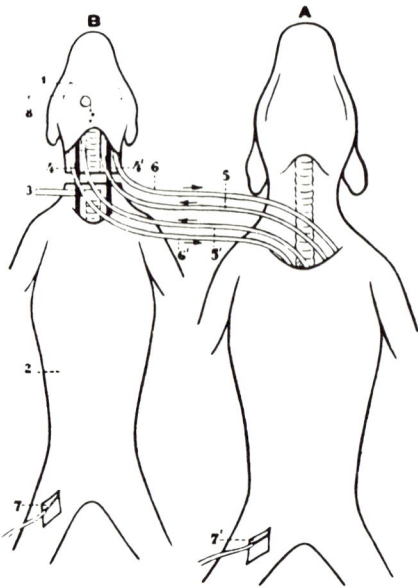

Figure 15. Scheme of the technique of perfusing the isolated head of one dog (B) by another (A). The head is connected to the trunk only by the vagus nerves.

illustrated in Fig. 16, was reflex in origin, for the effect could no longer be obtained after section of the vagi. Conversely, if the vagal nerves were intact, a fall of systemic pressure in dog (B) caused a reflex tachycardia. In 1925, Anrep and Starling (*4*) used the innervated heart-lung preparation, in which the head perfused by the heart-lung was connected to the trunk by the vagal nerves. The heart was thus kept under vagal restraint. In their first experiments they could not find any evidence of reflex changes of heart rate when the aortic pressure was raised; however, Anrep and Segall later succeeded (*3*) in confirming the results of Heymans and Ladon.

In 1926, I. deBurgh Daly and Verney (*44*) showed that an increase in the aortic pressure caused bradycardia; the technique employed did not, however, allow them to state whether the afferent endings responsible for the initiation of the reflex were restricted to the aorta or whether some lay in the heart itself. The next year they were able to show that both the left ventricle and the aortic arch appeared to be the site of afferent endings excited by a rise of pressure; when these endings were suitably stimulated, reflex bradycardia occurred (*45*). Kahn (*122*) used a sound, passed down the brachiocephalic artery, to dilate the origin of the vessel at its junction with the aortic arch. Distension of this part of the brachiocephalic artery caused reflex hypotension.

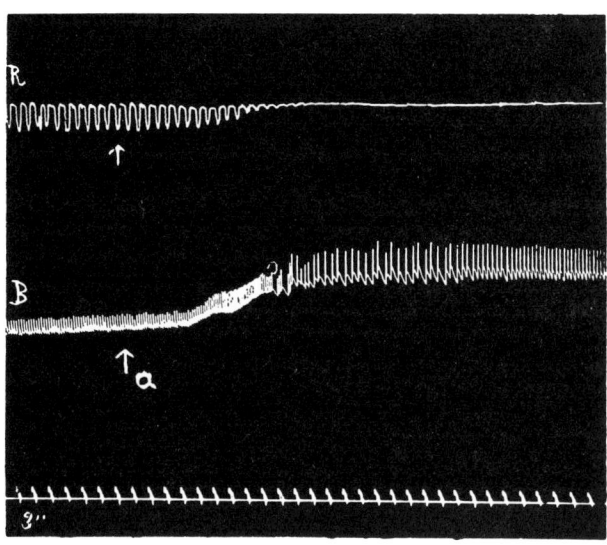

Figure 16. An increase in blood pressure in the trunk of B elicits bradycardia and apnea in A. From above downward, the record shows the respiratory movements of the larynx (R) of the isolated head of B, the systemic pressure of the trunk of B, and the time in 3-second intervals. At the arrow marked a, 0.1 mg. of epinephrine was injected intravenously into the trunk of B.

In their experiments of 1925 (*4*), Anrep and Starling showed that a rise of pressure in the heart and aorta caused a reflex vasodilatation. The head of a dog (B) was separately perfused by a heart-lung preparation made from another dog (A). The trunk of (B) was supplied by its natural circulation. By clamping the lower thoracic aorta the cardio-aortic pressure was artificially raised in the trunk of (B). This induced a reduction of the blood pressure in the perfused head. Both responses were abolished by section of the vagal nerves. These experiments constituted the first indisputable evidence of the vaso-regulatory function of the cardio-aortic nerves. In 1929, Heymans and Bouckaert (*101*) confirmed these results using a slightly different technique; they concluded that the vaso-dilatation occurred in the extracerebral blood vessels rather than in the brain proper. More recently (*113*), similar reflexogenic properties have also been established for the subclavian-carotid segment.

Baroreceptor Reflexes from the Carotid Sinus

The role of the carotid sinus mechanisms was not appreciated until 1923. But, ninety years before, Astley Cooper, the surgeon and pupil of John Hunter (*40*), had noted that occlusion of the common carotid arteries provoked a rise of systemic blood pressure; he ascribed it to the effects of cerebral anemia. This erroneous view that the change in systemic blood pressure acted by way of its direct effect on the medullary centers was subsequently reinforced by the observations and interpretations of a host of eminent investigators (*113*).

In 1866, Tschermak, a student of E. Hering, announced his "Vagus-druckversuch" (*191*). This test consisted of pressing firmly on the skin of the upper part of the neck (as we now know, over the carotid sinus), thus inducing cardiac slowing. Tschermak thought that he was directly stimulating the motor fibers in the vagal trunk (*192*). Concato's statement two years later, that pressure on the carotid bifurcation seemed to be more effective than pressure over the vagal trunk (*39*), seemed to pass unheeded. Even as late as 1925 Anrep and Starling wrote: "A mechanical rise in the blood pressure in the brain inhibits the vasomotor center and stimulates the cardio-inhibitory center."

But in the overwhelming mass of misleading evidence which accumulated between 1836 and 1926 were also the roots of modern concepts. In 1893, Bayliss stated that occlusion of the common carotid arteries did not markedly decrease the medullary blood flow because this was largely provided by the vertebral arteries (*9*). Pagano had noted in 1900 that the carotid bifurcation was particularly sensitive to irritant chemical agents such as silver nitrate, nicotine, and sodium carbonate—all of which caused reflex bradycardia on topical injection (*165*). On the other hand, he seemed to regard some degree of chemosensitivity as a property of all arteries:

"The vascular surface, the excitation of which can produce, indirectly, slowing or arrest of the heart is located between the origin of the primitive common carotid and its bifurcation. I could further say that, according to all evidence, the more sensitive area is that closest to the carotid bifurcation."

Also in 1900, Siciliano showed that changes in heart rate and blood pressure arose reflexly from the common carotid arteries and not directly from changes in blood supply to the brain.

"The normal pressure exerted on the walls of the common carotids is one of the factors contributing to the maintenance of the tonic state of the cardiac inhibitor nerves. I will only say a few words to clarify the protective action of the carotids with respect to the brain; it is evident that the specific sensitivity of these vessels explains better than any other hypothesis the auto-regulation of the cerebral circulation, in the sense that the mechanism on which it is dependent is located at the entrance of the brain, it does not involve the elements of the central nervous system, but it protects them against the dangers of anemia or hyperemia" (183).

Unfortunately, these fundamental statements of Pagano and Siciliano were contradicted in 1912 by Kaufmann (124), who obtained only negative results by distending the common carotid artery; the classic view again prevailed. In 1912, Sollmann and Brown (184, 185) came close to discovering the carotid sinus reflex when they found that tugging the cephalic end of the common artery caused bradycardia, even if the vessel had been previously ligated. But as late as 1923, in the laboratory of H. E. Hering, in which the carotid sinus reflex was to be discovered, Kisch and Sakai opposed the claims of Siciliano and Pagano, stating:

"Our experiments provide several lines of evidence to suggest that the previously described effect of carotid occlusion upon extra-cardiac nerves, is not of reflex origin secondary to reduced pressure in the vessel, but is predominantly due to hypaemia of the brain and more specifically of the brain areas supplied by the carotid arteries" (127, 128).

In 1923, "with one stroke confusion was replaced by order through the simple and convincing classical experiment of H. E. Hering" (129). Hering was the first professor of pathological physiology at Cologne from 1913 to his retirement in 1934. In his youth he was exposed to Knoll and Sherrington, but he was most strongly influenced by his distinguished father, E. Hering. His early interest, while with Knoll at

BLOOD VESSELS

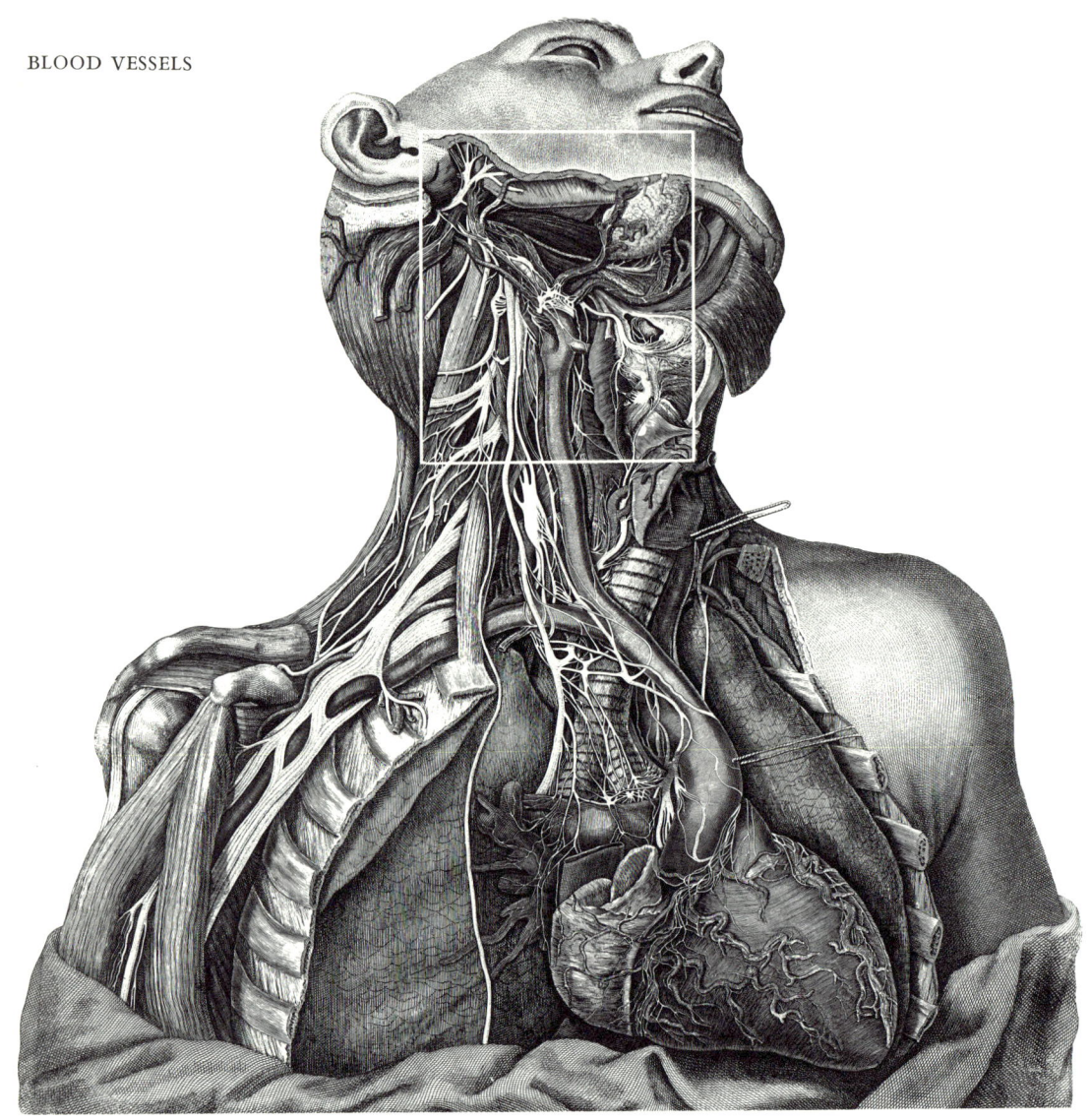

Figure 17a. Carotid artery with carotid sinus according to Scarpa (1794).

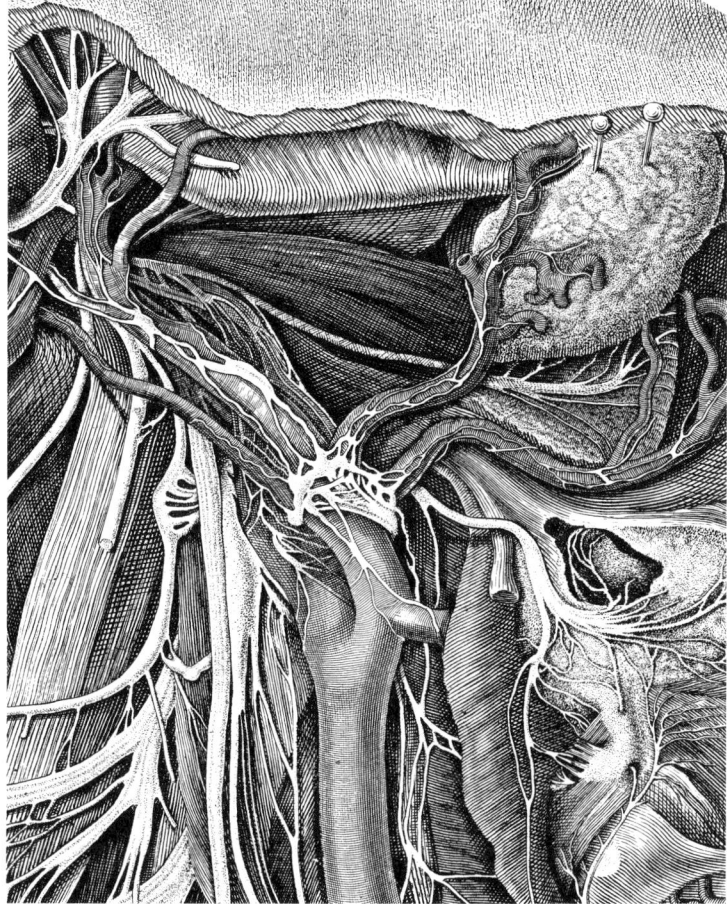

Figure 17b. Detail from area marked on Figure 17a.

VASOMOTOR CONTROL

Prague, centered around the mechanisms of various cardiac arrhythmias; when he moved to Cologne he directed his attention to the baroreceptors. He came to make his discovery because of his long-standing interest in the "Vagusdruckversuch" of Tschermak. In 1905, while performing this test on an old woman, he was struck by the fact that even light pressure with a finger on one of her carotid arteries was sufficient to evoke marked cardiac slowing. It seemed surprising to him that the vagus trunk could possibly be excited by such a delicate stimulus. In 1919, he showed that direct mechanical stimulation of the vagal trunk did not

BLOOD VESSELS

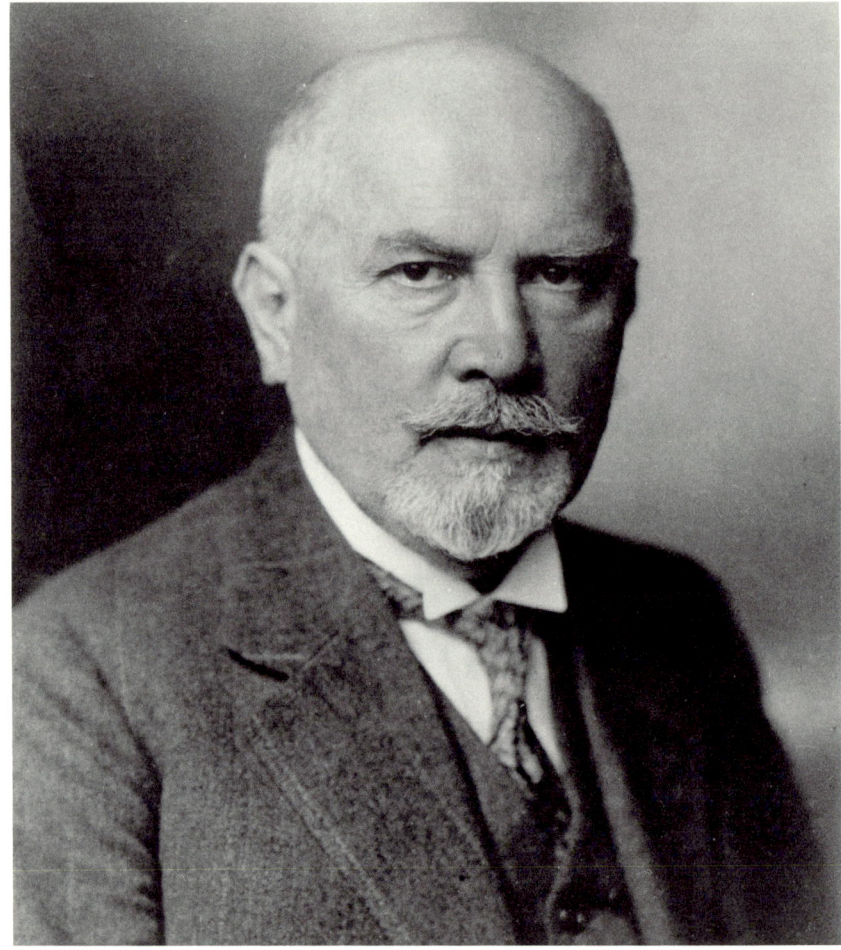

Figure 18. Heinrich Ewald Hering (1866–1936).

provoke bradycardia in the dog or the rabbit; on the contrary, he showed, in 1920, that digital compression of the larynx provoked bradycardia in the rabbit; he concluded that the "Vagusdruckversuch" might be a reflex phenomenon. In 1923, he localized the origin of the reflex to nerve endings in the region of the carotid bifurcation, particularly that of the carotid sinus. In 1924, he proved that the excitation of the carotid sinus wall in the dog caused not only reflex bradycardia but also reflex systemic hypotension. These effects were abolished by cutting the glossopharyngeal branch that Knoll had named "Sinusnerv." Hering performed the following experiments (*98*):

(1) He placed a small clip on the medial margin of the carotid sinus which caused mechanical stimulation but which did not occlude the vessels completely. The heart slowed and the blood pressure fell. After the injection of atropine, the reflex systemic hypotension still occurred.

(2) He stimulated the central end of the sinus nerve and obtained reflex bradycardia and hypotension. The hypotensive response persisted after atropine was injected.

(3) He induced the same reflex responses by tugging on the cephalic end of the common carotid artery.

(4) He introduced a sound into the cephalic end of the common carotid artery and stimulated the intimal wall of the sinus region and elicited the same reflex responses. All these reflex responses were abolished by cutting the sinus nerve.

VASOMOTOR CONTROL

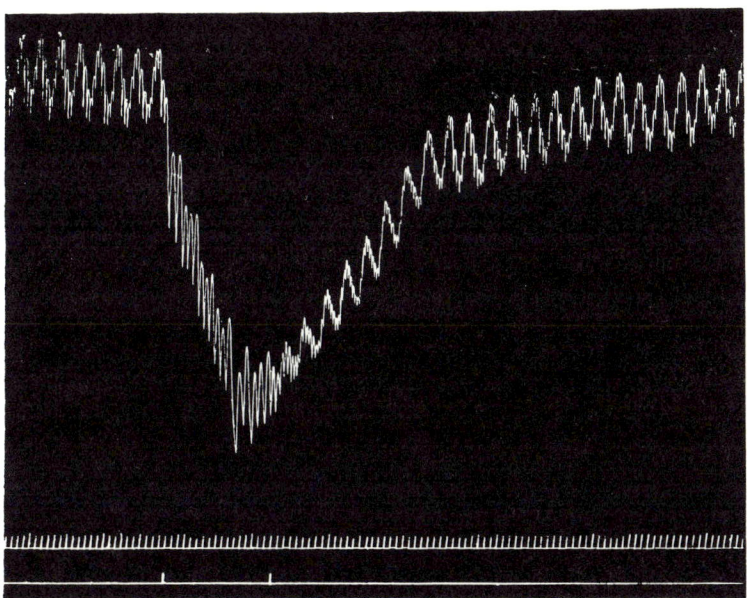

Figure 19. The effect of tugging on the closed common carotid artery by a weight of 64 grams. Upper record: blood pressure; middle record: time in seconds.

(5) He sectioned both sinus nerves and thereby discovered that this procedure caused systemic arterial hypertension. He also found that the nerve endings were tonically active. These fundamental observations have been confirmed and extended by E. Koch (*129*), C. Heymans (*100*), and others (*113*).

A continuous inhibitory influence of the baroreceptor mechanism on the vasomotor center is shown by the marked rise in systemic arterial blood pressure which follows their elimination. How then does the arterial blood pressure act on the baroreceptors? It has long been recognized that the arterial pressure affects the baroreceptors by deforming the arterial walls in which the receptors are located; if the deformation of the baroreceptive arterial walls, caused by a raised arterial pressure, is prevented, the baroreceptors no longer respond to the pressure changes (*91*). This observation raises the prospect that the response of the baroreceptive arterial wall to a given change in pressure may vary and thus

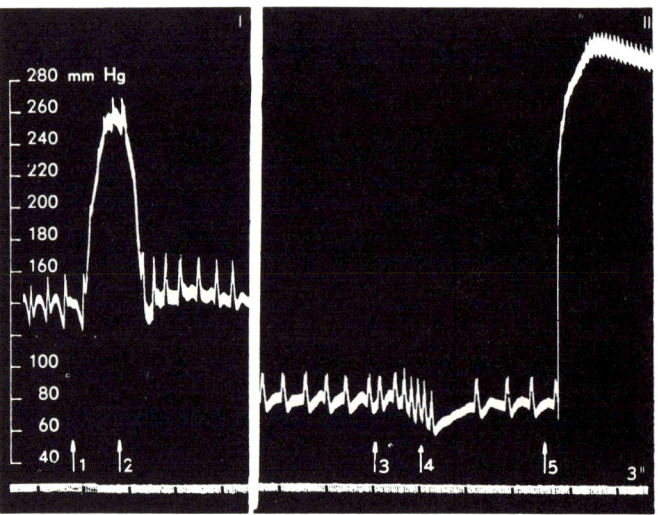

Figure 20. Effect of clamping and releasing common carotid arteries before and after infiltration of both carotid sinus areas with norepinephrine. Both vagi and aortic nerves cut. Blood pressure recorded at femoral artery. At 1, carotid arteries clamped; 2, carotid arteries unclamped. Between 2 and 3, carotid sinus areas infiltrated with 0.25 ml. of l-norepinephrine, 1 per cent. At 3, carotid arteries clamped; 4, carotid arteries unclamped. At 5, carotid sinus nerves sectioned.

play a role in the homeostasis of the blood pressure. More recently, it has been shown by C. Heymans, et al. (*110, 149*) that an increase in tension of the baroreceptive arterial walls, induced by local application of drugs such as epinephrine, norepinephrine, serotonin, or vasopressin, provokes a "resetting" of the baroreceptive mechanisms, thereby adjusting the blood pressure to lower levels. Decrease of intramural tension of the baroreceptive arterial walls, on the other hand, induced by local application of drugs such as papaverine, priscoline, or nitrite, provokes a "resetting" of the baroreceptive regulation mechanisms from normal to higher levels (*107, 109*).

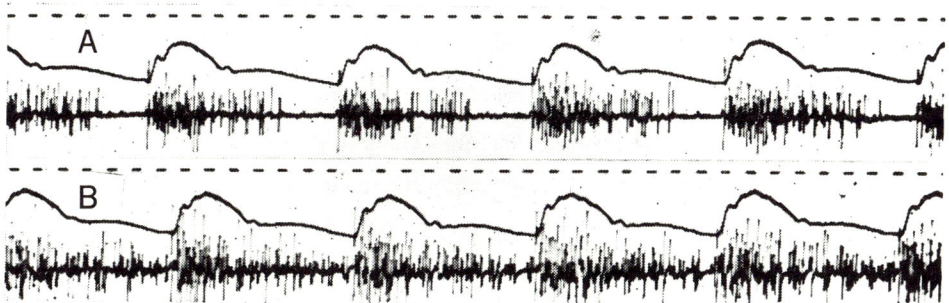

Figure 21. The increase in "impulse traffic" in the baroreceptive fibers following the application of epinephrine to the sinus wall. Blood pressure registered from the lingual artery. (A) Control. Mean blood pressure of 145 mm. Hg. (B) Four minutes after local application of 0.25 ml. of l-epinephrine, 1:1000. Mean blood pressure of 145 mm. Hg.

Action potentials recorded from the carotid sinus nerve have indicated that epinephrine, applied locally to the carotid sinus wall, stimulates stretch receptors "in series" with the contracting smooth muscles of the carotid sinus; stretching the vascular wall appears to stimulate receptors "in parallel" with the smooth muscles. The fibers of the latter receptor type are larger and have higher discharge rates than the "series" receptors. Presumably the interactions of these two types of receptors are of great importance for the "resetting" of the baroreceptor mechanisms.

BLOOD VESSELS

Experiments on the isolated carotid sinus preparation have also disclosed (*106, 107, 109*) that epinephrine and norepinephrine decrease the distensibility of the arterial wall to both steady and pulsatile pressures. Furthermore, an increased intramural tension of the carotid arterial wall, even when induced in the empty but normally innervated carotid sinus, is still able to provoke a stimulation of the baroreceptors and to cause, thereby, a reflex fall in the arterial pressure (*108*).

These experimental observations show that under normal conditions the degree of intramural tension, as well as the stretch or distortion of the baroreceptive arterial walls, depends not only on the level of arterial pressure, but also, and perhaps even more, on the resistance of the baroreceptive arterial walls to deformation by the intravascular pressure. Thus, a decrease in intramural tension could reset the pressure threshold for stimulation of the baroreceptors at higher levels, and a higher arterial pressure would then be necessary to evoke a response on the part of the mechanisms which buffer the arterial pressure.

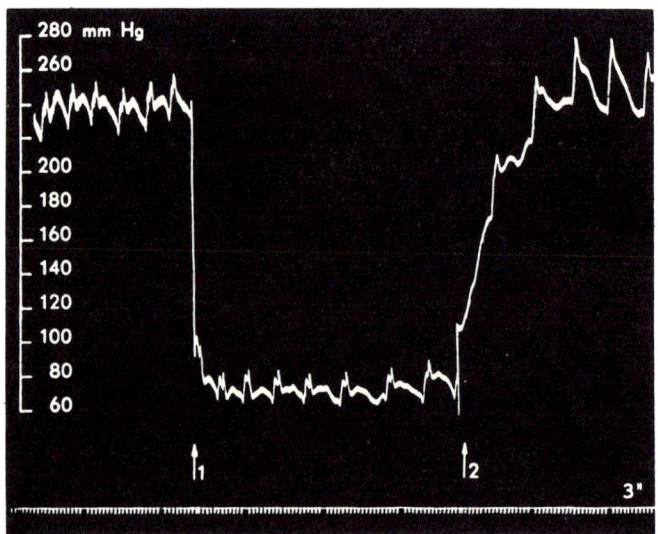

Figure 22. The effect of applying norepinephrine (0.2 mg.) to the walls of both empty carotid sinuses. The baroreceptors retain their innervation; the vagi and aortic nerves have been cut. Upon application of the norepinephrine (1), the systemic blood pressure drops reflexly from 240 to 70 mm. Hg. Section of both carotid sinus nerves (2) elicits an increase in systemic arterial blood pressure from 70 to 260 mm. Hg.

Such a situation may play a role in the genesis of arterial hypertension. Experiments by Matton in 1957 (*148*) support this suggestion. They show that, in chronic renal hypertension in dogs, the arterial pressure is "reset" from high to normal or low levels when the intramural tension and the pressure-response of the baroreceptive arterial walls are increased.

Experimental observations of McCubbin, Green, and Page (*150*) have also indicated that the baroreceptors are "reset" in the course of chronic hypertension. They measured baroreceptor responses by means of electro-neurograms in normotensive and chronically hypertensive dogs. They were able to show that the baroreceptor mechanisms are, indeed, reset to the hypertensive pressure level in chronic renal hypertension and that the buffer baroreceptive reflexes tend to maintain, rather than to prevent, the chronic phase of renal hypertension. Whether this is an example of receptor adaptation or a changed state of the vascular wall is not yet known.

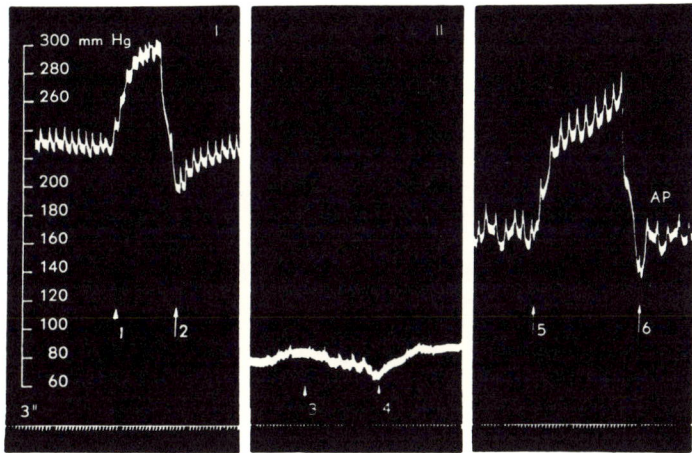

Figure 23. Resetting of the arterial blood pressure in a dog with chronic renal hypertension.

Panel I. Clamping (1) and unclamping (2) of both common carotid arteries. Reflex rise of systemic blood pressure. *Between Panels I and II.* Local application to carotid sinus of 0.1 mg. of norepinephrine. Fall in blood pressure from 240 to 80 mm. Hg. In Panel II, clamping (3) of common carotid arteries elicits no reflex increase in systemic blood pressure. *Between Panels II and III.* The carotid sinus pressure reflexes (5 and 6) have recovered.

BLOOD VESSELS

The general organization of the vasomotor pathways has been summarized in the first portion of this chapter. It is, however, pertinent to outline again the particular efferent channels of this organization which apply to baroreceptor reflex activity. It may also be noted in passing, that even though most analyses of the efferent pathways have been performed in connection with studies of the aortic and carotid baroreceptors, there is little doubt that the same paths are also used by the receptors within the cardio-pulmonary area and by the chemoreceptors.

The efferent pathways of these important reflexes have been studied mainly either by cutting the different vasomotor nerves or by registering their impulse activity. By these means, the important role of the splanchnic nerves in the regulation of the blood pressure was shown in 1864 by Ludwig and Thiry (*145*), in 1866 by Cyon and Ludwig (*41*), and subsequently by many others (*121, 120, 133*). Particularly impressive in this regard are the beautiful studies of Bronk and his co-workers (*23, 24*).

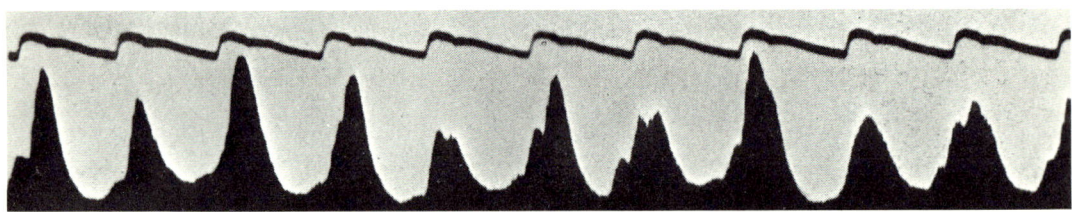

Figure 24. Volleys of cardiac-accelerator impulses synchronous with the pulse. Upper record, systemic arterial blood pressure.

In 1934, Bacq, Brouha, and Heymans (*8*) and Schneider (*179*) showed that baroreceptor vasomotor reflexes were completely abolished in dogs by excision of both paravertebral sympathetic chains. In cats, complete sympathectomy was not always successful in eliminating the baroreceptor vasomotor reflexes, possibly due, at least in part, to the rapid regeneration of the sympathetic pathways in this species (*8*) or to an aberrant outflow of constrictor fibers, as mentioned earlier.

Neither sympathetic nor parasympathetic *vasodilator* fibers participate actively in baroreceptor vasomotor reflexes (*19, 73, 34, 79*). It follows that the sympathetic *vasoconstrictor* nerves form the only efferent pathway to the vessels for the baroreceptor reflex. Since central inhibition of the vasomotor center, induced by the impulses from the baroreceptors, represents the only mechanism for the reflex, vasoconstriction can only occur in these reflexes as a consequence of either withdrawal of, or reduction in, the afferent baroreceptor impulses. This mechanism has been clearly displayed in records of impulse activity registered directly from the sympathetic nerves. In 1945, Gernandt, Liljestrand, and Zotterman (*87*), studying the efferent impulses in the splanchnic nerve, showed that they were greatly increased by a fall of systemic pressure, produced, e.g. by hemorrhage; conversely, they were almost completely abolished by an intravenous injection of a dose of epinephrine, which was sufficient to cause marked systemic hypertension. After section of the sino-aortic nerves the injection of epinephrine no longer abolished impulse activity in the splanchnic nerves, proving that the effect recorded in the intact animal was reflex in origin. Similarly, the splanchnic efferent impulse activity was greatly increased above its resting level upon section of the sino-aortic nerves. Dontas has recently made some similar observations (*52*).

VASOMOTOR CONTROL

The veins are also affected, both from the aortic and carotid baroreceptors and from receptors within the heart and adjacent vessels (*138, 51, 130*). It has been shown repeatedly since 1930 (*103*) that perfused innervated segments of the mesenteric veins constrict when the blood pressure is decreased in the carotid sinus and, conversely, that they dilate when carotid sinus pressure is increased. Alexander (*1*) has also pointed out that an increase in the central venous pressure evokes, per se, a reflex veno-dilatation; the afferent pathways of this reflex are vagal, while the efferent pathways are sympathetic. Finally, Rashkind and his co-workers noted that stimulation of the carotid sinus nerve in dogs caused a reduction in the venous return from the vena cava, a reduction in total peripheral resistance, and pooling of the blood in the periphery (*169*). The pooling was ascribed to increase in capacity of the post-arteriolar vessels, mainly the veins, due to a reflex reduction of venomotor tone. It seems valid to conclude that changes in the capacity of the venous reservoir, produced by shifts in baro- and chemoreceptor activity upon, e.g. bleeding, must be of considerable importance in organisms with depleted circulating blood volume.

BLOOD VESSELS

The baroreceptor vasomotor reflexes act on most organs, such as the kidneys, the spleen, the mesenteric blood vessels, and the limbs (*100, 105*). However, Heymans and Bouckaert (*102*) have shown that the cerebral vessels do not participate actively in the baroreceptor reflexes. Further, it is not known whether the above-mentioned parallel circuits are engaged to the same extent in the reflex.

In contrast to the intracranial vessels, the tone of the extracranial vessels may be modified considerably by changes of sinus pressure (*102, 178*). As early as 1870, Concato (*39*) had noted the reflex vasodilatation of the vessels of the face that occurs during stimulation of the carotid sinus area in man. More recently, Rein (*170*) showed that reflex vasoconstriction of the extracranial vessels, particularly of the external carotid artery and its branches, shifts the blood from the extra- to the intra-cranial vessels. Thus the extracranial vessels are involved in the reflexes that serve to protect the brain against variations in blood pressure, and to ensure a regular and stable cerebral blood flow.

The brain behaves as an organ which is in a state of high metabolic activity. Its blood supply depends essentially upon the mean blood pres-

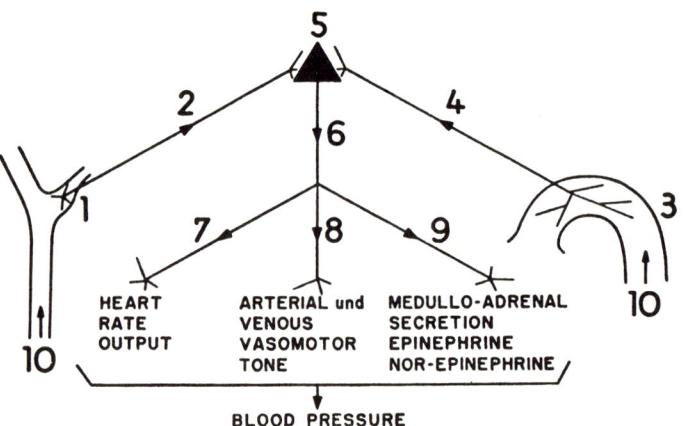

Figure 25. Schema of self-regulation of blood pressure.

1. Carotid sinus baroreceptors, 2. Carotid sinus nerves, 3. Aortic baroreceptors, 4. Aortic depressor nerves, 5. Cardiovascular centers, 6. Efferent pathways, 7. Vagosympathetic nerves to heart, 8. Vasomotor nerves to arteries and veins, 9. Sympathetic nerves to medullo-adrenal glands, 10. Arterial pressure acting on baroreceptive arterial walls.

sure and on local chemical factors (*177, 178*). Although fairly constant arterial blood pressure is of great importance, moderate alterations can be adequately counteracted by locally induced changes of vascular tone. Thus, the sino-aortic receptors are largely responsible for the regulation of blood pressure and cardiac output, but they effect this regulation by mechanisms which operate on the extracranial portions of the vascular system and which have little, if any, direct effect on the cerebral blood vessels themselves. A schematic representation of the self-regulation of the systemic blood pressure is shown in Fig. 25.

Other Baroreceptive Reflexes

Baroreceptor nerve endings have not only been demonstrated in the aortic arch and the carotid sinus area but also within the vessels of other tissues (*140, 50, 165*). Recently such receptors have been demonstrated in the common carotid artery (*89*) and in the thoracic and the mesenteric arteries (*105, 113*). These receptor areas do not seem to be involved, to any appreciable extent, in the homeostasis of the blood pressure, but they may play a role in local reflex adjustments of the blood supply.

More generalized effects on the cardiovascular system appear to be elicited from receptors situated within the heart (especially the atria), the caval veins, and the pulmonary circulation (*6, 151, 152, 166*). Their afferent fibers run in the vagal nerves. These receptors are under intensive study at present, but their precise influence on the circulation is still unclear. At least some of them may be concerned primarily with reflex adjustment of venous return, the cardiac output, and the heart rate (*113*).

Recent work has shown that at least some of the left atrial receptors may form the sensory endings of a reflex that controls blood volume (*85*). Experiments by Henry, et al. (*95*) have shown that negative pressure artificial respiration caused diuresis, presumably as an effect of the congestion of the thoracic vessels which is induced by this type of ventilation. Since this effect could be abolished by vagotomy, they concluded that cardiac or pulmonary vascular receptors of vagal origin, which are responsive to changes in pressure or to changes in distension of the vessels, were affected during the negative pressure ventilation. Further experimental observations substantiated their conclusions: as predicted, distension of a balloon introduced into the left atrium induced diuresis. Other experiments also indicated that the left atrium is the most impor-

BLOOD VESSELS

tant area for this reflex, since balloon distension of the left atrium did, in fact, increase the impulse activity of the atrial receptors (96). Gauer, et al. concluded that these receptors in the left atrium, i.e. in the low pressure part of the cardiovascular system, are largely responsible for the reflex control of diuresis and, thus, of blood volume (85). However, as mentioned earlier, slight reflex adjustments of the relationship between pre- and post-capillary resistance will shift the fluid balance between plasma and the interstitial spaces. It may be that the atrial receptors also affect this mechanism.

Chemoreceptor Reflexes

The carotid and aortic bodies contain epithelioid cells and nerve endings. C. Heymans discovered that these structures are sensitive to the

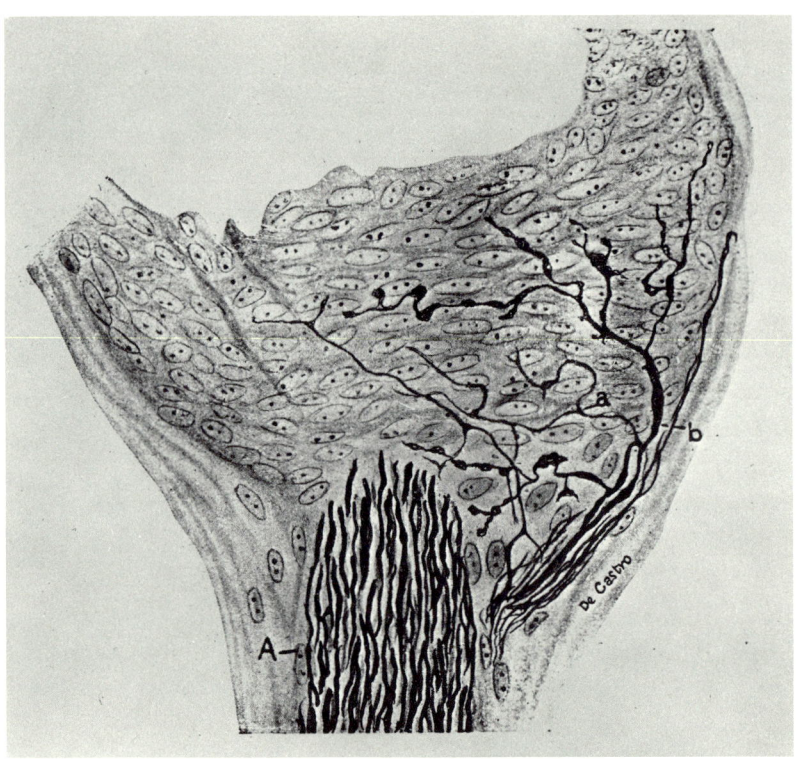

Figure 26. Sensory receptors in the adventitia of the internal carotid artery at the point of its origin in a mouse of two months.

chemical composition of the arterial blood (*105, 113*). Their sensory nerve endings are called chemoreceptors. The fibers of the carotid body are branches of the glossopharyngeal nerves, and those of the aortic body run in the aortic and vagal nerves. These chemoreceptors are sensitive to the Po_2, Pco_2, and pH of the blood, and also to several pharmacological stimulants.

Excitation of the chemoreceptors elicits reflex respiratory and circulatory reactions, such as hyperpnea, vasoconstriction, hypertension, and change in heart rate. The vasoconstriction, which also affects the veins, and the consequent hypertension are caused by the chemoreceptor activation of the sympathetic vasoconstrictor fibers. There is at present no evidence that any of the vasodilator fibers are involved in these reactions. The degree of reflex response to activation of the chemoreceptors is influenced by the type and depth of anesthesia (*105, 158, 159*). The chemoreceptor circulatory reflexes have also been shown to play a major role in the maintenance of arterial blood pressure after severe bleeding (*38, 135*).

Chemoreceptors have also been found in the pulmonary (*43, 48*) and coronary circulations (*196, 166*). Although these receptors are called chemoreceptors because they have been activated almost entirely by drugs, their adequate physiologic stimuli are not known. It may well be that under physiological circumstances these "chemoreceptors" are actually activated by some other mechanism, such as distension. Dawes and Comroe (*48*) identified two main groups of pulmonary chemoreflexes: the pulmonary depressor chemoreflex, which causes lowering of the systemic blood pressure and slowing of the heart, and the pulmonary respiratory chemoreflex, which gives rise to apnea, often followed by acceleration of breathing. The pulmonary chemoreflexes may be elicited by several chemical stimuli, such as ethylacetoacetate, amidines, guanidines, isothioureas, hydroxytryptamine, veratrum alkaloids, ATP, and others. The coronary chemoreflexes may also be stimulated by a variety of drugs and operate to lower the systemic blood pressure, the heart rate, and the respiratory frequency.

Chemoreceptors have also been identified in many other areas, and a role has been suggested for them in the reflex regulation of the blood pressure, heart rate, and respiration (*92, 165, 154*). It should be pointed out, however, that the experimental evidence for the existence of such specific chemoreceptors is not very convincing. Indeed, the reactions seem to arise from nonspecific and abnormal irritations (irritant drugs, noxious stimuli, ischemia, pain). However, it is not impossible that more specific local chemical or other stimuli, such as metabolites or shifts in pH, may induce other local or regional vasomotor reactions by way of centrally controlled vasomotor reflexes, e.g. the "nutritional reflex" of Fleisch and Hess (*64*).

Other Vasomotor Reflexes

It was observed long ago that stimulation of the central end of almost any nerve containing afferent fibers could induce a reflex change in blood pressure, and that increase in pressure was the usual response (*20, 5, 75*). This response also occurs on stimulation of the sensory nerves of the blood vessels (*140, 92, 165*). A reflex fall in blood pressure has been noted on central stimulation of a muscular nerve (*119*), or on afferent stimulation of an intercostal nerve (*22*). Not only are the heart and the resistance vessels involved, but the veins are involved as well (*118, 51*).

Undoubtedly, the sympathetic constrictor fibers constitute the most important, and probably the only, efferent vascular pathway. However, the afferent pathways are not yet established. It is unlikely that any important tissue baro- or chemoreceptors exist other than those described in the previous sections of this chapter. However, it is well known that stimulation of fibers such as those for pain and some other senses can influence the activity of the vasomotor fibers dramatically. It is indeed most probable that the afferent pathways from a number of receptors engaged in somatic sensations, especially the nociceptors, of which the pain fibers constitute the most important group, make reflex connections with vasomotor centers at various levels within the central nervous system (*58*). However, further analyses are needed to elucidate the exact types of somatoreceptors which can evoke vasomotor reflexes, whether some of these have an exclusively excitatory and others an exclusively inhibitory influence on the cardiovascular system, and at what levels within the central nervous system these receptors exert their main effects on the vasomotor fibers.

BIBLIOGRAPHY

1. ALEXANDER, R. S. Reflex alterations in venomotor tone produced by venous congestion. Circulat. Res., 4:49, 1956.
2. ANREP, G. V. A new method of crossed circulation. Proc. roy. Soc. B, 97:444, 1925.
3. ANREP, G. V., and H. N. SEGALL. The central and reflex regulation of the heart rate. J. Physiol. (Lond.), 61:215, 1926.
4. ANREP, G. V., and E. H. STARLING. Central and reflex regulation of the circulation. Proc. roy. Soc. B, 97:463, 1925.
5. AUBERT, H., and G. ROEVER. Ueber die vasomotorischen Wirkungen des Nervus vagus, laryngeus und sympathicus. Pflügers Arch. ges. Physiol., 1:211, 1868.
6. AVIADO, D. M., JR., T. H. LI, W. KALOW, C. F. SCHMIDT, G. L. TURNBULL, G. W. PESKIN, M. E. HESS, and A. J. WEISS. Respiratory and circulatory reflexes from the perfused heart and pulmonary circulation of the dog. Amer. J. Physiol., 165:261, 1951.
7. BACQ, Z. M., F. BREMER, L. BROUHA, and C. HEYMANS. Réflexes vasomoteurs chez le chat sympathectomisé non anesthesié. Arch. int. Pharmacodyn., 62:460, 1939.
8. BACQ, Z. M., L. BROUHA, and C. HEYMANS. Recherches sur la physiologie et la pharmacologie du système nerveux autonome. VIII. Réflexes vasomoteurs d'origine sino-carotidienne et actions pharmacologiques chez le chat et chez le chien sympathectomisés. Arch. int. Pharmacodyn., 48:429, 1934.
9. BAYLISS, W. M. On the physiology of the depressor nerve. J. Physiol. (Lond.), 14:303, 1893.
10. BAYLISS, W. M. On the local reactions of the arterial wall to changes of internal pressure. J. Physiol. (Lond.), 28:220, 1902.
11. BAYLISS, W. M. Further researches on antidromic nerve-impulses. J. Physiol. (Lond.), 28:276, 1902.
12. BAYLISS, W. M. On reciprocal innervation in vaso-motor reflexes and the action of strychnine and of chloroform thereon. Proc. roy. Soc. B, 80:339, 1908.
13. BAYLISS, W. M. The Vaso-motor System. London, Longmans, Green, 1923.
14. BERNARD, C. Influence du grand sympathique sur la sensibilité et sur la calorification. C.R. Soc. Biol. (Paris), 3:163, 1851.
15. BERNARD, C. De l'influence de deux ordres de nerfs qui déterminent les variations de couleur du sang veineux dans les organes glandulaires. C.R. Acad. Sci. (Paris), 47:245, 1858.
16. BERNARD, C. Leçons sur la physiologie et la pathologie du système nerveux. Paris, Baillière, 1858.

BLOOD VESSELS

17. BERNARD, C. An Introduction to the Study of Experimental Medicine. Tr. by G. H. Green. New York, Macmillan, 1927.
18. BERNHARDT, E. Anatomische und physiologische Untersuchungen über den Nervus depressor bei der Katze. Dorpat, Laakmann, 1868.
19. BERNTHAL, T., H. E. MOTLEY, F. J. SCHWIND, and W. F. WEEKS. The efferent pathway of chemoreflex vasomotor reactions arising from the carotid body. Amer. J. Physiol., 143:220, 1945.
20. BEZOLD, A. VON, and L. HIRT. Ueber die physiologischen Wirkungen des essigsauren Veratrin's. Untersuch. Physiol. Lab. Würzburg, 1:75, 1867.
21. BOZLER, E. Conduction, automaticity, and tonus of visceral muscles. Experientia, 4:213, 1948.
22. BRADFORD, J. R. The innervation of the renal blood vessels. J. Physiol. (Lond.), 10:358, 1889.
23. BRONK, D. W. The nervous mechanism of cardiovascular control. Harvey Lect., 29:245, 1933-34.
24. BRONK, D. W., L. K. FERGUSON, R. MARGARIA, and D. Y. SOLANDT. The activity of the cardiac sympathetic centers. Amer. J. Physiol., 117:237, 1936.
25. BROWN, G. L., and J. S. GILLESPIE. The output of sympathetic transmitter from the spleen of the cat. J. Physiol. (Lond.), 138:81, 1957.
26. BROWN-SÉQUARD, C. E. Experimental researches applied to physiology and pathology. Med. Exam. (Philadelphia), N.S. 8:481, 1852.
27. BROWN-SÉQUARD, C. E. Sur les résultats de la section et de la galvanisation du nerf grand sympathique au cou. C.R. Acad. Sci. (Paris), 38:72, 1854.
28. BROWN-SÉQUARD, C. E. Course of lectures on the physiology of the central nervous system. Philadelphia, 1860.
29. BÜCHERL, E., and M. SCHWAB. Der Sauerstoffverbrauch des ruhenden Skeletmuskels bei reflektorisch-nervoser Vasokonstriktion. Pflügers Arch. ges. Physiol., 254:337, 1952.
30. BULBRING, E. Correlation between membrane potential, spike discharge and tension in smooth muscle. J. Physiol. (Lond.), 128:200, 1955.
31. CALDONI, L. M. A., and F. CALDONI. Icones anatomicae quotquat sunt celebriones ex optimus neotericorum operibus summa diligentia depromptae et collectae. Venice, Joseph Picotti, vol. 3, Figure 250, 1801-3.
32. CANNON, W. B., and A. ROSENBLUETH. The Supersensitivity of Denervated Structures, a Law of Denervation. New York, Macmillan, 1949.
33. CELANDER, O. The range of control exercised by the "sympathicoadrenal system." Acta physiol. scand., suppl. 116, 1954.

34. CELANDER, O., and B. FOLKOW. Are parasympathetic vasodilator fibres involved in depressor reflexes elicited from the baroceptor regions? Acta physiol. scand., 23:64, 1951.
35. CHAUVEAU, A., and M. KAUFMANN. Expériences pour la détermination du coefficient de l'activité nutritive et respiratoire des muscles en repos et en travail. C.R. Acad. Sci. (Paris), 104:1126, 1887.
36. CHRISTIAN, P. Die funktionelle Bedeutung der Hirnrinde für die Kreislaufregulation. Arch. Kreisl.-Forsch., 21:174, 1954.
37. COHNHEIM, J. Untersuchungen über die embolischen Processe. Berlin, Hirschwald, 1872.
38. COMROE, J. H., JR. The location and function of the chemoreceptors of the aorta. Amer. J. Physiol., 127:176, 1939.
39. CONCATO, L. Sulla fisiologia e fisiopatologia del cuore. Riv. Clin. Bologna, 9:1, 1870.
40. COOPER, A. Some experiments and observations on tying the carotid and vertebral arteries, and the pneumo-gastric, phrenic, and sympathetic nerves. Guy's Hosp. Rep., 1:457, 1836.
41. CYON, E. DE, and C. LUDWIG. Die Reflexe eines der sensiblen Nerven des Herzens auf die motorischen-nerven der Blutgefässe. Arb. physiol. Anstalt Leipzig, p. 128, 1867.
42. DALE, H. H. Adventures in Physiology. London, Pergamon, 1953.
43. DALY, I. DE B., G. LUDANY, A. TODD, and E. B. VERNEY. Sensory receptors in the pulmonary vascular bed. Quart. J. exp. Physiol., 27:23, 1937.
44. DALY, I. DE B., and E. B. VERNEY. Cardiovascular reflexes. J. Physiol. (Lond.), 61:268, 1926.
45. DALY, I. DE B., and E. B. VERNEY. The localisation of receptors involved in the reflex regulation of the heart rate. J. Physiol. (Lond.), 62:330, 1927.
46. DASTRE, A., and J. P. MORAT. Recherches expérimentales sur le système nerveux vaso-moteur. Paris, Masson, 1884.
47. DAWES, G. S. The vaso-dilator action of potassium. J. Physiol. (Lond.), 99:224, 1941.
48. DAWES, G. S., and J. H. COMROE, JR. Chemoreflexes from the heart and lungs. Physiol. Rev., 34:167, 1954.
49. DE CASTRO, F. Sur la structure et l'innervation du sinus carotidien de l'homme et des mammifères. Nouveaux faits sur l'innervation et la fonction du Glomus caroticum. Trab. Lab. Invest. biol. Univ. Madrid, 25:331, 1928.
50. DELEZENNE, C. Démonstration de l'existence de nerfs vaso-sensibles régulateurs de la pression sanguine. C.R. Acad. Sci. (Paris), 124:700, 1897.
51. DONEGAN, J. F. The physiology of the veins. J. Physiol. (Lond.), 55:226, 1921.

52. DONTAS, A. S. Effects of protoveratrine, serotonin and ATP on afferent and splanchnic nerve activity. Circulat. Res., 3:363, 1955.
53. DORNHORST, A. C., and R. F. WHELAN. The blood flow in muscle following exercise and circulatory arrest: The influence of reduction in effective local blood pressure, of arterial hypoxia and of adrenaline. Clin. Sci., 12:33, 1953.
54. ECKHARD, C. Untersuchungen über die Erection des Penis beim Hunde. Beitr. Anat. Physiol., 3:123, 1863.
55. EINTHOVEN, W., A. FLOHIL, and P. J. T. A. BATTAERD. On vagus currents examined with the string galvanometer. Quart. J. exp. Physiol., 1:243, 1908.
56. ELIASSON, S., B. FOLKOW, P. LINDGREN, and B. UVNÄS. Activation of sympathetic vasodilator nerves to skeletal muscles in cat by hypothalamic stimulation. Acta physiol. scand., 23:333, 1951.
57. ELLIOTT, T. R. On the action of adrenalin. J. Physiol. (Lond.), 31:XX, 1904.
58. EULER, C. VON. Selective responses to thermal stimulation of mammalian nerves. Acta physiol. scand., suppl. 45, 1947.
59. EULER, U. S. VON. Noradrenaline: Chemistry, Physiology, Pharmacology and Clinical Aspects. Springfield, Ill., Thomas, 1956.
60. EULER, U. S. VON, and G. LILJESTRAND. Observations on the pulmonary arterial blood pressure Acta physiol. scand., 12:301, 1946.
61. EYSTER, J. A. E., and D. R. HOOKER. Vagushemmung bei Zunahme des Blutdruckes. Zbl. Physiol., 21:615, 1907.
62. EYSTER, J. A. E., and D. R. HOOKER. Direct and reflex response of the cardio-inhibitory centre to increased blood pressure. Amer. J. Physiol., 21:373, 1908.
63. FISHMAN, A. P. Respiratory gases in the regulation of the pulmonary circulation. Physiol. Rev., 41:214, 1961.
64. FLEISCH, A. Les réflexes nutritifs ascendants producteurs de dilatation artérielle. Arch. int. Physiol., 41:141, 1935.
65. FLEISCH, A., and P. WEGER. Die gefässerweiternde Wirkung der phosphorylierten Stoffwechselprodukte. Pflügers Arch. ges. Physiol., 239:363, 1937.
66. FLETCHER, W. M. John Newport Langley. In Memoriam. J. Physiol. (Lond.), 61:1, 1926.
67. FOG, M. Om Piatarteriernes Vasomotoriske Reaktioner. Kobenhaven, Munksgaard, 1934.
68. FOG, M. Cerebral circulation. I. Reaction of pial arteries to increase in blood pressure. Arch. Neurol. Psychiat., 41:260, 1939.
69. FOLKOW, B. Nervous control of the blood vessels. Physiol. Rev., 35:629, 1955.
70. FOLKOW, B. The nervous control of the blood vessels. In The Con-

trol of the Circulation of the Blood, supplemental volume, R. J. S. McDowall, Ed. London, Dawson, 1956.
71. FOLKOW, B., B. JOHANSSON, and B. ÖBERG. A hypothalamic structure with marked inhibitory effect on tonic sympathetic activity. Acta physiol. scand., 47:262, 1959.
72. FOLKOW, B., and S. MELLANDER. Aspects of the nervous control of the precapillary sphincters with regard to the capillary exchange. Acta physiol. scand., suppl. 175:52, 1960.
73. FOLKOW, B., and B. UVNÄS. The distribution and functional significance of sympathetic vasodilators to the hind limbs of the cat. Acta physiol. scand., 15:389, 1948.
74. FOX, R. H., and S. M. HILTON. Sweat gland activity, bradykinin formation and vasodilatation in human forearm skin. J. Physiol. (Lond.), 137:43P, 1957.
75. FRANÇOIS-FRANCK, C. A. Trajet cervical et cranien des filets sensibles du cordon cervical du sympathique. J. Physiol. Path. gén., 1:753, 1899.
76. FRANKLIN, K. J. A Monograph on Veins. Springfield, Ill., Thomas, 1937.
77. FRANKLIN, K. J. Joseph Barcroft 1872–1947. Oxford, Blackwell, 1953.
78. FREY, E. K., H. KRAUT, and E. WERLE. Kallikrein—Padutin. Stuttgart, Enke, 1950.
79. FRUMIN, M. J., S. H. NGAI, and S. C. WANG. Evaluation of vasodilator mechanisms in the canine hind leg; question of dorsal root participation. Amer. J. Physiol., 173:428, 1953.
80. FULTON, G. P., and B. R. LUTZ. The control of small blood vessels. Amer. J. Physiol., 133:P284, 1941.
81. GASKELL, P., and A. C. BURTON. Local postural vasomotor reflexes arising from the limb veins. Circulat. Res., 1:27, 1953.
82. GASKELL, W. H. On the changes of the blood-stream in muscles through stimulation of their nerves. J. Anat. (Lond.), 11:360, 1877.
83. GASKELL, W. H. Further researches on the vasomotor nerves of ordinary muscles. J. Physiol. (Lond.), 1:262, 1878–79.
84. GASKELL, W. H. The Involuntary Nervous System. London, Longmans, Green, 1920.
85. GAUER, O. H., J. P. HENRY, and H. O. SIEKER. Changes in central venous pressure after moderate hemorrhage and transfusion in man. Circulat. Res., 4:79, 1956.
86. GELLHORN, E. Analysis of autonomic hypothalamic functions in the intact organism. Neurology (Minneap.), 6:335, 1956.
87. GERNANDT, B., G. LILJESTRAND, and Y. ZOTTERMAN. Adrenaline apnoea. Acta physiol. scand., 9:367, 1945.
88. GOLTZ, F. Reflexlähmung des Tonus der Gefässe. Zbl. med. Wiss., 2:625, 1864.

89. Green, J. H. Baroceptor and Chemoceptor Control of the Circulation. Thesis, University of London, 1954.
90. Hallion, L., and C. A. François-Franck. Recherches expérimentales exécutées à l'aide d'un nouvel appareil volumétrique sur l'innervation vaso-motrice de l'intestin. Arch. physiol. norm. path., sér. 5, 8:478, 1896.
91. Hauss, W. H., H. Kreuzinger, and H. Asteroth. Über die Reizung der Pressorezeptoren im Sinus caroticus beim Hund. Z. Kreisl.-Forsch., 38:28, 1949.
92. Heger, P. Einige Versuche über die Empfindlichkeit der Gefässe. In Beiträge zur Physiologie Carl Ludwig ... gewidmet. Leipzig, Vogel, 1887, p. 193.
93. Henderson, Y. Production of shock by loss of carbon dioxide, and relief by partial asphyxiation. Amer. J. Physiol., 19:XIV, 1907.
94. Henle, J. Ueber die Contractilität der Gefässe. Wschr. ges. Heilk., 21:329, 1840.
95. Henry, J. P., O. H. Gauer, and J. L. Reeves. Evidence of the atrial location of receptors influencing urine flow. Circulat. Res., 4:85, 1956.
96. Henry, J. P., and J. W. Pearce. The possible role of cardiac atrial stretch receptors in the induction of changes in urine flow. J. Physiol. (Lond.), 131:572, 1956.
97. Hensel, H. Physiologie der Thermoreception. Ergebn. Physiol., 47:166, 1952.
98. Hering, H. E. Die Karotissinusreflexe auf Herz und Gefässe, vom normalphysiologischen, pathologisch-physiologischen und klinischen Standpunkt. Dresden, Steinkopff, 1927.
99. Hess, W. R. Die funktionelle Organisation des vegetativen Nervensystems. Basel, Schwabe, 1948.
100. Heymans, C. Le sinus carotidien et les autres zones vasosensibles réflexogènes. London, Lewis, 1929.
101. Heymans, C., and J. J. Bouckaert. Le sinus carotidien, zone réflexogène régulatrice du tonus vasculaire. C.R. Soc. Biol. (Paris), 100:202, 1929.
102. Heymans, C., and J. J. Bouckaert. Sinus caroticus and respiratory reflexes. I. Cerebral blood flow and respiration. Adrenaline apnoea. J. Physiol. (Lond.), 69:254, 1930.
103. Heymans, C., J. J. Bouckaert, and L. Dautrebande. Sinus carotidien et réflexes vénomoteurs mésentériques. C.R. Soc. Biol. (Paris), 105:217, 1930.
104. Heymans, C., J. J. Bouckaert, S. Farber, and F. J. Hsu. Influence réflexogène de l'acétylcholine sur les terminaisons nerveuses, chimio-sensitives, du sinus carotidien. Arch. int. Pharmacodyn., 54:129, 1936.

105. HEYMANS, C., J. J. BOUCKAERT, and P. REGNIERS. Le sinus carotidien et la zone homoloque cardioaortique. Paris, Doin, 1933.
106. HEYMANS, C., and A. L. DELAUNOIS. Fundamental role of the tone and resistance to stretch of the carotid sinus arteries in the reflex regulation of blood pressure. Science, 114:546, 1951.
107. HEYMANS, C., and A. L. DELAUNOIS. Action of drugs on pressure-response and distensibility of carotid sinus arterial wall. Arch. int. Pharmacodyn., 96:99, 1953.
108. HEYMANS, C., and A. L. DELAUNOIS. Action of norepinephrine on carotid sinus arterial walls and blood pressure. Proc. Soc. exp. Biol. (N.Y.), 89:597, 1955.
109. HEYMANS, C., A. L. DELAUNOIS, and A. L. ROVATI. Action of drugs on pulsatory expansion of the carotid sinus and carotid artery. Arch. int. Pharmacodyn., 109:245, 1957.
110. HEYMANS, C., and G. VAN DEN HEUVEL-HEYMANS. Action of drugs on arterial wall of carotid sinus and blood pressure. Arch. int. Pharmacodyn., 83:520, 1950.
111. HEYMANS, C., and A. LADON. Sur le mécanisms de la bradycardie hypertensive et adrénalinique. C.R. Soc. Biol. (Paris), 90:966, 1924.
112. HEYMANS, C., and A. LADON. Recherches physiologiques et pharmacologiques sur la tête isolée et le centre vague du chien. 1. Anémie, asphyxie, hypertension, adrénaline, tonus pneumogastrique. Arch. int. Pharmacodyn., 30:415, 1925.
113. HEYMANS, C., and E. NEIL. Reflexogenic Areas of the Cardiovascular System. London, Churchill, 1958.
114. HILLARP, N. A. Structure of the synapse and the peripheral innervation apparatus of the autonomic nervous system. Acta anat., suppl. 4, 1946.
115. HILTON, S. M. Experiments on the post-contraction hyperaemia of skeletal muscle. J. Physiol. (Lond.), 120:230, 1953.
116. HILTON, S. M., and G. P. LEWIS. The mechanism of the functional hyperaemia in the submandibular salivary gland. J. Physiol. (Lond.), 129:253, 1955.
117. HOLTZ, P., P. K. CREDNER, and G. KRONBERG. Über das sympathicomimetische pressorische prinzip des Harns ("Urosympathin"). Arch. exp. Path. Pharm., 204:228, 1947.
118. HOOKER, D. R. The veno-pressor mechanism. Amer. J. Physiol., 46:591, 1918.
119. HUNT, R. The fall of blood-pressure resulting from the stimulation of afferent nerves. J. Physiol. (Lond.), 18:381, 1895.
120. IZQUIERDO, J. J., and E. KOCH. Über den Einfluss der Nervi splanchnici auf den arteriellen Blutdruck des Kaninchens. Z. Kreisl.-Forsch., 22:735, 1930.

BLOOD VESSELS

121. JANSEN, W. H., W. TAMS, and H. ACHELIS. Blutdruckstudien. I. Zur Dynamik des Blutdrucks (nach experimentellen Untersuchungen an Mensch und Tier). Dtsch. Arch. klin. Med., 144:1, 1924.
122. KAHN, R. H. Die Blutdruckregler. Z. ges. exp. Med., 68:201, 1929.
123. KARPLUS, J. P., and A. KREIDL. Gehirn und Sympathicus. I. Mitteilung. Zwischenhirnbasis und Halssympathicus. Pflügers Arch. ges. Physiol., 129:138, 1909.
124. KAUFMANN, P. Zur Lehre von den zentripetalen Nerven der Blutgefässe. II. Mitteilung. Pflügers Arch. ges. Physiol., 147:35, 1912.
125. KELLY, W. D., and M. B. VISSCHER. Effect of sympathetic nerve stimulation on cutaneous small vein and small artery pressures, blood flow and hindpaw volume in the dog. Amer. J. Physiol., 185:453, 1956.
126. KETY, S. S., and C. F. SCHMIDT. The effects of altered arterial tensions of carbon dioxide and oxygen on cerebral blood flow and cerebral oxygen consumption of normal young men. J. clin. Invest., 27:484, 1948.
127. KISCH, B., and S. SAKAI. Die Änderung der Funktion der extrakardialen Herznerven infolge Änderung der Blutzirkulation. I. Mitteilung. Die Verstärkung der Wirkung peripherer Vagusreizung durch Verschluss des Aortenbogens oder der Bauchaorta und ihr Zusammenhang mit der Änderung der Schlagzahl bei Aortenverschluss. Pflügers Arch. ges. Physiol., 198:65, 1923.
128. KISCH, B., and S. SAKAI. Die Änderung der Funktion der extrakardialen Herznerven durch Änderung der Blutzirkulation. II. Der Einfluss des Carotidenverschlusses auf die Herzfrequenz und auf die Wirkung peripherer Vagusreizung. Pflügers Arch. ges. Physiol., 198:86, 1923.
129. KOCH, E. Die reflektorische Selbststeuerung des Kreislaufes. Dresden, Steinkopff, 1931.
130. KOCH, A., and M. NORDMANN. Mikroskopische Kreislaufbeobachtungen im Splanchnikusgebiet des Kaninchens mit gleichzeitiger Blutdruckverzeichnung. Z. Kreisl.-Forsch., 20:343, 1928.
131. KÖSTER, G., and A. TSCHERMAK. Ueber Ursprung und Endigung des N. depressor und N. laryngeus superior beim Kaninchen. Arch. Anat. Physiol. Anat. Abt., suppl., p. 255, 1902.
132. KÖSTER, G., and A. TSCHERMAK. Ueber den N. depressor als Reflexner der Aorta. Pflügers Arch. ges. Physiol., 93:24, 1903.
133. KREMER, M., and S. WRIGHT. The effects on blood-pressure of section of the splanchnic nerves. Quart. J. exp. Physiol., 21:319, 1932.
134. LAFFONT, M. De l'origine des nerfs vaso-dilateurs de la région buccolabiale. C.R. Soc. Biol. (Paris), 32:297, 1880.
135. LANDGREN, S., and E. NEIL. The contribution of carotid chemoceptor

mechanisms to the rise of blood pressure caused by carotid occlusion. Acta physiol. scand., 23:152, 1951.
136. LANDGREN, S., and E. NEIL. Chemoreceptor impulse activity following haemorrhage. Acta physiol. scand., 23:158, 1951.
137. LANDGREN, S., E. NEIL, and Y. ZOTTERMAN. The response of the carotid baroceptors to the local administration of drugs. Acta physiol. scand., 25:24, 1952.
138. LANDIS, E. M., and J. C. HORTENSTINE. Functional significance of venous blood pressure. Physiol. Rev., 30:1, 1950.
139. LANGLEY, J. N. The Autonomic Nervous System. London, Heffer, 1921.
140. LATSCHENBERGER, J., and A. DEAHNA. Beiträge zur Lehre von der reflectorischen Erregung der Gefässmuskeln. Pflügers Arch. ges. Physiol., 12:157, 1876.
141. LEWIS, T. The Blood Vessels of the Human Skin and Their Responses. London, Shaw, 1927.
142. LOEWI, O. Über humorale Übertragbarkeit der Herznervenwirkung. I. Mitteilung. Pflügers Arch. ges. Physiol., 189:239, 1921.
143. LOEWI, O. From the Workshop of Discoveries. Lawrence, Kansas, University of Kansas, 1953.
144. LOWER, R. Tractatus de Corde. Allestry, London, 1669.
145. LUDWIG, C., and L. THIRY. Ueber den Einfluss des Halsmarkes auf den Blutstrom. S. B. Akad. Wiss., Wien, Abt. 2, 49:421, 1864.
146. LUNDHOLM, L. The mechanism of the vasodilator effect of adrenaline. III. Influence of adrenaline, noradrenaline, lactic acid and sodium lactate on the blood pressure and cardiac output in unanesthetized rabbits. Acta physiol. scand., 43:27, 1958.
147. MAGENDIE, F. Leçons sur les phénomènes physiques de la vie. v. 3. Bruxelles, Etab. encycl., 1838.
148. MATTON, G. Pharmacological actions on the carotid sinus baroreceptors in arterial hypertension. Arch. int. Pharmacodyn., 110:474, 1957.
149. MAZZELLA, H., S. C. WANG, C. HEYMANS, and G. R. DE VLEESCHHOUWER. Mécanisme de l'action de la noradrénaline sur le sinus carotidien. Arch. int. Pharmacodyn., 89:122, 1952.
150. MCCUBBIN, J. W., J. H. GREEN, and I. H. PAGE. Baroceptor function in chronic renal hypertension. Circulat. Res., 4:205, 1956.
151. MCDOWALL, R. J. S. The Control of the Circulation of the Blood. London, Longmans, Green, 1938.
152. MCDOWALL, R. J. S., Ed. The Control of the Circulation of the Blood, supplemental volume. London, Dawson, 1956.
153. MELLANDER, S. Comparative studies on the adrenergic neurohormonal control of resistance and capacitance blood vessels in the cat. Acta physiol. scand., suppl. 176, 1960.

154. MIETKIEWSKI, E. W sprawie odruchowego dzialania chemiczenych czynikow ws wstrzasowych. Acta physiol. pol., 6:313, 1955.
155. MORUZZI, G. Problems in Cerebellar Physiology. Springfield, Ill., Thomas, 1950.
156. NASSE, C. F. Ueber das Verhältniss der Thätigkeit des Herzens zum Einfluss des Rückenmarks. Arch. med. Erfahr., 1:189, 1817.
157. NAWALICHIN, J. Ueber die Wirkung des verminderten Blutzuflusses zum Gehirn auf den Blutstrom im Aortensystem. Zbl. med. Wiss., 8:483, 1870.
158. NEIL, E. Chemoreceptor areas and chemoreceptor circulatory reflexes. Acta physiol. scand., 22:54, 1951.
159. NEIL, E. The carotid and aortic vasosensory areas. Their contribution to circulatory and respiratory adjustments occurring after haemorrhage. Arch. Middx. Hosp., 4:16, 1954.
160. OLIVER, G., and E. A. SCHÄFER. On the physiological action of extract of the suprarenal capsules. J. Physiol. (Lond.), 16:1, 1894.
161. OLMSTED, J. M. D. Charles-Édouard Brown-Séquard, a Nineteenth Century Neurologist and Endocrinologist. Baltimore, Johns Hopkins, 1946.
162. OLMSTED, J. M. D. Claude Bernard, Physiologist. New York, Harper, 1938.
163. OLMSTED, J. M. D. François Magendie. Pioneer in Experimental Physiology and Scientific Medicine in XIX Century France. New York, Schuman, 1944.
164. OWSJANNIKOW, PH. Die tonischen und reflectorischen Centren der Gefässnerven. Ber. sächs. Ges. (Akad.) Wiss., 23:135, 1871.
165. PAGANO, G. Sur la sensibilité du coeur et des vaisseaux sanguins. Arch. ital. Biol., 33:1, 1900.
166. PAINTAL, A. S. The conduction velocities of respiratory and cardiovascular afferent fibres in the vagus nerve. J. Physiol. (Lond.), 122:181, 1953.
167. PAINTAL, A. S. A study of ventricular pressure receptors and their role in the Bezold reflex. Quart. J. exp. Physiol., 40:348, 1955.
168. POURFOIS DU PETIT, F. Mémoire dans lequel il est demonstré que les nerfs intercostaux fournissent des rameaux qui portent des esprits dans les nerfs. Hist. Acad. roy. Sc. Paris, 1, 1727.
169. RASHKIND, W. J., D. H. LEWIS, J. B. HENDERSON, D. F. HEIMAN, and R. B. DIETRICK. Venous return as affected by cardiac output and total peripheral resistance. Amer. J. Physiol., 175:415, 1953.
170. REIN, H. Vasomotrische Regulationen. Ergebn. Physiol., 32:28, 1931.
171. RIGLER, R. Über die Ursache der vermehrten Durchblutung des Muskels während der Arbeit. Arch. exp. Path. Pharmak., 167:54, 1932.

172. ROBINSON, V. The Life of Jacob Henle. New York, Med. Life, 1921.
173. ROSENBLUETH, A. The Transmission of Nerve Impulses at Neuro-effector Junctions and peripheral Synapses. New York, Technology Press of M.I.T. and Wiley, 1950.
174. ROY, C. S., and J. G. BROWN. The blood-pressure and its variations in the arterioles, capillaries and smaller veins. J. Physiol., 2:323, 1879–80.
175. RUSHMER, R. F., and O. A. SMITH, JR. Cardiac control. Physiol. Rev., 39:41, 1959.
176. SCHIFF, M. Ueber den Einfluss der Nerven auf die Gefässe der Zunge. Arch. physiol. Heilk., 12:377, 1853.
177. SCHMIDT, C. F. The Cerebral Circulation in Health and Disease. Springfield, Ill., Thomas, 1950.
178. SCHMIDT, C. F., and J. P. HENDRIX. The action of chemical substances on cerebral blood-vessels. Proc. Ass. Res. nerv. ment. Dis., 18:229, 1938.
179. SCHNEIDER, D. Über die vasomotorische Benervung der Extremitäten. Arch. exp. Path. Pharmakol., 176:110, 1934.
180. SÉNAC, J. Traité de la structure du coeur. 2. éd. Paris, Méquignon l'aîné, 1783.
181. SEVERINI, L. La contrattilità dei vasa capillari in relazione ai due gas della scambio materiale. Perugia, 1881.
182. SEWALL, H., and D. W. STEINER. A study of the action of the depressor nerve, and a consideration of the effect of blood-pressure upon the heart regarded as a sensory organ. J. Physiol. (Lond.), 6:162, 1885.
183. SICILIANO, L. Les effets de la compression des carotides sur la pression, sur le coeur et sur la respiration. Arch. ital. Biol., 33:338, 1900.
184. SOLLMANN, T., and E. D. BROWN. The blood pressure fall produced by traction on the carotid artery. Amer. J. Physiol., 30:88, 1912.
185. SOLLMANN, T., and E. D. BROWN. The blood pressure fall produced by traction of the carotid artery. Amer. J. Physiol., 30:102, 1912.
186. SPALLANZANI, L. De fenomeni della circolazione osservata nel giro universale, de vai... Modena, 1773.
187. STELLING, C. Experimentelle Untersuchungen über den Einfluss des Nervus depressor auf die Herzthätigkeit und den Blutdruck. Dorpat, Laakmann, 1867.
188. STRICKER, S. Untersuchungen über die Gefässnerven-Wurzeln des Ischiadicus. S. B. Akad. Wiss., Wien, Abt. 3, 74:173, 1876.
189. SUTTON, D. C., and H. C. LUETH. Pain. Arch. intern. Med., 45:827, 1930.
190. THIRY, L. Ueber das Verhalten der Gefässnerven bei Störungen der Respiration. Z. med. Wiss., 722, 1864.

BLOOD VESSELS

191. TSCHERMAK, J. N. Zwei Beobachtungen uber die sogenannten Manege-Bewegungen in Folge von einseitiger Verletzung gewisser Hirntheile. (Jenaische Z., 1866). In his Gesammelte Schriften, v. 1, p. 769. Leipzig, Engelmann, 1879.
192. TSCHERMAK, J. N. Ueber mechanische Reizung des Nervus vagus beim Menschen. (Prager. Vierteljschr. 1868). In his Gesammelte Schriften, v. 1, p. 779.
193. UVNÄS, B. Sympathetic vasodilator outflow. Physiol. Rev., 34:608, 1954.
194. WALLER, A. V. Neuvième mémoire sur le système nerveux. C.R. Acad. Sci. (Paris), 36:378, 1853.
195. WEBER, E. H. Nutzen der Elasticität der Arterien. In Hildebrandt, Handbuch der Anatomie, 4th ed. Part III, 1831.
196. WHITTERIDGE, D. Afferent nerve fibres from the heart and lungs in the cervical vagus. J. Physiol. (Lond.), 107:496, 1948.
197. WIEDEMAN, M. P. Effect of venous flow on frequence of venous vasomotion in the bat wing. Circulat. Res., 5:641, 1957.
198. WOOD, J. E., J. LITTER, and W. W. WILKINS. The mechanism of limb segment reactive hyperemia in man. Circulat. Res., 3:581, 1955.
199. WRISBERG, H. E. De nervis arterias venasque comitentibus. Commentationes Soc. scient, Göttingen, 7:95, 1786.

VIII

Systemic Arterial Hypertension

IT is customary to divide the subject matter of science into what is basic or fundamental and what is applied, and the study of high blood pressure would commonly be relegated to applied science. But nature knows no such differences. The phenomena which have attracted men's attention belong equally to these two fields, and the method of science may be as well illustrated by the subject of high blood pressure as by any other, with two reservations. Because what we call disease is something that maims and kills, physicians must allay the fears of the sick, and thus from time to time pretend to them an understanding which they do not in fact possess. This topic, then, is characterized by prematurity of conclusion and fixity of ideas. Moreover, the growth of this subject is recent, and this account must to some extent suffer the lack of perspective common to all contemporary critiques.

The method of science is in essence the same whatever the range of phenomena it investigates. The first step is the recording of facts, the second their arrangement, the third their interpretation, and the fourth the testing of this interpretation, either by prediction or by experiment. It would be a mistake to think that progress is anything like orderly. Each individual's work and each phase of each individual's work may represent the whole of these processes. Nevertheless, the contributions of some to a particular facet of the whole represent their most important work. Another characteristic of science is that progress is marked by increasing precision. The observations that first excite wonder are usually made with the eye, either unaided or with its range enlarged by optical instruments. Later comes measurement; with measurement accuracy and the establishment of quantitative relationships. Moreover, science tends to advance as a whole, and understanding in one field promotes or stimulates understanding in another.

These processes occur in sequences, each contributor building on the foundations of his predecessor, so far as these foundations are solid, or rejecting them if they fail to stand the test. Each advance in knowledge represents to some extent a simplification. Nevertheless most advances are an oversimplification, and new data require modification, if not total repeal, of ideas that seemed an advance before.

Early Observations and Measurements of Arterial Pressure

That blood issued with unequal force from divided vessels must have been a common observation in the violent life of medieval and earlier times and seems to have been known to the more observant of artists. Thus, in the beheading of St. John the Baptist by Giovanni di Paolo (1403–83), there are three streams of blood, although similar in color, one dripping and the other two spurting in a smaller, peripheral and a larger, central jet from the severed neck. William Harvey's observations on the force with which blood emerged from a severed artery were among those that forced him to the revolutionary view that the blood moved in a circle.

"Lastly, as in the cutting of any arterie, the blood leaps out sometimes farther, sometimes nearer, you shall find the out-leaping to be just with the Arterial Diastole, at which time the heart strikes the breast, and at that time then when it appears that the heart is in its tention and contraction, it is in its Systole, and that the blood is thrust out with the same motion.

"From hence, this against the Common rule appears to be clear, that the Arterial Diastole is at the same time with the Systole of the heart, and that the arteries are fill'd and distended by reason of the immission and intrusion of blood made by the constriction of the ventricles of the heart; as likewise that the arteries are stretched, because they are fill'd like Baggs or Satchels, and are not fill'd because they are blown up like Bellows: and for the same cause do all the arteries of the body beat, by reason of the tention of the left ventricle of the heart, as the arterial vein from the tention of the right."

In Italy the new physics and mathematics were growing up under Galileo's leadership. Giovanni Borelli, though primarily a mathematician and physicist, interested himself in biology, and particularly in medicine. He emphasized the hydraulic properties of the circulation and believed that the heart acted like a piston. He calculated the force exerted by skeletal muscles and, arguing by analogy, reached the conclusion that the motive force of the heart considered by itself may be calculated as equal to that of supporting a weight of more than 3000 pounds.

However, little progress could be made until a method of measurement was introduced. This method was developed by the Rev. Stephen Hales, Rector of Farringdon in Hampshire and minister at Teddington in Middlesex, who, as we have seen in an earlier chapter, published in 1733 the second volume of *Statical Essays, Containing Haemastaticks* (60, 61).

"EXPERIMENT I. *In December I caused a mare to be tied down alive on her back, she was 14 hands high, and about 14 years of age, had a fistula on her withers, was neither very lean, nor yet lusty: having laid open the left crural artery about 3 inches from her belly, I inserted into it a brass pipe whose bore was one sixth of an inch in diameter; and to that, by means of another brass pipe which was fitly adapted to it, I fixed a glass tube, of nearly the same diameter, which was 9 feet in length: Then untying the ligature on the artery, the blood rose in the tube 8 feet 3 inches perpendicular above the level of the left ventricle of the heart: but it did not attain to its full height at once; it rushed up about half way in an instant, and afterwards gradually at each pulse 12, 8, 6, 4, 2, and sometimes 1 inch: when it was at its full height, it would rise and fall at and after each pulse 2, 3, or 4 inches; and sometimes it would fall 12 or 14 inches, and have there for a time the same vibrations up and down at and after each pulse, as it had, when it was at its full height; to which it would rise again, after forty or fifty pulses. . . .*

"*I measured the blood as it run out of the artery, and after each quart of blood was run out, I refixed the glass tube to the artery, to see how much the force of the blood was abated; this I repeated to the 8th quart, and then its force being much abated, I applied the glass tube after each pint had flowed out.*"

Hales then proceeded to measure various other quantities relating to the circulation, some of which have been described in Chapters II and VI.

The Physiological Mechanisms Regulating Arterial Pressure

The preceding account shows how profound an understanding Hales had of the working of the circulation. So had Thomas Young, physician to St. George's Hospital, author of the wave theory of light, and translator of the Rosetta stone, whose Croonian Lectures to the Royal Society

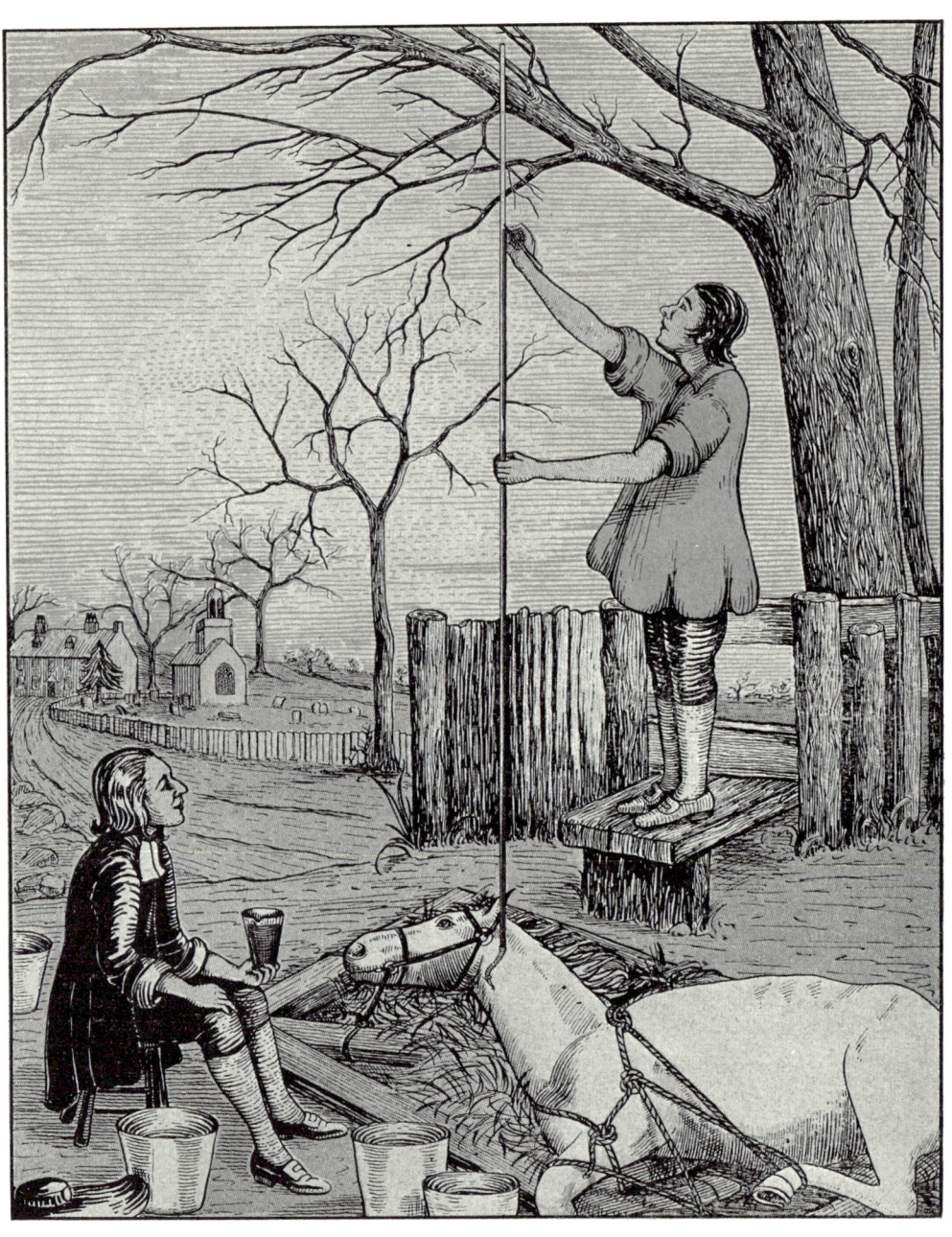

Figure 1. Stephen Hales and assistant measuring blood pressure in the horse.

in 1808 were "On the Functions of the Heart and Arteries" (*155*). However, it was Poiseuille, the inventor of the mercury manometer for measuring arterial pressure, who formalized the quantities concerned in 1846 (*129*). His contribution, now summarized in the familiar Poiseuille's equation, has formed the basis of quantitative thinking about blood pressure, whether it be "high" or "low."

The ways by which cardiac output is regulated and vascular diameter is adjusted, so that each organ receives blood at the rate and pressure appropriate to its needs, have been considered in other chapters of this book and will not be summarized here. Since Stephen Hales's day, the great advances have been the discovery of the vasomotor nerves, the baroreceptors regulating arterial pressure, and the existence of a variety of mechanisms for the chemical regulation of the circulation (*76*). Here we may ask two questions:

(1) Given that the vasomotor nerves have an important function and given that the baroreceptors work largely through them as affectors, how does the completely sympathectomized dog regulate its circulation so effectively that its activity seems almost unimpaired (*7*)? Does this suggest the existence of other regulating mechanisms which are as important as the sympathetic nerves and which are still almost entirely unknown?

(2) How does a man regulate his circulation at a resting arterial pressure of say 220 mm. Hg systolic and 130 mm. Hg diastolic, a level which is approximately double that usually found? Is it possible that the basic abnormality which causes the raised pressure represents a disturbance of one of these mechanisms which are as yet almost, or completely, unknown?

The Biological Significance of Arterial Pressure

The levels at which arterial pressure tends to be regulated differ in different species, which might be expected to have some biological meaning. It is possible that if this meaning were understood some light might be cast on the reasons why arterial pressure is regulated at different levels in certain maladies in man. To the writer's knowledge this has never been systematically explored, although it was touched on by August Krogh. Krogh (*88*) realized more clearly than any of his predecessors that the real business of the circulation is transacted in the capillaries, where exchange obeys the physical laws that govern diffusion across semipermeable membranes. Clearly, arterial pressure must be high enough to exceed colloid osmotic pressure of plasma. In its turn, colloid osmotic pressure must be high enough to prevent filtration edema.

BLOOD VESSELS

"... *the functional capacity of an anatomical structure may depend on its size just as much as upon its form. I would like to draw your attention to the example of this rule which we have, I believe, in this case. It might be imagined that a circulatory system like that of a mammal might be reproduced in any desired dimensions, but it is at least not improbable that the giraffe is not very far removed from the limit at which, in an animal living on land, the unavoidable increase in hydrostatic capillary pressure can be compensated by increasing the colloid osmotic pressure of the blood, which, in its turn, must be limited by the consequent increase in viscosity and perhaps by other factors.*"

Interestingly enough, the arterial pressure in the giraffe has only recently been measured. Warren, et al. (*149*) found that the arterial pressure ranged from 282/150 to 344/194 mm. Hg.

High Blood Pressure in Man

Although isolated observations had been made before, the continuous unfolding of knowledge and understanding in hypertension began with Richard Bright. Bright was educated in Edinburgh and was appointed assistant physician to Guy's Hospital in 1820. He was the first of a long line of physician-pathologists at Guy's Hospital, and, together with his contemporaries Addison and Hodgkin, performed autopsies as a matter of course, and thus made unique contributions to the natural history of disease. (It is of interest that the physicians at Guy's continued to do their own autopsies till the 1930's.) In 1827, Bright published his *Reports of Medical Cases Selected with a View to Illustrating the Symptoms and Cure of Disease by a Reference to Morbid Anatomy* (*21*). In this he described meticulously a series of patients observed over twelve years in which coagulable urine was associated with dropsy. "I have never yet examined the body of a patient dying with dropsy attended with coagulable urine in whom some obvious derangement was not discoverable in the kidneys." He noted three types of kidney; one he thought was degenerative, the other two might be different stages of the same disease.

In his *Tabular View of the Morbid Appearance in 100 Cases Connected with Albuminous Urine* (*22*), Bright wrote:

SYSTEMIC ARTERIAL HYPERTENSION

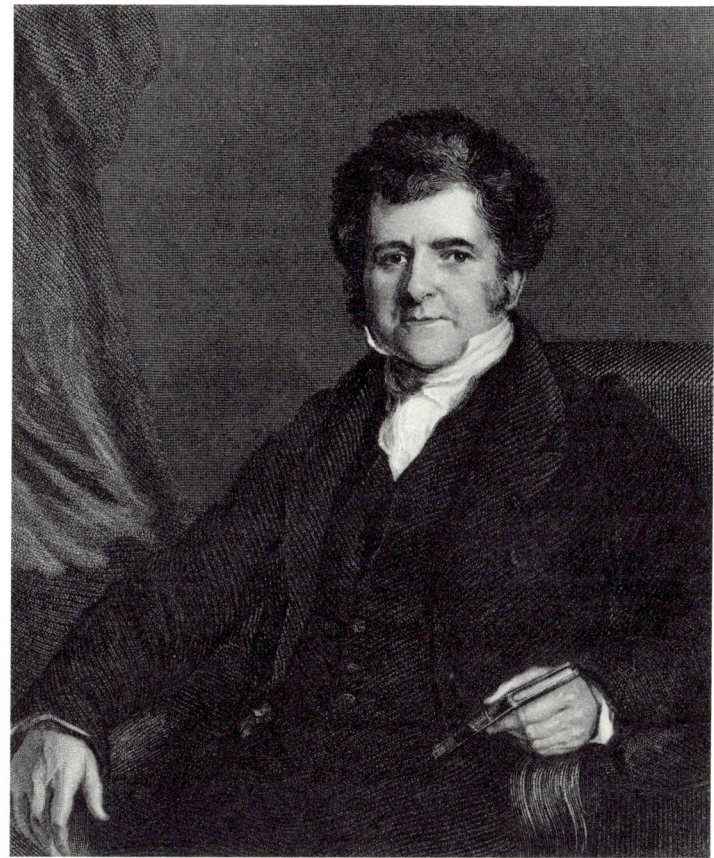

Figure 2. Richard Bright (1789–1858).

"*The obvious structural changes in the heart have consisted chiefly of hypertrophy with or without valvular disease; and what is most striking, out of fifty-two cases of hypertrophy, no valvular disease whatsoever could be detected in thirty-four: but in eleven of these thirty-four, more or less, disease existed in the coats of the aorta; still, however, leaving twenty-two without any probably organic cause for the marked hypertrophy generally affecting the left ventricle. This naturally leads us to look for some less local cause, for the unusual efforts to which the heart has been impelled; and the two most ready solutions appear to be, either that the altered quality of the blood affords irregular and unwonted stimulus to the organ immediately; or, that it so affects the minute and capillary circulation, as to render greater action necessary to force the blood through the distant sub-divisions of the vascular system."*

BLOOD VESSELS In Britain, clinicians were occupied, for the next thirty or forty years, in attempting to classify Bright's disease and in enquiring whether the cause was single or multiple. Samuel Wilks (*151*), also of Guy's Hospital, wrote, "Amongst these were two very remarkable extreme conditions—the one a kidney large and white, often double the natural size, and associated with a very considerable dropsy of the whole body; the other kidney hard and contracted, often only half the usual size, chronic in its character, and often destitute of symptoms." These two varieties, the large, white kidney and the small, white kidney, were later distinguished by Bartels (*9*) as being characteristic of chronic parenchymatous and chronic interstitial nephritis; they are now considered as the end stages of the types II and I of nephritis of Ellis (*119*), types B and A of Longcope (*119*).

The next landmark in the study of hypertension was the paper by George Johnson, who described hypertrophy of the muscular coats of the small arteries in the kidney and subsequently of other organs in Bright's disease. In 1868 he wrote,

"It cannot be supposed that the great hypertrophy of the left ventricle, which is often found in cases of chronic Bright's disease, is a direct result solely of the resistance offered by the renal arteries. We must look for the cause of this hypertrophy rather in the fact that the blood, in consequence of degeneration of the kidney, being contaminated by urinary excreta and otherwise deteriorated, is impeded in its transit through the minute arteries throughout the body. We have evidence of such an impediment in the full, hard, throbbing pulse, which is a very common phenomenon in the advanced stage of chronic Bright's disease. Dr. Sanderson, in his recently published 'Handbook of the Sphygmograph' (p. 80), states that in cases of chronic Bright's disease with hypertrophy of the left ventricle, the sphygmograph affords decided evidence of increased arterial pressure. Still more conclusive evidence of an impediment to the circulation is afforded by the existence of hypertrophy of the muscular walls of the arteries in various tissues and organs. Dr. Hughlings Jackson lately did me the favour to bring me a kidney, some vessels from the brain, and a portion of pia mater, from a man who had died with a contracted granular kidney. There had been

headache and other cerebral symptoms during life, and after death we found that, not only were the walls of the renal arteries hypertrophied, but also, though in a less degree, those of the brain and pia mater" (*82*).

This paragraph is interesting not only for its content but for its reference to contemporary workers. Dr. Sanderson (subsequently Sir John Burdon-Sanderson—the first professor of physiology at Oxford, later Regius Professor of Medicine and Osler's immediate predecessor) we shall meet again in connection with the sphygmograph. Hughlings Jackson was Physician to the London Hospital and the National Hospital, and a dominant figure in neurology then and subsequently.

In 1872, Sir William Gull of Guy's Hospital and H. G. Sutton of the London Hospital published their paper, *The Pathology of the morbid state commonly called Chronic Bright's Disease with contracted kidney* ("*arteriocapillary fibrosis*") (*57*). This paper confirmed Johnson's observations on the widespread alteration in the small arteries, but differed as to the nature of the alteration. They concluded:

"... *the arterioles throughout the body in that condition usually called chronic Bright's disease with contracted kidney, are more or less altered. That this alteration is due to a 'hyalin-fibroid' formation in the walls of the minute arteries, and a 'hyalin-granular' change in the corresponding capillaries. That this change occurs chiefly outside the muscular layer, but also in the tunica intima of some arterioles. . . . This morbid change in the arterioles and capillaries is the primary and essential condition of the morbid state called chronic Bright's disease with contracted kidney.*"

The latter conclusion was based on their finding three forms of the disease:

"(*1*) *Kidneys often much contracted, heart much hypertrophied, minute arteries and capillaries proportionately thickened by 'hyalin-fibroid' formation.* (*2*) *Kidneys little contracted, but heart much hypertrophied, minute arteries and capillaries much thickened by hyalin-fibroid substance.* (*3*) *Kidneys healthy, whilst heart much hypertrophied and minute arteries and capillaries much thickened by hyalin-fibroid substance.*"

Gull's insight is illustrated by the following quotation from a clinical lecture given in 1872:

SYSTEMIC ARTERIAL HYPERTENSION

BLOOD VESSELS

"It is always dangerous to rest in a narrow pathology; and I believe that to be a narrow pathology which is satisfied with what you now see before me on this table. In this glass you see a much hypertrophied heart and a very contracted kidney. This specimen is classical. It was, I believe, put up under Dr. Bright's own direction, and with a view of showing that the wasting of the kidney is the cause of the thickening of the heart. I cannot but look upon it with veneration, but not with conviction. I think, with all deference to so great an authority, that the systemic capillaries, and, had it been possible, the entire man, should have been included in this vase, together with the heart and the kidneys; then we should have had, I believe, a truer view of the causation of the cardiac hypertrophy and of the disease of the kidney" (56).

Meanwhile in Germany, Bright's observation of the association between left ventricular hypertrophy and kidney disease had also been observed by Ludwig Traube (*145*), who, less discerningly than Bright, Johnson, and Gull and Sutton, attributed the raised pressure purely to the change in the kidney.

"The shrinking of the renal parenchyma has, therefore, two-fold consequences. It will act, first, by decreasing the blood volume which flows out in a given time from the arterial system into the venous system. It will, secondly, act by decreasing the amount of liquid which at the same time is removed from the arterial system as urinary secretion. As a result of both these conditions, particularly because of the latter, as is clear from what has just been stated, the mean pressure of the arterial system must increase. Consequently again, an increase in resistances is produced which oppose the emptying of the left ventricle."

Ewald (*36*), examining chiefly the small vessels of the pia mater, confirmed Johnson's finding of hypertrophy of the media, while Jores (*83*), in a characteristically thorough investigation, emphasized change in the arterial intima, particularly a fatty-hyaline thickening, which he found not only in the kidney but in arteries of the organs generally except heart and skeletal muscle.

Such were the chief contributions of simple observation during life and after death. Bright used the simplest tools. The kidneys were not examined microscopically, though, according to Hale-White, in 1842 Bright began a microscopic examination of the kidneys (*59*); no account of this was ever published. "Most commonly when the urine has been exposed to the heat of a candle in a spoon, before it rises quite to the boiling point it becomes clouded, sometimes simply opalescent, at other times almost milky." Johnson, and Gull and Sutton, used the microscope, but often without fixation of tissues, and with very imperfect methods of staining.

Bright and his successors noted that the pulse was hard in the disease they described, and Traube gave a comprehensive list of signs by which left ventricular enlargement could be recognized during life. However, the most important new data were to come from actual measurement of arterial blood pressure in man.

SYSTEMIC ARTERIAL HYPERTENSION

Measurement of Arterial Pressure in Man

Unlike the situation in lower animals, almost the whole of our knowledge of the behavior of blood pressure in man has been based on indirect methods of measurement. Although Faivre (*38*), in 1856, used Poiseuille's (*128*) manometer to measure arterial pressure directly during limb amputation, and the recent developments of membrane manometers have made possible direct measurement for considerable periods without sacrifice of an artery, these methods have yet to contribute materially to our understanding of high blood pressure in man.

The first indirect instrument was that of Hérisson (*71*) in which a membrane covering a cup containing mercury was pressed on the radial artery to obliterate it; the pressure on the graduated tube leading out of the cup was then read. In this instrument, estimation of arterial pressure was secondary (and incidentally, inaccurate); its real purpose was to estimate the amplitude of the pulse.

The first instrument specifically designed to measure arterial pressure was that of Vierordt (*146*) in which weights were added to a scale pan placed on a lever which pressed on a button overlying the radial artery; obliteration of the pulse was shown by the writing point attached to the lever ceasing to move. In 1863, Marey of Paris (*100*) introduced the first practical instrument. The purpose of his instrument was to measure the amplitude, duration, and compressibility of the pulse. This latter was done by altering the tension on the spring by the screw P and thus was a very crude quantitative assessment. Mahomed's sphygmograph was a modification in which the pressure on the button overlying the radial artery was adjusted by a thumbscrew, the pressure itself being recorded in ounces troy weight on the adjacent dial. It was thus the first quantitative instrument. These clumsy instruments were the forerunners of other more practical devices, e.g. that of von Basch (*10*) which was designed to compress the radial artery until the pulse could no longer be felt. Modern practice stems from Riva-Rocci's method, of 1896 (*134*). The larger 10–15 cm. wide cuff was introduced by von Recklinghausen in 1901 (*132*), and the auscultatory method by Korotkoff in 1905 (*87*).

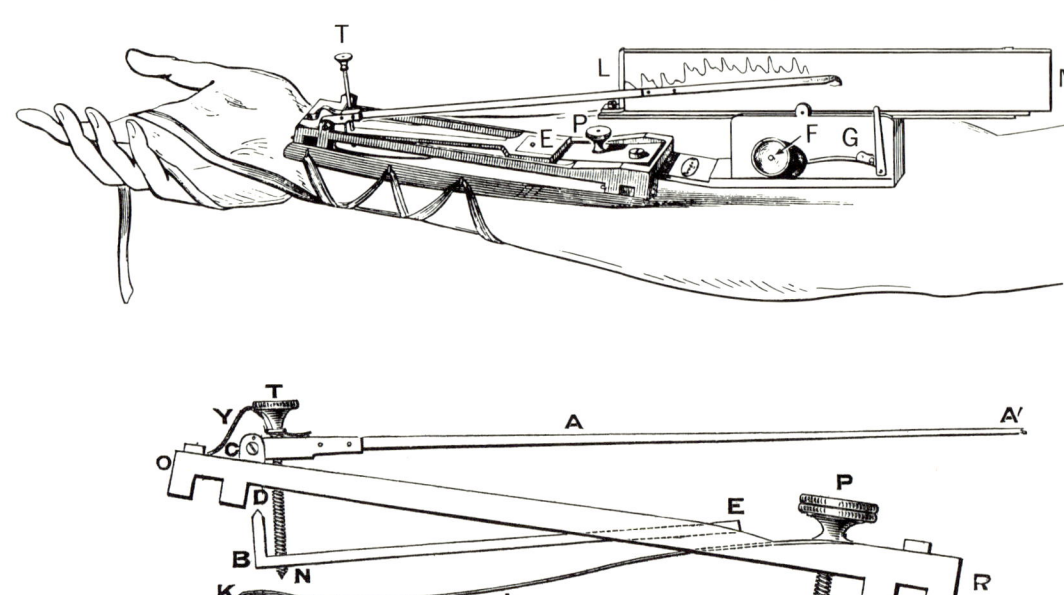

Figure 3. Marey's sphygmograph applied to the arm above, and the arrangement of levers below.

The button K rests on the radial pulse, the tension of its spring being adjustable by the screw P; compressibility is thus estimated by the extent to which the screw must be turned until the writing point ceases to move. AA′ is the writing lever, the axis of which is at C; K the spring; B the lever by which the movements of K are transmitted to A; D its knife edge; T an adjusting screw for varying the distance between K and D according to the pressure required; P an adjusting screw for permanently adjusting the spring at the proper obliquity; FG the box in which the clockwork is contained; LM the traveler.

Primary Hypertension Versus Bright's Disease

The first man systematically to estimate arterial pressure was Mahomed, whose work is little known. He perceived clearly what others later established more fully. Frederick Henry Horatio Akhbar Mahomed was the grandson of an Indian physician formerly in the service of the East India Company. His grandfather had settled in Brighton, in what is now the Queen's Hotel, and set up a shampooing and vaporbath business there; his clientele included the cream of Regency Society, who undoubtedly were in great need of his skill. He later became Shampoo Surgeon to their Majesties George IV and William IV. Frederick Akhbar Mahomed (he always omitted his two middle names) entered Guy's Hospital as a student in 1869. As has been noted, Marey of Paris had introduced his sphygmograph in 1863, and Burdon-Sanderson (23) had made an extended study of its use. Mahomed improved it while he was still a student, and his efforts won him the Pupil's Physical Society prize of 1870. His improvements were published in 1872 (94). Mahomed qualified as a medical practitioner in 1872. His second post was that of resident medical officer to the London Fever Hospital, where he continued his researches with the sphygmograph and published his first classical paper *The etiology of Bright's disease and the prealbuminuric stage* (95). In this much misquoted paper Mahomed summarized the results of his estimations of the tension of the pulse (in ounces) made during his resident appointments, particularly in patients developing acute nephritis following scarlet fever. He wrote:

"The observations I have now to bring before you are briefly these: 1st. That previous to the commencement of any kidney change, or to the appearance of albumin in the urine, the first condition observable is high tension in the arterial system. . . . The series of cases to which I especially desire to draw your attention this evening are all of one type. Their characteristic features are these: they all occur in patients recovering from scarlet fever."

He then described seven cases in which the observation had been made.

Mahomed not only made the first observation of high arterial tension in acute nephritis; he observed that it began before albumin appeared in the urine. This is what he meant by the prealbuminuric stage of Bright's

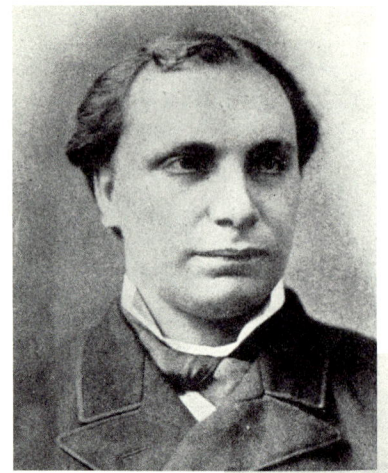
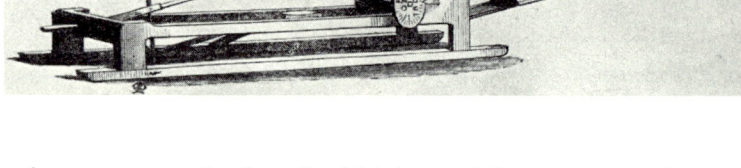

Figure 4. Frederick Akhbar Mahomed (1849–84) and his sphygmograph.

disease. In the same paper he described high arterial pressure in eclampsia, and noted that it occurs in cirrhosis of the kidneys.

Mahomed became medical tutor at St. Mary's in 1875, medical registrar at Guy's in 1878, and assistant physician to Guy's in 1881. He died of typhoid fever at the age of thirty-five.

When the problem of "arteriocapillary fibrosis" was discussed at the Pathological Society in 1877, Gull and Sutton confessed their inability to recognize the early stages of the malady during life. Mahomed suggested, "It is very common to meet with people apparently in good health who have no albumin in the urine or any other sign of organic disease, who constantly present a condition of high arterial tension when examined by the aid of the sphygmograph" (*96*).

In 1879, Mahomed published two papers (*97, 98*) analyzing 100 cases of granular kidneys and relating the findings during life to those after death. Only 26 had "the ordinary symptoms of Bright's disease, namely albuminuria and dropsy" and these were found to have "a yellow or mixed contracted kidney." The remainder had a "red contracted kidney," often unaccompanied by albuminuria during life and came

[500]

under treatment for "symptoms of cerebral haemorrhage, heart disease, lung disease and sundry medical and surgical diseases." It was with this latter group that Mahomed dealt. He used the old term Bright's disease and not the new "arteriocapillary fibrosis" because "it would be wrong to rob the name of Bright of half its glory." He left little doubt that the condition he was describing differed from the other half of Bright's disease in which there was albuminuria and anasarca. "The symptoms consist essentially in the signs of high arterial tension taken together with the absence of albuminuria." His papers contain a remarkable number of accurate observations on the condition now commonly called essential hypertension.

SYSTEMIC ARTERIAL HYPERTENSION

"My first contention is that high pressure is a constant condition in the circulation of some individuals and that this condition is a symptom of a certain constitution or diathesis."

Mahomed also found hypertension in young persons and discussed "the recognition of the diathesis in young persons during health, and previous to structural change."

"These persons appear to pass on through life pretty much as others do and generally do not suffer from their high blood pressures, except in their petty ailments upon which it imprints itself. . . . As age advances the enemy gains accession of strength . . . the individual has now passed forty years, perhaps fifty years, of age, his lungs begin to degenerate, he has a cough in the winter time, but by his pulse you will know him. . . . Alternatively headache, vertigo, epistaxis, a passing paralysis, a more severe apoplectic seizure, and then the final blow.

"Of this I feel sure, that the clinical symptoms and the pathological changes resulting from high arterial pressure are frequently seen in cases in which very slight, if any disease is discoverable in the kidney. The observations provide strong evidence of Gull and Sutton's work. It appears to me that these clinical, and their pathological, observations must stand or fall together; that one is the pathological, the other the clinical aspect of the same condition."

In 1881 (99) he published personal observations of 61 cases of "Chronic Bright's disease without albuminuria" seen during life, and the results of post mortem examinations of 21 of them. He divided his cases into clinical groups, of which the largest included patients with heart failure and cerebral hemorrhage, and he observed the common occurrence of bronchitis in many. He described three stages in chronic Bright's disease: first, the functional stage, limited to high blood pressure without organic change in vascular system or kidneys; second, chronic Bright's disease without albuminuria and with the pathological changes of arteriocapillary fibrosis; and third, chronic Bright's disease with nephritis, which he states is "the natural but by no means the invariable termination of the disease," death occurring more commonly from heart failure or cerebral hemorrhage.

"The disease may commence as an acute infection and afterwards become chronic. . . . What has been the cause in one case may be the result in another; thus, general disorder may cause high arterial pressure and this, in its turn, kidney changes; while on the other hand, kidney changes may be primary and acute and they may in their turn produce impurity of blood and this general pressure. But whether we read the tale backwards or forwards, it is the same tale in the end."

Thus Mahomed, combining for the first time measurement of arterial pressure (although somewhat crudely) with clinical and pathological observation, anticipated by thirty-three years the better known work of Volhard and Fahr.

Mahomed's work, although more thorough and penetrating, was long overlooked, and credit for the recognition of primary hypertension is commonly given to Huchard, von Basch, and Allbutt. Huchard, professor of medicine in Paris, recognized clearly that hypertension might occur independently of nephritis. He wrote:

"It has been wrongly assumed that chronic hypertension only appears following interstitial nephritis. The opposite is true; arterial hypertension is the cause of arteriosclerosis; it precedes by a varying time interval the evolution of different diseases (heart disease and arterial nephritis, etc.) which are in turn secondary to vascular sclerosis."

Huchard named the condition presclerosis.

Von Basch, professor of medicine in Vienna (Fig. 5), developed a much better implement for measuring arterial pressure, and at first regarded 135–165 mm. Hg as the normal range; later he regarded 150 mm. Hg as abnormal. Influenced by Traube, he regarded the high

SYSTEMIC
ARTERIAL
HYPERTENSION

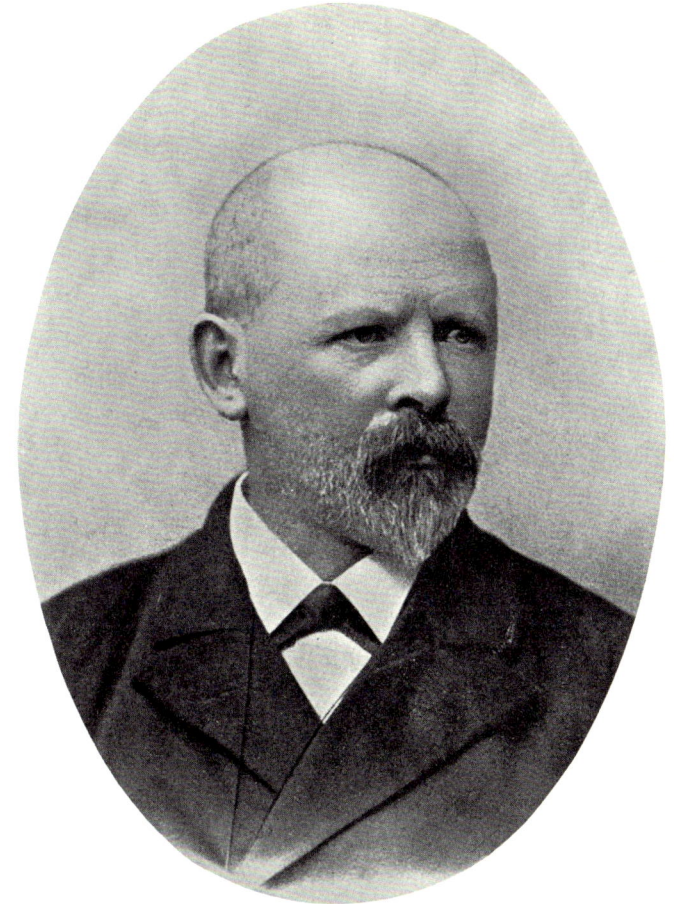

Figure 5. Samuel S. K. von Basch and his sphygmomanometer.

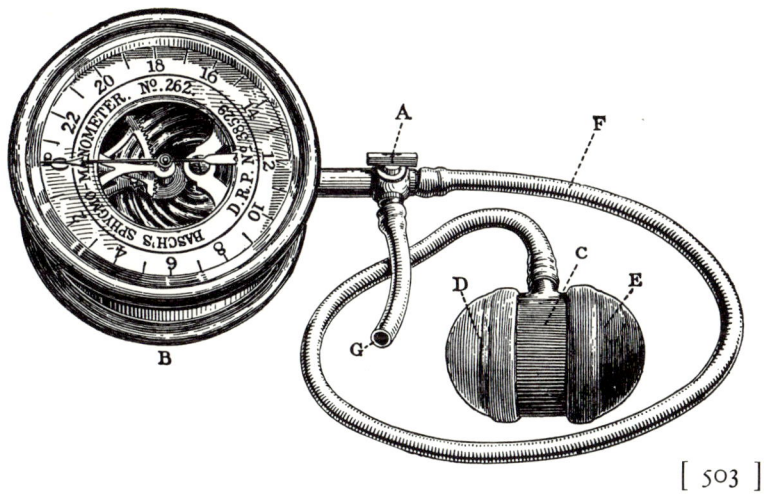

arterial pressure as due to arteriosclerosis, and those patients with pressures just above normal he classed as "latent arteriosclerosis."

At the same time, Allbutt, Regius Professor of Physic at Cambridge, had observed the occurrence of raised arterial pressure in the absence of albuminuria. In 1895 (*2*), he described five cases under the term "senile plethora." In 1915 (*3*), he wrote:

> "*Thus gradually I became convinced that cases, such as we are considering, must be divided, first, into Bright's disease . . . secondly, into the class to which soon afterwards I gave the name Hyperpiesis, a malady in which at or towards middle life blood pressures rise excessively, a malady having a course of its own and deserving the name of a disease; and thirdly, into at least one other class of arterial degeneration, one not typically associated with rise of blood pressure, a class in which indeed the blood pressure does not exceed, or scarcely exceeds, the rise common to almost all persons in later life; a series of which the course, symptoms, and issues are altogether different.*"

To this third class Allbutt gave the name "decrescent" arteriosclerosis. Allbutt's classification has been expanded and modified; yet in its bare outline it remains acceptable.

One of the most important systematic studies was that of Janeway (*81*), professor of medicine of Columbia University, who, impressed with the importance of disease of heart and vessels in causing death and disability, termed the condition "hypertensive cardiovascular disease."

Classification of Hypertension and Nephritis

Throughout this period, the classification of renal lesions of Bright's disease had dominated men's minds. This culminated in Volhard and Fahr's "Die Brightsche Nierenkrankheit" in 1914 (*148*). Volhard, the physician, and Fahr, the pathologist, divided Bright's disease into three, namely the degenerative diseases or nephroses, the inflammatory diseases or nephritides, and the arteriosclerotic diseases or scleroses. The latter was subdivided into the simple benign sclerosis, and the "Kombinationsform," or nephritis superimposed on simple sclerosis. Later they revised their view of the "Kombinationsform," which represented the endstage of the malignant course (*37*). Volhard was particularly responsible for demonstrating that essential hypertension might follow either the benign or the malignant course. In the benign form, characterized

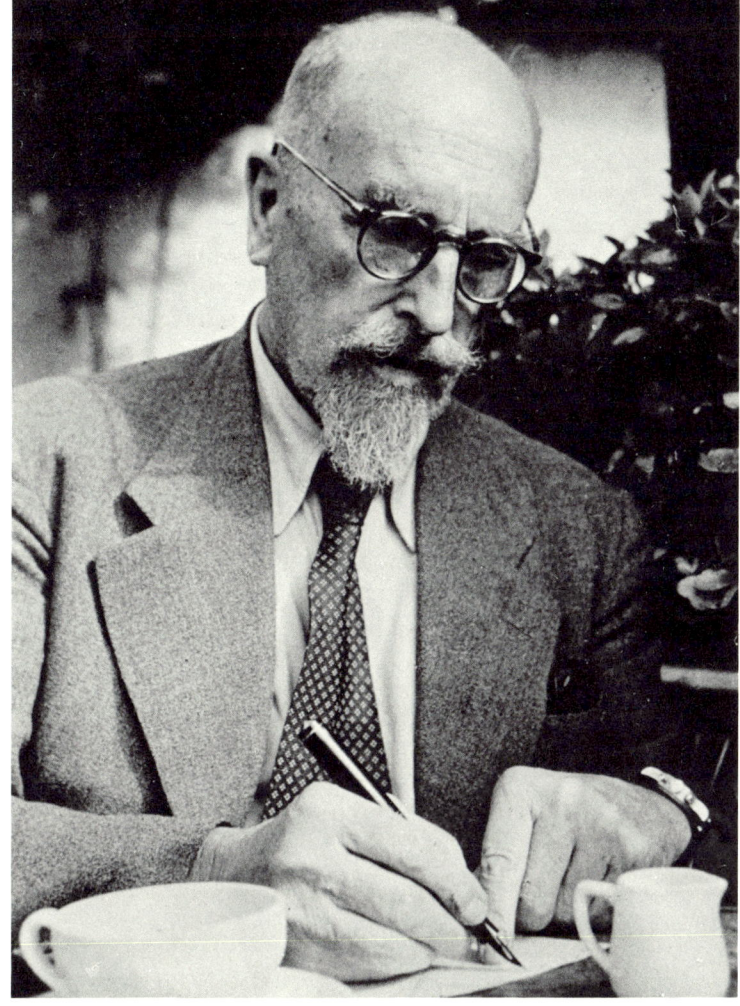

Figure 6. Franz Volhard (1872–1950).

by high blood pressure and varying degrees of enlargement of the heart, the condition might remain unchanged for years, the patient eventually dying of heart failure, intercurrent disease, or apoplexy, renal function remaining unimpaired throughout. The onset of the malignant form was heralded by the changes in the fundus oculi first recognized by von Graefe (*52*) and named by Liebreich (*92*) "retinitis albuminurica";

BLOOD VESSELS

renal function might then be unimpaired, but soon protein and red cells appeared in the urine, the kidney failed, and the patient died, usually within the year, of uremia.

Subsequent work has shown that neither nephritis nor nephrosis are strict entities. For example, the kidney of polyarteritis nodosa (*29*) has been differentiated from nephritis. The Kimmelstiel-Wilson kidney of diabetes, as well as the kidney of disseminated lupus, masquerade as nephrosis, though both are complicated in their later stages by high blood pressure.

Volhard, in particular, advanced further in his concept of hypertension. In the 1931 edition of Bergmann and Staehelin's "Handbuch der inneren Medizin" (*147*), his article, 1826 pages long, states his concept of two forms of hypertension, red and white. Red hypertension, which is identical with Frank's essential hypertension, he regarded as due to elastosis of the prearterioles, which thus became less distensible by the arterial pulse. This change was attributed to the effects of age on a certain genetic constitution. This condition was stable, the patient remaining unchanged for years and dying eventually of heart failure, apoplexy, or intercurrent disease. Kidney function remained more or less intact throughout, and after death the kidney showed simple sclerosis. Opposed to this was pale hypertension, or "Bösartige Sklerose," characterized clinically by retinitis, albuminuria, a gross hypertension, and a rapid decline in renal function, leading to death in uremia.

> "*It can be seen that the 'malignant' cases of subacute nephritis, of secondary contracted kidneys and of true contracted kidneys generally have the highest blood pressure, just as the blood pressure in malignant sclerosis exceeds the pressure in the benign type.*
>
> "*In contrast to the benign sclerosis, we have never seen either a transient rise in blood pressure, or pure 'systolic hypertension' in the malignant type. On the contrary, the diastolic pressure is usually markedly increased, often reaching values of 120 and 130, or even 160–180 mm. Hg.*"

Volhard thought that pale hypertension was due to the action of a renal pressor substance released through renal ischemia; the renal ischemia, in turn, could come about if, in red hypertension, the pre-arterioles contracted sufficiently, or if, in nephritis, arterial spasm or organic disease reduced the renal blood flow. He thought that the acute arteriolar necroses, which Fahr, in 1919, had shown to characterize the malignant phase (*148*), were due to vascular spasm induced by the supposed renal pressor substance. The necroses occurring in the kidney reduced renal blood flow still further, thereby promoting the release of the pressor substance, and leading to the vicious circle which determines the progressive downhill course of the patient with Bright's disease.

Since Volhard's masterly analysis of the relationship between benign and malignant hypertension, the cause of the malignant phase has provoked much discussion. In 1935, Derow and Altschule (*31*) showed that "malignant hypertension is a syndrome which may occur: (a) with no evidence of previously existing hypertension; (b) as the end stage of essential hypertension . . .; (c) as the end stage of a miscellaneous group of conditions characterized by hypertension secondary to acute, subacute or chronic glomerular nephritis, pyelonephritis, adrenal tumour, pituitary basophilism, periarteritis nodosa, hyperemesis gravidarum, chronic lead poisoning, etc." They repeated this suggestion in 1941 (*32*) and stated that "the mechanism by which the benign course of primary or secondary hypertension is suddenly and dramatically transformed into the rapid, progressive, downhill course of the syndrome of malignant hypertension is not understood."

In 1934, while investigating cerebrospinal fluid pressure in hypertension, I obtained evidence that the retinopathy of the malignant phase was associated with a relatively high cerebrospinal fluid pressure, which in turn seemed to be due to a high diastolic arterial blood pressure (*113*). More conclusive evidence for a relationship between the malignant phase and the level of the blood pressure (*46*) came in 1938 when Goldblatt demonstrated the occurrence of arteriolar necroses in animals in which hypertension had been produced by narrowing the renal arteries (*47*). These lesions were identical with those in man, both in histological appearance and in distribution, except that they were absent from the kidney whose renal artery had been clamped. For a while, the etiology of the arteriolar necroses was in doubt. Goldblatt, finding lesions only in dogs with severe renal artery constriction, attributed them to a combination of high intravascular pressure and renal failure. On the other hand, Child (*24*) observed them in a dog whose pressure exceeded 300 mm. Hg for the last two months of its life and whose blood urea nitrogen was 17 mg./100 ml. on the day of death. Wilson and Pickering (*154*), finding the lesions only in those rabbits with the highest pressures, and noting their absence from the clamped kidney, attributed them to the high level of intra-arterial pressure. Strong evidence for this view was provided by Wilson and Byrom's observation that, in rats, constriction of one renal artery produced gross hypertension and the arteriolar and glomerular necroses of malignant hypertension in the *intact* kidney; these lesions did not occur in the kidney with the clamped renal artery (*152*).

Thus, both the clinical and histological characteristics of the malignant phase seemed to be due, though in an uncertain manner, to the severity of the hypertension. It was accordingly suggested (*116*) that the difference between the benign and malignant courses reflected different intensities of hypertension, the former characterizing a less, the latter a more severe, degree. This hypothesis provided an explanation for Derow and Altschule's dilemma. Moreover, it was possible to predict that, if the arterial pressure could be reduced sufficiently and for long enough, the malignant could be converted to the benign course. Clinical and histological support for this hypothesis has since been provided (*126*). Experience with the potent hypotensive drugs has supplied the most convincing evidence. Nevertheless, some workers, notably Perera (*110, 111*) and McMichael (*85*), do not accept this explanation of the nature of the malignant phase. They have described patients in whom retinal lesions, with or without progressive uremia, develop in the absence of hypertension. In the writer's experience, neuroretinitis and uremia, quite dissociated from hypertension, have occurred in polyarteritis nodosa and disseminated lupus. Neuroretinitis has also been found associated with normal blood pressure in temporal arteritis (*26*), and in gastro-intestinal hemorrhage (*107*). It is probable that there is a pathological process common to all these causes of neuroretinitis, perhaps focal anoxia of the retina. At any rate, the occurrence of neuroretinitis in patients without high arterial pressure does not exclude the intensity of hypertension as the major determinant of the neuroretinitis in patients who manifest no other etiologic abnormality than an unusually high arterial blood pressure.

Summary of the Natural History of Hypertension

A century and a quarter of observation by the bedside and in the deadhouse, later supplemented by measurement of arterial pressure during life, has shown that high blood pressure can occur in two sorts of ways. In the first, called secondary hypertension, high pressure is associated with a specific disease to which it is believed to be secondary; in some diseases, such as pheochromocytoma, unilateral renal disease, Cushing's syndrome, and coarctation of the aorta, surgery has demonstrated that this assumption is true; in others such as acute nephritis, in which Mahomed demonstrated the temporal precedence of raised pressure, evidence is wanting. In the second group, called primary hypertension, there is no associated disease to which the high pressure can be attributed. The recognition of this condition was slow and it has received a bewildering succession of names: "chronic Bright's disease without albuminuria" (*98*), "presclerosis" (*78*), "latent arteriosclerosis" (*10*), "hyperpiesia" (*2*), "essentielle hypertonie" (*40*), "hypertensive cardiovascular disease" (*81*), and "hypertensive disease" (*50*). Primary hypertension may follow the benign or the malignant course, the end-stage of the malignant form being remarkably similar to the end-stage of secondary hypertension. The nature of the malignant phase has been discussed.

Two major questions emerge. What is the mechanism by which the arterial pressure becomes raised in these several morbid conditions? What is the nature of primary or essential hypertension? To answer these questions three lines of enquiry have been pursued: first, the production of high pressure in experimental animals; second, an analysis of the circulatory changes in man; and third, an attempt to study the genetic and environmental factors concerned in producing primary hypertension.

Experimental Hypertension

Since the publication of Claude Bernard's *Experimental Medicine*, one of the most respected methods of elucidating causal sequences in human disease has been that of animal experiment. However, as Lewis has pointed out, the method has many potential fallacies, and it is essential that any conclusions so drawn should be provisional, and conditional on the final proof being obtained in man himself.

In the experimental production of hypertension, progress depended on the development of simple and reliable methods of estimating arterial pressure in the unanesthetized animal and of producing hypertension.

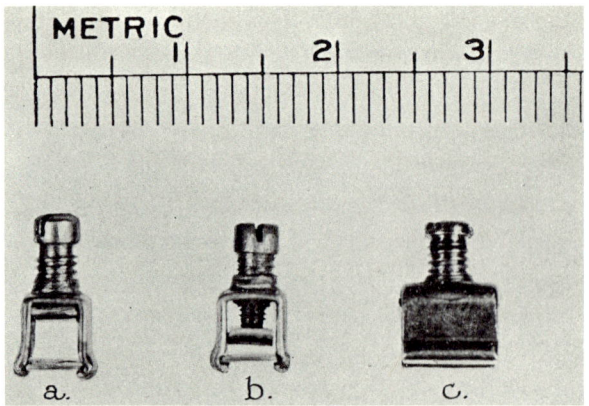

Figure 7. The Goldblatt clamp.

The first reliable method of measuring arterial pressure to be widely used was the carotid loop of van Leersum (*90*), by which a carotid was enclosed in a tube of skin, and the pressure required in an encircling cuff to stop the pulse was measured. The second was the modification of von Recklinghausen's capsule for compressing the dilated central artery of the ear of a rabbit, introduced by Grant and Rothschild (*54*). The third was direct puncture of the femoral artery in trained dogs, as used by Goldblatt in all his later work. It is only in recent years that a satisfactory method of measuring the blood pressure in the tail of the unanaesthetized rat has been devised.

Following Hering's demonstration of the importance of the baroreceptors of the carotid sinus and aortic arch in regulating arterial pressure (*70*), his pupils Koch and Mies (*86*) showed that prolonged hypertension could be produced by sectioning the four nerves, in two stages, in rabbits, cats, and dogs. This work was greatly extended by Heymans and Bouckaert (*74*). It was naturally suggested that failure of the nerves was responsible for raised pressure in essential hypertension (*76*). However, Gammon (*43*) and Pickering, Kissin, and Rothschild (*122*) showed that the carotid sinus nerves are functioning in essential hypertension and found no evidence that they were more or less stimulated than normal.

Arteriolar necroses have never been produced in this type of hypertension and cardiac enlargement is slight, which facts are perhaps correlated with the absence of hypertension when the animal is asleep or quiet (74). In fact, these animals are peculiar chiefly because of the absence of a mechanism to restrain arterial pressure from rising very high. It has not been generally recognized that the conditions which the experimenter commonly imposes to measure arterial pressure constitute a pressor stimulus of not inconsiderable size.

SYSTEMIC ARTERIAL HYPERTENSION

The greatest single advance in the experimental production of a condition resembling that of hypertension in man was the convincing demonstration by Goldblatt, Lynch, Hanzal, and Summerville (49) that a gross and persistent hypertension could be produced in dogs by constricting both renal arteries, or one if the other kidney had been removed.

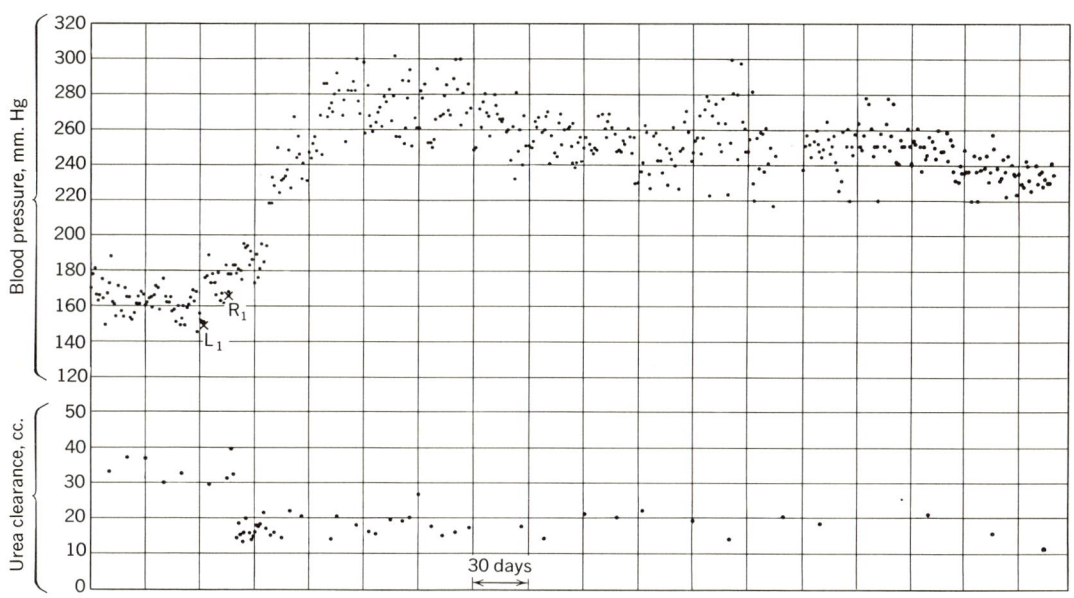

Figure 8. The production of persistent hypertension by renal ischemia in the dog. Each point represents a value for systolic blood pressure. L_1, severe constriction of left main renal artery; R_1, severe constriction of right main renal artery. Although the urea clearance fell to about 50 per cent of normal, at no time did non-protein nitrogen products accumulate in the blood.

BLOOD VESSELS

"In the investigation here reported the working hypothesis adopted was that ischemia limited to the kidneys may be the initial condition in the pathogenesis of the hypertension that is associated with nephrosclerosis. If this be true, then renal ischemia, no matter how produced, should be followed by elevation of blood pressure. This report deals with the effect on the blood pressure of dogs of experimentally produced ischemia limited to the kidneys. The simplest method for this purpose being obviously constriction of the main renal arteries, this was the method chosen."

In their original papers, Goldblatt and his colleagues showed that if renal artery constriction was not too severe, a stable hypertension unaccompanied by more than mild renal impairment was produced, in these respects resembling benign nephrosclerosis in man. Subsequently, Goldblatt showed that, with severe constriction, retinal changes and arteriolar changes resembling those in malignant hypertension could occur. Cardiac hypertrophy is also pronounced (116). Goldblatt (48) has remained steadily of the opinion that essential hypertension in man is similarly due to renal ischemia occasioned either by stenosis of a main artery, which is rare, or by organic changes in the smaller renal arteries down to the size of the afferent glomerular arteries, which is common. The strongest evidence for Goldblatt's view is Moritz and Oldt's (103) paper demonstrating that with increasing age arteriosclerosis advances in all organs of the body, but that its advance in the kidney is particularly associated with high arterial pressure. Most, however, still agree with Bell's conclusion (12) that in early cases of hypertension there may be no vascular changes in the kidney, and that the arterial and arteriolar changes that are invariable in the later phases are the consequences of hypertension rather than its cause. However, no one has yet succeeded in producing elastosis or fatty hyaline intimal thickening experimentally, and so the problem remains, as yet, unresolved.

Mechanism of Renal Hypertension

At first sight it would seem a simple matter to identify precisely the chain of events that begins with renal artery constriction and ends with persistently raised arterial pressure associated with cardiac hypertrophy and, in severe cases, the phenomena of the malignant phase. And yet such remains obscure.

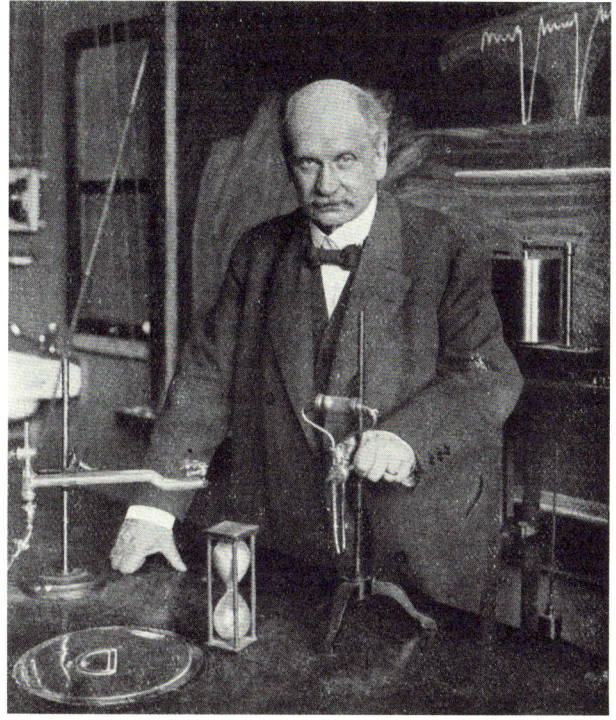

Figure 9. Robert Tigerstedt (1853–1923).

SYSTEMIC
ARTERIAL
HYPERTENSION

The first set of facts established beyond reasonable doubt is that constricting the renal artery can elevate arterial pressure if the kidney is deprived of all nervous connections by transplanting it to the neck (*17*), or to the groin (*44*), and that the blood pressure declines if, after a few hours or days, the constriction is removed. Again persistent hypertension can be produced by renal artery constriction when the animal has been deprived of its sympathetic nerves by bilateral paravertebral ganglionectomy (*75, 4, 41*). Clearly, then, it would seem that the mechanism is humoral, and since, as Goldblatt (*45*) showed, removal of the ischemic kidney quickly abolished hypertension, it would seem that the kidney itself is the source of a pressor agent.

Renin was discovered by the well-known Finnish physiologist Robert Tigerstedt, working with Bergman in Stockholm in 1898 (*144*). They showed that saline extracts of fresh rabbit kidney or of an alcohol dried

[513]

BLOOD VESSELS

powder produced a prolonged rise of pressure when injected into rabbits lightly anaesthetized with urethane. They named the active principle renin. They showed that renin could only be extracted from the cortex of the kidney, that it was destroyed at 56°C., precipitated by half-saturated ammonium sulphate, did not dialyse, had little action on the heart, but raised the pressure in the pithed cat. All these observations have since been confirmed (*119*).

Let us now return to 1936. At that time Prinzmetal came to work with me. We had quite independently obtained evidence that human essential hypertension was due to vasoconstriction not effected through the vasomotor nerves, and had failed to raise arterial pressure in man by transfusing blood from patients with hypertension. We were thus led to search for a pressor substance, suspecting that it might have unusual qualities. With Kissin (*121*), I had satisfied myself that epinephrine was not concerned. Prinzmetal and Friedman (*130*) also confirmed Harrison, Blalock, and Mason's (*68*) observations that saline extracts of ischemic kidney of dogs with hypertension raised the pressure of unanaesthetized dogs when injected intravenously into them (this was an odd effect because the peak rises occurred twenty minutes after injection). Renin seemed the strongest candidate. Yet its existence was suspect. No contemporary textbook of physiology even listed renin in the index. Only Bingel and his co-workers (*14*, *15*) had succeeded in repeating the work of Tigerstedt and Bergman. All this was the more odd because the discovery of renin was announced only four years after that of epinephrine, and Tigerstedt was no less respected than Schäfer. Yet the composition of epinephrine had been elucidated and it was believed to be the chemical transmitter of sympathetic impulses; despite the connection between the kidney and hypertension, renin had been forgotten. This anomaly has never been fully explained. However, it is worth recording that in the cat anaesthetized with urethane, Heller and I had failed to obtain pressor effects with renal extracts, and Prinzmetal and I also completely failed. Saline extracts of fresh rabbit kidney were depressor and often killed unanaesthetized rabbits; it was only when we used saline extracts of alcohol dried kidney in unanaesthetized rabbits that we achieved success. In 1938, we reported complete confirmation of Tigerstedt and Bergman's findings (*123*, *124*). The other authors who, quite independently, in that year arrived at a similar conclusion also encountered difficulties.

Landis, Montgomery, and Sparkman (*89*), using a colloid mill to grind the kidney with saline, found their extracts sometimes pressor, sometimes depressor. They observed that the mill got hot and that pressor extracts were obtained more often in summer than winter. They therefore heated saline extracts to 56°C. for twenty minutes and found that the precipitate carried with it the depressor material, leaving active pressor extracts.

Hessel, a pupil of Volhard, had with Hartwich claimed to have confirmed the existence of renin in 1932 (*73*). But their method was to autolyse renal press-juice, and their pressor material was totally unlike renin and probably consisted in a mixture of putrifactive amines. In 1938 (*72*), Hessel prepared renin whose properties agreed with those described by Tigerstedt and Bergman. Thus, by 1938 the existence and main properties of renin were firmly established.

In 1938, Fasciolo, Houssay, and Taquini had also shown that renal

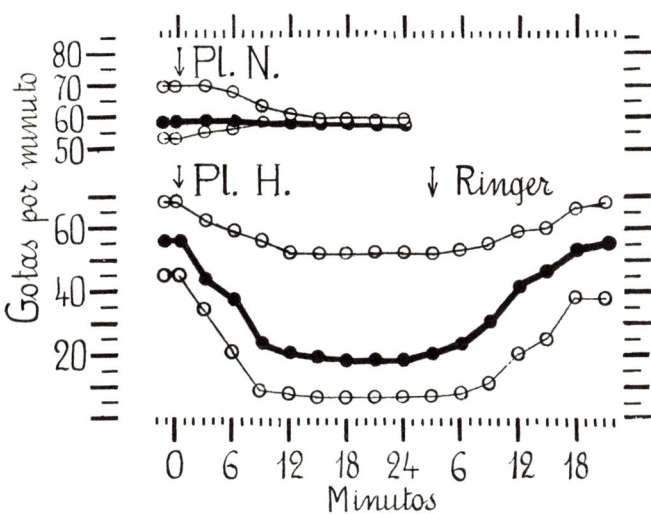

Figure 10. Vasoconstrictor action of renal venous blood from hypertensive dogs on the vascular system of the toad, according to the Läwen-Trendelenburg method. (Pl. N), venous blood plasma from normal kidneys; (Pl. H.), venous blood plasma from ischemic kidneys of hypertensive dogs. The fine lines represent the maximum and minimum vasoconstriction observed with each type of plasma; the heavy line between these limits represent the average effects.

[515]

venous blood from dogs with hypertension produced a greater vasoconstriction in the Läwen-Trendelenburg toad preparation than did that from normal dogs (*39*). In 1939, Braun-Menéndez, Fasciolo, Leloir, and Muñoz showed that the pressor substance in renal vein blood was soluble in 75 per cent acetone, was thermostable, and was dialysable (*19*). It was thus quite unlike renin. They named this substance hypertensin and went on to show that a substance having similar properties was obtained by incubating renin with plasma. Quite independently, and in the same year, Page (*105*) and Page and Helmer (*106*) had found that renin was inactive when perfused in saline through the rabbit's ear but that activity was restored by blood. They also showed that incubating renin with plasma produced a new substance which they named angiotonin. Each of these groups of workers demonstrated that in this reaction renin acts as enzyme and a plasma protein as substrate. The discoveries of 1938 and 1939 are interesting in that they show how the tide of ideas drives quite independent groups of workers to the same conclusions. And since this work is concerned with ideas, it may not be out of place to recall that I too was on the brink of joining the 1939 party. For I had been struck with the similarity in the chemical properties of renin with those of enzymes and with the slow onset and long duration of the pressor response. Yet the single anomalous observation which confronted the other workers and drove them to the truth was absent, and I made no decisive experiments.

The purification of renin has been energetically pursued by Haas, Lamfrom, and Goldblatt (*58*), but apart from its being a protein with specific chemical properties its composition is not yet known. More success has attended angiotensin (hypertensin, angiotonin). This substance has been isolated and its chemical structure ascertained by two groups of workers. In 1954, Skeggs, Marsh, Kahn, and Shumway, working at the Veterans Hospital, Cleveland, isolated two products from incubating hog renin with horse serum, hypertensin I and II (*140*). Lentz, Skeggs, Woods, Kahn, and Shumway (*91*, *139*) showed subsequently that hypertensin II consists of the following eight amino acids, in this order:

aspartic – arginine – valine – tyrosine – isoleucine – histidine – proline – phenylalanine

Hypertensin I is a decapeptide, with two additional amino acids, histidine and leucine, added to the phenylalanine end of the chain.

Skeggs, Kahn, and Shumway (*138*) have also shown that hypertensin I is inactive when perfused through the rat's kidney but is quickly broken down in plasma to hypertensin II by an enzyme which they have partially purified. The activity of hypertensin II is lost when the phenylalanine molecule is interfered with.

In 1956, Peart (*108*), working in my laboratory at St. Mary's and at Mill Hill, isolated two forms of hypertensin from ox serum incubated with rabbit renin. The more abundant was a decapeptide, and he and Elliott (*34*) showed that it had the following amino-acid composition:

aspartic – arginine – valine – tyrosine – valine – histidine – proline – phenylalanine – histidine – leucine.

Thus, the two decapeptides, isolated from horse and ox serum, respectively, are identical except for the fifth amino acid from the aspartic end. The final step was taken by Schwyzer and his colleagues, who, beginning in 1956, have synthesized both isoleucine[5] and valine[5] deca- and octa-peptides (*137*). Independently Schwarz, Bumpus, and Page synthesized the isoleucine[5] octapeptide (*136*).

Weight for weight, angiotensin is twice as active in raising arterial pressure as norepinephrine, and molecule for molecule the octapeptide is eleven times as active. It is thus by far the most powerful pressor substance known. Whether or not it is concerned in the pathogenesis of hypertension, it is, from the point of view of pure science, a substance of exceptionally great interest and promise.

Angiotensin has a rather general vasoconstrictor action similar to that of norepinephrine. It probably does not act directly on the heart. In man it raises diastolic pressure more than systolic, decreases blood flow through the hand and kidney, and decreases the glomerular filtration rate; it is markedly anti-diuretic and decreases sodium chloride output (*109*). In the dog, it is also anti-diuretic, while in the rabbit it is anti-diuretic in small doses but diuretic in large doses (*79*).

Whether or not renin plays a part in hypertension, it has always seemed probable to me that it is concerned in the economy of the normal body. The renin-hypertensin system has remarkable and unusual properties. Renin is located in, or close to, the glomerulus (*13, 25*). It seems to be released by lowering the intra-arterial pressure either locally in the kidney or generally (*62*, *80*). Renin only acts when it has entered the circulation and has released hypertensin, so that although the original release takes place in the kidney, the agent itself has equal access to all organs receiving blood. The rise of arterial pressure, like that due to norepinephrine, is effected by a vasoconstriction that is fairly uniformly spread, and owing little if anything to cardiac effect. In the rabbit and rat there is in addition an effect on renal tubular function, though this has not yet been demonstrated in dog or man. If one regards the renin-hypertensin system as part of the homeostatic mechanism of the body, and if one accepts the provisional hypothesis that the structures appreciating a change set up mechanisms that tend to oppose that change, then it would seem that the renin-hypertensin system's function would have something to do with maintaining the renal circulation and perhaps particularly intraglomerular blood pressure, on which the whole formation of urine depends (*117*). Such a suggestion is at the present stage no more than speculation. But if this hypothesis is wrong it may at least stimulate experiment that will disprove it, and in doing so substitute one that is more in accord with fact.

The observations of the Buenos Aires group in 1938 and 1939 seemed to leave little doubt that the release of renin from the kidney was the mechanism by which renal artery constriction raised arterial pressure. They went further. In 1942, Dell'Oro and Braun-Menéndez assayed the blood of the dog for renin (*30*). They were unable to demonstrate any in the blood of normal dogs, but found considerable amounts in renal venous blood and less in femoral arterial blood one or two days after constricting the renal artery. The rises in arterial pressure and of femoral artery renin produced by intravenous infusion of renin were not dissimilar. Subsequently a number of disparate facts have emerged, the most important of which is the observation of Taggart and Drury (*143*) and of Drury, Flasher, Gordon, and Dorough (*33*) that tachyphylactic extinction of the response to renin does not reduce the hypertension induced by renal artery constriction. These important observations have not yet been repeated.

The remaining controversial evidence will be found reviewed elsewhere (*119*). It may be summed up as follows. It seems extremely probable that the rise of blood pressure in the first days or weeks after renal artery constriction is due to the release of renin from the kidney. Thus the bulk of the evidence favors an increased content of renin in the renal venous blood and kidney; continuous infusion of renin produces a sustained hypertension of similar magnitude (*16*); the pressure returns to normal at a similar rate when the kidney is excised or renin infusion stopped. However, it seems clearly established that whether or not renin is concerned in the early stages, in the later stages another mechanism takes over and may be sufficient in itself to maintain the high pressure. This sequence first became clear when, by chance, it was found that, in prolonged hypertension, excision of the sole ischemic kidney did not abolish hypertension (*118*); after still longer periods, even removal of the renal artery clamp is ineffective (*28*). At this stage, those who found renin in the renal vein blood in the early stages now fail to do so (*20*); the renin content of the kidney is normal (*125*). It is possible that the new mechanism is represented by a change in the level at which the buffer nerves are set, so that they now regulate arterial pressure at a new and higher level, in the same way, and as efficiently, as they regulated it at a lower level before. The evidence for this is that the rate of discharge of impulses up the sinus nerves is approximately the same as in an animal without hypertension (*93*).

The persistence of hypertension after excision of the sole ischemic kidney at two months or more after renal artery constriction, particularly when contrasted with the quick return of the arterial pressure to normal after excision of the kidney at one week, was the first clear-cut example of what now seems a general phenomenon. In man, excision of a unilaterally diseased kidney or of a pheochromocytoma or repair of coarctation of the aorta tend to leave residual high pressures. Thus, it seems that if hypertension has lasted long enough, the removal of the original cause may not reverse it, irrespective of the nature of the prime cause. The vicious circle by which hypertension leads to renal artery disease which in turn produces hypertension, postulated by Volhard (*147*) and supported experimentally by Wilson and Byrom (*153*), is wholly inadequate to explain these phenomena. This quite unexpected behavior of the circulation—to call it an adaptation would be to avoid the issue—is one of the most challenging issues today and demonstrates clearly that the development of ideas concerning the circulation need not by any means have ended.

The Mechanism of High Blood Pressure in Man

If we look at the problem of high arterial pressure in man from the vantage point reached by our survey of experimental hypertension, it is not surprising that the main problems remain unanswered. Yet thirty years ago it seemed to the self-confident eye of a young man, trained in physiological methods, that it would be a simple matter of experimental analysis to decide which order of vessels was disturbed, the nature of the disturbance, and its proximate cause. Our failure to answer the last two of these questions is probably not entirely a matter of inadequate techniques, nor of poverty of ideas, for there have been many, but rather that as yet no one has had an idea of the right kind or size to unlock the whole complex mechanism.

Let us first take the problem of persistent hypertension as exemplified by chronic nephritis, chronic pyelonephritis, and essential hypertension. The successive methods that have been developed for measuring cardiac output have shown that this value does not systematically differ from that found in normal subjects at rest (55). Austrian found a low viscosity of the blood in nephritis (6) and the writer (114) found normal values in essential hypertension. Clearly, therefore, the elevated blood pressure is due to vascular narrowing. From Poiseuille's equation, which gives a fair idea of the dimensions involved even though it does not apply in detail to the circulation, it may be deduced that the increased resistance is due either to increased length of the resistance vessels, or to their decreased diameter. The latter assumption is universally made, though to the writer's knowledge without any valid evidence for excluding the factor of length. The vessels concerned are generally believed to be those contributing most to resistance, namely, the small arteries and arterioles (133); measurements of pressure in digital arteries (104) and capillary pressure (35) suggest that this is the case.

This can be judged by organ blood flow. The first observations directed to this end were those of Prinzmetal and Wilson (131) and the writer (114) in 1936. These authors independently showed that the blood flow through the resting forearm was of the same order in subjects with persistent hypertension as in those with normal pressures. In 1938, Grant and Pearson (53) showed that the plethysmographic method these authors had used included hand blood flow. In 1942, Abramson and

Fierst (1), eliminating the hand circulation, showed that forearm blood flow tended to be a little higher in hypertensive than in normotensive subjects and that this increase was related quantitatively to the systolic pressure. Muscle blood flow would therefore seem to be a little increased.

The blood flow through other tissues is summarized in Table I.

TABLE I
Comparison of Rates of Blood Flow Through Tissues of Normal Subject and Patient with Essential Hypertension (119)

	Normal Subject ml./min.	Patient ml./min.
Cardiac Output	5,900	5,900
Muscle	800	1,360
Kidney	1,300	800
Liver, including gut	1,400	1,400
Brain	810	810
Other organs	1,590	1,530

From this table it may be seen that at rest the pattern of organ blood flow is very similar in the subjects with persistent hypertension and those with normal blood pressures, except that muscle is better perfused and the kidney is less well perfused in those with the high pressures.

If vasoconstrictor sympathetic tone is removed from the hand vessels, the blood flow does not exceed that found in normal subjects under similar conditions (114). It is clear, then, that the hand vessels are subject to an increase in peripheral resistance of non-nervous origin, and of such an order that if generally distributed it would account for the pressures observed. Subsequent observations have shown that the same is true of the kidney (51) and the brain (67). As has been mentioned, the available evidence suggests that the baroreceptors discharge at a rate in hypertension which is not very different from that in health. It would seem, therefore, that in persistent hypertension the ordinary nervous control of the distribution of blood is superimposed on a fairly general increase of vascular resistance which is not of nervous origin.

Organic vascular narrowing is not generally regarded as a sufficient cause. In the first place, though such changes are common in all patients with raised pressures of long duration, their distribution affects the organs too unequally to account for the pattern of blood flow observed. Second, in tissues such as the forearm and the kidney, the extent of vasodilatation that can be induced is thought to be too great to be consistent with anatomical vascular narrowing. Third, in some cases, though not, as we shall see, in all, arterial pressure can be reduced to nearly normal limits by removing a unilaterally diseased kidney, or, as in Cushing's syndrome, all or most of the adrenal glands. It would be difficult to account for such a fall in any other way than by terminating a functional vascular narrowing.

The search for vaso-active substances in blood and urine has been long and arduous. Despite many alleged successes, none has stood the test of time; though it should be noted that Kahn, Skeggs, Shumway, and Wisenbaugh (*84*), who now have the isolation of hypertensin to their credit, claim to have obtained evidence of abnormal amounts of hypertensin in the blood in essential hypertension. However, Peart, who holds a similar distinction, has not yet been able to do so (personal communication).

No differences between the behavior of the circulation in chronic nephritis and essential hypertension has yet been demonstrated. Is the agent identical in the two cases? No answer can yet be given. It is, however, worthwhile to draw attention to the fact demonstrated in the last section, namely that in the rabbit, when hypertension is produced by renal artery constriction, there comes a time when removing the kidney does not abolish the hypertension. It seems that another mechanism has taken over from the kidney and is enough to maintain the pressure. There is now abundant evidence that similar events occur in man. Thus excision of a unilaterally diseased kidney reduces arterial pressure in only half of the patients, and then not fully to the expected level (*120*). Again, excision of a pheochromocytoma may leave persistent hypertension, though the urinary excretion of catechol amines returns to normal (*63*). Finally, repair of coarctation leaves a value for arterial pressure which, though reduced, is yet above that found in normal subjects of similar age (*27*). Can it be that the hypertension in both chronic nephritis and essential hypertension is maintained by some mechanism that is common to the two conditions even though the remote causes of the rise of pressure were quite different? This question cannot be answered. That it is not an irrelevant one is evident from the following small fragment of evidence. In patients with pheochromocytoma, the blood flow through the hand from which sympathetic tone has been removed is greatly reduced (*8*). A similar reduction in blood flow occurs when norepinephrine, with or without epinephrine, is infused into normal subjects. These observations are part of the consistent evidence which suggests that the hypertension in patients with pheochromocytoma is produced by the release into the blood stream of excessive amounts of these humoral substances. In those patients in whom hypertension persists after removal of the tumor, the hand circulation behaves very much as in essential hypertension and chronic nephritis, i.e. blood flow through the hand is within the normal range when vasomotor tone is abolished from the vessels of the hand.

SYSTEMIC ARTERIAL HYPERTENSION

The case of pheochromocytoma has just been mentioned. In such patients, the pattern of the circulation during an attack is different from that of essential and nephritic hypertension, and is the same as that produced by infusion of norepinephrine and epinephrine. These substances are excreted in large amounts in the urine in the disease. When the tumor or tumors are removed, the attacks cease and catechol amine excretion returns to normal. This is evidence for the raised arterial pressure during the attacks being due to the release of pressor amines from the tumor.

Acute nephritis presents a problem. Hand blood flow, with vasomotor tone off, tends to be higher during the phase of hypertension than when hypertension has subsided (*115, 5*). Moreover, the order of magnitude of the increase is that expected from the rise in pressure alone. Thus there is no evidence of non-nervous vascular narrowing. Interestingly enough, hypertensin infused into normal subjects increases arterial pressure and also increases blood flow through the hand from which nervous tone has been removed (*109*). It would seem, therefore, first, that the agent producing hypertension is not the same in acute nephritis as in chronic nephritis, and second, that in acute nephritis the pressor mechanism could involve the renin-hypertensin system. But Mahomed's evidence for the temporal precedence of hypertension over proteinuria suggests that perhaps the kidney lesion of acute nephritis is part of some as yet unidentified general vascular disturbance.

Thus, for human high blood pressure, there would seem to be at least three patterns of circulation.

BLOOD VESSELS

In the first, that of pheochromocytoma, the circulation shows changes similar to those induced by intravenous infusion of norepinephrine, and the evidence is conclusive in showing that this substance, with varying amounts of epinephrine, is discharged in excess from the tumor.

In the second, that of acute nephritis, a pressor substance is involved, and hypertensin would in some respects, at least, fill the bill.

In the third, that characteristic of essential and chronic nephritic hypertension, we have evidence of a vascular narrowing of non-nervous origin that is fairly uniformly distributed, perhaps affecting the muscle vessels rather less, and the kidney vessels rather more, than vessels elsewhere. Anatomical changes of the blood vessels may contribute to the increased resistance but are unlikely to be the sole factor concerned. An analysis of the pattern of the circulation in human hypertension, and a comparison with the patterns evoked by injection or infusion of known pressor substances, seemed the logical way to venture into the unknown when I first began working on this problem in 1930. I have no doubt that the knowledge so gained has been worth gaining. After all, is not this the essence of pure or basic or fundamental research—knowledge for its own sake? Nevertheless, such is my defection from the cause of so-called pure science that I confess I am disappointed with the harvest: I now know that no comparisons can be more than suggestive, for they differ in at least one important factor—time. As we have seen, time changes the behavior of the animal, as exemplified by the effects of excising the ischemic kidney in the rabbit (118). Assay of the relevant substances in the blood is the only valid method of answering the question.

In patients with chronic hypertension, the baroreceptors seem to have adapted to the new level of blood pressure; moreover, the absence of symptoms, even in quite severe hypertension, suggests that the mechanisms which regulate organ blood flow during activity are intact.

Genetic and Environmental Factors

The problem of classification which, as we have seen, predominated during the first century of our story, was an essential preliminary to the study of mechanism and of the genetic and environmental factors concerned in causation. However, classifications exercise a fascination all their own. Once a label has been fixed to a patient, treatment and prognosis are a matter of routine. Lists of causes have also been a popular method of assessing a candidate's competence and thus are a popular vehicle of teaching. It has become implicit in the minds of teachers and students that each of these "diseases" represents a specific morbid entity with a unique or "specific" cause.

SYSTEMIC ARTERIAL HYPERTENSION

Such is the background to our present account of the evolution of ideas concerning genetic and environmental factors in the pathogenesis of "essential hypertension," which in simple terms signifies a group of patients who have high pressures without a specific organ lesion to which the cause of this high pressure can be assigned.

The first really careful study of epidemiological factors in essential hypertension was that of Wilhelm Weitz in 1923, then in charge of the Polyklinik at Tübingen (*150*). Weitz studied 82 patients in whom a diagnosis of essential hypertension had been made and 267 patients of similar age attending for complaints other than cardiovascular ones. He was able to exclude environmental causes which were then held to be important. For example, hard physical work seemed to have no relevance. He found no undue tendency to elevated pressures in psychotic patients. Tobacco and alcohol were excluded by the occurrence of the disease in women (who in those days, in that part of the world, did not smoke) and by its lack of association with the habitual drunkards well known to the hospital authorities. He was able to identify only one factor, inheritance. He found a family history of death from stroke or heart disease in 76.8 per cent of the parents of his patients with hypertension but only in 30.3 per cent of the parents of his controls. Recognizing the possible fallacies in family history, he measured the arterial pressures in 93 brothers and sisters of patients with essential hypertension and in 359 controls of similar age. He found the percentage of subjects with hypertension increased with age but, for a given age, was greater in the patients' relatives than in the controls. He argued that essential hypertension was a condition which manifested itself with age, and that it became apparent at different ages in different families. Accepting 160 mm. Hg as the dividing line between normal and abnormal, and restricting himself to siblings who were older than the patient, and in whom the disease should have appeared if it were going to, he found that half had pressures above and half had pressures below 160 mm. Hg, giving a ratio between

BLOOD VESSELS

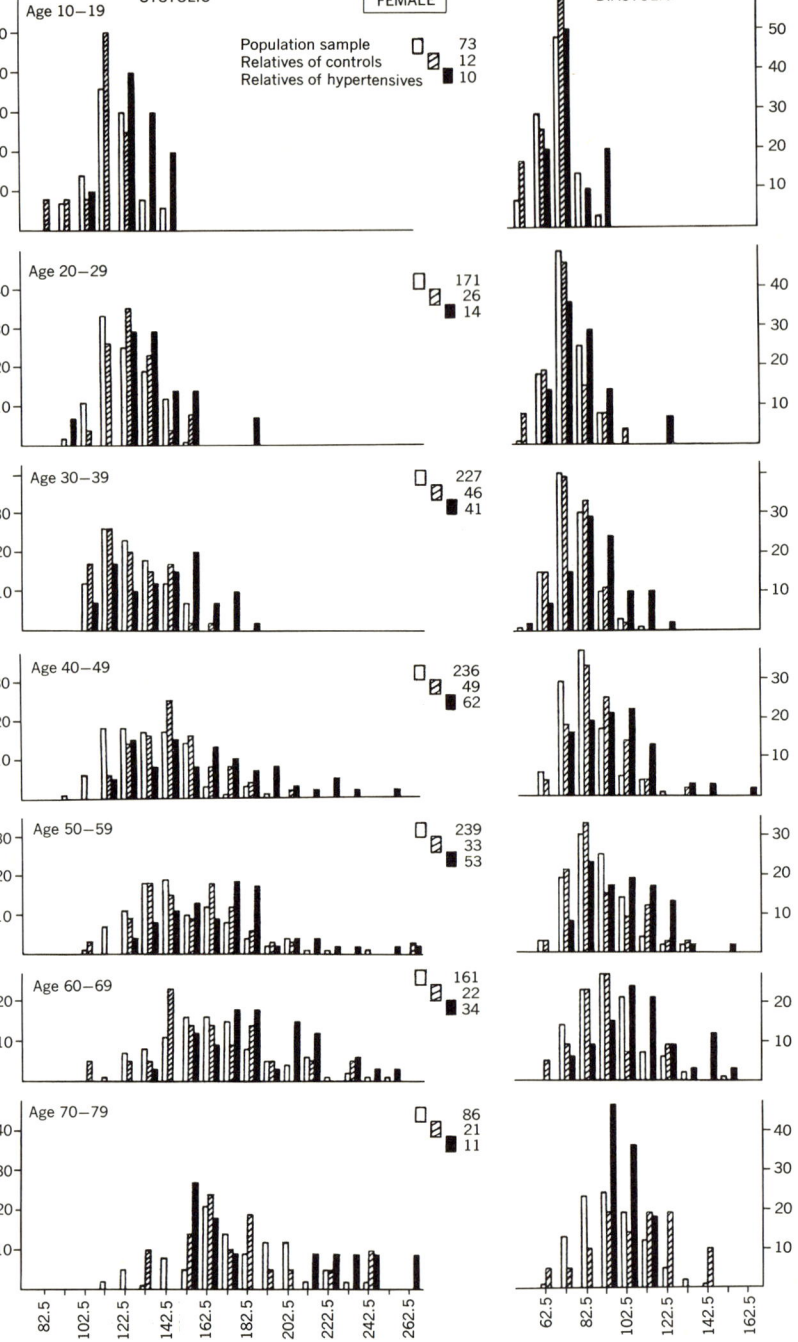

affected and unaffected of 1 to 1. This is the ratio which would be expected if the disease were inherited as a Mendelian dominant, a conclusion reinforced by its appearance in three successive generations. Weitz's facts were confirmed, with his conclusions of Mendelian dominant inheritance supported, by Robert Platt (*127*) of Manchester, who studied family histories, and by Søbye, from Tage Kemp's department of genetics at Copenhagen, who measured arterial pressure in relatives and controls (*141*).

It is difficult to exaggerate the theoretical importance of such a conclusion. In the first place, the presence or absence of the disease would be determined primarily by events taking place at the time of union of sperm and ovum. In the second place, since it is believed that a single gene controls the synthesis of specific enzyme molecules, Mendelian dominant inheritance would imply a specific chemical abnormality, the identification of which would be largely a matter of ingenuity, luck, and perseverance. However, a critical appraisal of the evidence showed it to be far from watertight. Family histories contain several sources of error and in fact guide to vascular disease rather than to hypertension. The blood pressure surveys were scarcely adequate, in that the study of the population at large had been rather cursory and no study of control relatives had been made.

These considerations induced Hamilton, Pickering, Roberts, and Sowry (*64, 65, 66*) to seek more conclusive evidence. It seemed clear that measurement of arterial pressure was the only valid observation. A single measurement under, as far as possible, comparable circumstances was therefore made in three groups of subjects: (1) a sample of the population at large, believed to be representative; (2) first degree relatives of patients with essential hypertension; and (3) first degree relatives of patients without essential hypertension. It took approximately two years

---

Figure 11. Frequency distribution of systolic and diastolic pressures for females in the second to eighth decades of the three samples. *White rectangles:* population sample; *hatched rectangles:* first degree relatives of propositi without hypertension; *black rectangles:* the first degree relatives of propositi with hypertension. The pressures are arranged in groups of 10 mm. Hg. The height of each rectangle denotes the percentage of subjects in that decade of each sample having that range of pressure. The figures in the center show the number of subjects in each decade.

BLOOD VESSELS

to gather the data. Their analysis and interpretation took another two years, since the final conclusion was, for this subject and at that time, revolutionary; though, as we shall see, it might have been anticipated from general biological principles.

The results were briefly as follows. In the population sample, the frequency distribution curves of arterial pressure gradually move upward and spread out as age advances. At no age is there a clear division, or even a suggestion of a division, into "normal" and "high" at 160 mm. Hg systolic or at any other pressure. This point is more clearly brought out in the studies made by Bøe and others on the bulk of the inhabitants of Bergen (*18*); with blood pressure plotted on a logarithmic scale the frequency distribution curves are essentially normal.

The frequency distribution curves for arterial pressure in the relatives of subjects without hypertension are indistinguishable from those of the population sample. Those for relatives of subjects with essential hypertension are similar in shape but are shifted upwards (to the right); moreover, they are shifted by about the same amount at all ages. In fact, blood pressure rises with age at the same rate in the relatives of subjects with hypertension as in the rest of the population, but the relatives tend to have higher pressures at all ages. By adopting Fraser Roberts's suggestion of a "score" to adjust for the effects of age and sex on the population at large, it was found that the greater the deviation of the patient's blood

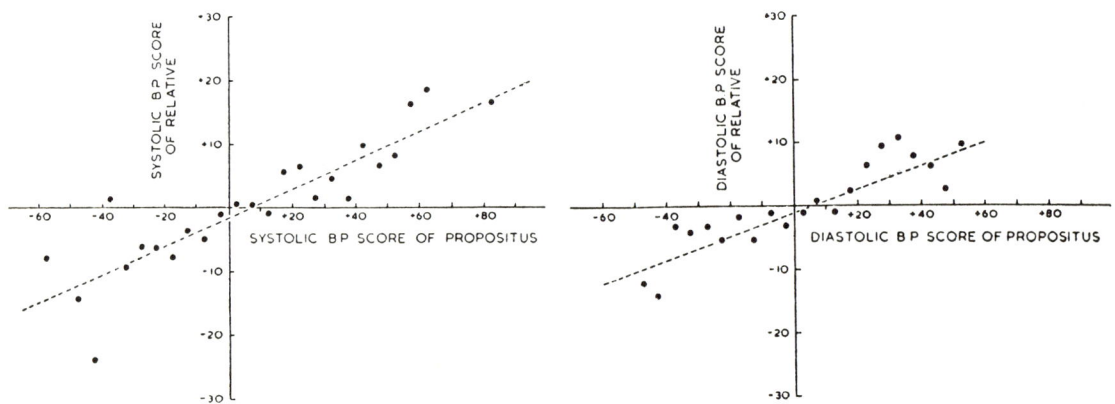

Figure 12. Relationship between blood pressure scores of relatives and of propositi. *Left:* Systolic scores. *Right:* Diastolic scores.

pressure from the norm for that age and sex in the population sample, the greater was the average deviation of the blood pressure of their first degree relatives. This suggested that it was not hypertension itself but the degree of hypertension that was inherited.

These observations have received a very important extension by Miall and Oldham (*101, 102*). They took as propositi a one in ninety sample of the population of a Welsh mining valley and measured their blood pressures and those of their first degree relatives. Later they did the same in a Welsh agricultural valley. Using the same age-adjusted score, they showed that there is a linear relationship between blood pressures of relatives and blood pressures of propositi. Moreover, the regression coefficient of blood pressure of relatives on those of propositi, about 0.2, was almost exactly the same as Hamilton and others had found in their hypertensive families. It seems that blood pressure is inherited as a graded character over the whole blood pressure range, whether this has hitherto been regarded as hypotension, normotension, or hypertension.

These results are similar to those found by Francis Galton for height

SYSTEMIC ARTERIAL HYPERTENSION

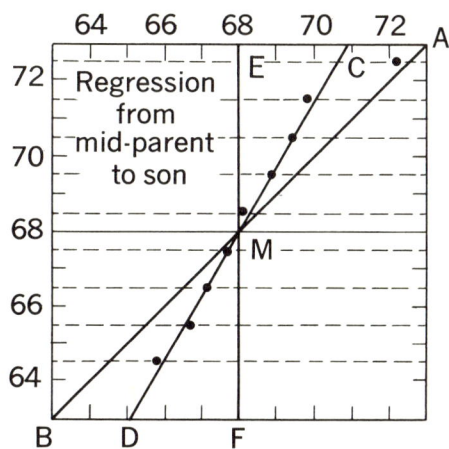

Figure 13. Stature of mid-parent (up) plotted against mean heights of their children. Female height adjusted to male by multiplying by 1.08. AB would be the expected line if heights of children were identical with those of parents. The line CD is 2/3 of the distance towards it.

"*The value of two-thirds will therefore be accepted as the amount of the Regression, on the average of many cases, from the Mid-Parental to the Mid-Filial stature, whatever the Mid-Parental stature may be.*"

(*42*), which he showed is inherited as a graded character over the whole range ordinarily met. He, too, had to make adjustments because of sex differences, though height is unaffected by age from maturity to senility. Figure 13 shows the relationship he found between heights of midparent (mean of father's and adjusted mother's heights) and the mean heights of their children.

Now the resemblance between first degree relatives is greater for height than for blood pressure, the regression coefficients being about 0.4 and 0.2, respectively. The discrepancy is partly accounted for by diurnal variability in blood pressure. But, since it is thought that environmental factors (particularly nutrition) partly determine height, it seems also likely that environmental factors partly determine blood pressure. It is one of the great future tasks of epidemiology to find out what these environmental factors are and to try and assess their contributions. From what was said earlier, the factors most naturally suspect are those which greatly raise arterial pressure, such as those which operate through the mind.

Miall and Oldham's recent careful studies (*102*) have provided suggestive evidence that, in a given population, arterial pressure tends to be lower in those who do heavy work than in those who do light work, and to be lower in both men and women with large families than in those with small. These observations are directly contrary to the advice commonly tendered by doctors, in all ignorance, to patients. To an admirer of the late Wilfred Trotter, this again poses his question: "Has the Intellect a Function?"

From the standpoint of biometrics, there are no such entities as "normotension" and "hypertension" any more than there are entities for height of "normomacria" and "hypermacria." (These would be the words which doctors educated in the Greek tongue would have used to express heights below and above, say, 5 feet 9 inches, if they had found any correlation between height and mortality.) In fact, just as there are people of short, medium, and tall stature, so there are people with low, medium, and high blood pressure. In both cases, inheritance is concerned, and in both the inheritance is graded. In height, age is only concerned during youth and old age; in blood pressure, it is concerned throughout. Environmental factors are concerned in both, though the actual factors are almost certainly quite different in the two instances.

However, the main differences between height and arterial pressure are in their effects. Height has not much influence on expectation of life, nor are very tall people particularly susceptible to disease, except possibly pulmonary tuberculosis. On the other hand, high blood pressure carries a decreased expectation of life. Here, too, the relationship is quantitative or graded (*119*). High blood pressure is also associated with cardiac hypertrophy and a variety of vascular diseases. Again the relationship is quantitative. But, at the highest pressures a new vascular lesion appears, the acute fibrinoid arteriolar necrosis that characterizes and determines the malignant phase. These relationships between blood pressure, heart size, and type and kind of vascular disease seem to be the same whatever the underlying cause of the raised pressure, bearing in mind of course that age is also a factor in producing vascular disease and that certain diseases such as pyelonephritis also are associated with their own particular vascular lesions in the kidney.

Conclusion

It seems that high blood pressure may be provoked in a variety of ways; for example, by a disturbance of the kidneys, by a disturbance in the adrenal cortex (Cushing's syndrome) and by overproduction of norepinephrine and epinephrine (pheochromocytoma). In the last instance alone have we a detailed understanding of mechanism. In addition to these specific disturbances, genetic and environmental factors also determine arterial pressure, and they would seem to be the chief, or the only, factors concerned in the etiology of primary or essential hypertension. The environmental factors concerned have not yet been fully identified; the magnitude of their contribution is unknown. Inheritance seems to be graded as it is in height, and its contribution can be assigned a probability value. Moreover, it seems that whatever the cause, high blood pressure, once initiated, tends to be self-perpetuating, through a mechanism that is not fully apparent. Finally, it would seem that, in its effects on the circulation, high blood pressure acts in a graded or quantitative manner, until the highest pressures are reached, when a new set of phenomena, those of the malignant phase, become manifest.

This account will have served its purpose if it has illustrated how a consideration of the so-called abnormal may display gaps in knowledge that will not be appreciated if scientific method is confined to a consideration of so-called normal behavior. In other words, it may illustrate that knowledge is unitary. It may also illustrate that the proper distinction between pure and applied science is not so much the range or kind of knowledge, but that in pure science knowledge is won, in applied science it is used.

BIBLIOGRAPHY

1. ABRAMSON, D. I., and S. M. FIERST. Resting blood flow and peripheral vascular responses in hypertensive subjects. Amer. Heart J., 23:84, 1942.
2. ALLBUTT, T. C. Senile plethora or high arterial pressure in elderly persons. Abstr. Trans. Hunter. Soc., 77:38, 1895.
3. ALLBUTT, T. C. Diseases of the Arteries Including Angina Pectoris. London, Macmillan, 1915.
4. ALPERT, L. K., A. S. ALVING, and K. S. GRIMSON. Effect of total sympathectomy on experimental renal hypertension in dogs. Proc. Soc. exp. Biol., 37:1, 1937.
5. ARNOTT, W. M., and G. D. MATTHEW. The nature of the arteriolar hypertonicity in acute glomerulo-nephritis. Quart. J. Med., N.S., 8:353, 1939.
6. AUSTRIAN, C. H. The viscosity of the blood in health and disease. Johns Hopk. Hosp. Bull., 22:9, 1911.
7. BACQ, Z. M., L. BROUHA, and C. HEYMANS. Recherches sur la physiologie et la pharmacologie du système nerveux autonome. VII. Réflexes vasomoteurs d'origine sino-carotidienne et actions pharmacologiques chez le chat et chez le chien sympathectomisés. Arch. int. Pharmacodyn., 48:429, 1934.
8. BARNETT, A. J., R. B. BLACKET, A. E. DEPOORTER, P. H. SANDERSON, and G. M. WILSON. The action of noradrenaline in man and its relation to phaeochromocytoma and hypertension. Clin. Sci., 9:151, 1950.
9. BARTELS, C. Structural diseases of the kidney and the general symptoms of renal affections. In H. von Ziemssen, Ed. Cyclopaedia of the Practice of Medicine. Tr. by R. Southey and R. Bertolet. Vol. 15, p. 3. London, Sampson Low, 1877.
10. BASCH, S. VON. Ueber latente Arteriosclerose und deren Beziehung zu Fettleibigkeit, Herzerkrankungen und anderen Begleiterscheinungen. Vienna, Urban and Schwartzenberg, 1893.
11. BATTY SHAW, A. Frederick Akhbar Mahomed and his contribution to the study of Bright's disease. Guy's Hosp. Rep., 101:153, 1952.
12. BELL, E. T. The pathological anatomy in primary hypertension. In

E. T. Bell, Ed. Hypertension, p. 183. Minneapolis, University of Minnesota Press, 1951.
13. BING, J., and B. WIBERG. Localisation of renin in the kidney. Acta path. microbiol. scand., 44:138, 1958.
14. BINGEL, A., and R. CLAUS. Weitere Untersuchungen über die blutdrucksteigernde Substanz der Niere. Dtsch. Arch. klin. Med., 100:412, 1910.
15. BINGEL, A., and E. STRAUSS. Ueber die blutdrucksteigernde Substanz der Niere. Dtsch. Arch. klin. Med., 96:476, 1909.
16. BLACKET, R. B., A. DEPOORTER, G. W. PICKERING, A. L. SELLERS, and G. M. WILSON. Hypertension produced in the rabbit by long continued infusions of renin. Clin. Sci., 9:223, 1950.
17. BLALOCK, A., and S. E. LEVY. Studies on the etiology of renal hypertension. Ann. Surg. 106:826, 1937.
18. BØE, J., S. HUMERFELT, and F. WEDERVANG. The blood pressure in a population. Acta med. scand., suppl. 321, 1957.
19. BRAUN-MENÉNDEZ, E., J. C. FASCIOLO, L. F. LELOIR, and J. M. MUÑOZ. La substancia hipertensora de la sangre del rinon isquemiado. Rev. Soc. argent. Biol., 15:420, 1939.
20. BRAUN-MENÉNDEZ, E., J. C. FASCIOLO, L. F. LELOIR, J. M. MUÑOZ, and A. C. TAQUINI. Renal Hypertension. Tr. by L. Dexter. Springfield, Ill., Thomas, 1946.
21. BRIGHT, R. Reports of Medical Cases Selected with a View of Illustrating the Symptoms and Cure of Diseases by a Reference to Morbid Anatomy, 2 vols. London, Longman, 1827.
22. BRIGHT, R. Tabular view of the morbid appearances in 100 cases connected with albuminous urine. With observations. Guy's Hosp. Rep., 1:380, 1836.
23. BURDON-SANDERSON, J. Handbook of the Sphygmograph. London, Hardwicke, 1867.
24. CHILD, C. G. Observations on the pathological changes following experimental hypertension produced by constriction of the renal artery. J. exp. Med., 67:521, 1938.
25. COOK, W. F., and G. W. PICKERING. The location of renin within the kidney. J. Physiol. (Lond.), 143:78P, 1958.
26. COOKE, W. T., P. C. P. CLOAKE, A. D. T. GOVAN, and J. C. COLBECK. Temporal arteritis: a generalized vascular disease. Quart. J. Med., N.S., 15:47, 1946.
27. COUNIHAN, T. B. Changes in the blood pressure following resection of coarctation of the aortic arch. Clin. Sci., 15:149, 1956.
28. DANIEL, P. M., M. M. L. PRICHARD, and J. N. WARD-MCQUAID. Removal of the clip on the renal artery in rabbits with experimental chronic hypertension. Quart. J. exp. Physiol., 39:101, 1954.

BLOOD VESSELS

29. Davson, J., J. Ball, and R. Platt. The kidney in periarteritis nodosa. Quart. J. Med., N.S., 17:175, 1948.
30. Dell'Oro, E., and E. Braun-Menéndez. Dosaje de renina en la sangre de perros hipertensos por isquemia renal. Rev. Soc. argent. Biol., 18:65, 1942.
31. Derow, H. A., and M. D. Altschule. Malignant hypertension. New Engl. J. Med., 213:951, 1935.
32. Derow, H. A., and M. D. Altschule. The nature of malignant hypertension. Ann. intern. Med., 14:1768, 1941.
33. Drury, D. R., J. Flasher, D. B. Gordon, and M. E. Dorough. Renin substrate and renal hypertension, including a one-stage method for evisceration in the rabbit. Amer. J. Physiol., 164:630, 1951.
34. Elliott, D. F., and W. S. Peart. Amino-acid sequence in a hypertensin. Nature, 177:527, 1956.
35. Ellis, L. B., and S. Weiss. The measurement of capillary pressure under natural conditions and after arteriolar dilatation; in normal subjects and in patients with arterial hypertension and with arteriosclerosis. J. clin. Invest., 8:47, 1929.
36. Ewald, C. A. Ueber die Veränderungen kleiner Gefässe bei Morbus Brightii und die darauf bezüglichen Theorien. Virchows Arch. path. Anat., 71:453, 1877.
37. Fahr, T. Ueber Nephrosklerose. Virchows Arch. path. Anat., 226:119, 1919.
38. Faivre, J. Études expérimentales sur les lésions organiques du coeur. Gaz. méd. Paris, 11:712, 1856.
39. Fasciolo, J. C., B. A. Houssay, and A. C. Taquini. The blood-pressure raising secretion of the ischaemic kidney. J. Physiol. (Lond.), 94:281, 1938.
40. Frank, E. Bestehen Beziehungen zwischen chromaffinem System und der chronischen Hypertonie des Menschen? Ein kritischer Beitrag zu der Lehre von der physio-pathologischen Bedeutung des Adrenalins. Dtsch. Arch. klin. Med., 103:397, 1911.
41. Freeman, N. E., and I. H. Page. Hypertension produced by constriction of the renal artery in sympathectomized dogs. Amer. Heart J., 14:405, 1937.
42. Galton, F. Natural Inheritance. London, Macmillan, 1889.
43. Gammon, G. D. The carotid sinus reflex in patients with hypertension. J. clin. Invest., 15:153, 1936.
44. Glenn, F., C. G. Child, and G. J. Heuer. Production of hypertension by constricting the artery of a single transplanted kidney; an experimental investigation. Ann. Surg., 106:848, 1937.

45. GOLDBLATT, H. Studies on experimental hypertension. V. The pathogenesis of experimental hypertension due to renal ischemia. Ann. intern. Med., 11:69, 1937.
46. GOLDBLATT, H. Studies on experimental hypertension. VII. The production of the malignant phase of hypertension. J. exp. Med., 67:809, 1938.
47. GOLDBLATT, H. Studies on experimental hypertension. XII. The experimental production and pathogenesis of hypertension due to renal ischemia. Amer. J. clin. Path., 10:40, 1940.
48. GOLDBLATT, H. The renal origin of hypertension. Physiol. Rev., 27:120, 1947.
49. GOLDBLATT, H., J. LYNCH, R. F. HANZAL, and W. W. SUMMERVILLE. Studies on experimental hypertension. I. The production of persistent elevation of systolic blood pressure by means of renal ischemia. J. exp. Med., 59:347, 1934.
50. GOLDRING, W., and H. CHASIS. Hypertension and Hypertensive Disease. New York, Commonwealth Fund, 1944.
51. GOLDRING, W., H. CHASIS, H. A. RANGES, and H. W. SMITH. Effective renal blood flow in subjects with essential hypertension. J. clin. Invest., 20:637, 1941.
52. GRAEFE, A. VON. Nachträgliche Bemerkung über Sclerotico-chorioideitis posterior. Albrecht v. Graefes Arch. Ophthal., 1 (2. Abt.), 307, 1854–55.
53. GRANT, R. T., and R. S. B. PEARSON. The blood circulation in the human limb; observations on the differences between the proximal and distal parts and remarks on the regulation of body temperature. Clin. Sci., 3:119, 1938.
54. GRANT, R. T., and P. ROTHSCHILD. A device for estimating blood-pressure in the rabbit. J. Physiol. (Lond.), 81:265, 1934.
55. GROLLMAN, A. The Cardiac Output of Man in Health and Disease. London, Bailliere, Tindall and Cox, 1932.
56. GULL, W. W. Chronic Bright's disease with contracted kidney (arterio-capillary fibrosis). Brit. med. J., II:673, 1872.
57. GULL, W. W., and H. G. SUTTON. On the pathology of the morbid state commonly called chronic Bright's disease with contracted kidney. ("Arterio-capillary fibrosis"). Med.-chir. Trans., 55:273, 1872.
58. HAAS, E., H. LAMFROM, and H. GOLDBLATT. Isolation and purification of hog renin. Arch. Biochem., 42:368, 1953.
59. HALE-WHITE, W. Richard Bright and his discovery of the disease bearing his name. Guy's Hosp. Rep., 1:1, 1921.
60. HALES, S. Statical Essays: vol. 1, Containing Vegetable Staticks; or an Account of Some Statical Experiments on the Sap in Vegetables. London, Innys and Manby, 1731.

61. HALES, S. Statical Essays: vol. 2, Containing Haemastaticks; or an Account of Some Hydraulick and Hydrostatical Experiments made on the Blood and Blood-vessels of animals. London, Innys and Manby, 1733.
62. HAMILTON, A. S., and D. A. COLLINS. The homeostatic rôle of a renal humoral mechanism in hemorrhage and shock. Amer. J. Physiol., 136:275, 1942.
63. HAMILTON, M., J. W. LITCHFIELD, W. S. PEART, and G. S. C. SOWRY. Phaeochromocytoma. Brit. Heart J., 15:241, 1953.
64. HAMILTON, M., G. W. PICKERING, J. A. F. ROBERTS, and G. S. C. SOWRY. The aetiology of essential hypertension. 1. The arterial pressure in the general population. Clin. Sci., 13:11, 1954.
65. HAMILTON, M., G. W. PICKERING, J. A. F. ROBERTS, and G. S. C. SOWRY. The aetiology of essential hypertension. 2. Scores for arterial blood pressures adjusted for differences in age and sex. Clin. Sci., 13:37, 1954.
66. HAMILTON, M., G. W. PICKERING, J. A. F. ROBERTS, and G. S. C. SOWRY. The aetiology of essential hypertension. 4. The role of inheritance. Clin. Sci., 13:273, 1954.
67. HARMEL, M. H., J. H. HAFKENSCHIEL, G. M. AUSTIN, C. W. CRUMPTON, and S. S. KETY. The effect of bilateral stellate ganglion block on the cerebral circulation in normotensive and hypertensive patients. J. clin. Invest., 28:415, 1949.
68. HARRISON, T. R., A. BLALOCK, and M. F. MASON. Effects on blood pressure of injection of kidney extracts of dogs with renal hypertension. Proc. Soc. exp. Biol. (N.Y.), 35:38, 1936.
69. HARVEY, W. Exercitatio anatomica de motu cordis et sanguinis in animalibus. Frankfurt. W. Fitzeri. 1628.
70. HERING, H. E. Die Karotissinusreflexe auf Herz und Gefässe vom normal-physiologischen, pathologisch-physiologischen und klinischen Standpunkt. Dresden, Steinkopff, 1927.
71. HÉRISSON, J. Le Sphygmomètre: Instrument qui traduit à l'oeil toute l'action des artères. Paris, Crochard, 1834.
72. HESSEL, G. Über Renin. Klin. Wschr., 17:843, 1938.
73. HESSEL, G., and A. HARTWICH. Experimentelle Untersuchungen zur Kreislaufwirkung Korpereigener Stoffe; chemische Eigenschaften des blutdrucksteigernden Prinzips in Nierenautolysaten. Zbl. inn. Med., 53:626, 1932.
74. HEYMANS, C., and J. J. BOUCKAERT. Modifications de la pression artérielle après section des quatre nerfs frénateurs chez le chien. C.R. Soc. Biol. (Paris), 117:252, 1934.
75. HEYMANS, C., J. J. BOUCKAERT, L. ELAUT, F. BAYLESS, and A. SAMAAN. Hypertension artérielle chronique par ischémie rénale chez le chien totalement sympathectomisé. C.R. Soc. Biol. (Paris), 126:434, 1937.

76. HEYMANS, C., J. J. BOUCKAERT, and P. REGNIERS. Le sinus carotidien et la zone homologue cardio-aortique. Paris, Doin, 1933.
77. HOUSSAY, B. A., and A. C. TAQUINI. Actión vasoconstrictora de la sangre venosa del rinon isquemlado. Rev. Soc. argent. Biol., 14:5, 1938.
78. HUCHARD, H. Maladies du coeur et des vaisseaux. Paris, Doin, 1889.
79. HUGHES-JONES, N. C., G. W. PICKERING, P. H. SANDERSON, H. SCARBOROUGH, and J. VANDENBROUCKE. The nature of the action of renin and hypertensin on renal function in the rabbit. J. Physiol. (Lond.), 109:288, 1949.
80. HUIDOBRO, F., and E. BRAUN-MENÉNDEZ. The secretion of renin by the intact kidney. Amer. J. Physiol., 137:47, 1942.
81. JANEWAY, T. C. A clinical study of hypertensive cardiovascular disease. Arch. intern. Med., 12:755, 1913.
82. JOHNSON, G. I. On certain points in the anatomy and pathology of Bright's disease of the kidney. II. On the influence of the minute blood-vessels upon the circulation. Med.-chir. Trans., 51:57, 1868.
83. JORES, L. Ueber die Arteriosklerose der kleinen Organarterien und ihre Beziehungen zur Nephritis. Virchows Arch. path. Anat., 178:367, 1904.
84. KAHN, J. R., L. T. SKEGGS, JR., N. P. SHUMWAY, and P. E. WISENBAUGH. The assay of hypertensin from the arterial blood of normotensive and hypertensive human beings. J. exp. Med., 95:523, 1952.
85. KINCAID-SMITH, P., J. MCMICHAEL, and E. A. MURPHY. The clinical course and pathology of hypertension with papilloedema (malignant hypertension). Quart. J. Med., 27:17, 1958.
86. KOCH, E., and H. MIES. Chronischer arterieller Hochdruck durch experimentelle Dauerausschaltung der Blutdruckzügler. Krankheitsforschung, 7:241, 1929.
87. KOROTKOFF, N. S. On methods of studying blood pressure. Izv. voennomed. Akad., 11:365, 1905.
88. KROGH, A. The Anatomy and Physiology of Capillaries. Rev. ed. London, Oxford University Press, 1929.
89. LANDIS, E. M., H. MONTGOMERY, and D. SPARKMAN. The effects of pressor drugs and of saline kidney extracts on blood pressure and skin temperature. J. clin. Invest., 17:189, 1938.
90. VAN LEERSUM, E. C. Eine Methode zur Erleichterung der Blutdruckmessung bei Tieren. Arch. ges. Physiol., 142:377, 1911.
91. LENTZ, K. E., L. T. SKEGGS, K. R. WOODS, J. R. KAHN, and N. P. SHUMWAY. The amino acid composition of hypertensin II and its biochemical relationship to hypertensin I. J. exp. Med., 104:183, 1956.
92. LIEBREICH, R. Ophthalmoskopischer Befund bei morbus Brightii. v. Graefes Arch. Ophthal., 5:265, 1859.

BLOOD VESSELS

93. McCubbin, J. W., J. H. Green, and I. H. Page. Baroceptor function in chronic renal hypertension. Circulation Res., 4:205, 1956.
94. Mahomed, F. A. The physiology and clinical use of the sphygmograph. Med. Times & Gaz., 1:62, 1872.
95. Mahomed, F. A. The etiology of Bright's disease and the pre-albuminuric stage. Med.-chir. Trans., 57:197, 1874.
96. Mahomed, F. A. 3. On the sphygmographic evidence of arterio-capillary fibrosis. Trans. path. Soc., 28:394, 1877.
97. Mahomed, F. A. Some of the clinical aspects of chronic Bright's disease. Guy's Hosp. Rep., 3rd ser., 24:363, 1879.
98. Mahomed, F. A. On chronic Bright's disease, and its essential symptoms. Lancet, I:46, 1879.
99. Mahomed, F. A. Chronic Bright's disease without albuminuria. Guy's Hosp. Rep., 3rd ser., 25:295, 1881.
100. Marey, E. J. Physiologie médicale de la circulation du sang,... Paris, Delahaye, 1863.
101. Miall, W. E., and P. D. Oldham. A study of arterial pressure and its inheritance in a sample of the general population. Clin. Sci., 14:459, 1955.
102. Miall, W. E., and P. D. Oldham. Factors influencing arterial blood pressure in the general population. Clin. Sci., 17:409, 1958.
103. Moritz, A. R., and M. R. Oldt. Arteriolar sclerosis in hypertensive and non-hypertensive individuals. Amer. J. Path., 13:679, 1937.
104. Oppenheimer, E. T., and M. Prinzmetal. Role of the arteries in the peripheral resistance of hypertension and related states. Arch. intern. Med., 60:772, 1937.
105. Page, I. H. On the nature of the pressor action of renin. J. exp. Med., 70:521, 1939.
106. Page, I. H., and O. M. Helmer. A crystalline pressor substance (angiotonin) resulting from the reaction between renin and renin-activator. J. exp. Med., 71:29, 1940.
107. Pears, M. A., and G. W. Pickering. Changes in the fundus oculi after haemorrhage. Quart. J. Med., N.S. 29:153, 1960.
108. Peart, W. S. The isolation of a hypertensin. Biochem. J., 62:520, 1956.
109. Peart, W. S., G. W. Pickering, and P. H. Sanderson. Unpublished data.
110. Perera, G. A. Development of hypertensive manifestations after the disappearance of hypertension. Circulation, 10:28, 1954.
111. Perera, G. A. The accelerated form of hypertensin—a unique entity? Trans. Assoc. Amer. Physic., 71:62, 1958.
112. Pettigrew, T. J. Medical Portrait Gallery. London, Fischer, 1838–40.
113. Pickering, G. W. The cerebrospinal fluid pressure in arterial hypertension. Clin. Sci., 1:397, 1934.

114. PICKERING, G. W. The peripheral resistance in persistent arterial hypertension. Clin. Sci., 2:209, 1936.
115. PICKERING, G. W. Observations on the mechanism of arterial hypertension in acute nephritis. Clin. Sci., 2:363, 1936.
116. PICKERING, G. W. The relationship of benign and malignant hypertension. J. Mt. Sinai Hosp., 8:916, 1942.
117. PICKERING, G. W. The circulation in arterial hypertension. Lecture I. Brit. med. J., II:1, 1943.
118. PICKERING, G. W. The role of the kidney in acute and chronic hypertension following renal artery constriction in the rabbit. Clin. Sci., 5:229, 1945.
119. PICKERING, G. W. High Blood Pressure. London, Churchill, 1955.
120. PICKERING, G. W., and R. H. HEPTINSTALL. Nephrectomy and other treatment for hypertension in pyelonephritis. Quart. J. Med., N.S., 22:1, 1953.
121. PICKERING, G. W., and M. KISSIN. The effects of adrenaline and of cold on the blood pressure in human hypertension. Clin. Sci., 2:201, 1936.
122. PICKERING, G. W., M. KISSIN, and P. ROTHSCHILD. The relationship of the carotid sinus mechanism to persistent high blood pressure in man. Clin. Sci., 2:193, 1936.
123. PICKERING, G. W., and M. PRINZMETAL. Some observations on renin, a pressor substance contained in normal kidney, together with a method for its biological assay. Clin. Sci., 3:211, 1938.
124. PICKERING, G. W., and M. PRINZMETAL. Experimental hypertension of renal origin in the rabbit. Clin. Sci., 3:357, 1938.
125. PICKERING, G. W., M. PRINZMETAL, and A. R. KELSALL. The assay of renin in rabbits with experimental renal hypertension. Clin. Sci., 4:401, 1942.
126. PICKERING, G. W., A. D. WRIGHT, and R. H. HEPTINSTALL. The reversibility of malignant hypertension. Lancet, II:952, 1952.
127. PLATT, R. Heredity in hypertension. Quart. J. Med., N.S., 16:111, 1947.
128. POISEUILLE, J. L. M. Recherches sur la force du coeur aortique. Paris, Didot, 1828.
129. POISEUILLE, J. L. M. Recherches expérimentales sur la mouvement des liquides dans les tubes des très petits diamètres. Mem. Acad. Sci. (Paris), 9:433, 1846.
130. PRINZMETAL, M., and B. FRIEDMAN. Pressor effects of kidney extracts from patients and dogs with hypertension. Proc. Soc. exp. Biol. (N.Y.), 35:122, 1936.
131. PRINZMETAL, M., and C. WILSON. The nature of the peripheral resistance in arterial hypertension with special reference to the vasomotor system. J. clin. Invest., 15:63, 1936.

BLOOD VESSELS

132. RECKLINGHAUSEN, H. VON. Ueber Blutdruckmessung beim Menschen. Arch. exp. Path. Pharmak., 46:78, 1901.
133. REIN, H. Vasomotorische Regulationen. Ergebn. Physiol., 32:28, 1931.
134. RIVA-ROCCI, S. Un nuovo sfigmomanometro. Gazz. med. Torino, 47:981, 1896.
135. ROTHSCHUH, K. E. Geschichte der Physiologie. Berlin, Springer, 1953.
136. SCHWARZ, H., F. M. BUMPUS, and I. H. PAGE. Synthesis of a biologically active octapeptide similar to natural isoleucine angiotonin octapeptide. J. Amer. Chem. Soc., 79:5697, 1957.
137. SCHWYZER, R. Synthese von Polypeptidwirkstoffen. Chimia, 12:53, 1958.
138. SKEGGS, L., JR., J. R. KAHN, and N. P. SHUMWAY. The preparation and function of the hypertensin-converting enzyme. J. exp. Med., 103:295, 1956.
139. SKEGGS, L., JR., K. I. LENTZ, J. R. KAHN, N. P. SHUMWAY, and K. R. WOODS. The amino acid sequence of hypertensin II. J. exp. Med., 104:193, 1956.
140. SKEGGS, L., JR., W. H. MARSH, J. R. KAHN, and N. P. SHUMWAY. The existence of two forms of hypertensin. J. exp. Med., 99:275, 1954.
141. SØBYE, P. Heredity in essential hypertension and nephrosclerosis. A genetic-clinical study of 200 propositi suffering from nephrosclerosis. Op. dom. Biol. hered. Hum. Kbh., vol. 16, 1948.
142. STEPHEN HALES—Father of Hemodynamics. Medical Times, November, 1944.
143. TAGGART, J., and D. R. DRURY. The action of renin on rabbits with renal hypertension. J. exp. Med., 71:857, 1940.
144. TIGERSTEDT, R., and P. G. BERGMAN. Niere und Kreislauf. Skand. Arch. Physiol., 8:223, 1898.
145. TRAUBE, L. Ueber den Zusammenhang von Herz- und Nieren-Krankheiten. Gesammelte Beiträge zur Pathologie und Physiologie. Vol. 2. Berlin, Hirschwald, pp. 290–353, 1871.
146. VIERORDT, K. Die bildliche Darstellung des menschlichen Arterienpulses. Arch. physiol. Heilkunde., 13:284, 1854.
147. VOLHARD, P. Nieren und ableitende Harnwege. In G. von Bergmann and R. Staehelin, Eds. Handbuch der inneren Medizin, Vol. 6, Part 1. Berlin, Springer, 1931.
148. VOLHARD, F., and T. FAHR. Die Brightsche Nierenkrankheit. Klinik, Pathologie und Atlas. Berlin, Springer, 1914.
149. WARREN, J. W., J. D. PATTERSON, JR., J. T. DOYLE, O. H. GAUER, E. N. KEEN, M. MCGREGOR, and R. H. GOETZ. Circulation and respiration in the giraffe. Circulation, 16:947, 1957.

150. WEITZ, W. Zur Ätiologie der genuinen oder vaskulären Hypertension. Z. klin. Med., 96:151, 1923.
151. WILKS, S. Cases of Bright's disease, with remarks. Guy's Hosp. Rep., 2nd ser., 8:232, 1853.
152. WILSON, C., and F. B. BYROM. Renal changes in malignant hypertension; experimental evidence. Lancet, I:136, 1939.
153. WILSON, C., and F. B. BYROM. The vicious circle in chronic Bright's disease. Experimental evidence from the hypertensive rat. Quart. J. Med., N.S., 10:65, 1941.
154. WILSON, C., and G. W. PICKERING. Acute arterial lesions in rabbits with experimental renal hypertension. Clin. Sci., 3:343, 1938.
155. YOUNG, T. On the functions of the heart and arteries. Croonian Lecture. Phil. Trans. Roy. Soc. Med., (Part I), p. 1, 1809.

Part Three

SPECIAL CIRCULATIONS

IX

Renal Physiology

THE story of renal physiology can well begin where the story of Harvey leaves off—with the introduction of the microscope, which extended the range of observation and discovery into realms undreamt of by the discoverer of the circulation.

A double-lens magnifier may have been invented before the time of Roger Bacon (*c.* 1214–94), but it first emerged from historical obscurity in the 1590's, when Dutch spectacle makers greatly improved the art of grinding lenses. Knowledge of the Dutch two-lens system reached Galileo in about June, 1609. The Paduan physicist devised a lead tube fitted at one end with a planoconvex lens and fitted at the other with a planoconcave lens, bringing the instrument to an optical efficiency which it could not have hitherto possessed. By appropriate focusing, Galileo's tube could be used either as a telescope or microscope, and it was, of course, to the first purpose that Galileo himself put it with greatest effect, as he described in *Sidereus Nuncius* published in 1610. This short pamphlet recorded more world-shaking discoveries than any other book of whatever length ever written. But Galileo also used his tube as a microscope, and in 1610 he observed the legs and eyes and other anatomical features in minute animals such as insects.

Much labor and skill were required to grind good lenses, however, and through the first half of the seventeenth century the use of the microscope was limited to a small, intimate, and wealthy coterie of Italians who called themselves the *Accademia dei Lincei* (Companions of the Lynx). One of the achievements of the Lincei was the work entitled the *Apiarium*, published in 1625 by Prince Frederigo Cesi and Francesco Stelluti, containing descriptions of every bee and wasp known to the Lincei, including some American species. This was the first recorded treatise on microscopic anatomy. Another achievement was the discovery, by Cesi in 1625, of the spores of a fern, previously thought to

SPECIAL
CIRCULATIONS

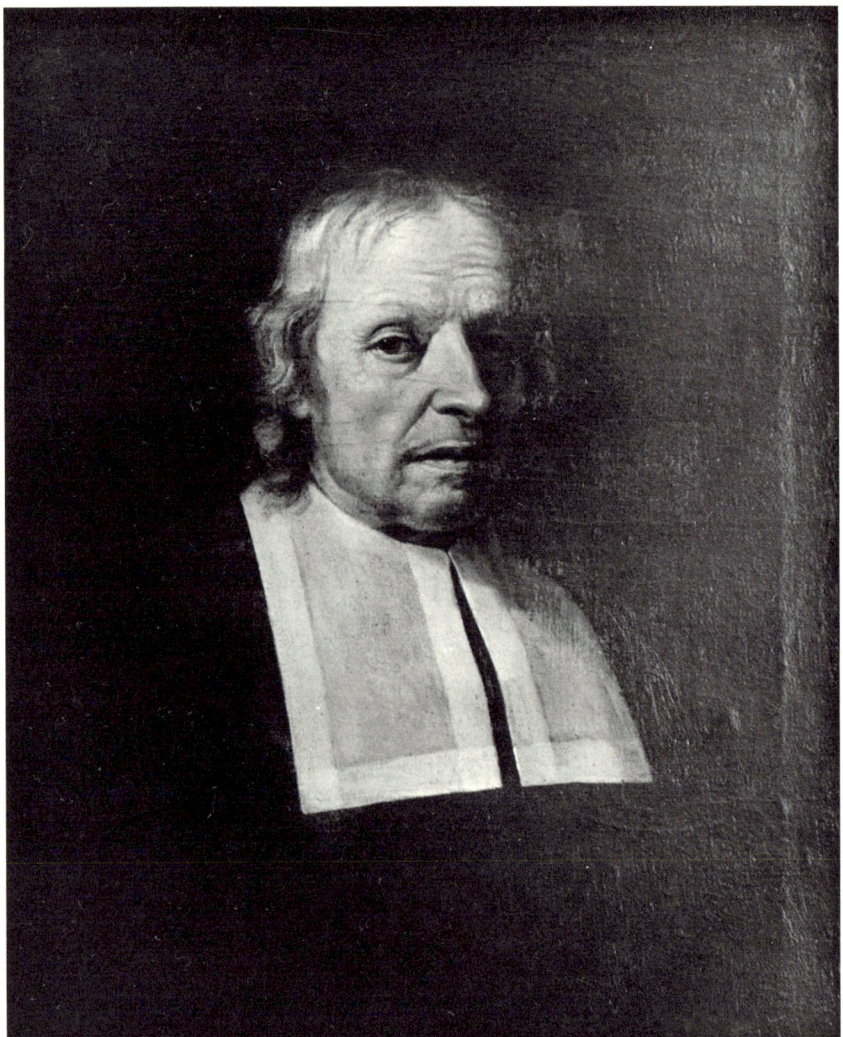

Figure 1. Marcello Malpighi (1628–94).

be seedless, which were perhaps the first objects wholly beyond the range of unaided vision to be revealed by the microscope (72).

Galileo's "trunk" or "cylinder" was probably known north of Italy well before 1620, but it was not until the middle of the century that it was used, to the great enrichment of all biology, by Marcello Malpighi of Italy, Robert Hooke (1635–1703) and Nehemiah Grew (1641–1712) of London, Jan Swammerdam (1637–80) of Amsterdam, and Antony van Leeuwenhoek (1632–1723) of Delft.

The Malpighian Corpuscle

RENAL PHYSIOLOGY

Of the five men named, the one who was destined to have the most immediate influence on medical science was Malpighi. Born near Bologna in 1628, the year in which Harvey's book was published, Malpighi at first undertook the study of philosophy at the University of Bologna, but after six years turned to medicine and obtained his degree in 1653. A man of delicate fiber and modest to the point of timidity, he was plagued throughout his life by frail health and family misfortunes, and was perhaps as much impelled into the study of nature by personal adversity as by his inquiring spirit, even though the latter was indeed extraordinary. He was appointed to the chair of Medicine at Bologna in 1656 at the age of twenty-eight. In that same year he was enticed to the University of Pisa, where Ferdinand II, Grand Duke of Tuscany, created for him a special chair of Theoretical Medicine (meaning Physiology). After three years he returned to Bologna, only to move to the chair of Medicine in the University of Messina in 1662. Finally he returned to Bologna in 1666, where he served in the chair of Medicine until his death at the age of sixty-six (*19*).

Malpighi's autobiographical notes suggest that from youth he had been amusing himself with a microscope (*41*). Shortly after completing his medical training, he turned to the study of the fine structure of animal and vegetable tissues, with such success that five sciences now claim him for their own—botany, embryology, comparative anatomy, pathology, and microscopic anatomy. It is, however, his work in microscopic anatomy, an area wherein he had no peer for nearly two centuries, that justifies his inclusion with Harvey as one of the founders of modern medicine.

In 1660, Malpighi discovered the capillaries while observing the dilated lung of the living frog. This discovery is recorded in the second of two letters addressed to his friend, Giovanni Alphonso Borelli (1608–79), professor of mathematics at the University of Pisa. The letters were published in 1661 under the title *De pulmonibus observationes anatomicae*. Here he told how he had been following the arteries

[547]

SPECIAL CIRCULATIONS

and veins in the lung of the dog, but without solving the mystery of how the blood gets from one to the other, until he turned (as was his custom) to the study of other animals and happened to examine the dilated lung of the living frog. If relying on the naked eye alone, he said,

> "*I might have believed that the blood itself escaped into an empty space and was gathered up again by a gaping vessel. . . . But an objection to this view was afforded by the movement of the blood being tortuous and scattered in different directions and by its being united again in a determinate part [or vessel]. My doubt was changed into certainty . . . [when] by the help of our more perfect glass . . . there appears a network made up of the continuations of the two vessels. . . . Hence it was clear to the senses that the blood flowed away from the tortuous vessels and was not poured into spaces, but was always contained within tubules, and that its dispersion is due to the multiple winding of the vessels*" (*19*).

Eight years later van Leeuwenhoek observed the capillaries in the fish and the Amphibia and gave a fuller description of them, but it was Malpighi who supplied the missing link in Harvey's "circulation" three years after Harvey's death (*28, 4, 6*).

With lenses that magnified perhaps no more than twenty- or thirty-fold Malpighi saw the red corpuscles of the blood in the mesenteric vessels of the hedgehog in 1665 (*De omento, pinquedine, et adiposis ductibus*), although he believed them to be globules of fat, an error which was corrected by van Leeuwenhoek in 1674. Three other short tracts, published in 1665, dealt with the sensory nature of the papillae of the tongue and skin and the general structure of the brain, respectively. (The important work of Thomas Willis, *Cerebri anatome: cui accessit nervorum descriptio et usus*, published in 1664, was not known to Malpighi.) In his major work, *De viscerum structura exercitatio anatomica*, published in 1666, Malpighi gave a detailed and (except for the brain) fairly accurate account of the structure of the spleen, kidneys, liver, and cerebral cortex.

The information available to Malpighi when he began his studies of the kidneys was meager indeed. Aristotle held that the bladder was the chief site of urine formation and that the kidneys were not essential for life—they existed "not of actual necessity, but as matters of greater finish and perfection." Galen improved on this interpretation to the extent of recognizing that urine is formed in the kidneys and that the ureters serve to convey it from these organs to the bladder. Vesalius depicted the structure of the kidneys quite fancifully, as hollow organs each divided by a sieve-like membrane into two compartments, into one of which blood was conducted by the renal artery and vein, while from the other the ureter carried the perfected urine to the bladder. Highmore, in his *Corporis humanis disquisitio anatomica* of 1651, corrected these errors to the extent of showing that the organ consisted of an outer, parenchymatous part, and an inner, fibrous part, but within the latter he conceived that the arteries and veins anastomose to form "spaces" which communicate with the renal pelvis.

RENAL PHYSIOLOGY

Shortly before Malpighi began his studies, Lorenzo Bellini (1643–1704), a nineteen-year-old student of Borelli's, had been set by his mentor to the task of examining the kidneys of a deer. In his *Exercitatio anatomica de structura et usu renum* (1662) Bellini dealt primarily with the structure and divisions of the renal pelvis, but he reported that the great bulk of the kidney is composed, not of solid fibrous strands, as Highmore had said, but of hollow tubes or canaliculi extending radially from the papillae to the cortex. Following Borelli's mechanical-physiological theories, Bellini proposed that the clear or aqueous fluid of the blood drains off into these canaliculi to form the urine, the rest escaping from the kidney by the renal vein, the separation of the two fluids being effected according to the size and configuration of the particles (*19, p. 110*). Bellini worked without a microscope and could not distinguish between the radially arranged collecting ducts and the renal tubules proper, and it would have been impossible for him to discover the relation between the tubules and the renal blood supply.

Malpighi evidently knew of Bellini's work, but in that portion of *De viscerum structura* (*39*) which deals with the kidney he started, as it were, from scratch, and with only the most general references to the work of others. Here we follow the excellent translation by Dr. Joseph M. Hayman, Jr. (*40*):

"*For a long time* [*Malpighi said in his introduction*] *the kidneys have been the subject of varying opinions, some even having regarded them as superfluous and unnecessary, a thought which is certainly not a tribute to Nature. More*

[549]

SPECIAL CIRCULATIONS

recently, however, because of their wonderful structure, and because of the very necessary function attributed to them, they have attained a place among the important parts of the body. So many different views regarding their composition are held by anatomists that there is little agreement.

"The ancients conceived of a sieve which provided a means for separating the urine. Many have been satisfied with the name 'parenchyma.' In the meantime, the idea of fibers for drawing out the fluid pleased some, and this idea was strengthened by the similar structure of the heart. Among subsequent writers the existence of fibers in the kidney appeared doubtful and unlikely, whereupon they announced that when the substance of the kidney was cut, certain little canals were to be seen. Later some have contended that the substance of the kidney is complex, parenchyma certainly, and fibers. And still more recently it has been stated in a very elaborate work [by Bellini?] that the substance of the kidney consists of a single fibrous substance, permeated by little canals. This was determined from cut sections in which, everything but vessels having been excluded, it was evident that the body of the kidney consists of nothing but a collection of little canals or channels which increase in size uninterruptedly from the external surface toward the center.

"The fact that the human mind has pondered these and similar ideas about the kidneys through the ages stimulated me to further investigation, or at least to the confirmation of the statements of others. Study with me, then, a few things in the spirit of truth alone, so that we may establish the manner of Nature's operations in the individual viscera as I have revealed it in the liver and other organs. For this essay which I plan will perhaps shed light upon the structure of the kidney. Do not stop to question whether these ideas are new or old, but ask, more properly, whether they harmonize with Nature. And be assured of this one thing, that I never reached my idea of the structure of the kidney by the aid of books, but by the long, patient and varied use of the microscope. I have gotten the rest by the deductions of reason, slowly, and with an open mind, as is my custom."

Malpighi went on to describe the gross anatomy of the kidney in a variety of animals—specifically he mentioned cattle, sheep, the bear, dog, cat, turtles, and birds—while his dissections of adult animals were supplemented in some instances by studies of the newborn and even the embryo. He noted that in many species the kidney has distinct subdivisions which give to the surface of the organ a lobulated appearance

—in the bear, for example, "presenting the appearance of a bunch of cherries"—the surrounding space being filled with fat. These subdivisions are not confined to the surface, but extend to the interior in some animals. In the human fetus they form a variable number of lobules between which lie the major blood vessels.

On making a cut through the kidney, the outermost part—half a finger's breadth—can be distinguished at first glance by its color, which is generally redder than the rest of the organ. Where other anatomists had held this outer part to be coagulated blood or parenchyma, Malpighi showed that it is composed of almost innumerable little worm-like vessels (the renal tubules) which he sometimes called "fibers" and sometimes "canaliculi" (he used the word *tubulos* only to identify Bellini's ducts), and he spoke of the mass of canaliculi as having a "fibrous structure." He admitted that he was never able to demonstrate any continuity between the convoluted canaliculi in the outer part of the kidney and the straight tubules in the papilla, "either on account of my clumsiness, perchance, or on account of the crudity of my instruments"; but it seemed to him that reason and sense, aided by research, confirm that this continuity exists.

Concerning the outer part of the kidney, he wrote,

"It must be added, however, that there is considerable difficulty in believing that this whole part of the kidney is absolutely fibrous, and that nothing (except blood vessels) is present besides this fibrous [tubular] material. For in all kidneys which up to this time I have been able to get, I have detected a number of very small glands [i.e., Malpighian corpuscles or glomeruli]. These I have observed in quadrupeds, turtles, and always in man himself. In order to see these glands, black fluid mixed with spirit of wine should be injected through the renal artery until the whole kidney swells, and the exterior grows black. If now the capsule of the kidney be removed, the glands immediately meet the naked eye, attached as they are to the arteries which bifurcate in different directions, the glands being dyed with the same color as the arteries. And when the kidney is sectioned in the same manner as before, longitudinally, between the bundles of the urinary vessels and the narrow spaces formed by them, one will see these same innumerable glands attached like apples to the blood vessels, the latter swollen with the black liquid and stretched out into the form of a beautiful tree. . . .

SPECIAL
CIRCULATIONS

"These glands, situated in the outer part of the kidney, are almost innumerable, and probably, as I think, correspond in number to the urinary vessels [*tubules*] by which the mass of the kidney is formed. . . .

"As to the structure of the glands, a distinct outline cannot be obtained on account of their minute size and translucency. They appear, however, spherical, precisely like fish eggs: and when a dark fluid is perfused through the arteries they grow dark, and one would say that all around them are the extreme ends of the blood vessels, which run along like creeping tendrils, so that they appear as it were crowned, with this reservation, however, that the part which is fastened to the branch of the artery grows black; the rest retains its former color.

"The glands are connected with the branches of the arteries in the following manner. They spring from the deeper branches of the arteries and in some instances from the superficial branches which are bent inward and continued into intricate branchlets. That they are attached directly to these vessels is clearly demonstrated by the perfusion of colored fluid through the renal artery, for the glands and the connected arteries are stained with the same color, so that the eye very easily perceives their connection.

"The glands are also connected with the veins, which follow the ramifications of the arteries; for when the veins are filled with ink, although the glands may not be filled with the same fluid, nevertheless the color seems to be worked in toward them, so that nothing intervenes between the glands and the ends of the veins. It is probable that the liquid injected through the veins by force, having overcome their valves, clings to the mouths of the glands and is shut out from their different passages.

"To these arguments it may be added that the glands are at first white and almost translucent, then red, which certainly happens because of the blood of the arteries which is poured out. Moreover, it is known from the usual custom of Nature that the radicles of the veins take their origin from the same place in which the terminal arteries end, whence, although the senses do not perceive the connection, reason, nevertheless, sufficiently prevails."

(Notice how the argument from "reason" had recourse, not to the time-honored parenchyma, but by implication, at least, to Malpighi's capillaries.)

Malpighi was unable to demonstrate whether or not these "glands" are connected with the ureter: he was never able to inject the urinary tubules by perfusion of the arteries or veins, although neither was he able to inject the tubules from the ureter. But from experiments involving the ligation of the renal vein and ureter in the dog he inferred that such was the case, since the urine, he argued, is derived from the blood in the arteries, and "the ends of the arteries lie open [sic] in these very numerous glands," and, since the urine passes into the pelvis through the canaliculi of the kidney, "there must of necessity be granted a continuity and communication between them, for otherwise no secreted fluid would be strained out from the arteries into the pelvis." (The word "open" should not here be given its earlier, and later, connotation of "draining freely.")

Malpighi's detailed discussion included the structure of the medulla and a description of how the canaliculi converge on the pelvis, to drain into the latter through one or more papillae (he noted that in man there are usually twelve), so that the urine enters the pelvis through the papillae and not through the pores in the walls of the pelvis—an important part of his physiological theory. He described quite accurately the general course of the arteries and veins and how these undergo multiple branching to end in the "glands," as well as describing the relation of the ureter to the pelvis.

On the function of the kidneys, he said,

"If, indeed, as is probably agreed by all, the material of the urine is derived from the arteries, and since it is clear from the evidence above that the ends of the arteries lie open in these very numerous glands . . . there must of necessity be granted a continuity and communication between them, for otherwise no secreted fluid would be strained out from the arteries into the pelvis. . . .

"But by what means this is accomplished is most obscure. It is reasonable to assume that this is wholly the result of the work of the glands: but since the minute and simple structure of the openings within the glands escapes us, we can only postulate some things in order to give a satisfactorily probable answer to this question. It is obvious that this mechanism accomplishes the work of separation of the urine by its internal arrangement. But whether this arrangement is similar to those devices which we make use of here and there for human needs, and in imitation of which we built rough contrivances, is doubtful. . . . And since the manifestation of Nature's working is most varied, we may discover mechanisms which are unknown to us and whose operations we cannot understand.

SPECIAL
CIRCULATIONS

"I marvel at this, that so many different substances are separated through these glands by the process of Nature, for water with salty, sulphurous and similar particles goes through, and in disease the remains of abscesses, and sometimes the defiled particles of the whole body are separated from the parts of the blood which are retained. These blood particles are many, and not all of one form. Nevertheless, as I think, Nature has made the structure of these glands very small and most simple, so that we cannot doubt that those things which are excreted through the urinary vessels go together into one mass, so that the particles of salt and other substances entering in turn form one great body of definite shape. And whatever is of larger size or of different shape does not enter the little pores and small spaces of the excreting body, and is not excreted."

All this is essentially the theory of filtration through selective pores, as proposed by Borelli and Bellini. Malpighi's pathology was the pathology of his day, involving the "violent agitation" and "thinning" and "thickening" and other "diseases of the blood." In addition, "the little glands of the kidney suffer from all the diseases peculiar to glands, which for the sake of brevity in our studies we omit." However, on one problem in pathology, the formation of stone, he was ahead of his time:

"The ureter, expanded into the pelvis, is affected by worms and particularly by calculi, for if one of the saline or tartar particles which are continually flowing out is ensnared by the pelvis it fosters the beginning of a stone. For it is clear that it would meet the particles that pass through and detain those like itself, so that the stone grows from all these particles which are massed together. On this account perchance Nature has added the pelvic fat, so that its interior surface may be continually kept smooth."

One of the regrettable episodes in the history of physiology is that Malpighi failed to identify the nature of the "glands" at the beginning of the urinary canaliculi, and failed to observe that they consisted of a tuft of the very capillaries which he had discovered in the lung of the frog. It is true that he saw the capillaries in the living animal and identified them as such in consequence of the regular coursing of the blood through their visible extent; the dense, contracted tuft of the capillaries in the Malpighian corpuscle is difficult to identify as such in the exsanguinated kidney. Yet his use of the arterial injection method must have occasionally afforded him a well-injected capillary vessel, visible under the same microscope by means of which he had seen the capillaries in the lung.

Throughout the last year of his life, according to his friend and physician, George Baglivi, Malpighi was subject to vomiting and palpitations of the heart, and to the excruciating pain of renal calculi (frequently passing stones into the urine), in addition to occasional attacks of gout. He suffered an apoplectic stroke in June, 1694, and died on November 28 of that year, at the age of sixty-six. At autopsy Baglivi found the heart generally enlarged, particularly the wall of the left ventricle. The left kidney was normal, but the right was enlarged and the pelvis dilated from long-standing calculus obstruction (*12*).

In closing his biography of Malpighi, Michael Foster wrote:

"All the deeper problems of physiology turn on the mutual action of the tissues and the blood, as the stream of the latter sweeps among the elements of the former. Harvey shewed that the blood did sweep through the tissues, Malpighi shewed what the tissues were and how the blood swept through them. And thus the way was opened for those inquiries into the ways in which the blood acts on the tissue and the tissue acts on the blood, inquiries the results of which are the pride of modern times and the hope of times to come" (*19*).

The Glomerular Capillaries

After Malpighi, nearly two centuries passed before any further notable advance was made in renal anatomy or physiology. The identification of the glomerular capillaries as such is attributed to Frederik Ruysch (1638–1731) in 1729. Ruysch was professor of anatomy at Leyden and Amsterdam, and was most famous for his excellent method of injecting blood vessels—the recipe for the injection material that he used long remained a secret (*21*). In his *Thesaurus anatomicus* X, No. 86 (1729), a catalogue of his anatomical museum which in his "heavy old age" he was then offering for sale, he described Malpighi's glands as consisting of the "twisted terminal extremities of arterioles. When the renal arteries are filled most carefully, these are separated or expanded, like a ball [glomer] of thread." He added, "it must be noted that twistings of this sort of the blood vessels are never formed in other viscera."

SPECIAL CIRCULATIONS

Ruysch was, however, anything but clear on this point, because in another catalogue item (No. 149) he wrote, "the ducts called Bellini's ducts are also entirely filled because of a filling of the arterioles" (i.e., after arterial injection), and elsewhere (No. 88) he referred to the injected "kidney of a youth on the interior surface of which many glandiform round particles [Malpighian glands] appear that feign to be glandules. These, however, as I said above, are nothing but twisted arterioles, some of which separated here, degenerate into Bellini's ducts [*in ductus Bellinos degenerant*]." Quoting the last statement, Bowman (*3*) noted that "This was the principal ground for the famous, but now exploded theory, of the existence of exhalant arteries with open mouths, which in the secreting glands opened directly into the excretory canals."

Schumlansky, in a dissertation published in 1782, had concluded, as did Malpighi, that the corpuscle and tubule were connected, but Huschke in 1828 and Johannes Müller in 1830 could still deny this connection, Huschke asserting that the tubules terminate in free, blind extremities and that Malpighi's corpuscles are concerned only with the blood vessels.

Bowman's Secretory Hypothesis

These few observations bring us to the classic paper in renal anatomy, and indeed one of the classics of medical science, *On the structure of and use of the Malpighian bodies of the kidney, with observations on the circulation through the gland*, published by William Bowman in 1842 (*3*). At the time of publication Bowman was only twenty-six years old, a demonstrator in anatomy at King's College and Assistant Surgeon to the King's College Hospital, London. Bowman worked before the introduction of aniline dyes and the microtome, and depended entirely on teasing kidney tissue apart under a dissecting microscope. His instrument had a magnifying power of some 300-fold, whereas Malpighi's had no more than one-tenth this power; but, more importantly, Bowman brought to the problem the double injection method (potassium bichromate followed by lead acetate) recently introduced by Doyère. An additional reason for his success was his resort to comparative anatomy—as with Harvey in his studies of the circulation and Malpighi in his studies of the kidney, Bowman examined many different kinds of

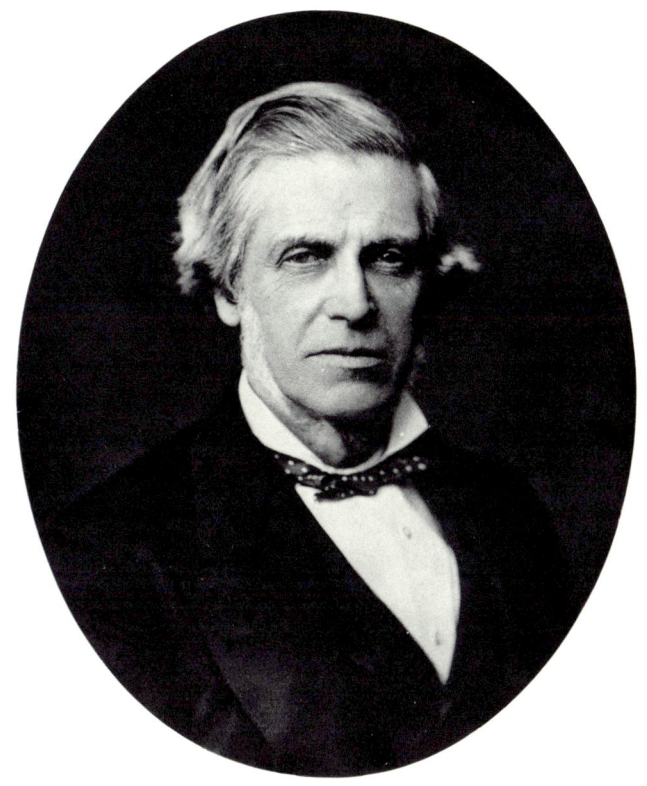

Figure 2. William Bowman (1816–92).

animals before arriving at his conclusions. Not only the kidney of man but that of the badger, dog, lion, cat, mouse, squirrel, guinea pig, horse, parrot, tortoise, boa, frog, and common eel came under his scrutiny. This approach not only afforded him perspective, it also introduced him to the loose, easily dissected kidney of the fish, frog, and other cold-blooded animals, where he found an organ better suited to his ends than was the more compact, encapsulated kidney of the mammal. Above all, however, Bowman's work was characterized by extraordinary care and visual acuity.

Among his signal achievements were an accurate description of the glomerular capillary tuft, that it is divided into lobules, that this tuft hangs free in the spherical capsule which today we call Bowman's

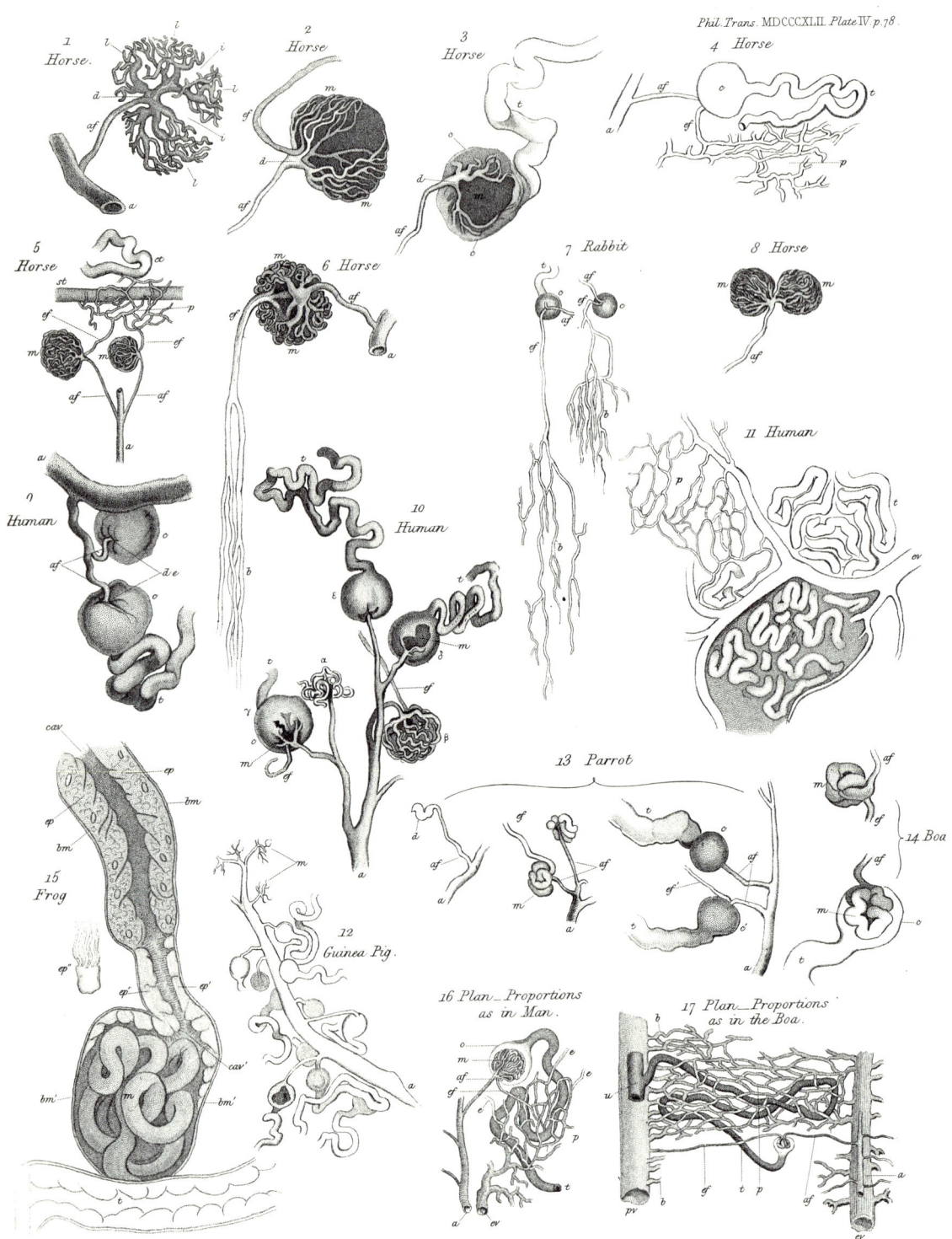

capsule, and that the space within this capsule communicates freely with the lumen of the tubule so that any fluid separating from the capillaries drains freely down the latter. He first recognized the definitive nature of the basement membrane of the tubule and showed that the spherical capsule investing the glomerulus is a continuation and bulbous expansion of this basement membrane. He correctly described the tubule as a single layer of nucleated epithelial cells lining the basement membrane. His technique did not permit him to follow the nephron in the mammalian kidney through its tortuous convolutions and its long, hair-pin extension into the medullary pyramid; nevertheless he concluded that there is one glomerulus attached to each tubule, and that each tubule is continued as a unit until, with many others, it joins the system of collecting ducts.

Bowman correctly described the relation of the efferent arteriole to the glomerular tuft, and the formation, from the efferent arteriole, of the peritubular capillary plexus, and he showed that the peritubular capillaries are closely applied to the basement membrane of the tubule, with frequent anastomoses between adjacent capillaries (53). In his words,

"All the blood of the renal artery (with the exception of a small quantity distributed to the [renal] capsule, surrounding fat, and the coats of the larger vessels) enters the capillary tufts of the Malpighian bodies; thence it passes into the capillary plexus surrounding the uriniferous tubes, and it finally leaves the organ through the branches of the renal vein."

This short summary does scant justice to a quite detailed and magnificent study. Bowman's paper inevitably contained some errors: in the lower animals he observed cilia in the "neck" where the glomerular capsule joins the tubule, and he incorrectly inferred that cilia are also present in the mammals. And at a magnification of 300 and without the use of dyes he was led to conclude that the glomerular tuft contains only one cell type—capillary endothelium. But these errors are slight in comparison with the many features of the nephron and its blood supply which he did correctly describe for the first time.

Figure 3. Plate from Bowman illustrating his observations on the comparative anatomy of the kidney.

As for the mechanism of urine formation, Bowman was inevitably impressed with the structure of the glomerulus:

SPECIAL CIRCULATIONS

"It would indeed be difficult to conceive a disposition of parts more calculated to favour the escape of water from the blood, than that of the Malpighian body. A large artery breaks up in a very direct manner into a number of minute branches, each of which suddenly opens into an assemblage of vessels of far greater aggregate capacity than itself, and from which there is but one narrow exit. Hence must arise a very abrupt retardation in the velocity of the current of blood. The vessels in which this delay occurs are uncovered by any structure. They lie bare in a cell [Bowman's capsule] from which there is but one outlet, the orifice of the tube. This orifice is encircled by cilia, in active motion, directing a current towards the tube [sic]. These exquisite organs must not only serve to carry forward the fluid already in the cell, and in which the vascular tuft is bathed, but must tend to remove pressure from the free surface of the vessels, and so to encourage the escape of their more fluid contents. Why is so wonder-

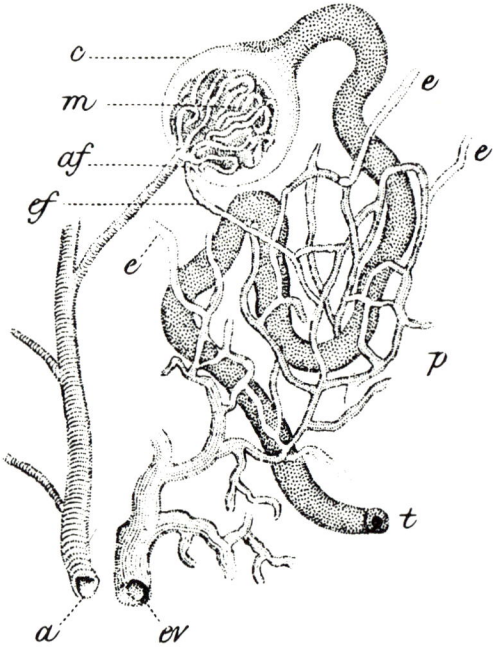

Figure 4. The nephron of the human kidney according to Bowman. Enlarged from Figure 3.

ful an apparatus placed at the extremity of each uriniferous tube, if not to furnish water, to aid in the separation and solution of the urinous products from the epithelium of the tube?"

If the last sentence is ambiguous, it is because the contemporary theory of "secretion" is ambiguous:

"This theory, in its widest sense, supposes the epithelium of secreting surfaces either to pass through constant stages of renovation and decay, or else to remain, during a longer period, as a permanent organic form, assimilating and rejecting.... In many cases the epithelial particles [cell contents] appear to be cast off entire when their growth is complete, and thus to form the secretion; in other instances, they seem to lose their substance by a more gradual process, and to waste or dissolve away on the surface of the membrane, as fresh particles are deposited below; in other examples still, there is reason for believing that they are a long persistent structure....

"Applying this theory to the kidney, it may be considered highly probable that the epithelium of the uriniferous tubes is continually giving up its effete particles, and undergoing a gradual decay. This view harmonizes in a striking manner with what has been before advanced as to the use of the Malpighian bodies. If the peculiar urinous particles were poured out at once, they must be in a dissolved state from the first, and could need no further aqueous current to carry them off; but if they are deposited in a more or less solid form, as a part of an organized tissue, they will require (being sparingly soluble) an additional and extraneous source of water, by which, when their formation is complete, they may be taken up and conveyed from the gland."

By "urinous products" Bowman was referring to all urinary constituents, and specifically to urea, uric acid, and salts which he had previously mentioned. He seemed to contradict himself at a later point when he said that various foreign substances may transude through the bare capillaries in the tuft, but the general argument was that only in the case of foreign substances, or in disease, did excretion involve passage through the tuft of anything but water. Conscious that he was here arguing in a circle, he added:

"It may possibly be considered by some, that, in the preceding observations on the use of the aqueous element of the urine, and on the nature of secretion in general, I have been endeavoring to illustrate a doubtful hypothesis by speculation

SPECIAL CIRCULATIONS

more doubtful still, obscurum per obscurius. *But I rest my view on the function of the Malpighian bodies principally on anatomical grounds, and the other considerations have been introduced in connection with it, rather in consequence of the interest they appear to me to add to it, than because I am fully satisfied of their validity. Undoubtedly both questions are worthy of being separately handled, and require a much wider and more elaborate investigation than seems to have been given to them."*

There was prescience in his final statement:

"Parallel lines of inquiry into the anatomical varieties of the Malpighian bodies and uriniferous tubes, and into the chemistry of their secretion, in the different tribes of animals and in various stages of their development, could scarcely fail either to confirm or to confute what has now been advanced."

Ludwig's Filtration-Reabsorption Hypothesis

Bowman's secretory theory of renal function remained without support in experimental evidence, and it was scarcely off the press before it was challenged by the wholly independent thesis of Carl Ludwig. Destined to become, with Johannes Müller and Claude Bernard, one of the three great physiologists of the nineteenth century, Ludwig was the innovator of many modern physiological methods, such as the kymograph and the graphic record. He invented the mercury gas pump and initiated the study of blood gases and pulmonary exchange; he invented the stromuhr for measuring blood flow, and first conceived of the perfusion of isolated organs; he discovered the ganglionic cells in the interauricular septum and the secretory nerves to the salivary glands, and showed that secretion was accompanied by metabolic changes in the secretory cells; he was the first to propound a mechanical theory of lymph formation; and he and his pupils laid the systematic foundations of the dynamic physiology of the circulation and its nervous control. The list could go on indefinitely—the excellent *In Memoriam* written by William Stirling (*78*) is a cross-section of nineteenth-century physiology. To Ludwig and Bernard may be attributed the establishment of experimental physiology as a critical method of investigation centered around controlled observations in which secondary variables are minimized.

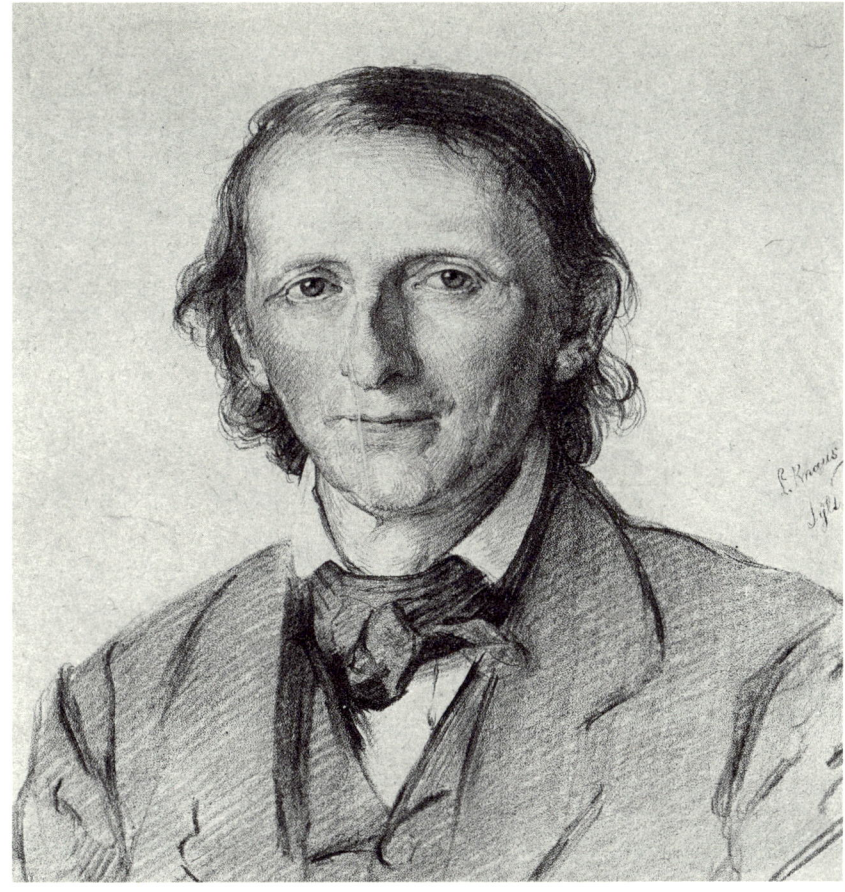

Figure 5. Carl F. Ludwig (1816–95).

Appointed privat-dozent in Physiology at Marburg in 1842 and professor of comparative anatomy in 1846, Ludwig moved to Zurich as professor of anatomy and physiology in 1849, and in 1855 went to Vienna as professor of physiology and zoology in the Josephinum, a school for military surgeons. In 1865 he was appointed chief of the newly created Institute of Physiology at Leipzig, the first of its kind in the world, where he remained until his death. During the twenty and more years that he directed the Leipzig Institute, over two hundred investigators from all over the world came under his influence, to work on

SPECIAL CIRCULATIONS

almost as many different problems and to carry away something of his methods and philosophy. Ludwig's role in physiological science was long obscured by his method of publication, because it was his custom to suggest a problem to the student, to work with him, at least in the early stages, and to write the paper for him, and then publish the work under the student's name (*5, 34, 68*). Indeed, one commentator said that sometimes the student sat on the window sill while Ludwig and his faithful assistant, Salvenmoser, did the work (*20, p. 555*). But however substantial the contribution of the student, something of Ludwig was in every manuscript; and the story is told that when one of his colleagues entered a remonstrance on this policy, Ludwig smiled and pointed to the top of the paper where there appeared the name of the Institute, saying, "That is enough."

Ludwig's era was one of intense debate over the doctrine of vitalism, which held that a mystical power, neither physical nor chemical in nature, is active in living organisms, and here alone, and that this vital force is a necessary condition for vital phenomena. At the beginning of the century there were perhaps more vitalists than mechanists in the biological sciences; by the middle of the century, however, the tide had turned in favor of "molecular physiology" (*18*). Ludwig was among the leaders of the antivitalist group, which then or later included Claude Bernard, Du Bois-Reymond, E. W. Brücke, Helmholtz, Karl Vogt, Mosso, Jacques Loeb, and Max Verworn. Du Bois-Reymond denied Aristotelian "final causes" in all such matters as the nature of force and matter, the origin of motion, the origin of life, the purposeful character of natural phenomena, the origin of sensation, thought, and speech, and the freedom of the will; and summed up his view in the phrase, *Ignorabimus, dubitemus* (where we do not know, let us be cautious) (*20, p. 535*). The effort to explain physiological phenomena solely by reference to the laws that operate in the domain of inorganic nature was first expounded fully in Ludwig's celebrated *Lehrbuch der Physiologie des Menschen* (*37*), in the introduction to which (1851) he wrote, "The task of a scientific philosophy is to determine the functions of the animal body and deduce them as a necessity from its elementary composition" (*68*).

This mechanistic philosophy was also the keynote of Ludwig's theory of urine formation. It has been generally assumed that Ludwig's work on the kidney was undertaken with full knowledge of Bowman's work, but this assumption stems from the fact that Ludwig's theory is usually dated from his essay in Wagner's *Handwörterbuch der Physiologie* of 1844. Actually, the evidence is quite to the contrary. On the occasion of his appointment as privat-dozent at Marburg in 1842, Ludwig delivered in Latin two little-known inaugural addresses, presumably in September or October. These were translated by him into German and printed in pamphlet form in 1843, with a Foreword dated November 1, 1842 (*35*). The writer has been unable to find out when Bowman's paper, which was read on February 17, appeared in print, although it was reviewed in the Lancet for April 16, presumably immediately after it was published. Therefore, it was possibly in circulation for some six months before Ludwig's inaugural addresses were given, but for several reasons it seems very unlikely that Ludwig had seen it. First, he referred to the opinions of other anatomists (Berres, Krause, Cayla, Huschke, J. Müller, R. Wagner, Weber, Henle—the Marburg papers have no bibliography and were apparently translated into German hastily, and poorly, from his Latin manuscripts), but only twice did he refer to Bowman's work (he misspelled the name, *Bowmann*), once in connection with the fact that the arteriole undergoes star-shaped division inside the glomerulus, when he said, "In the viewpoint most recently appearing on this subject Bowmann had lined up with the opinion of Berres and Krause; Cayla supports the older view of Huschke"; and again when he remarked that he agreed with Bowman on the point that there is only one *vas efferens* to each glomerulus. These are trivial points in both Bowman's and Ludwig's work. Second, though many of Bowman's observations could have been marshalled to support Ludwig's theory in the strongest way, he did not use one of them for this purpose, nor did he mention Bowman's "secretory" theory. Third, it is clear that he must have carried out most if not all of his time-consuming anatomical studies and experiments before the summer of 1842. The writer therefore believes that at the time of the Marburg addresses Ludwig had only fragmentary knowledge of Bowman's work, which had come to him by word of mouth or by letter during the preparation of his inaugural addresses. By 1843, however, when he probably wrote the essay for Wagner's Handwörterbuch (*36*), he outlined Bowman's theory quite completely and criticized the lat-

SPECIAL CIRCULATIONS

ter's "secretory" theory, arguing instead that everything in the plasma is filtered through the glomerulus except the proteins, fats, and associated "metals." Ludwig's ideas were further developed in his own *Lehrbuch* published in 1856 and 1861 (*37, 38*), and as investigation progressed his theory was fortified or modified in details, particularly in papers by his pupils, Goll, Hermann, and Ustimovitsch. Our emphasis here will be on the Marburg addresses.

In the first of these he described his anatomical observations on the kidney of the dog, rabbit, pig, horse, and man, observations almost as extensive as those of Bowman, even if not as detailed. He described many injection studies, in which he used albumin, dyes, wax, isinglass solution, lead chromate, indigo, ink, and a fine suspension of cinnabar, and he arrived at the same general anatomical conclusions as Bowman. Specifically, he concluded that the blood does not escape directly into the renal tubules in the glomeruli but passes through by way of their capillaries into the efferent arterioles; and he asserted that all the blood passing through the kidney must traverse the glomeruli except where the tips of (some) interlobular arterioles discharge into the subcapsular venous plexus. He correctly noted that there are many anastomoses between the capillaries in any one lobule of the glomerular tuft, and that the efferent arteriole breaks up into a tightly knit plexus of capillaries around the convoluted tubules, a large proportion of these capillaries passing more or less directly to the veins. He also noted that from this plexus larger capillaries descend with the straight tubules in their course toward the medulla, forming multiple loops which return on their course before becoming confluent and discharging into the veins. (Bowman had missed both the glomerular anastomoses and the long capillary loops of the cortical capillaries.) He agreed with Bowman and other anatomists that the tubules never end freely, or interconnect with each other.

In the second Marburg address Ludwig reviewed the available (if meager) information on the chemical composition of the serum and the urine, and emphasized the relatively high concentrations of urea, sulphates, and phosphates in the latter. Joining the anatomical and chemical evidence with hemodynamic and many other arguments, he arrived at his hypothesis of glomerular filtration and tubular reabsorption.

This hypothesis, in brief, is that the glomerular capillaries, like capillaries elsewhere in the body, are permeable to practically all substances in the blood except the proteins, lipids, and formed elements. Under the hydrostatic pressure of the blood in these capillaries, a substantial quantity of protein- and cell-free fluid is separated from the blood by a simple physical or mechanical process of filtration, the volume of this filtrate being sufficient to account for all the constituents of the urine.

Since many substances (urea, sulphates, phosphates) are present in the urine in higher concentration than in the plasma, the volume of filtrate formed per unit time must be considerably larger than the volume of urine excreted; hence a considerable fraction of the filtrate must be reabsorbed by the tubules. With respect to this reabsorptive process, Ludwig recognized that the blood in the peritubular capillaries is derived from the efferent glomerular arterioles and hence has traversed the glomeruli and must now have a relatively low hydrostatic pressure; also he conceived that in the separation of the glomerular filtrate the blood is "concentrated" by loss of water and solutes. Consequently between the relatively dilute fluid in the tubules and the "concentrated" blood in the peritubular capillaries an endosmotic force exists which will cause water (and other substances to which the tubules are permeable, such, perhaps, as sodium chloride) to return from the filtrate into the capillaries, thus concentrating all residual substances in the final urine.

Apart from the "naked" nature of the capillary tuft in the glomerulus and the great expanse of these vessels, which would result in a slower movement of the blood through them, Bowman gave no reason why they should be "ideally" suited for the separation of "water" from the blood. Ludwig used the anatomy of the capillary tuft with better logic when he visualized its function in terms of hydrostatic pressure and semipermeability: his hypothesis of the physical filtration through these capillaries of a protein-free fluid sufficient in amount to remove from the blood all the urinary constituents was truly an intellectual tour de force. Though resting on no foundation other than a knowledge of anatomy, not as good as Bowman's, but bolstered by a keen appreciation of hemodynamics wholly absent from Bowman's approach, it had the supreme glory that it is true. But his proposition that this filtrate is subsequently elaborated into the final urine by the endosmotic absorption of water into the "concentrated" peritubular capillary blood, although equally ingenious for its day, proved in time to be wholly inadequate.

In the first instance, Ludwig spoke of "concentrated" blood leaving

RENAL PHYSIOLOGY

the glomerulus without spelling out in what respect the blood is "concentrated." It has been implied that he was thinking in terms of the osmotic pressure of the plasma proteins, but in the strict sense this was not possible, because the fact that the plasma proteins possess significant osmotic pressure vis-à-vis a protein-free solution was first suspected and demonstrated by Starling in 1896 (76) in connection with the absorption of fluids from the "connective tissue spaces"; Starling again investigated the osmotic pressure of the proteins in 1899 (77) in connection with the minimal arterial pressure at which glomerular filtration can occur.

In 1842, however, Ludwig could have had only the vaguest idea of what solutes contributed to endosmosis, and it is probable that he had in mind the total solids, including the proteins. In this sense the plasma was some four times as concentrated as the average urine, and would, of course, be further concentrated in the glomerulus. Add to this last fact his correct inference that the hydrostatic pressure of the blood must be higher in the glomerulus than in the peritubular capillaries, and his theory of physical filtration by the glomeruli and endosmotic reabsorption by the tubules is rationalized. This theory sufficed to explain changes in the flow and concentration of the urine in relation to hydropenia, water diuresis, cold weather, fever, glucosuria, uricosuria, saline diuresis, etc., the reciprocal relation between the concentrations of glucose or "extracted material" and of urea in the urine (Lecanu's law), and the strange phenomenon of "dry urine" (semi-solid uric acid) in snakes and birds.

After the Marburg papers, which Ludwig wrote when he was not yet twenty-six years old, increasing knowledge of the phenomenon of osmotic pressure came from the work of Traube (1867), Pfeffer (1877), de Vries (1888), and others, until van't Hoff (1884–87) formulated the analogy between gases and solutions, and Arrhenius (1887) published the theory of electrolytic dissociation. Not until 1881 did Hoppe-Seyler (13) point out that the urine may have a greater osmotic pressure than the blood, and that this hyperosmotic state cannot be attained by endosmosis, which operates only to equalize osmotic pressure. (The first accurate measurements of the osmotic pressure of urine in the dog were reported by Dreser (13) in 1891, in man, by Korányi (31, 32) in 1894–98.)

Since there were available to Ludwig no measurements of the total osmotic pressure of either blood or urine, much less of the plasma proteins, we may be indulgent on this point—he could scarcely be expected to anticipate by forty-six years the development of the theory of solution, which was to constitute the outstanding achievement of (physical) chemistry in the nineteenth century. But if the theory of solution militated against him in respect to the composition of the urine, it favored him in respect to the composition of the glomerular filtrate. In 1896 Tammann (*79*) calculated that the osmotic pressure of the plasma was some 5840 mm. Hg; since the maximal pressure in the glomeruli was probably not above 1 per cent of this figure, Tammann's calculation confirmed Ludwig's hypothesis that essentially all the osmotically active substances in the plasma (exclusive of the proteins and their salts) must be present in the capsular fluid in the same concentration (per kg. of water) as in the plasma, if the formation of this fluid is effected by simple physical filtration. (Tammann considered the osmotic pressure of the plasma proteins to be negligible.)

Ludwig carefully avoided attributing any steps in urine formation to "vital activity" on the part of the glomeruli or tubules. It was, as he later said, an "audacious" hypothesis, and justified the closing sentence of his second paper: "Thus we see in these relationships [between glomeruli and tubules] a simplicity, a harmony which stands second to no natural process in beauty."

In elaborating on his hypothesis in the second edition of his *Lehrbuch* (1861) (*38*), Ludwig added little beyond the provisional admission that the tubular epithelium may be chemically reactive. He recognized that some protein may be filtered, and suggested that its absence from the urine may be attributable to "chemical" processes within the kidney; and he admits that sodium chloride may be reabsorbed into the blood by a force analogous to a "chemical" one, thus accounting for the difference in the relative quantities of sodium chloride and urea in the blood and urine.

In the filtration hypothesis the *vis a tergo* behind urine formation is, of course, the blood pressure. In 1854, Goll (*22*), working in Ludwig's laboratory, showed that changes in systemic pressure are in general accompanied by parallel changes in urine flow; in 1862, Hermann (*27*), one of Ludwig's pupils, showed that the maximal ureteral pressure against which the kidney will excrete urine is about 40 mm. Hg less than the mean arterial pressure. Bernard had reported his discovery of the

RENAL
PHYSIOLOGY

SPECIAL CIRCULATIONS

vasomotor nerves in 1851–53, and in 1859 he had shown that, when the splanchnic nerves in anesthetized animals are cut, the urine flow increases on the operated side, a phenomenon which he attributed to increased renal blood flow. Pursuing the implications of Bernard's work, Ustimovitsch (*80*), another one of Ludwig's pupils, in 1870 showed that urine formation ceases when the arterial pressure is reduced to some 40 mm. Hg or less; he confirmed that denervation of the kidney (in the anesthetized animal) increases the urine flow and that stimulation of the renal nerve decreases it—which results are all explicable in terms of vasodilatation or vasoconstriction of the renal arterioles and consequent changes in glomerular pressure.

Beyond introducing the filtration-reabsorption hypothesis, the experiments of Ludwig and his pupils forced recognition of the role of the renal nerves and renal arterioles in controlling the renal circulation. But these experiments failed to prove the filtration-reabsorption hypothesis because in none of them was it established whether the important factor in urine formation was the perfusion pressure or the blood flow to the glomeruli and tubules.

Heidenhain's Secretory Hypothesis

It was partly on this lack of distinction between pressure and flow that Ludwig's hypothesis was challenged in 1874 by Rudolph Peter Heinrich Heidenhain, professor of physiology at Breslau and the outstanding student of the time in the physiology of glandular secretion. Heidenhain's extensive experience with the histologic changes in the cells concerned with the secretion of saliva, milk, the gastric and intestinal fluids, etc., led him to view all "secretory" phenomena in terms of cellular activity, and it was thus that he interpreted urine formation (*26, 24*).

Heidenhain's secretory theory of renal function stemmed in the first instance from his observations on the excretion of indigo carmine (sodium sulphindigotate, indigodisulphonic acid), a dye used by Chrzonszczewsky in 1864 to visualize the biliary capillaries. He found that when this dye was injected intravenously into rabbits in which urine formation had been arrested by cervical cord transection or hemorrhage, it could be seen in the cells and lumen of the renal tubules, when no color could be discerned in Bowman's capsule. He argued, therefore, that the dye is secreted from the blood directly into the tubu-

RENAL
PHYSIOLOGY

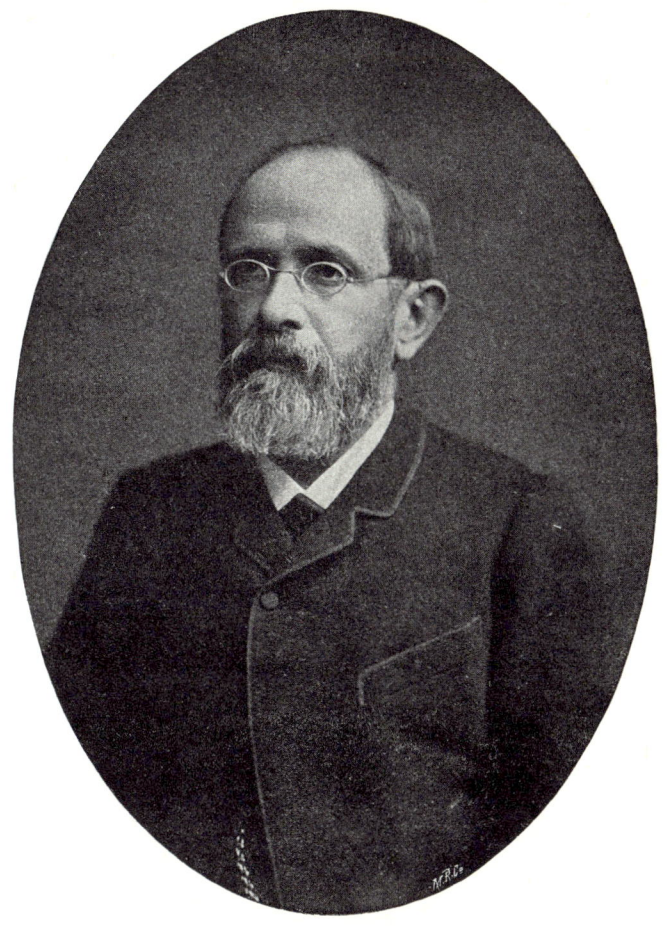

Figure 6. Rudolph P. H. Heidenhain (1834–97).

lar urine, independently of any glomerular activity. Heidenhain's observations on indigo carmine set off a controversy which continued until recent years, even though his experiments failed to establish the tubular excretion of this dye in particular, or the role of tubular excretion generally, in the formation of urine. The presence of indigo carmine or any other dye in the tubular lumen at a time when it is not "visible" in Bowman's capsule does not exclude the possibility of filtration in dilute (and not visible) solution and subsequent concentration in the tubular urine by the reabsorption of water; and the presence of dye,

SPECIAL CIRCULATIONS

distributed either diffusely or in the form of granules, in the tubule cells does not establish tubular excretion because it may gain access to the cells from either the blood or the urine and this by active transport (in Heidenhain's sense) or by simple diffusion and concentration (e.g., the vital stain, neutral red).

Among the experiments which seemed to support Heidenhain's position were those of Moritz Nussbaum (1850–1915), who in 1878 sought to arrest glomerular filtration in the frog by ligating the arterial supply to the kidney, leaving the renal-portal system intact. Under these conditions no bladder urine was normally formed, but urine excretion was restored by the intravenous injection of urea. From these experiments Nussbaum concluded that the tubules of the frog can excrete both indigo carmine and urea (55, 56).

In another direction, it was known to Ludwig that total occlusion of the renal vein led to cessation of urine formation, a fact which he attributed to increased intrarenal pressure and collapse of the tubules. On the other hand, Heidenhain argued that partial occlusion of the renal vein should increase glomerular pressure and hence urine flow, and

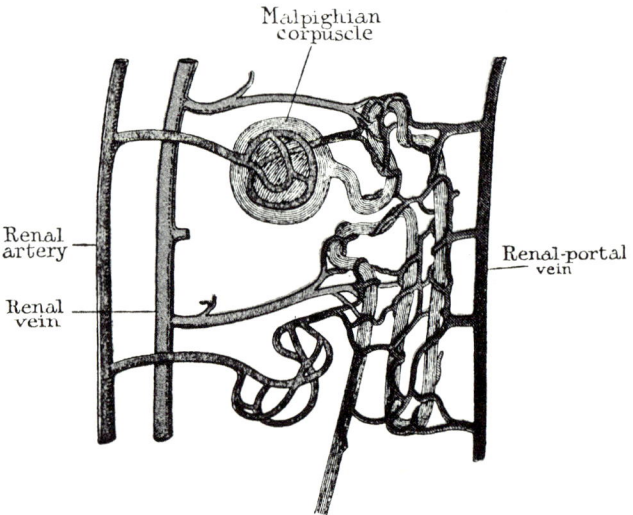

Figure 7. The afferent blood supply of the frog's kidney showing the capillary anastomosis between the efferent vessels from the glomerulus and the renal-portal system.

pointed out that an increase in urine flow rarely occurred under the conditions of his experiments.

Later, in 1883, Heidenhain calculated that the volume of filtrate required to contain all the urea a man excretes in one day would be of the order of 70 liters, of which, by Ludwig's hypothesis, some 68 liters must be reabsorbed, figures that seemed to require an impossibly large blood flow to the kidney (25). Mustering these and many other arguments, Heidenhain took the position that the urine is formed entirely by secretion, some substances (water and perhaps sodium chloride and other salts) being secreted by the glomerular tuft, others by the tubular epithelium. In his view, the important determinant in urine formation is the volume of blood perfusing the glomerular tuft and peritubular capillaries, because this volume determines the quantity of secreted substances and of oxygen delivered to the secretory cells. At no point did this theory admit of physical filtration, in Ludwig's sense, nor was the hydrostatic pressure of the blood per se important.

Nussbaum's experiments (which suffered from technical pitfalls) served at best to show that the glomerulus in the frog is the chief site of water excretion, while Heidenhain's experiments only suggested that "secretion" may involve not only the discharge of local metabolic products by secretory cells but also the transport of foreign, non-metabolized substances (such as indigo carmine) across the cell (tubular "excretion") from blood to urine. But for neither of the two views—Ludwig's filtration-reabsorption hypothesis or the Bowman-Heidenhain secretory hypothesis—was there unequivocal experimental evidence. Nor were they mutually exclusive. However, such was the force of Heidenhain's arguments that the secretory theory of urine formation remained the most popular until the second decade of the twentieth century.

Cushny and the "Modern View"

By World War I a large literature had accumulated on renal function, some writers favoring Ludwig's filtration-reabsorption hypothesis, others the secretory interpretation. Ludwig's view was pre-eminently mechanistic, as opposed to the theory of selective, secretory processes operating in the glomerulus and more particularly in the tubules, which, so far as was known, could be attributed only to an unidentifiable "vital" activity of the cells. It was after some years of controversy between the

SPECIAL CIRCULATIONS

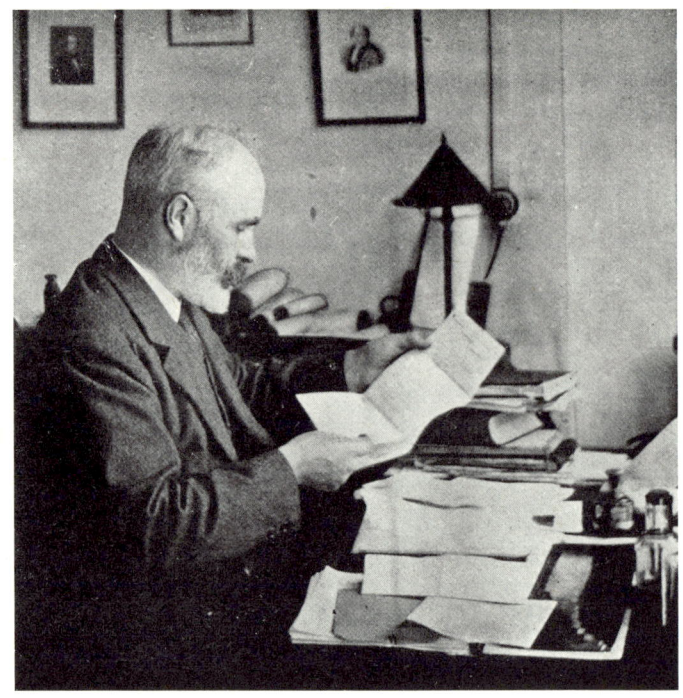

Figure 8. Arthur Robertson Cushny (1866–1926).

mechanistic and vitalistic interpretations of renal function that the mechanists gained qualified support with the publication of Cushny's *The Secretion of the Urine* in 1917 (*8*).

Arthur Robertson Cushny received his medical degree from the University of Aberdeen in 1889 and spent the next few years in various European laboratories. In 1893 he was called to the chair of Materia Medica and Therapeutics at the University of Michigan, to fill the post left vacant by John J. Abel who had moved to the chair of Pharmacology in the newly opened Johns Hopkins Medical School. It was from Michigan that Cushny published his *Textbook of Pharmacology and Therapeutics* (1899), the first such text to be published in English. In 1905 he returned to England to fill the newly created chair of Pharmacology at University College, London, the first of its kind in that country, and in

1918 he went as professor of pharmacology to Edinburgh, a chair which he held until his death in 1926 (*1, 10*).

Cushny had become interested in renal physiology through studying the intestinal tract. In 1897–98 at Ann Arbor he and George Barclay Wallace (1874–1948) (who was to hold the third chair of Pharmacology in the United States (1902–46), at what is now New York University-Bellevue Medical Center) had been studying the action of saline cathartics. They had found that sulphates and phosphates are not readily absorbed through the intestinal epithelium, and they attributed the catharsis induced by these salts to the osmotic pressure they produced in the intestinal contents (*83*). It was a simple notion, but, against the background of the last decade of the nineteenth century, a profound one, and the Wallace-Cushny paper has the historical interest that (except for Ludwig's theory of glomerular filtration) it presents the first complete explanation of a pharmacological (or physiological) phenomenon in terms of modern physical chemistry. From the phenomenon of catharsis it was a short step for Cushny (*7*) to argue in 1902 that the diuresis which follows the intravenous administration of sulphate and phosphate salts is similarly a result of the fact that these salts are not absorbed by the renal tubules and that they prevent the tubular reabsorption of water—a little later Hans Meyer in Germany could refer to saline diuresis as "diarrhea of the tubules."

In the decade after Cushny returned to London (1905–15) British physiology had come into the pre-eminent position which it was long to occupy. The studies of Walter Holbrook Gaskell, Charles Scott Sherrington, John Scott Haldane, Frederick Gowland Hopkins, Keith Lucas, Henry Hallett Dale, and many others, were bearing a rich harvest in molecular physiology. Notable among those who were inclined toward mechanistic interpretation were Ernest Henry Starling and his brother-in-law William Maddock Bayliss, who dominated the medical sciences at University College in that era. Cushny could scarcely have failed to be influenced by these two adventurous leaders in the application of chemistry to physiology.

In the interval since his work with Wallace, Cushny had published only three papers on renal physiology, but just prior to 1916 he had been gathering and sorting material for a monograph on this subject, to be published with other monographs on physiology under the editorship of

Starling. In 1916 he was invited to give the Sidney Ringer lecture at University College, a circumstance which doubtless accelerated both completion of this difficult task and integration of his views. Perhaps we are indebted to both Starling and the Sidney Ringer lectureship committee for *The Secretion of the Urine*.

When the manuscript was ready for publication, Colonel Starling was with the British Expeditionary Force in Egypt. Cushny sent the paper to Starling with a prefatory note:

"*The growth in the literature of the kidney has been extraordinary since the time when you and I began to work on it, and this increase in bulk has not gone along with an improvement of quality, but rather the reverse. No other organ of the body has suffered so much from poor work as the kidney, and in no other region of physiology does so much base coin pass as legal tender. It was therefore necessary to sift thoroughly this mass of printed matter of over 6000 pages, and I have read it carefully and, as far as might be, sympathetically, though I must confess that my patience has been sorely tried by some papers in which the depth bore no proportion to the length . . .*

"*It is often complained that the physiology of the kidney given in the textbooks is made up of a wrangle between the two great views of its activity; on the other hand, it may be argued that the many isolated observations need to be correlated with each other, and this can only be done by welding them with some definite view of renal function. I have not avoided the controversy, but I have at any rate given the ascertained facts apart from the discussion, so that they at least may remain, whatever theory of kidney activity may survive. The different views are presented, and one is advocated which differs in some respects from any that has been accepted hitherto, and which embraces some of the features of each of its precursors. Since it has been developed gradually from the work of many, it would not be fair to attach to it the name of any one investigator, and I have therefore called it ' the modern view '. . . .*

"*You will probably complain that instead of presenting the facts and following them to the theoretical principle to which they point, I have first stated the theory and then discussed how far each set of observations can be brought into accord with it . . . [but] the facts are so multitudinous that unless the student were first given some general scheme on which he could arrange them, he would be lost in detail and might fail to appreciate where the path was leading*" (8, p. viif).

Writing shortly after the beginning of this century, Max Verworn, professor of physiology at the University of Bonn, said: "By the second half of the nineteenth century [that is, in the heyday of Müller, Ludwig, Helmholtz, Bernard, etc.] the doctrine of vital force was definitely and finally overthrown to make way for the triumph of the natural method of explaining vital phenomena, which down to the present time has continued to spread and flourish with an unparalleled fertility" (*81*). Verworn was apparently not versed in renal physiology because, if we accept Cushny's interpretation, what he found in 6000 dusty pages was shot through and through with vitalism. If at times Cushny unfairly charges those with whom he does not agree with vitalism on grounds no better than suspicion, the selective, secretory operations envisioned in the Bowman-Heidenhain theory certainly still carried the older implications.

RENAL PHYSIOLOGY

Bowman had never used the expression, but Heidenhain had said that in both the glomerulus and the tubules the "diffusate" from the plasma is driven onwards and expelled into the lumen by the "active force" of the cells. It may be questioned how far Heidenhain's "active force" involved immaterial forces, but charitable as we may be, it cannot be denied that once we posit tubular excretion, particularly of foreign substances, we have only opened a door on greater mysteries, for how many such substances are excreted by the tubules? how do the tubules know just which ones to excrete? just when to abstract them from the blood? and by how much? Tubular excretion, Cushny said, would seem to endow "the renal cell with powers of discrimination of a very high order. Not only is it able to distinguish foreign substances in the plasma from the ordinary constituents and to eliminate the intruders, but it is capable of detecting, and is aroused to activity by, quantitative aberrations in the composition of the blood" (*8*, p. 41f). Admittedly, such multiplicity of function is apt to become elastic and, running riot, escape from all rules to become a rule unto itself.

"The Bowman-Heidenhain theory, if fact, amounts to little more than the statement that the kidney secretes the urine by the vital activity of its cells. It has the advantage that no possible conjunction of conditions can be imagined which cannot be attributed to some special activity of unspecified cells, whose activity is governed by no known laws and whose anatomical position in the organ can be

SPECIAL CIRCULATIONS

arranged to suit the circumstances. But such a nebulous statement of the renal function, while it offers a facile explanation of all possible observations, in reality explains nothing. As a defensive position it is impregnable, but it offers no point from which an advance may be made" (8, p. 42).

With respect to Ludwig, Cushny (who did not refer to the Marburg papers) limited favorable comment to one sentence:

"Ludwig held that the capsule [glomerulus] was a simple filter, which allowed all the constituents of the plasma to pass through it except the proteins, and that in the tubules this filtrate was elaborated into the urine by the return of much of the fluid into the blood through a process of diffusion" (8, p. 43).

This is a rather summary dismissal, inasmuch as physiology was indebted to Ludwig not only for the basic concept of filtration as a purely physical process but also for subsidiary propositions such as the role of glomerular blood pressure in the formation of this filtrate, the role of the peritubular capillaries in its reabsorption, and the potential role of the renal arterioles and renal nerves in controlling the renal circulation—as well as for engaging in battle with vitalism (as was Cushny himself) at a time when vitalistic doctrines were very much more in vogue than they were in London in the early part of this century. But Cushny, warmed up to give battle, not only sought to oust Bowman and Heidenhain but went after Ludwig's head: "Ludwig's theory," he said, "possesses only historical interest, no one at the present time supposing that the secretion of urine can be explained by purely physical forces" (8, p. 43). The notion of tubular reabsorption by "endosmosis" into the "concentrated" blood in the peritubular capillaries is, of course, where Ludwig came to grief. As Hoppe-Seyler had pointed out, and as Cushny emphasized again, endosmosis cannot explain the formation of urine of greater osmotic pressure than the blood. And so condemning both "the uncompromising vital secretion of Heidenhain" and Ludwig's theory of tubular reabsorption, Cushny sought emancipation in what he called the "modern view,"

"which accepts the general scheme of filtration and reabsorption of Ludwig, but, appreciating the inadequacy of the known physical forces, supplements them as far as necessary [sic] by the ' vital activity ' postulated by Heidenhain" (8, p. 44).

Vitalism, damned in the first part of this sentence, is readmitted to quasi-scientific status at the end; and shortly we shall see it escape from quotation marks to be confined only by dialectic chains.

With meager credit to Ludwig, Cushny accepted the hard core of Ludwig's hypothesis, that the initial step in urine formation is the separation in the glomerulus of a fluid which, except for the presumed absence of plasma proteins and formed elements to which the glomerular capillaries are impermeable, contains all the filterable constituents of the plasma in the same concentration as these are present in the plasma water. This process is purely physical and is performed by the hydrostatic pressure of the blood (and hence at the expense of the heart) in accordance with the Ludwig-Starling principle of filtration applicable to capillaries generally. That all microsolutes must pass freely into the filtrate follows from the fact, first pointed out by Tammann (79) in 1896, that their combined osmotic pressure is over 5000 mm. Hg, a force exceeding by one-hundred-fold the available hydrostatic pressure in the glomerulus.

Cushny rejected the possibility of tubular excretion in part because it offered "a facile explanation of all possible observations [and] in reality explains nothing," and in part because its proponents had advanced no incontrovertible evidence for its existence (although admittedly the evidence, even on indigo carmine, was ambiguous). Having rejected tubular excretion, the unavoidable corollary of the filtration hypothesis was, as Ludwig had held, that the volume of filtrate formed per unit time must be large enough to remove from the blood all the constituents destined to be excreted in the urine, a volume far in excess of the urine volume. It followed that not only a large fraction of the filtered water but also most of the filtered glucose, amino acids, sodium, potassium, chloride, sulphate, and uric acid must be reabsorbed by the tubules. It is in consequence of the reabsorption of water that waste products, such as creatinine, urea, etc., appear in the urine in many times the concentration in which they are present in the plasma. But since different substances are concentrated to a different extent, relative to the plasma, it must be accepted that they are reabsorbed in varying degree: substances which need to be conserved by the organism (sodium, chloride, glucose, amino acids, etc.) are perhaps reabsorbed completely or nearly so, while some waste products, such as creatinine, are possibly not reabsorbed at all. Cushny believed that substances in the first group are completely reabsorbed so

SPECIAL CIRCULATIONS

long as the plasma concentration is below a certain critical threshold concentration, and therefore he called them "threshold" substances, a term first used by Bernard in describing the excretion of glucose. Waste products, such as creatinine, which are rejected by the tubules regardless of plasma concentration, he called "no-threshold" substances.

At first sight the process whereby water and the many "threshold" substances are reabsorbed might appear to be extraordinarily complex, but Cushny resolved this difficulty by a simplifying assumption: namely, that what the tubules reabsorb is a fluid of constant composition, a "perfected Locke's fluid" containing glucose, amino acids, and similar food substances, with sodium, potassium, chloride, urea, urate, and phosphate in approximately the proportions in which they are "best adapted to the tissues":

"The formation of the glomerular filtrate is due to a blind force. The absorption in the tubules is equally independent of any discrimination, for the fluid absorbed is always the same, whatever the needs of the organism at the moment" (*8, p. 48*).

Cushny does not refer to Claude Bernard's thesis of the constancy of the internal environment, but we may note that by constantly abstracting a "perfected Locke's fluid" from a filtrate of variable composition and returning this fluid to the blood the tubules operate automatically to maintain the constancy of composition which that body fluid normally has, while insuring the excretion of all superfluous or deleterious substances.

The reabsorption of a "perfected Locke's fluid" as a single operation would truly have been another physiologic tour de force, equaling Ludwig's hypothesis of glomerular filtration, had it proved to be true, or even theoretically possible. Subsequent observations showed that it is not true, and in retrospect we can ask, is it conceivably possible? How could the tubules absorb a "fluid" containing many substances (the number would obviously have to be much larger than Cushny supposed), each in its proper quantitative relation to reabsorbed water, without distinguishing them from each other and from foreign substances, and without (in the proximate step) operating on or engaging each substance separately —which is simply "specific" tubular "activity" reversed in direction? Indeed, in the absence of any imagined mechanism to explain the reabsorption of this "perfected fluid" Cushny was forced to say it "depends on the vital activity of the [tubular] epithelium" (*8, p. 44*). Thus having rejected Heidenhain's tubular secretion because of its vitalistic implications in one paragraph, he reinvokes vitalism in tubular reabsorption two paragraphs later—though this vital activity is now reduced to the attractively constant and presumably definable dimensions of a "perfected fluid." "The chief attraction of the original Ludwig theory lay in its eliminating altogether the unknown vital activity of the cell. The modern theory accepts this activity as necessary . . ." but it possesses the advantage over the Bowman-Heidenhain theory in that

"it reduces the kidney to a machine instead of postulating for it the capacity of a highly trained analytical chemist. One part of the kidney filters off the plasma colloids, another part absorbs a fluid of unchanging composition. The kidney exercises no discrimination . . . just as a muscle exercises no discrimination. . . . The kidney loses somewhat in dignity and romance when it is thus represented as merely a hard-working organ . . . so devoid of judgment that in some conditions it acts to the prejudice of the organism by removing the diluent instead of the poison" (*8, pp. 55-6*).

If Cushny's position concerning "vital activity" seems inconsistent, it is inconsistent; the difficulty lies in the paradox that though we name the things we know, we do not necessarily know them because we name them.

A second paradox presented by *The Secretion of the Urine* is that though the process of glomerular filtration remained central in Cushny's theory, he failed to see the importance of measuring this process reliably and precisely. On the premise that each liter of plasma contains 300 mg. of urea, each liter of urine 20 gm., and assuming that no urea is reabsorbed, he calculated that in man about 62 liters of filtrate must be formed each day to deliver this urea into the urine, from which 61 liters of water are reabsorbed (*8, p. 48*). The magnitude of this operation did not seem impossible to him, as it had seemed to Heidenhain. (Actually, the true filtration rate is twice this value since some 50 per cent of the filtered urea is reabsorbed.) He recognized that phlorizin probably "poisoned" the tubules and prevented the reabsorption of glucose and possibly other substances; he believed that the absorbing power of the tubules may possibly be decreased or increased by various drugs; and that the presence

SPECIAL CIRCULATIONS

of any unabsorbable substance (sulphate, phosphate, urea, glucose) in the tubular fluid will limit reabsorption of water and other substances, and produce diuresis. And lastly he believed that the rate (velocity) at which the filtrate passes down the tubules will influence the amount of reabsorption. It was possibly because of these logically reasonable variables —and because urea was the only "no-threshold" substance known to him—that the author of the "Modern Theory" did not visualize the possibility of measuring accurately the central operation of glomerular filtration and failed to bring this problem to focus anywhere in his monograph.

However, despite Cushny's failure to make a quantitative approach to this problem, despite his a priori prejudice against tubular excretion and his unsupported premise of the reabsorption of a "perfected Locke's fluid," and despite the nominal readmission of "vital activity" in the reabsorption of this "perfected fluid," *The Secretion of the Urine* remains an important event in the history of renal physiology. It brought hitherto unsupported speculation and indiscriminate experimentation within the restraints of a critical theory; and it served, as its author hoped it would, both as an advanced post from which others might proceed against the remaining ramparts of vitalism and as a guide and powerful stimulus to students of renal physiology. For these reasons it can be said that it ushered in the period of modern renal physiology.

Richards's Experiments: Fact Replaces Theory

Cushny had attempted to reduce the multitudinous and contradictory data on renal function to philosophical order at a time when the *sine qua non* of philosophical order—a foundation of established fact—was lacking. Except as supported inferentially by observations of a second order of cogency, his hypothesis was without experimental substantiation, and consequently his position frequently seems dogmatic.

It remained for Alfred Newton Richards and his co-workers at the University of Pennsylvania to lay the experimental foundations of the filtration-reabsorption hypothesis. Richards had trained in chemistry at Yale University under the influence of R. H. Chittenden, and he entered the area of renal physiology through biochemistry and pharmacology. When the *Journal of Biological Chemistry* was founded by Christian A. Herter and John J. Abel in 1905, he became assistant editor;

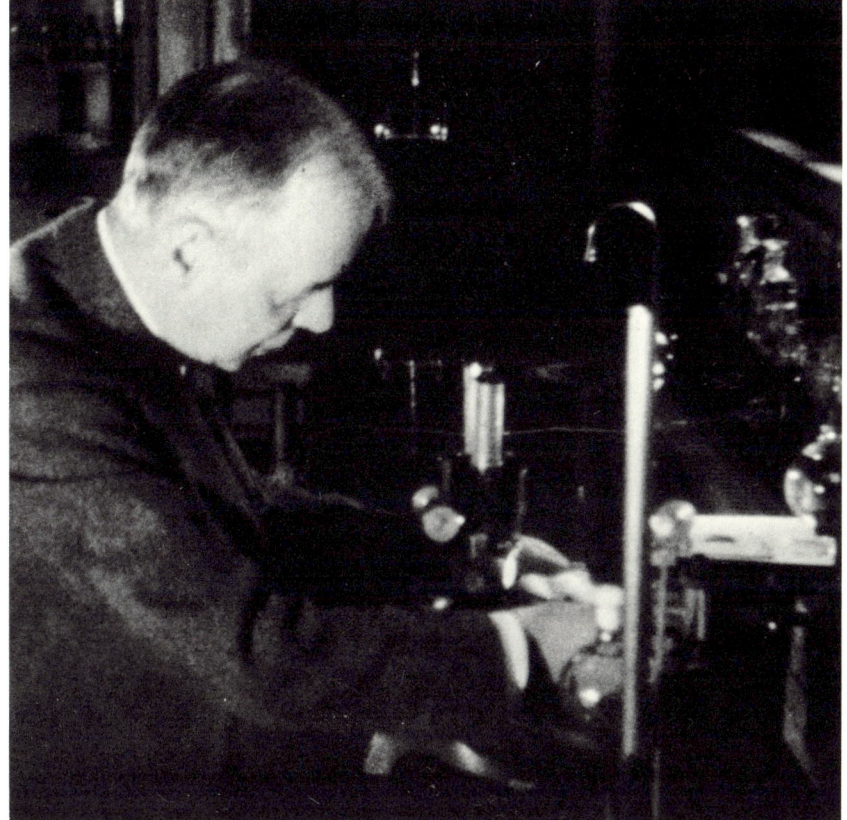

Figure 9. Alfred Newton Richards (1876–   ).

subsequently (1911–14) he served as managing editor of that journal until Donald D. Van Slyke took over. During the latter years the business of the Journal was conducted in two rooms of Richards's laboratory at the University of Pennsylvania. It has been said by his friends that he had little time to do anything but edit, but *that* he did damn well.

In these busy years Richards started the first course in experimental pharmacology at Columbia's College of Physicians and Surgeons; in 1908 he reorganized the course at Northwestern University Medical School and taught it practically singlehanded for two years; and he repeated the process at Pennsylvania in 1910. During this time he also studied the action of HCN on metabolism with George B. Wallace, investigated the manifestations of chloroform poisoning with John Howland, and started experiments on the perfusion of the kidney with Cecil K. Drinker and Oscar H. Plant.

SPECIAL CIRCULATIONS

It was while teaching experimental pharmacology at Columbia, between 1904 and 1908, that Richards became interested in the isolated mammalian heart as a means of studying the action of drugs on this organ. With John Howland, he had been working on the problem of toxemia in children, particularly as it related to detoxification, presumably by the liver—the paper by Howland and Richards (29) on delayed necrosis of the liver caused by chloroform, a by-product of that study, remains a classic in the field. While pursuing these investigations it had occurred to Richards that an adequate perfusion technique, one better than any hitherto described, might unlock the answers to many problems. By the time that he moved to Pennsylvania as professor of pharmacology in 1910, he had formulated a plan for a perfusion pump which avoided any contact between blood and metal. In the summer of 1911, Cecil K. Drinker (1887–1956), then a medical student, began working with Richards, and after graduation in 1913 he stayed on as assistant for a year. Drinker's help and interest were a large factor in carrying forward the development of a successful pump by which, in 1913, they kept the isolated brain of a cat alive for two hours, and, in 1914, they carried out a successful experiment on the isolated dog kidney.

When Drinker left in 1914 to take up his internship at Peter Bent Brigham Hospital in Boston, Oscar H. Plant (1875–1939), who had joined Richards's staff in 1911 and had worked in some of the early perfusion experiments, embarked with him on experiments with the perfused rabbit kidney, with special reference to the diuretic action of caffeine. Underlying these experiments was the question of whether the action of this drug was to be explained by its vascular action and an increase in filtration, or by stimulation of secretory activity, as was suggested by its power to increase oxygen consumption and its known stimulating action on other structures. With a constant output pump, Richards and Plant thought that they could eliminate vascular action and settle the question of secretion. Their experiments revealed no parallelism between perfusion pressure and urine flow, so long as the volume flow remained constant, while caffeine caused diuresis even when the rate of blood flow remained constant (*64*).

These experiments seemed contradictory, but they pointed the way to tackling the Ludwig-Heidenhain controversy. In the next year Richards and Plant (*65, 66*) conducted experiments on the rabbit kidney perfused *in situ*, in which they showed that changes in perfusion pressure, induced by splanchnic stimulation, epinephrine, nitroglycerin, or compression of the renal vein, were accompanied by parallel changes in the rate of urine formation. This urine was generally moderately concentrated with respect to urea and creatinine, and dilute with respect to chloride; it was also shown that if the perfusion pressure is at such a level that compression of the renal vein does not decrease blood flow, then an increase in venous pressure does in fact increase urine flow, thus answering one of Heidenhain's strongest arguments against Ludwig.

Subsequently Richards and Plant applied the volume recorder or oncometer, which had been introduced into renal physiology by Roy and Cohnheim in 1883, to the excised dog and rabbit kidney during perfusion. They observed that the addition of minimally effective doses of epinephrine to the perfusing blood caused an increase in perfusion pressure simultaneously with a small increase in kidney volume (*65, 66*). Conversely, when the kidney was perfused at constant pressure, epinephrine might cause a decrease in blood flow simultaneously with an increase in kidney volume. Since an increase in perfusion pressure at constant flow requires vasoconstriction in the organ, and vasoconstriction of other organs is accompanied by a decrease in volume, they sought an explanation for the paradoxical behavior of the kidney in the unique features of its circulation. They proposed that epinephrine in the concentrations studied acts predominantly on the efferent glomerular arterioles, causing an increase in intraglomerular pressure and distention of the glomeruli, with consequent increase in kidney volume and some increase in urine formation. The unique hemodynamic possibilities of independent or at least differential control of the afferent and efferent arterioles was noted by Starling in 1912 and was foreseen as early as 1856 by Ludwig, who had recognized the functional importance not only of the afferent and efferent arterioles but also of the muscles in "the roots of the renal vein."

Then, in April of 1917, World War I began, and these experiments,

SPECIAL CIRCULATIONS

except for preliminary reports, remained unpublished. In August of that year Richards went to England to serve as a member of the scientific staff of the British Medical Research Committee. After American troops became embroiled in gas warfare early in 1918 he went to Chaumont, France, to equip and conduct a physiological laboratory for the newly established Chemical Warfare Service of the United States Army. He had met Cushny in London and the two had become close friends, and it was in the milieu of the Cushny renal renaissance that Richards returned home by way of London in December of 1918. He and Plant began to write up their experiments on the perfused kidney, which generally supported the Ludwig-Cushny hypothesis. In the spring of 1920 Richards was invited to give a Harvey Lecture. This is an invitation no scientist can easily decline. Founded at the New York Academy of Medicine in 1905 to present to physicians and research workers the results of investigations in all areas of medical science, it was and has remained America's most distinguished lectureship. Richards accepted, but with some misgivings since he had for discussion only the perfusion experiments, which served to bolster the filtration hypothesis, and the epinephrine paradox, for which he and Plant had only an unsubstantiated theory. Worse, immediately after accepting the Harvey Society invitation he came down with acute appendicitis. In the ensuing enforced vacation, he reread Cushny's monograph and a paper by August Krogh (1874–1949) (33) on the capillary circulation, and pondered the problem of how to get evidence as to whether or not the glomeruli swelled under the action of epinephrine. In Krogh's paper, which described the direct observation of the capillaries in the tongue and muscles of the frog, Richards saw a possible new approach to this problem: why not examine a frog's kidney under the microscope and, treating it with epinephrine, possibly obtain direct evidence on how this drug worked? It might be possible to confirm the efferent action of epinephrine and to present in his Harvey Lecture a demonstrated fact rather than an hypothesis. When he returned to the laboratory in the early autumn he suggested the experiment to Carl Frederic Schmidt (1893–   ), who had come as an instructor to his department in 1919.

Heidenhain and others had searched for dyes in the capsular fluid in the kidneys and tubular urine of living frogs and other animals, but apparently with little regard for the glomerular circulation. Now Richards and

Schmidt (67), using reflected light to examine the ventral surface of the kidney in a pithed or anesthetized animal, found circular arrangements of capillaries which were patently glomeruli, and in which the movement of red cells could be discerned. In some glomeruli the blood moved with bewildering rapidity through a maze of pathways; in others, the stream was slower and involved fewer capillary channels. In some glomeruli the tuft appeared to fill the capsular space, in others it did not. The blood flow in a few capillaries might be more active than in others in the same glomerulus, a single capillary passing in the course of a short time from a state of abundant flow to one of sluggish or wholly arrested circulation. And different glomeruli might show variable activity from time to time. When constriction proximal to the capillary tuft occurred, the red cells generally moved out of the capillaries, leaving the tuft all but empty.

The question that had led to these experiments, the action of epinephrine, was examined by introducing this agent into the blood. Large doses led to a decrease in the number of active glomeruli, or to a decrease in the number of patent capillary loops in a single glomerulus, though the susceptibility of different vessels was not the same. Cessation of blood flow could here be attributed to constriction proximal to the glomerular tuft. Minimally effective doses, however, caused the capillary tuft to become engorged with cells, the velocity of flow to decrease, and the tuft to swell, which changes were consonant with efferent arteriolar constriction. It proved to be impossible, however, to measure the diameter of the efferent arteriole, and since a similar effect could have been produced by accelerated inflow of blood into the glomerulus, this approach did not afford a final answer to the epinephrine paradox.

From their observations on the frog kidney Richards and Schmidt came to speak of "intermittence of glomerular activity," and to conclude that in the normal kidney not all the glomeruli are active at any one moment. As they noted, the effect of their observations was "to reintroduce into considerations of renal physiology the conception held by Hermann and doubtless by Ludwig that the extent of the filtration surface in the kidney is variable and a factor which must be of major importance in the adjustment of renal function to excretory requirement." Although final publication of the perfusion experiments had been delayed by World War I, these and the direct observations on the glomerular circulation were reviewed by Richards in his Harvey Lecture of February 26, 1921 (*59*).

SPECIAL CIRCULATIONS

The visualization of the living frog's kidney proved to be an important turning point in the Philadelphia investigations, because this direct approach was to lead to the micropuncture studies for which Richards's laboratory is justly famous. In 1921 Schmidt turned from renal to respiratory physiology, and in 1922 he left Philadelphia to join the staff of the Peking Union Medical School in China. Joseph Treloar Wearn (1893–   ), who had come to Philadelphia in 1921 from a senior residency at the Peter Bent Brigham Hospital, had meanwhile chosen to work on the kidney. Richards showed Wearn how to prepare a frog for examination, asked him to perfect himself in the technique, and to go on looking at it; but to report if he had any ideas. Leaving Wearn to acquire skill and to develop fresh ideas, Richards wandered off with the problem of the epinephrine paradox uppermost in his mind.

Micropuncture of Glomerulus, Final Proof of Filtration

Profitable is the course of science when a man is moved, by whatever considerations, to drift a bit, to leave his laboratory and mingle with colleagues working on seemingly unrelated experiments. It was at the Philadelphia meeting of the American Association of Anatomists at the Wistar Institute, in April, 1921, that Richards met Robert Chambers, then demonstrating his micromanipulator, with the needle of which he was able to perform exquisite dissections or injections in single cells. It occurred to Richards that he could test the theory of the epinephrine paradox by using Chambers's technique to apply the drug directly to the efferent arterioles of the frog glomerulus. On discussing the matter with Wearn, the latter countered with the suggestion that they puncture a glomerulus, withdraw some fluid from the capsule, and test it for protein —since the cardinal point in the Ludwig-Cushny hypothesis was that the capsular fluid was protein-free. The first micropipette in Philadelphia was thus used to collect glomerular fluid (*84*) and not to test the epinephrine paradox, which because of technical difficulties was never put to the micropipette test.

Thus began another chapter in renal physiology. Fifteen years elapsed before all the definitive papers on the composition of glomerular and

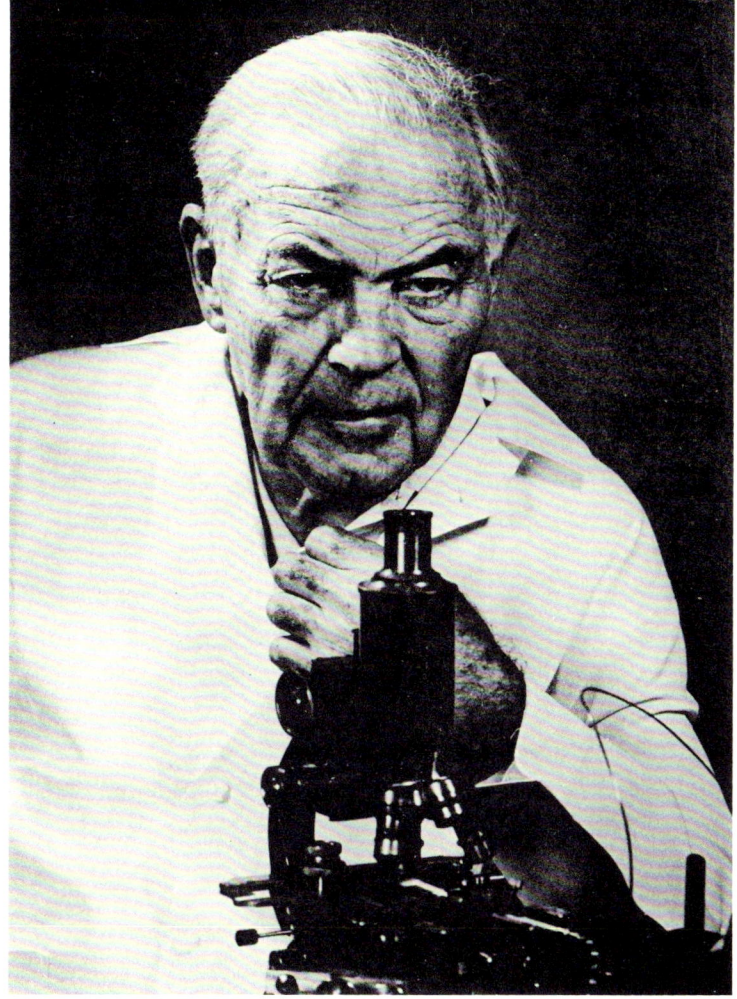

Figure 10. Robert Chambers (1881–1957).

tubular urine in the Amphibia were published from the Philadelphia laboratories. In 1923 Wearn left Philadelphia to rejoin the Department of Medicine at Harvard, but not before he and Richards had demonstrated that the glomerular fluid is essentially free of protein (down to the lower

SPECIAL CIRCULATIONS

limit of the analytical method) but contains sugar and chloride, when the simultaneous bladder urine is free of these substances; and that indigo carmine, phenol red, and methylene blue are present in the capsular fluid after these dyes have been injected intravenously.

In subsequent years Arthur M. Walker, Leonard Bayliss, John B. Barnwell, James Bordley III, R. C. Bradley, Phyllis A. Bott, T. Findley, Jr., J. M. Hayman, Jr., J. P. Hendrix, C. L. Hudson, Hugh Montgomery, J. A. Pierce, B. B. Westfall, and others participated in these studies, patiently developing microanalytical methods which were applied to the quantitative examination of the capsular fluid of the frog, mud-puppy (Necturus), and, in a few instances, the snake. It was shown that, in respect to all constituents for which analytical methods had been developed, the capsular fluid has the composition to be expected of a protein-free filtrate. By puncturing a tubule where it presented itself in a vulnerable position in the transilluminated kidney, and blocking it proximally and distally with a droplet of mercury, they were able to perfuse limited segments of the nephron and to demonstrate significant segmental differences in function (*60–63*).

In 1926, Joseph Marchant Hayman, Jr. (1896–   ), working in the Philadelphia laboratory, showed that the systolic pressure in the afferent glomerular arteriole in the frog averaged 85 per cent of the simultaneous aortic pressure; that in the glomerular capillaries, 54 per cent (*23*). In almost all instances the glomerular capillary pressure exceeded 10 cm. H_2O, the average osmotic pressure of the proteins in frog's plasma as determined by Harvey Lester White (1896–   ) (*85*). These findings placed Ludwig's filtration theory on a firm hemodynamic basis. Hayman also confirmed that under the action of epinephrine or caffeine the glomerular capillary pressure could be influenced quite out of proportion to the effect on aortic pressure, as predicted by Ludwig, Starling, and Richards and Plant.

Subsequently Walker in the Philadelphia laboratories succeeded in applying the micropuncture technique to the mammalian kidney, in which, because of its compactness, the task is exceedingly difficult. In collaboration with Bott of Philadelphia and Jean Oliver and Muriel C. McDowell (*82*) of the Long Island College of Medicine, experiments were made with guinea pigs, white rats, and opossums, with results which, with respect to the composition of glomerular fluid and the division of function between the proximal and distal segments of the tubule, were consistent with those obtained in the earlier work with Amphibia.

The micropuncture technique not only established the filtration hypothesis beyond any doubt, but also laid the foundations for our knowledge of segmental function in the nephron. For twenty years a man and his pupils studied frogs and mudpuppies! It seems unlikely that the immediate future will see a comparable series of investigations, concentrating on one objective, sustained for so long a period, and involving as many technical difficulties, as is represented in this work. Richards has remarked that the major credit should not come to him, but rather it should go to the many investigators who carried out the bulk of the actual work. True enough, perhaps, but one of the rough spots of modern medical research is that many young men, interested, willing, and competent, come and go through our laboratory portals, spending at the most two or three years in research before launching into a career in which they are all too frequently engulfed by other professional or administrative duties. It can be no other way because clinical medicine needs them, and the clinical and preclinical research departments cannot always contain them. Despite its disadvantages this system of transient apprentices continues to produce a large fraction of both our medical researchers and our good clinicians. As for credit, however, through these twenty years someone had to maintain continuity, esprit de corps, high standards of performance, perspective, critical acuity, and courage when the going was particularly rough; and, probably in many instances, to reduce complicated series of data to a comprehensible paper. Like Ludwig, Richards's name is on every paper in the small type that reads *From the Laboratory of Pharmacology of the University of Pennsylvania*.

Tubular Excretion: Marshall's Experiments

At first thought it would seem that the micropuncture technique would have afforded an answer to the vexing question of tubular excretion, but this answer could not come from observations on the concentration of any one substance at any point along the nephron. As the urine passes down the tubule, various substances (creatinine, urea, phosphate)

SPECIAL CIRCULATIONS

are concentrated to a variable degree and it is impossible on the prima facie evidence to determine, for any particular substance, whether this progressive concentration is attributable solely to the reabsorption of water by the tubule, or complicated by the tubular reabsorption or tubular excretion of the substance under consideration. An answer to this question requires knowledge of the extent of filtration and reabsorption of water itself (either in individual nephrons or in the kidney as a whole), and this knowledge can only be obtained by reference to the degree of concentration of some standard of reference which itself undergoes neither tubular addition nor subtraction on its way to the bladder. Agreement as to the qualifications, in this respect, of several candidate substances was not to come for a decade after the micropuncture studies were begun, and consequently the field was, for a time, left open for the continuation of the "wrangle" (to use Cushny's term) over tubular excretion which Cushny had deplored.

Among those who held to the possibility of tubular excretion were Eli Kennerly Marshall, Jr. and his co-workers at the Johns Hopkins Medical School. Marshall had trained in organic chemistry at the Johns Hopkins University, taking his degree in this subject in 1911. After three years of teaching biochemistry at the medical school, he transferred to pharmacology as an associate under John J. Abel, and obtained his M.D. degree in 1917. Leaving Baltimore in 1919 to take the chair of Pharmacology at Washington University, he returned to Hopkins as professor of physiology in 1921, and moved to the chair of Pharmacology and Experimental Therapeutics in 1932.

In the summer of 1912 Marshall went to Halle to work with Abderhalden, in conformity with the current opinion that in order to be accredited as a good scientist one had to spend some time in the laboratory of one of the Continental masters. In Abderhalden's laboratory he worked on the hydrolysis of proteins, amino acid separation, and enzymatic reactions, but found spare time to browse in the library, where he came across Takeuchi's demonstration of urease in the soy bean. He conceived that the urea-urease system might be a good one for the study of reaction rates, and on returning to Baltimore in the fall of 1912, he procured some soy beans with this goal in mind. The problem of reaction rates was, however, soon subordinated to the use of urease for the specific, quantitative determination of urea in urine and blood (*42, 43*),

RENAL
PHYSIOLOGY

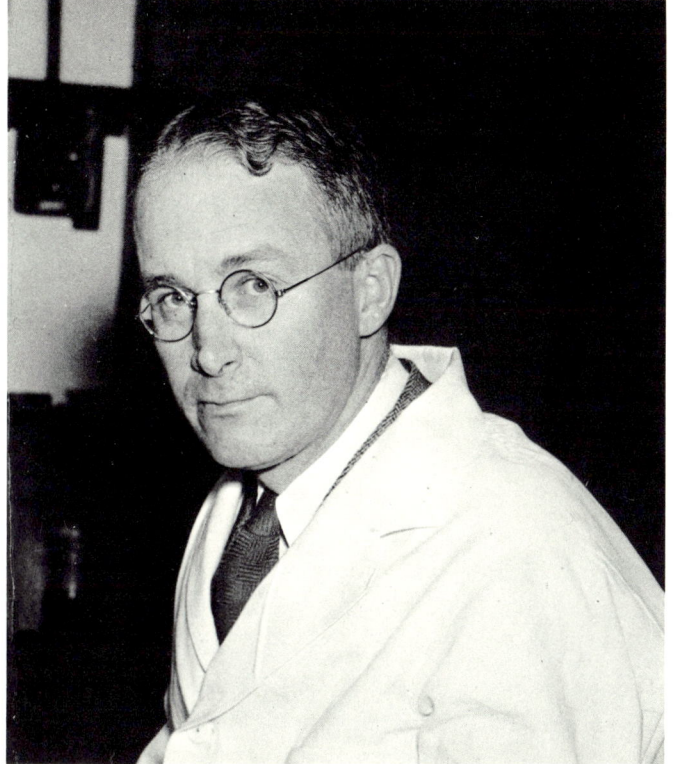

Figure 11. Eli Kennerly Marshall (1889–   ).

his attention having been called to the importance of developing such a method by Leonard G. Rowntree.

In 1914, Marshall and David Melvin Davis (1886–   ) undertook a study of the distribution of urea in various tissues of the body; they found that this compound was distributed uniformly throughout the body water, and that the rate of excretion in the dog is proportional to its concentration in the blood (*48*). Very little money was then available for research, and not wanting to waste fifty cents on two normal dogs they used the carcasses of two dogs which had been adrenalectomized by Samuel Crowe and George Wislocki, only to discover that the concentration of urea in the tissues was markedly elevated. This led them to study the influence of the adrenals on the kidney, and, because of the

SPECIAL CIRCULATIONS

anatomical proximity of the adrenals to the renal hilus, this in turn led to a study by Marshall and Alfred Conrad Kolls (1891–   ) of the influence of the renal nerves on the excretion of urea, creatinine, and water. These experiments had to be set aside when World War I came and Marshall undertook the study of war gases in New Haven in the summer of 1917. While at New Haven, he read Cushny's monograph and came to the opinion that some of the results which he and Kolls had obtained were incompatible with Cushny's simple filtration-reabsorption hypothesis.

The war over, and gas warfare no longer of interest, Marshall returned to Baltimore, and, in 1919, he and Kolls published a report of their pre-war experiments. By this time he had become convinced that, despite the technical inadequacy of all experiments from Heidenhain's time on, which purported to demonstrate tubular excretion, Cushny's summary dismissal of this process was arbitrary and unwarranted. It was inevitable that in the further exploration of this problem Marshall should turn to phenol red (phenol sulphonephthalein), firmly established at Johns Hopkins in 1910 as a clinical kidney function test by the studies of Leonard George Rowntree (1883–   ) and John Timothy Geraghty (1876–1924) (69). In 1923, while working with James Leonard Vickers (1899–1953), Marshall showed that when phenol red is administered intravenously to dogs in which urine excretion had been abolished by reduction of blood pressure to below 40 mm. Hg, as much as 35 per cent of the injected dye was taken up by the kidneys. The dye was concentrated in the renal cortex, and on microscopic examination of teased preparations, it appeared to be located in the cells of the convoluted tubules and to be absent from the urine. Proceeding from the knowledge that certain phenols and dyes are partially (though reversibly) bound to plasma proteins, and on the principle that the bound fraction is not available for filtration into a protein-free glomerular fluid, Marshall and Vickers examined the protein-binding of phenol red in dog plasma by ultrafiltration through collodion membranes and found only 37 to 41 per cent of the total phenol red to be filterable. Assuming a maximal renal blood flow of 5 cc. min. per gm. of kidney, they calculated that filtration could not account for all the phenol red excreted from known plasma concentrations even if 100 per cent of the plasma were filtered through the glomeruli (50). (Cushny rather hyperbolically dismissed these observations as possibly representing "diffusion from a dying cell" (*9, 2nd ed., p. 78*).) In the interim deHaan had independently demonstrated that phenol red and other dyes are extensively bound by plasma proteins, but he had concluded that the dye-protein complex is filtered through the glomeruli, the protein to be reabsorbed by the tubules while the dye is excreted in the urine. Marshall and Vickers correctly rejected this hypothesis in favor of the view that, in addition to filtration, tubular excretion, coupled with the continuous diffusion of free dye from the capillaries into the tubule cells, could account for the high rate of excretion. As opposed to the numerous qualitative observations recording merely the presence of a dye in the tubule cells, and despite the fact that Marshall and Vickers did not wholly exclude dead space errors and other technical hazards, their paper remains the first convincing evidence of tubular excretion in the mammal.

These experiments were followed up by Marshall and Marian M. Crane (*47*), in 1924, who demonstrated that (as was now well established) the rate of excretion of urea in the mammal increases in proportion to the plasma urea concentration, a result to be expected if urea is excreted entirely by glomerular filtration with no tubular reabsorption, and if the filtration rate remains constant. As the plasma concentration of phenol red is raised, however, the rate of excretion ultimately levels off and approaches a constant, maximal value, a result incompatible with exclusive filtration but explicable in terms of filtration plus tubular excretion, the latter process becoming "saturated" at higher plasma concentrations. They showed that a similar limitation applies to the excretion of urea in the bull frog (*R. catesbiana*), and they concluded that where urea is probably excreted solely by filtration in the dog (and other mammals), phenol red in the dog and frog, and urea in the latter, are excreted by the tubules, in addition to being filtered. The experiments reported by Marshall and his co-workers (*46*) on phenol red and urea cannot be explained otherwise, and have generally been considered by the writer as constituting the first unassailable demonstration of the participation of tubular excretion in urine formation.

At about the same time Edward Brice Cooper Mayrs (1891–   ) (*51*) adduced good evidence for the tubular excretion of uric acid in the chicken, where the rate of excretion is inconceivably greater than can be explained by filtration alone at any plausible value for the filtra-

SPECIAL CIRCULATIONS

tion rate. Mayrs's work was done in Cushny's laboratory in Edinburgh, and it is said that Cushny was very annoyed—in any case, he later disposed of the chicken in a rather pointless footnote (*9, 2nd ed., p. 122*).

Here, in effect, the matter rested for several years, the "wrangle" over tubular excretion continuing unabated. As the micropuncture studies initiated by Wearn and Richards in the Amphibia got under way, the Philadelphia investigators, with what seemed to many to be only reasonable conservatism, sought to explain urine formation in terms of the filtration-reabsorption hypothesis without invoking tubular excretion. The debate acquired a sort of bipolar character, with one focus in Baltimore, positively charged in favor of the tubular excretion of phenol red in the mammal and of both phenol red and urea in the frog, the other in Philadelphia, negatively (or at least very skeptically) charged with respect to the frog and mudpuppy. On the periphery, investigators leaned to the north or south according to their geographic loyalties or the latest but still conflicting arguments in the rapidly multiplying literature (*45, 70, 16, 17*).

The Goosefish Tubule Must Excrete

In the fall of 1925 the writer was engaged in a study of the composition of the body fluids of fish, this work having been started in the summer at the Mount Desert Island Biological Laboratory at Salisbury Cove, Maine, and continued during the winter by commuting from Charlottesville to the New York Aquarium. Marshall, with whom I had worked on mustard gas in 1917 (I had also collected urine with him and Kolls in 1919), one day asked me what I was doing, and when I told him that I was working on fish he exclaimed with vehemence, "Fish? My God, man! Don't you know that fish are *lower* than frogs?" I recall he made it clear that I could never be a proper "physiologist" unless I shifted my interests upward in the vertebrate scale.

Marshall, however, having studied urine formation in the frog, rabbit, and dog, had come to recognize that conclusions with respect to renal function cannot be safely transferred from one class of vertebrates to another. He was thus the first to realize that a systematic, comparative study of renal function in all classes of vertebrates was essential to the proper understanding of this complicated problem. This motive led him, in the fall of 1925, to the library in search of information on the com-

RENAL PHYSIOLOGY

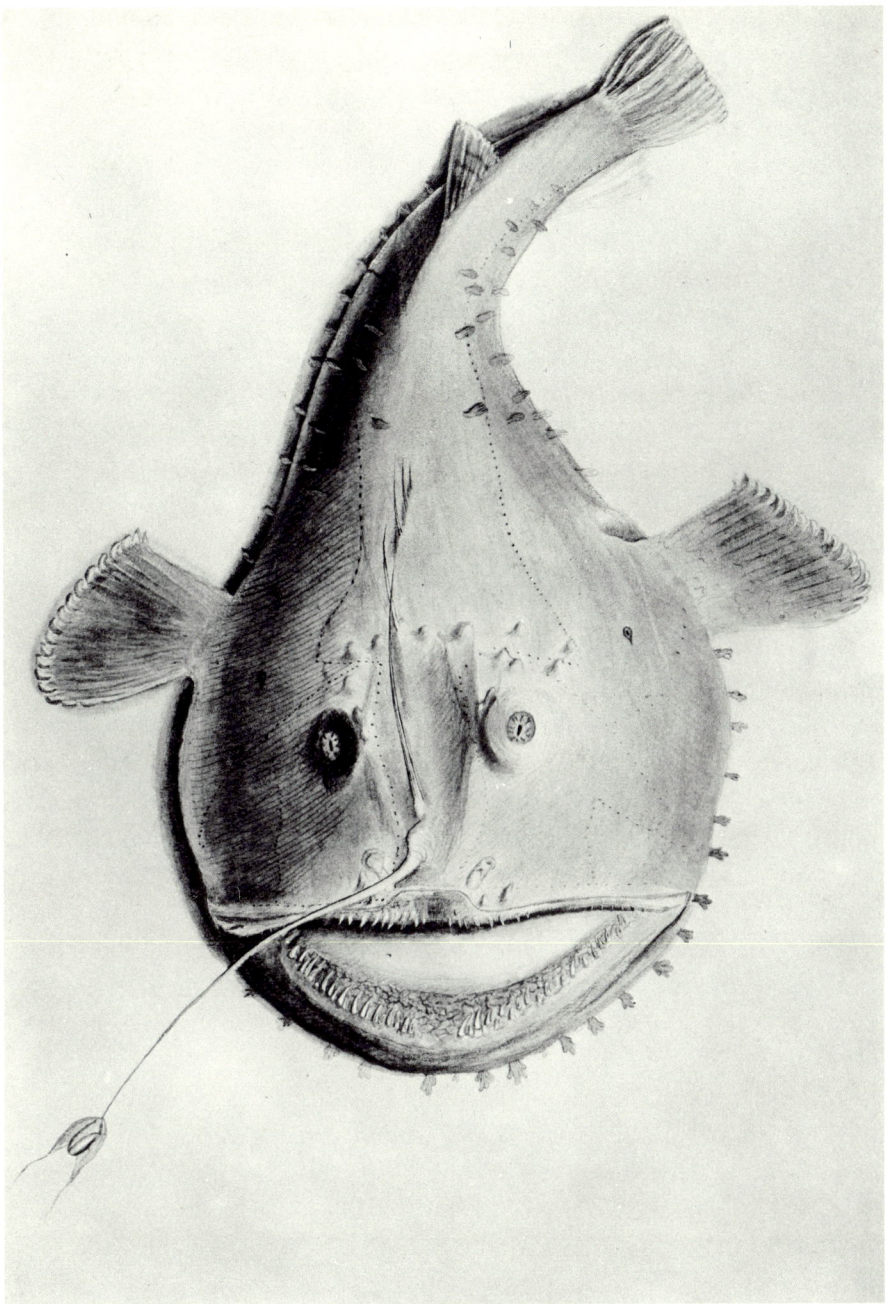

Figure 12. *Lophius piscatorius* by Edward Tyson.

SPECIAL CIRCULATIONS

parative physiology of the kidney, and in Winterstein's *Handbuch der vergleichender Physiologie* he came upon references to papers by A. Huot (1897), F. Guitel (1900), and J. Audige (1910), wherein it was reported that in certain marine teleosts the kidney is entirely aglomerular, made up wholly of blind tubules; and, what was even worse for those who argued against tubular excretion, these tubules were supplied only with venous blood from the renal-portal system, the arterial supply to the glomeruli, characteristic of all glomerular vertebrates, having disappeared along with the glomeruli (75). If such a fish could excrete urine, it must be entirely by tubular excretion. That, specifically, the kidney of *Lophius piscatorius* (goose fish, angler fish, monk fish) was aglomerular had been stated by Audige; and that this kidney did in fact excrete urine had been demonstrated by Burian in 1909, and this urine had been subjected to limited chemical analysis by Willy Denis of Folin's laboratory working at Woods Hole in the summer of 1913 (11). All that was required to demonstrate that tubular excretion alone could subserve the ends of homeostasis in at least one vertebrate was to clip together the respective papers by Audige and Denis; but instead Marshall sought to confirm and to extend these observations in detail. He learned from Warren Harmon Lewis (1870–   ), then at the Carnegie Institution at Hopkins, that *Lophius* could be procured at Salisbury Cove—*Lophius* is mostly mouth, but the tail supplies what are said to be two delicate filets, of which Lewis was fond; and he knew *Lophius* was available in Frenchman's Bay because it was his custom to buy *Lophius* steaks at the Bar Harbor fish market.

The low Baltimore opinion of the class Pisces then changed, and in the summer of 1926 Marshall joined the Salisbury Cove laboratory, where he obtained a *Lophius* kidney. In the following winter he and Allan Lyle Grafflin (1906–   ), then a second year medical student at Hopkins, examined it by serial sections and with the utmost care, confirming, except for minor details, Audige's description of its aglomerular nature (49). Work on the aglomerular pipefish and sea horse was undertaken independently by John Graham Edwards (1890–   ), who had been an instructor in Marshall's department and who in the fall and winter of 1926 worked at the Aquarium of the Zoological Station in Naples (14, 15). In the summer of 1927 Marshall and Grafflin extended their studies from the anatomical to the physiological realm on live *Lophii*, and it soon became clear that the aglomerular kidney, consisting entirely of blind tubules homologous with the second half of the proximal segment in other vertebrates, can excrete nearly all the characteristic constituents of fish urine: creatinine, creatine, uric acid, magnesium, sulphate, potassium, and chloride; and, among foreign substances, iodide, nitrate, thiosulphate, thiocyanate, indigo carmine, neutral red, and phenol red, along with such water as is needed to carry the urinary solutes out of the body. It could not, however, excrete glucose or ferrocyanide, or, as Raymond Nicholas Bieter (1900–   ) (2) showed in 1931, protein: these substances gain access to the urine only through the glomeruli. (*Lophius* is

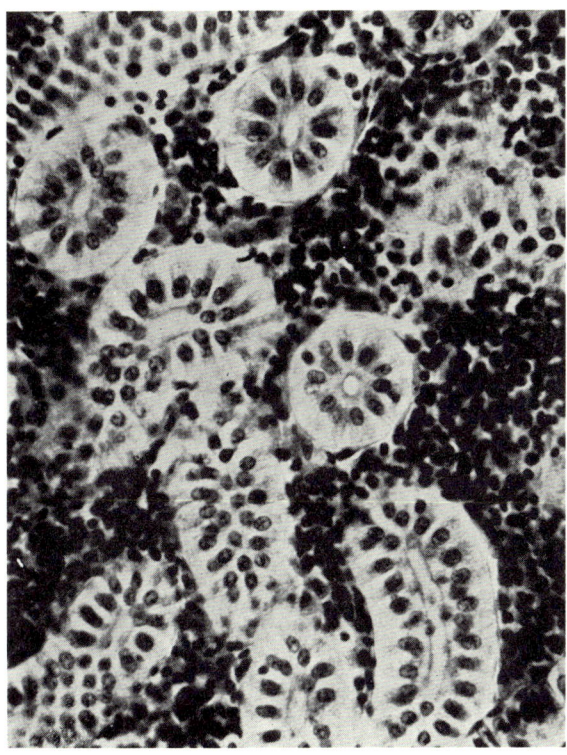

Figure 13. Aglomerular kidney of toadfish, *Opsanus Tau*. The aglomerular tubules, which consist entirely of the proximal segment, are nearly separated from each other by lymphoid tissue. The tubules are composed of cuboidal cells which are essentially uniform throughout the kidney.

<small>SPECIAL
CIRCULATIONS</small>

available off the English and Continental coasts, and one wonders what the consequences would have been had Bowman or Ludwig laid their hands on one. Perhaps neither of them would have published their epoch-making papers!)

Thus, by 1930, the reality of tubular excretion had been firmly established in principle—but only in principle. As Richards remarked at a Woods Hole seminar during the discussion of a paper delivered by Marshall on the formation of urine in the aglomerular fish, "I am glad that at last Marshall has found an animal that fits in with his theory!" In this there was as much cogency as rhetoric—to demonstrate tubular excretion in a strange, ugly fish out of the sea, or even to demonstrate tubular excretion of urea in the frog, or of phenol red in the dog and rabbit, opened, rather than closed, a chapter in the history of renal physiology. Conceivably the situation with respect to tubular excretion might be different in a multitude of different animals and for a multitude of different substances, a particular substance possibly being reabsorbed by the tubules in one animal (uric acid in man) and excreted by the tubules in another (uric acid in the chicken). Each species and each substance had to be put to the test of direct examination (46).

As noted above, the demonstration of tubular reabsorption or excretion requires, in the first instance, measurement of the central operation of glomerular filtration. For this measurement one needs some substance which is completely filterable at the glomerulus and which undergoes neither addition or subtraction by the tubules on its way to the bladder. Then, knowing the quantity of this substance in each cc. of plasma (p) and the rate of its excretion per unit time (UV), the simple calculation of the plasma clearance supplies the volume of plasma filtered per unit time (46). The simultaneous determination of the clearance of any other substance will then afford direct information on whether, in the net operations of the tubules, the excretion of the latter is accompanied by tubular reabsorption or excretion.

Measurement of Filtration Rate

In the nature of the problem, the question of whether a particular substance is suitable for measuring the filtration rate can only be determined by the comparison of a variety of simultaneous clearances under a variety of conditions, including plasma concentration and urine flow, and it was not until the 'thirties that general agreement was reached on the use of inulin in man, and inulin or exogenous creatinine in the dog and most other mammals, for this purpose. With this measurement available, problems of tubular transport, both in reabsorption and excretion, rapidly came under exact examination in many laboratories, and renal physiology began to develop into its present status as a precise and highly critical discipline.

It can fairly be said that a larger body of quantitative knowledge is available today on the multitudinous operations of the normal and diseased kidney than on any other organ of the body. This knowledge is expanding so rapidly that it is doubtful if it will ever again be possible to encompass within one volume any reasonably comprehensive discussion and complete bibliography of the subject. As always, increasing precision of measurement leads not to permanence and stability but only opens new roads of discovery and invites revision of theory. Of the two, discovery by hard, cold observation is the more important: Thomas Henry Huxley spoke of "the great tragedy of science—the slaying of a beautiful hypothesis by an ugly fact—which is so constantly being enacted under the eyes of philosophers" (*30*). The renal physiologist of the present day feels little pressure to achieve philosophical order—a new but well substantiated fact, however paradoxical, appeals to the physiologist with an eloquence that transcends the most enticing theory. Happily the tragedy described by Huxley at worst injures the dogmatist; otherwise it is the phoenix of progress whereby observation and theory emerge together out of the ashes of past error.

The writer has sometimes reminded his students that once upon a time, when men sought an appeal to "authority," they confidently turned to the Book of Genesis. Then times changed and, in medical science at least, Galen took over. In recent years authority has reposed in the last number of the "Journal of Scientific Investigation." Now, with more caution, men turn hopefully to the multitudinous abstracts printed in advance by the many scientific societies meeting every year, all over the United States and all over the world—abstracts that for the most part will not be "read" before any society and scarcely any of which even represents a completed manuscript. But neither is authority here—it lies (if it exists at all) in papers not yet dreamt of, to be written by men not yet conceived.

BIBLIOGRAPHY

SPECIAL CIRCULATIONS

1. ABEL, J. J. Arthur Robertson Cushny and pharmacology. J. Pharmacol., 27:265, 1926.
2. BIETER, R. N. Albuminuria in glomerular and aglomerular fish. J. Pharmacol., 43:407, 1931.
3. BOWMAN, W. On the structure and use of the Malpighian bodies of the kidney, with observations on the circulation through that gland. Philos. Trans. Roy. Soc., 132:57, 1842.
4. BROWNE, T. Sir Thomas Browne's Works Including His Life and Correspondence 1:364. Ed. by Wilkin. London, Pickering, 1835.
5. BRUNTON, L. Ludwig's and other theories of the secretion of urine and the action of diuretics. Proc. roy. Soc. Med., 5: Therap. and Pharmacol. Sect., 133, 1912.
6. COLE, F. J. Henry Power on the circulation of the blood. J. Hist. Med., 12:291, 1957.
7. CUSHNY, A. R. On diuresis and the permeability of the renal cells. J. Physiol. (Lond.), 27:429, 1902.
8. CUSHNY, A. R. The Secretion of the Urine. London, Longmans, Green, 1917.
9. CUSHNY, A. R. The Secretion of the Urine, 2nd ed. London, Longmans, Green, 1926.
10. DALE, H. H. Arthur Robertson Cushny—1866–1926. Proc. roy. Soc. B, 100:xix, 1926.
11. DENIS, W. Metabolism studies on cold-blooded animals. II. The blood and urine of fish. J. biol. Chem. 16:389, 1913.
12. DONLEY, J. A note on the last illness and the post-mortem examination of Marcellus Malpighi. Ann. med. Hist., 3:238, 1921.
13. DRESER, H. Ueber Diurese und ihre Beeinflussung durch pharmakologische Mittel. Arch. exper. Path. Pharmak., 29:303, 1892.
14. EDWARDS, J. G. Studies on aglomerular and glomerular kidneys. I. Anatomical. Amer. J. Anat., 42:75, 1928.
15. EDWARDS, J. G., and L. CONDORELLI. Studies on aglomerular and glomerular kidneys. II. Physiological. Amer. J. Physiol., 86:383, 1928.
16. EKEHORN, G. Einige allgemeine Bemerkungen zu den verschiedenen Auffassungen über die Grundzüge der Nierenfunktion. Virchows Arch. path. Anat., 286:409, 1932.
17. EKEHORN, G. Die Bedeutung der Untersuchungen über die renalen Ausschwemmungsgrade der Farbstoffe. Virchows Arch. path. Anat., 295:256, 1935.
18. FOSTER, M. Physiology. Encyclopaedia Britannica (9th ed.), 19:22d, 1885.

19. FOSTER, M. Lectures on the History of Physiology during the Sixteenth, Seventeenth and Eighteenth Centuries. Cambridge, England, Cambridge University Press, 1901.
20. GARRISON, F. H. An Introduction to the History of Medicine. 4th ed. Philadelphia, Saunders, 1929.
21. GARRISON, F. H. Garrison and Morton's Medical Bibliography. 2nd ed. London, Grafton, 1954.
22. GOLL, F. Ueber den Einfluss des Blutdruckes auf die Harnabsonderung. Z. rat. Med. N. F., 4:78, 1854.
23. HAYMAN, J. M., JR. Estimations of afferent arteriole and glomerular capillary pressures in the frog kidney. Amer. J. Physiol., 79:389, 1927.
24. HEIDENHAIN, R. Mikroskopische Beiträge zur Anatomie und Physiologie der Nieren. Arch. mikr. Anat., 10:1, 1874.
25. HEIDENHAIN, R. Die Harnabsonderung. In L. Hermann. Handbuch der Physiologie, 5:279. Leipzig, Vogel, 1883.
26. HEIDENHAIN, R., and A. NEISSER. Versuche über den Vorgang der Harnabsonderung. Pflügers Arch. ges. Physiol., 9:1, 1874.
27. HERRMANN, M. Ueber den Einfluss des Blutdruckes auf die Secretion des Harns. S. B. Akad. Wiss., Wien. Math.-Naturwiss. Cl. 2. Abt., 45:317, 1862.
28. HILLEMANN, H. H. Comparative physiology of the kidney. J. Amer. med. Ass., 157:531, 1955.
29. HOWLAND, J., and A. N. RICHARDS. An experimental study of the metabolism and pathology of delayed chloroform poisoning. J. exp. Med., 11:344, 1909.
30. HUXLEY, T. H. Discourses, biological and geological. In his Collected Essays, 8:244, New York, Appleton, 1897.
31. KORANYI, A. v. Physiologische und klinische Untersuchungen über den osmotischen Druck thierischer Flüssigkeiten. Z. Klin. Med., 33:1, 1897.
32. KORANYI, A. v. Physiologische und klinische Untersuchungen über den osmotischen Druck thierischer Flüssigkeiten. Z. Klin. Med., 34:1, 1898.
33. KROGH, A. The supply of oxygen to the tissues and the regulation of the capillary circulation. J. Physiol. (Lond.), 52:457, 1919.
34. LOMBARD, W. P. The life and work of Carl Ludwig. Science, 44:363, 1916.
35. LUDWIG, C. Beiträge zur Lehre vom Mechanismus der Harnsecretion. Marburg, Elwert, 1843.
36. LUDWIG, C. Nieren und Harnbereitung. In R. Wagner. Handwörterbuch der Physiologie 2:628. Braunschweig, Vieweg, 1844.
37. LUDWIG, C. Lehrbuch der Physiologie des Menschen. 1. Aufl. 2:274, Leipzig, Winter, 1856.

SPECIAL
CIRCULATIONS

38. LUDWIG, C. Lehrbuch der Physiologie des Menschen. 2. Aufl. 2:373, 427. Leipzig, Winter, 1861.
39. MALPIGHI, M. De viscerum structura exercitatio anatomica. Bologna ex typ. J. Montij, 1666.
40. MALPIGHI, M. Malpighi's "Concerning the structure of kidneys." Tr. by J. M. Hayman, Jr. Ann. med. Hist., 7:242, 1925.
41. MALPIGHI, M. Encyclopaedia Britannica (9th ed.), 15:337d, 1883.
42. MARSHALL, E. K., JR. A rapid clinical method for the estimation of urea in urine. J. biol. Chem., 14:283, 1913.
43. MARSHALL, E. K., JR. A new method for the determination of urea in blood. J. biol. Chem., 15:487, 1913.
44. MARSHALL, E. K., JR. The secretion of urine. Physiol. Rev., 6:440, 1926.
45. MARSHALL, E. K., JR. The secretion of phenol red by the mammalian kidney. Amer. J. Physiol., 99:77, 1932.
46. MARSHALL, E. K., JR. The comparative physiology of the kidney in relation to theories of renal secretion. Physiol. Rev., 14:133, 1934.
47. MARSHALL, E. K., JR., and M. CRANE. The secretory function of the renal tubules. Amer. J. Physiol., 70:465, 1924.
48. MARSHALL, E. K., JR., and D. M. DAVIS. Urea: its distribution in and elimination from the body. J. biol. Chem., 18:53, 1914.
49. MARSHALL, E. K., JR., and A. L. GRAFFLIN. The structure and function of the kidney of Lophius piscatorius. Bull. Johns Hopkins Hosp., 43:205, 1928.
50. MARSHALL, E. K., JR., and J. L. VICKERS. The mechanism of the elimination of phenolsulphonephthalein by the kidney—a proof of secretion by the convoluted tubules. Bull. Johns Hopkins Hosp., 34:1, 1923.
51. MAYRS, E. B. Secretion as a factor in elimination by the bird's kidney. J. Physiol. (Lond.), 58:276, 1924.
52. MÖLLER, E., J. F. MCINTOSH, and D. D. VAN SLYKE. Studies of urea excretion: II. Relationship between urine volume and the rate of urea excretion by normal adults. J. Clin. Invest., 6:427, 1929.
53. NICOLAI, J. A. H. Disquisitiones circa quorundam animalium venas abdominales praecipue renales. Berlin, Diss., 1823.
54. NICOLAI, J. A. H. Untersuchungen über den Verlauf und die Vertheilung der Venen bei einigen Vögeln, Amphibien und Fischen, besonders die Venen der Nieren betreffend. Isis von Oken, 18:404, 1826.
55. NUSSBAUM, M. Ueber die Secretion der Niere. Pflügers Arch. ges. Physiol., 16:139, 1878.
56. NUSSBAUM, M. Fortgesetzte Untersuchungen über die Secretion der Niere. Pflügers Arch. ges. Physiol., 17:580, 1878.

57. ORAVISTO, K. J. Investigations into the excretion mechanism of indigo carmine in normal human kidney. Ann. Chir. Gynaec. Fenn., 46:Suppl. 2, 1957.
58. PETERS, J. P., and D. D. VAN SLYKE. Quantitative Clinical Chemistry. Baltimore, Williams and Wilkins, 2 vols., 1931–32. I. Interpretations. Chap. V., p. 335ff. Urea.
59. RICHARDS, A. N. Kidney function. Harvey Lect., 16:163, 1920–21.
60. RICHARDS, A. N. Methods and Results of Direct Investigations of the Functions of the Kidney. Baltimore, Williams and Wilkins, 1929.
61. RICHARDS, A. N. Urine formation in the Amphibian kidney. Harvey Lect., 30:93, 1934–35.
62. RICHARDS, A. N. Physiology of the kidney. Bull. N.Y. Acad. Med., series 2, 14:5, 1938.
63. RICHARDS, A. N. Processes of urine formation. The Croonian Lecture. Proc. roy. Soc. B, 126:398, 1938.
64. RICHARDS, A. N., and O. H. PLANT. Urine formation by the perfused kidney: preliminary experiments on the action of caffeine. J. Pharmacol., 7:485, 1915.
65. RICHARDS, A. N., and O. H. PLANT. Urine formation in the perfused kidney. The influence of alterations in renal blood pressure on the amount and composition of urine. Amer. J. Physiol., 59:144, 1922.
66. RICHARDS, A. N., and O. H. PLANT. Urine formation in the perfused kidney. The influence of adrenalin on the volume of the perfused kidney. Amer. J. Physiol., 59:184, 1922.
67. RICHARDS, A. N., and C. F. SCHMIDT. A description of the glomerular circulation on the frog's kidney and observations concerning the action of adrenalin and various other substances upon it. Amer. J. Physiol., 71:178, 1924.
68. ROSEN, C. Carl Ludwig and his American students. Bull. Inst. Hist. Med., 4:609, 1936.
69. ROWNTREE, L. G., and J. T. GERAGHTY. An experimental and clinical study of the functional activity of the kidneys by means of phenolsulphonephthalein. J. Pharmacol., 1:579, 1910.
70. SHEEHAN, H. L. The deposition of dyes in the mammalian kidney. J. Physiol. (Lond.), 72:201, 1931.
71. SHEEHAN, H. L. The renal elimination of phenol red in the dog. J. Physiol. (Lond.), 87:237, 1936.
72. SINGER, C. The earliest figures of microscopic objects. Endeavour, 12:197, 1953.
73. SMITH, H. W. Lectures on the Kidney. Lawrence, Kans., University of Kansas, 1943.
74. SMITH, H. W. The Kidney: Structure and Function in Health and Disease. New York, Oxford University Press, 1951.

SPECIAL
CIRCULATIONS

75. SMITH, H. W. From Fish to Philosopher. Boston, Little, Brown, 1953.
76. STARLING, E. H. On the absorption of fluids from the connective tissue spaces. J. Physiol. (Lond.), 19:312, 1896.
77. STARLING, E. H. The glomerular functions of the kidney. J. Physiol. (Lond.), 24:317, 1899.
78. STIRLING, W. In Memoriam—Carl Ludwig. Med. Chron. n.s., 3 (Apr.-Sept.):178, 1895.
79. TAMMANN, G. Die Thätigkeit der Niere im Lichte der Theorie des osmotischen Drucks. Z. phys. Chem., 20:180, 1896.
80. USTIMOVITSCH, C. Experimentelle Beiträge zur Theorie der Harnabsonderung. Arb. physiol. Anstalt Leipzig, 5:199, 1870.
81. VERWORN, M. Physiology. Encyclopeadia Britannica (9th ed.), 21: 554b, 1911.
82. WALKER, A. M., P. A. BOTT, J. OLIVER, and M. C. MACDOWELL. The collection and analysis of fluid from single nephrons of the mammalian kidney. Amer. J. Physiol., 134:580, 1941.
83. WALLACE, G. B., and A. R. CUSHNY. On intestinal absorption and the saline cathartics. Amer. J. Physiol., 1:411, 1898.
84. WEARN, J. T., and A. N. RICHARDS. Observations on the composition of glomerular urine, with particular reference to the problem of reabsorption in the renal tubules. Amer. J. Physiol., 71:209, 1924.
85. WHITE, H. L. On glomerular filtration. Amer. J. Physiol., 68:523, 1924.
86. WINTON, F. R. Modern Views on the Secretion of Urine. Boston, Little, Brown, 1956.

X

The Splanchnic Circulation

THE current stock of ideas basic to an understanding of splanchnic physiology has evolved from an unthinkably long and complex process of trial and error. Recognition of animal parts that are discrete and unchanging and the realization of their relevance to antecedents and effects must have required thousands of centuries during which men developed the means of communicating with one another.

Language involves the use of concepts, i.e., abstractions that clarify the interconnections within a group of data and that serve as a basis for the inference of new and previously unsuspected correlations. Hence, the technique of logical thought grew up with speech, providing man with a method equally effective in self-enlightenment and self-deception. Excessive speculation and error in assigning cause and effect were inevitable in the absence of an adequate knowledge of the physical world. Since error has a continuing and pervasive influence upon thought, any study of concept formation must be as much concerned with fallacious concepts as with sound ones.

Unfortunately, the origin and growth of physiological concepts, whether true or false, can hardly ever be precisely defined. Occasionally an original insight may be so impressive that both the circumstances in which it was conceived and the man responsible are remembered. More frequently, however, new ideas emerge imperceptibly from the interplay of the thought and experiences of many men or out of the context of certain facts as self-evident deductions that seem worthy of little notice. Recognition comes later when the record may have been lost or confused. As a rule, however, there is no written record whatever and reliance must be placed upon legends, customs, religious practices, social organizations, artifacts, and the more durable monu-

SPECIAL
CIRCULATIONS

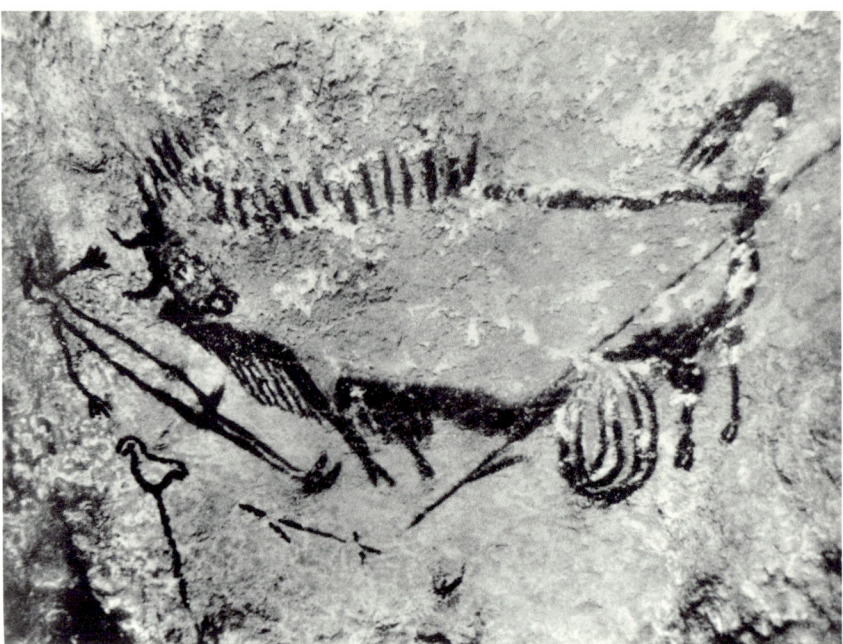

Figure 1. Paleolithic painting in the cave at Lascaux showing the evisceration of a bison by a spear. The hunting scene shown here is one of the most remarkable examples of Upper Paleolithic art not only because a figure of man has been included but also because the effort to portray the viscera is realistic in concept and technique.

ments of man's making as sources of information. Although the invention of writing resulted in more accurate documentation, the techniques that had been evolved in the perpetuation of an oral tradition and that were used at first in writing resulted in considerable obscurity. It is possible that the poetic figures of contrast and proportional metaphor were a help to logic (*163*) but mnemonic devices, colorful allusions, and riddling rhymes play hob with any effort to work out precise attribution and characterization. What is more, an explicit interest in physiology is a relatively recent phenomenon; early references to function tended to be casual and incidental to more engrossing topics. In time, however, concern with physiology, and with circulatory physiology in particular, did develop. The splanchnic vasculature occupied a special place because of its close association with organs known to be necessary for life. In fact, an analysis of the growth of ideas regarding the splanchnic circulation affords an excellent means of tracing the rise of physiology in general. Of course, much must be conjectural. Even the more recent creation of an extensive literature in the hands of generations of disciplined and critical investigators has not eliminated the possibility of error in selecting and interpreting material relevant to the evolution of concepts.

During the half million years or more in which man has fashioned tools and used fire, he has gradually extended his command and understanding of himself and other living things. The progressive refinement of the techniques employed in hunting, fishing, and the preparation of animal parts for food, clothing, shelter, and a thousand other purposes, certainly indicates an equivalent growth in the knowledge of anatomy and physiology. All this is evident not only in the meager traces of man's old dwelling places and in the character of the countless stone tools, weapons, and ornaments that fill our museums, but also in the paintings that adorn the walls of caves in the south of France, in Spain, Africa, and other parts of the world. These beautiful murals clearly prove that Paleolithic man, living more than 30,000 years ago, possessed a knowledge of animal structure that could have been gained only by hours of careful dissection (45). In the cavern of Lascaux, located on the Vézère not far from Perigeux, the crudely sketched figure of a man falls before a bison whose abdomen has been opened by a spear thrust. The spear remains in the wound and reddish loops of intestine have tumbled out. This seems to be the earliest known attempt to portray an abdominal viscus and its vasculature (109). The careful representation of red blood may be particularly significant. It is generally believed that cave art served a religious function, presumably indicating an interpretation of life as a manifestation of the divine. Such a view seems implicit also in the careful ritualistic disposal of the dead that began even earlier. The staining of the dead with red ochre (41) suggests, too, the equation of the life-force with blood (and by extension with any red material), a view that was to find expression through the ages in diverse ways—from animal and human sacrifice by blood-letting to establishment of kinship by blood exchange.

These notions, both true and false, persisted even after the remarkable

SPECIAL CIRCULATIONS

leap forward that occurred during the Neolithic Revolution, approximately 10,000 years ago. At that time, technical advances in stone working and in social organization were associated with the epoch-making biological discoveries in the Middle East that freed man from the insecurities of a life devoted to food gathering and made of him a farmer and a herdsman. Within two or three millennia these advances brought in their train the development of large urban communities and ultimately the complex civilizations of the Tigris-Euphrates, Indus, and Nile valleys.

The Seat of Divination

In each instance, civilization developed among a settled people, supported by farming and dependent upon increasingly elaborate systems of irrigation and flood control. The planning, supervision and power necessary for the construction and operation of these works and for the maintenance of adequate communications, supply, and other appurtenances of city life seem to have rested in the hands of a clearly defined managerial class. In both Egypt and Mesopotamia, priestly and governmental responsibilities were fused or at least closely allied. In the absence of an understanding of Indus script we know very little about the contemporary civilization of Harappa and Mohenjo-daro, but that little suggests an even more pervasive sacerdotal authority (*137*). Religious sanctions seem to have provided the most effective means of assuring a wholehearted communal collaboration at all levels. Priests skilled in enlisting spiritual assistance served also in the regulation of commerce and the trades and in setting the times for planting and harvesting, for flood and festival. In doing so, they were forced to devise efficient methods of chronology, computation, and accounting that soon raised the curtain upon written history. Their records disclose a constant preoccupation with supernatural powers manifest in life and in every natural force. Seen as a garment of spirit, the body is of little moment except insofar as it may reflect or serve divinity. The viscera—and specifically the liver—were regarded as vitally important in this connection. In Mesopotamia, the liver became, as Plato (*138*) noted, the "seat of divination"; in Egypt, the liver and other viscera were specially prepared for the use of the dead in the afterlife.

MESOPOTAMIA AND EGYPT

A complete and confident dependence upon the prophetic arts persisted throughout antiquity. No decision could be made and no new departure embarked upon without examination of the omens apparent in an astonishing variety of natural phenomena. The flight and behavior of birds, the character of thunder and lightning, the courses of the stars, and the configuration of animal viscera were all believed to reveal the mysterious purposes of the supernatural. An expert knowledge of these matters required a long and arduous training, for which few were adequately equipped. Although independent practitioners of seercraft (both amateur and professional) were always active, divination was mainly a function of an organized priesthood. Certainly this was already the case in Mesopotamia when writing was invented. In all probability, the practice had its roots deep in the past, long before man became successful in manipulating his environment, as a logical response to a world of uncertainty in which divine powers were constantly immanent and generally malevolent. Perhaps it was from the act of propitiation by animal sacrifice that divination based upon the appearance of the entrails (extispicy) and the liver (haruspicy) was derived. Haruspicy, along with astrology and the interpretation of such ephemera as dreams, the movements of incense smoke in the wind, and the spread of oil droplets upon water, was developed by the priests of Sumer, Akkad, Mari, and Babylonia to a remarkable degree of complexity and sophistication.

Large collections of tablets bearing cuneiform inscriptions that deal with haruspicy have been unearthed at numerous sites throughout Mesopotamia (*86, 99, 127, 128, 147*). These texts disclose a well-organized body of belief and ritual which was already considered ancient in the third millennium before Christ. The inscriptions were written in what was even then an antique tongue, presumably indicating a continuity with the past through a tradition like that evident in the modern use of Latin in academic and ecclesiastical documents. A prescribed rite was followed in examining the entrails. The diviner, or *bārūm*, stood at the foot of the lamb or kid (an adult was rarely used) secured on its back upon an altar with its head to the north. (The belief that the victim's left, or east, side was unfavorable proved remarkably durable.

THE SPLANCHNIC CIRCULATION

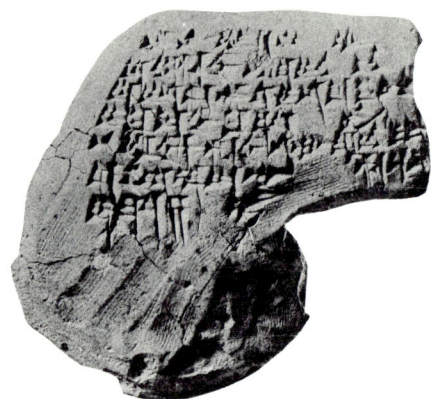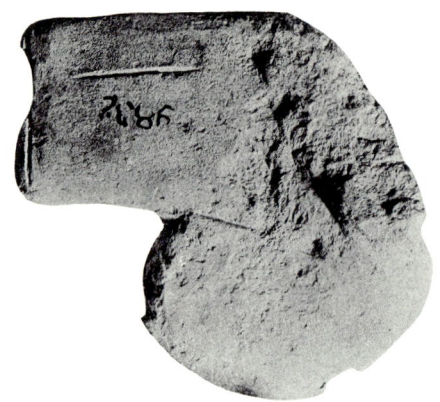

Figure 2. Baked clay tablet bearing cuneiform inscription describing the appearance of the liver of a sacrificial lamb. In this instance, the text describes the findings on the specific occasion when the stairs collapsed upon the king's entry into the temple. The tablet is constructed here in a shape resembling that of the liver, but in the majority of instances the tablet is rectangular.

The Romans called it the *pars hostilis* as opposed to the *pars familiaris* and it echoes still in modern English in such words as *sinister* and *dexterity*.) An assistant cut a jugular vein with appropriate invocations and at the moment of death opened the abdomen and thorax by carefully specified incisions. The external appearance, color, markings, and movements made just prior to death were noted. The sternum and viscera were studied in sequence and special attention was devoted to the liver, every small irregularity of its surface, lobation, color, and configuration having significance. The most important parts bore names drawn from daily life in a highly complex community, suggesting that organized haruspicy developed after the urban revolution. For instance, a feature apparently identical with the incisura umbilicalis was referred to as the "door of the palace," the porta hepatis as the "gate," the ventral surface of the lower border of the left lobe as the "road," and the large left lobe was likened to the "blinkers" worn by a harnessed ass. The word for the liver itself, *kabittu*, from the root *kbi*, "to be heavy," probably indicates a much older recognition. It should be stressed that interpretation did not depend solely upon the inspiration of the *bārūm*. Intensive

THE SPLANCHNIC CIRCULATION

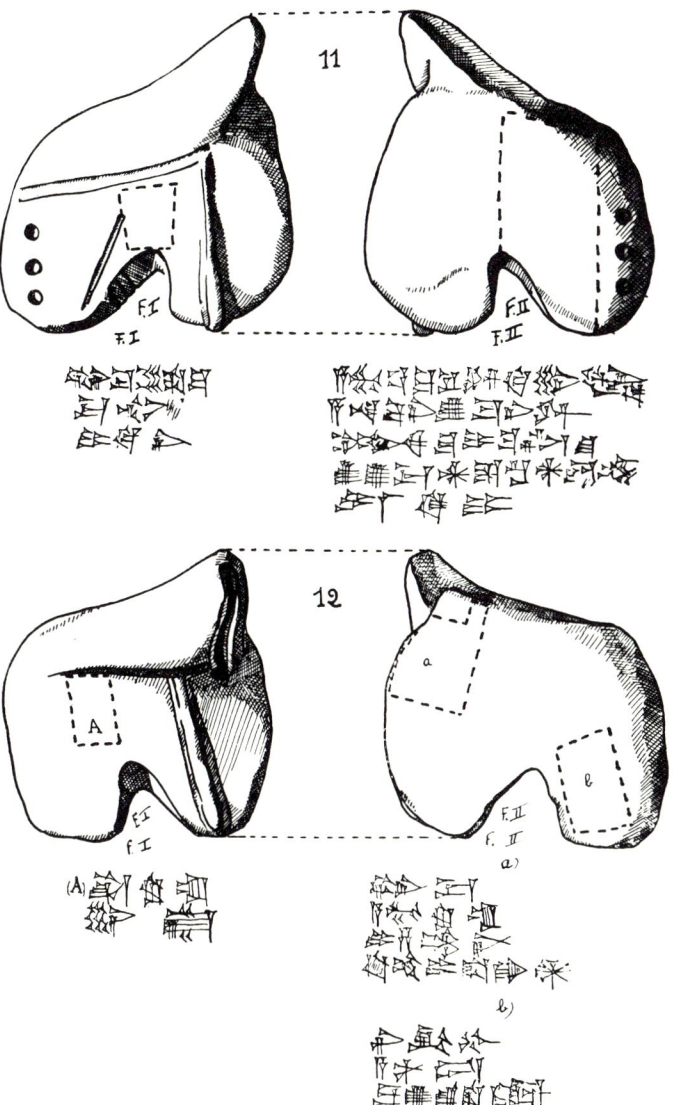

Figure 3. Liver models from Mari showing the appearance of the liver and the cuneiform inscriptions upon them. The upper figures show the configuration observed when the army of Isma-Dagan was taken prisoner. The lower figures indicate (at A on the left) the point at which a swelling of the portal vein might be seen and which is referred to in the text as "the wind in the door." The inscription on the superior aspect of the organ (lower right) states, "If Amurru is diminished, the liver will appear thus."

SPECIAL
CIRCULATIONS

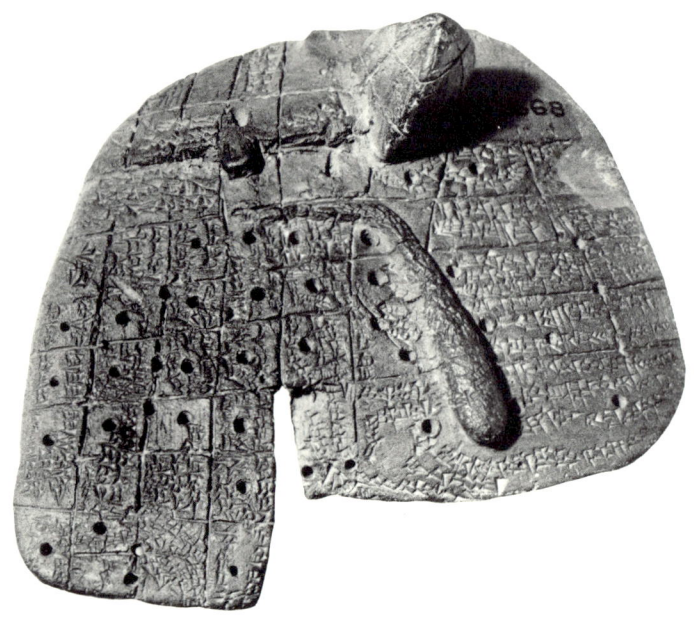

Figure 4. Baked clay model of Babylonian liver in the British Museum. This large model, approximately the size of a grapefruit, is covered with numerous inscriptions, each relating to a specific prediction, appropriate to the point at which it is placed.

training was needed for proficiency in mantic techniques based upon a codified experience.

For centuries, unusual appearances of the liver were carefully recorded and compared with actual events, in order to develop reliably predictable correlations. The thousands of tablets recovered in recent years are mere remnants of the large libraries in which these data were preserved. Not infrequently, exceptional livers were modeled in clay and the notable features indicated in writing. More than fifty have been found in various sites, the oldest from Mari going back almost to 2000 B.C. (*54, 86, 99, 115, 127, 128, 147*). The inscriptions report observations ("When 'such an event' occurred, the liver appeared thus") and inferences ("If the liver appears thus, 'such-and-such an event' will take place"). The models were also used for purposes of instruction. One large and unique example from North Babylonia, now in the British Museum, seems to have been a kind of textbook. A large number of cuneiform labels and perforations denote a variety of predictions appropriate to changes in each part. The system perpetuated by these devices endured for more than a thousand years and was ultimately to affect profoundly the development of Western thought in many spheres.

Although Mesopotamia seems to have had a seminal influence upon the development of civilization in the Nile valley, Egyptian attitudes toward the viscera were conditioned by an indigenous religious outlook which focused upon life after death rather than upon magical control of the physical world. The techniques of mummification were perfected by the time of the New Kingdom (*c.* 1580–1090 B.C.), after more than a thousand years of experimentation during which it had been discovered that removal of the viscera retards putrefaction (*54, 69*). Even as early as the burial of Queen Hetep-heres (*c.* 2650 B.C.) the viscera were preserved separately in a compartmented alabaster box. In later burials the box was replaced by four urns, or Canopic jars, one at each of the four corners of the sarcophagus. The heart—considered by Egyptians as the seat of the soul and intelligence—was usually removed, washed with palm wine, bandaged and returned to the body cavity on completion of the prolonged ritualistic process of dehydration with natron (sodium sesquicarbonate) and treatment of the body tissues with various aromatic resins. The liver, lungs, stomach, and intestines were placed in separate jars closed by tops shaped in early times in the likeness of human heads. Later these tops were modeled in the more distinctive features of each of the tutelary genii or Sons of Horus. Thus the lungs were protected by Hapy (ape-headed), the stomach by Duamutef (falcon), and the intestines by Qebhsenuef (jackal). The liver alone was kept in a human-headed urn guarded by Imsety.

Despite the extensive experience with human anatomy and the continuing contact with the East, haruspicy was never taken up officially in Egypt. Instead, the practice moved toward the West by way of Syria and the Middle East (*115, 183*). Many tablets and liver models like those found in Mesopotamia have been unearthed at Boghaz-keui in Turkey, the site of the capital of the Hittite Empire (*22*). There is no evidence of a similar interest in the liver in the leavings of the Minoan or Mycenean civilizations, but elsewhere throughout the Middle East haruspicy became a decisive instrument of policy-making. The texts indicate that almost every act of the leaders in the Eastern city-states and in the more

THE SPLANCHNIC CIRCULATION

SPECIAL
CIRCULATIONS

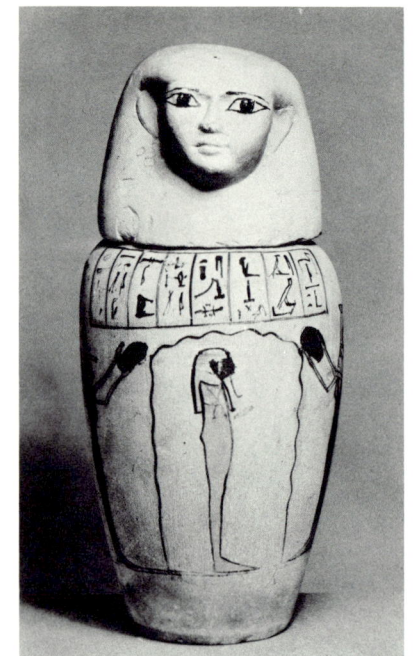
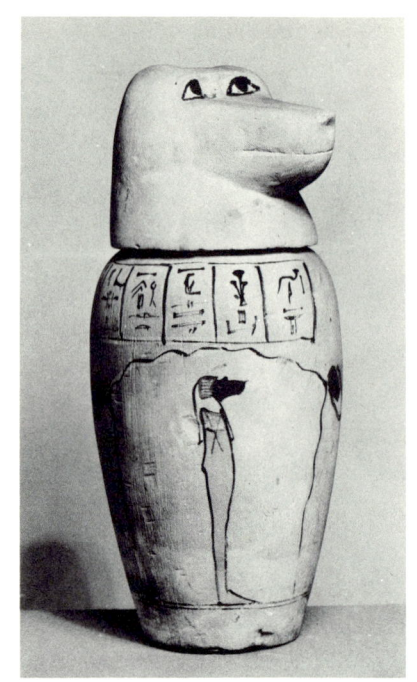
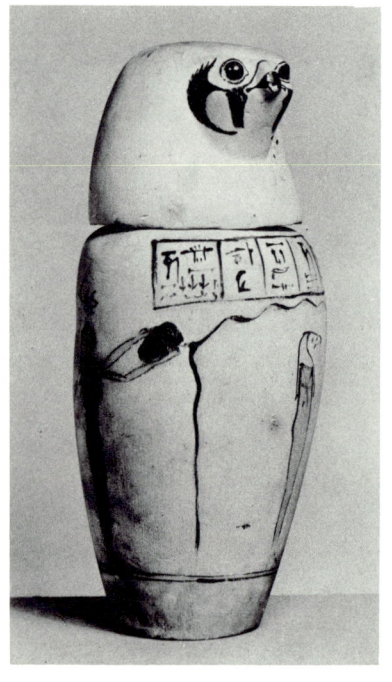
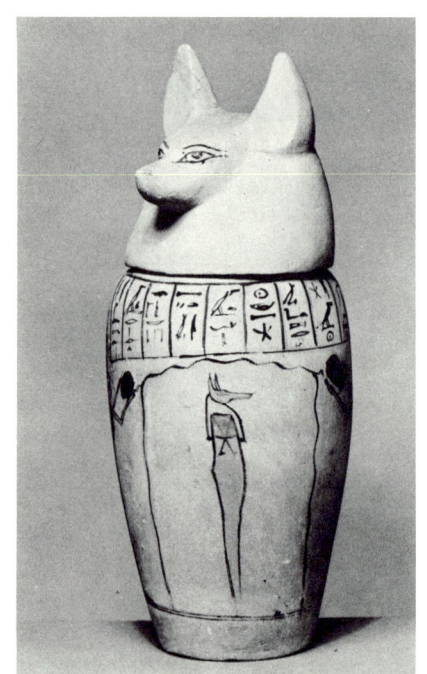

[616]

extensive imperial organizations was governed by haruspicy. At some time in the dark ages that followed the collapse of the ancient kingdoms (*c.* 1000 B.C.) before the onslaught of barbarian invaders armed with iron, divination from entrails was transmitted to the Western World.

GREECE AND ITALY

In classic times the Greeks believed that haruspicy was among the many benefits conferred by Prometheus upon Mankind (*3*). Oracular prophecy was, of course, exceedingly important, but the diviner or haruspex occupied a privileged position and often exerted a vital influence in decisions of life and death. The entrails were always consulted before battle, and fighting was delayed until the moment indicated by appropriate signs. Herodotus (*96*) wrote, for instance, of the Spartans at Plataea patiently suffering many casualties while waiting until "the victims became favorable" after repeated sacrifices before beginning the battle. Professional diviners, presumably trained in a family craft or by apprenticeship, employed technical terms and conventions that apparently stemmed from the East. The Greek practitioners were obviously skilled and respected (Herodotus noted that the Persians employed them), but they never gained the recognition accorded the Etruscans. Indeed, throughout the Mediterranean world, haruspicy ultimately came to be known as the "Etruscan discipline."

According to tradition, which modern scholarship and archaeology cannot verify, the Etruscans were an Eastern people (*132*). Their civilization was far advanced when Rome was founded, and it was ultimately taken over by its mighty neighbor. From the Etruscans Rome received the questionable benefits of the haruspicy and gladiatorial games. The use of the haruspices was traced by the Romans themselves to the time of Tarquinius Superbus, and the practice became increasingly important in deciding matters of public policy after the Second Punic War

Figure 5. Canopic jars of limestone. The lids represent the four sons of Horus and include Imsety (human-headed—containing the liver), Hapy (ape—lungs), Duamutef (falcon—stomach), and Qebhsenuef (jackal—intestines). The picture on each jar shows the protecting goddesses pouring the purifying water over the deity. The inscriptions are ancient magical formulas assuring the aid of the goddesses against all enemies of the son of Horus within the jar, i.e., the organ identified with each one.

SPECIAL
CIRCULATIONS

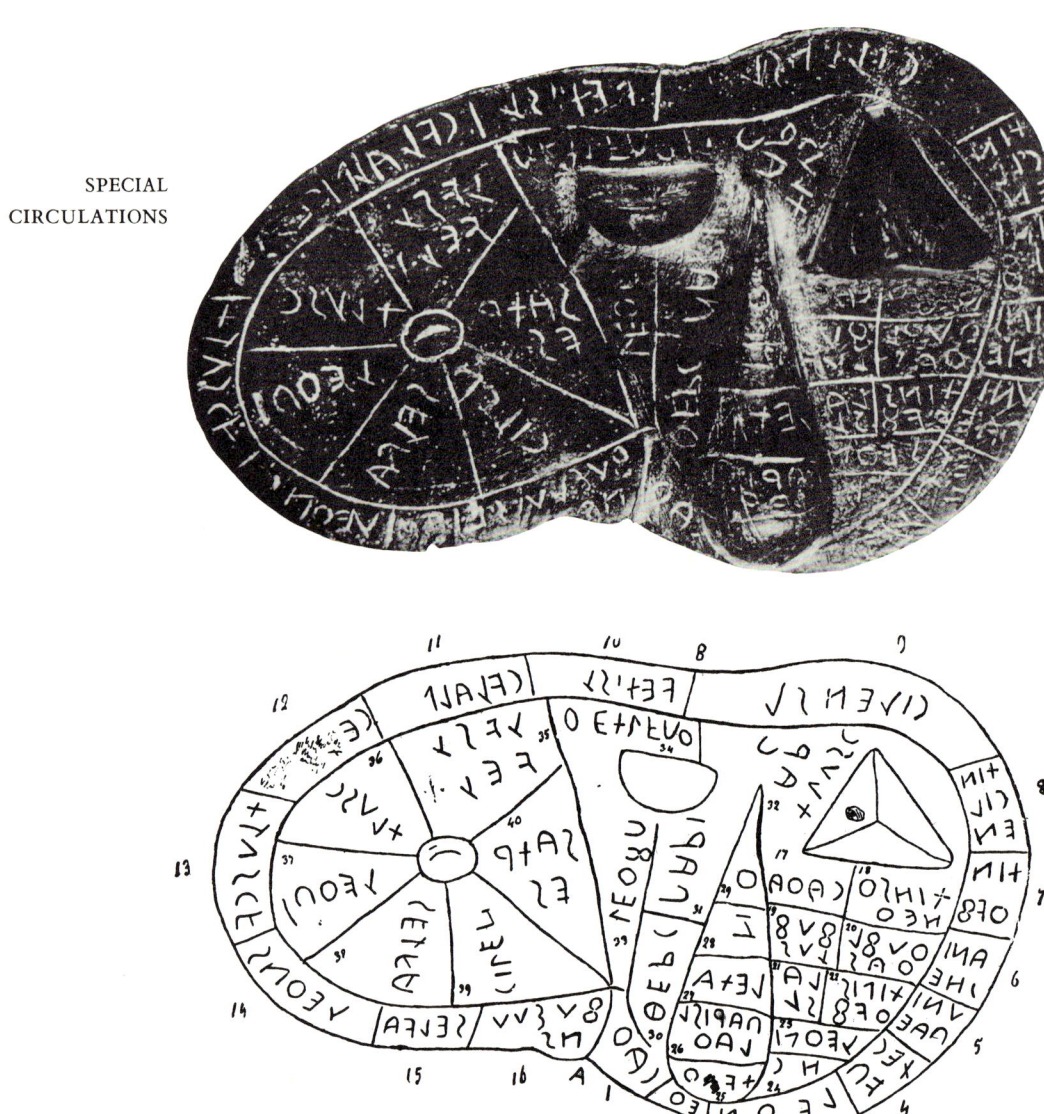

Figure 6. Etruscan liver model in bronze. On the under surface (A) of this sheep's liver, appropriately shaped prominences indicate the pyramidal lobe, the caudate lobe, and the gallbladder. Over these features and over the flat surface the names and the appropriate cosmic positions of the deities are laid out, each in his appropriate space as though within a temple enclosure oriented to the points of the compass. These markings are more clearly shown in (B).

in 218 B.C. (*134*). The official religious organizations of Rome varied from time to time, but they usually included the pontiffs to regulate ritual and a college of augurs to evaluate the auspices. The latter appeared to depend upon collegiate bodies in Etruria to train and provide haruspices to serve the state. These men were active not only at the seat of the government but also in the army and the colonies (*171–173*).

The "libri haruspini" are lost, but references in many works and lucky finds of liver models throw some light upon the so-called "science." These models have proved particularly valuable. One is a large bronze model of a sheep's liver (12.6 cm. long) found in 1877 near Settino in Italy and kept today in the Civic Museum of Piacenza (*105*). Markings on the inferior surface, upon which the gallbladder and the pyramidal and caudate lobes stand out in high relief, appear to define the "sacred circular space" oriented with respect to the sky and compass as it would be in the open abdomen with the liver edge turned anteriorly and craniad. The names of Etruscan deities are inscribed, each in his proper cosmic position, above the sacred space and over the various outstanding structural features. A similar model is held by the recumbent figure of a haruspex upon the lid of an alabaster urn found in the ruins of the Etruscan center of Volterra just outside Siena. It has been suggested that such models were used for the instruction of novices; it is also possible that they were used by the haruspex in checking his findings. The livers of goats, oxen, even dogs and chickens, were examined under various circumstances, but as in Mesopotamia, the sheep's liver was resorted to most often. Unlike the *bārūm*, the Etruscan haruspex stood at the head of the victim, but the similarity of the Etruscan and Mesopotamian terminology otherwise strongly suggests a derivative relationship.

Haruspicy was employed at first by the Romans only for important occasions touching upon the welfare of the state or the problems of the powerful. In the last days of the Republic the haruspices were consulted more frequently. Indeed, Cicero (*43, 134*) claimed that nearly everybody used them in his day (*Extis enim omnes feres utentur*). With the advent of the Church and religious opposition to the practice, however, haruspicy fell into desuetude. Perhaps St. Ansano (*101*), the patron saint of Siena, who usually holds in his right hand the entrails used in divining, is a transmogrified haruspex of ancient Volterra, the last vestige of

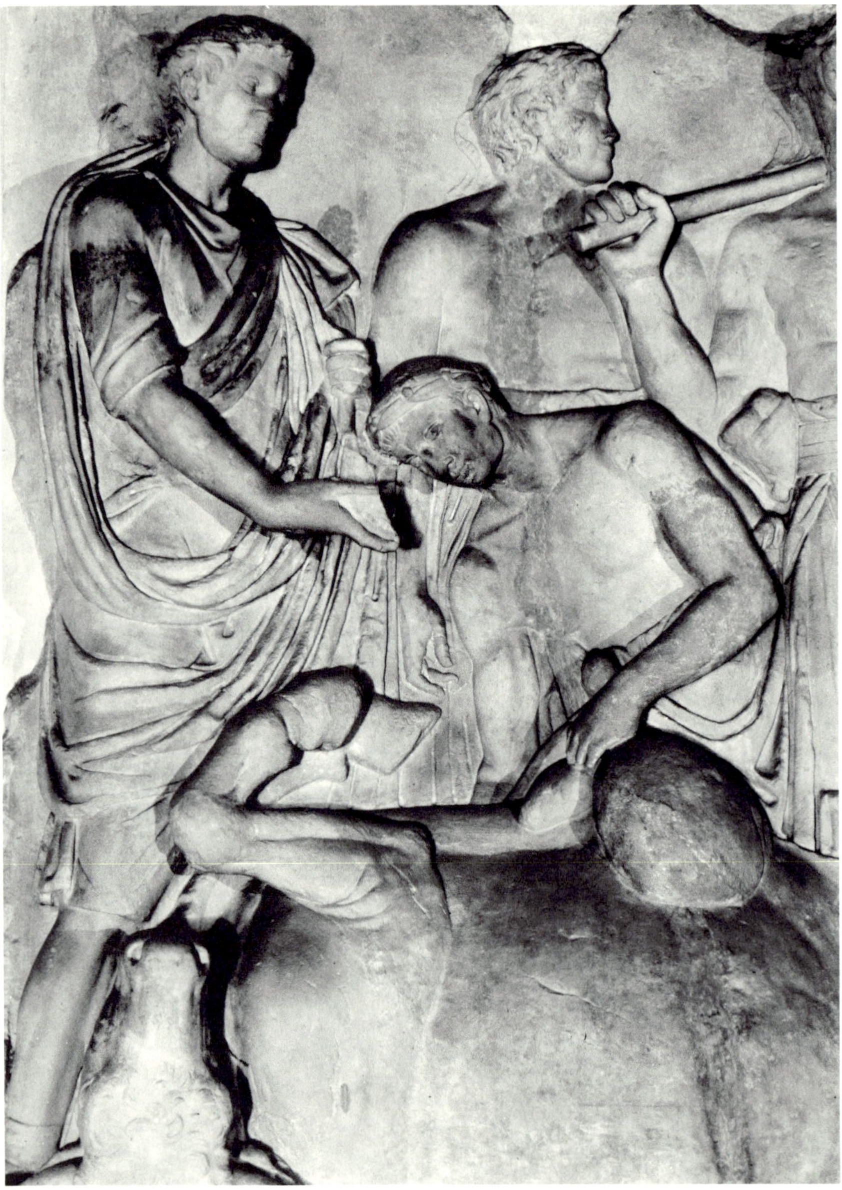

SPECIAL CIRCULATIONS

Figure 7. Haruspicy in the Forum before the Temple of Jupiter Capitolinus (from a sculpture in the Louvre). The haruspex (presumably Etruscan) stands at the head and on the left of the slaughtered ox while his assistant exposes the liver for examination. He holds in his left hand his staff of office and in his right what appears to be a liver model.

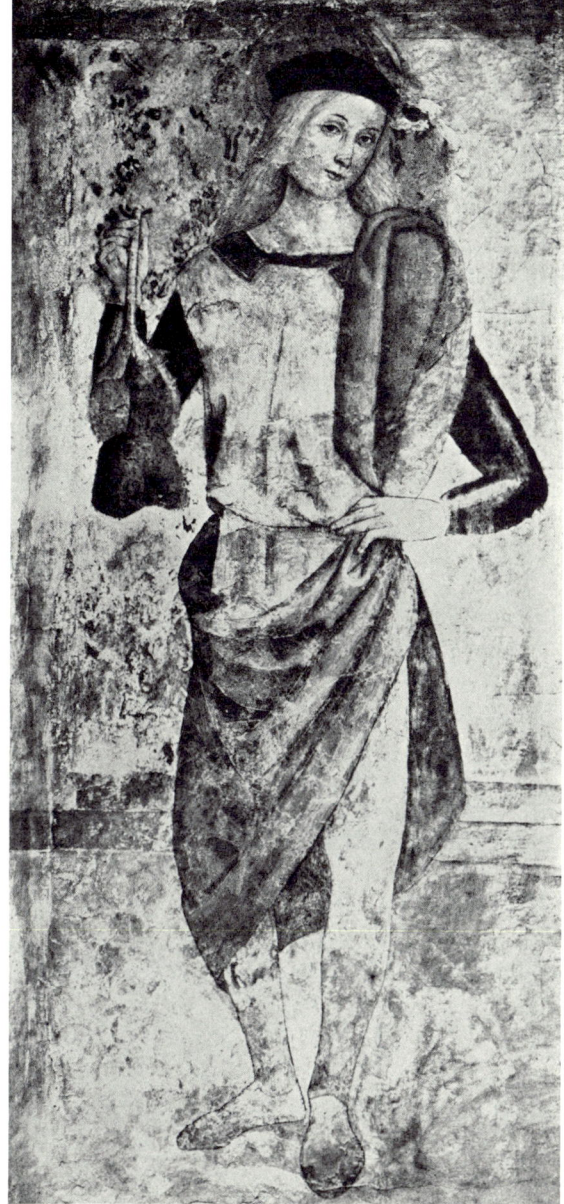

Figure 8. Saint Ansano of Siena, from a fresco by Tiberio d'Assisi. The saint holds in his hand the lungs and liver, the viscera traditionally used by the Etruscan haruspex. These viscera are usually referred to as emblems of the saint's martyrdom.

a once potent and popular craft. Unlike astrology, haruspicy has vanished from the West, but within the present century the Kayan, a tribal society of central Borneo, have been found to consult the liver of a pig for aid in settling disputes (*70*).

SPECIAL CIRCULATIONS

ROLE IN CONCEPT FORMATION

It is difficult to say why the liver was chosen as an instrument of augury. The early recognition of the importance of blood to life may well have been most influential. The liver is obviously engorged with blood at death and bleeds profusely when it is cut. An additional explanation may lie in the difficulty experienced by early man (and by primitive peoples in modern times) in localizing the seat of intelligence and emotion (*130*). Abdominal visceral sensations, palpitation, panting, sighing, yawning, speech, dreams, and hallucinations call attention variously to the upper abdomen, thorax, and head. If thought can produce overt changes in respiration and in heart rate it is not unreasonable to believe that it may also affect the appearance of the liver and other viscera. It is but one step from this to the belief that the liver of a sacrificial victim may disclose the mind of the deity taking possession at the moment of death. If this is so, structure is temporary and fluid, simply reflecting "the power of thought" and having no relevance to the function or need of the body. Thus, with haruspicy, the first steps essential to an understanding of the splanchnic circulation—the recording and collation of careful observations—were made in the wrong direction. The false emphasis upon the prime position of the liver in the body was to exert a detrimental influence upon the subsequent construction of valid concepts even after supernatural causation had been rejected and the need for interpretation in terms of animal physiology rather than theology had been realized. This distortion in perspective dominated discussions of physiology throughout Greco-Roman times, receiving its final authoritative expression in the work of Galen. It was not corrected until Harvey's discovery of the circulation substituted the heart for the liver at the center of the circulatory system.

The Hellenic Contribution

The intellectual reorientation that first made meaningful conceptualization of function possible took place during the troubled period following the destruction of the ancient Eastern empires in the last centuries of the second millennium B.C. Haruspicy was practiced little, if at all, by the civilized city-states of Crete, Greece, and the Aegean littoral. The conquerors who sacked Knossos, Tiryns, and Pylos worshipped Olympian deities with whom they maintained a respectful but distant relationship, unaided by the darker sciences (*87*, *91*). The Greeks of the classic age appear to have sprung from a cattle-culture, in which animals were regarded as goods, not gods, in which the supernatural was considered an intrusion rather than an essence, and in which a large aristocratic governing class went its way freely and without regimentation (*114*). Possibly this background provides an explanation for the novel point of view that permitted freedom of speculation with regard only for logical circumstances. Or perhaps the phenomenon may be traced to disillusion. Webster (*180*) argues that the precisely mathematical and angular abstractions so typical of Protogeometric and Geometric vasepainting during the dark age represent not so much a decadence in artistic taste and ability as it does a reaction to defeat.

THE SPLANCHNIC CIRCULATION

> "*Obviously it is an art stripped down to essentials just as life was stripped down to essentials with the collapse of the Mycenean palaces. The essential here is perhaps a belief in human reason, in human capacity to reduce things to simple and clear patterns so that they become manageable—a purely human operation when all the mystery and magic of the kings had failed. Seen like this the Protogeometric vasepainter takes his place not only as the forerunner of later developments in art, mathematics and philosophy but also as the colleague of the poet who sees life in similar rational and human terms.*"

By 600 B.C. a well-established social order of independent Greek city-states had grown up in the Aegean area out of the remnants of the Mycenean Empire, inheriting its language (as we know now that Ventris has deciphered the linear B script) as well as its traditions. The new intellectual approach appeared first in the major centers along the Asiatic coast of the Aegean, in Ionia, Caria, and Lydia, and soon spread to the Greek colonies in Italy, Sicily, and Africa (see map, Chapter 1). Throughout the sixth century B.C. the problems of knowledge and existence were attacked by a sequence of original thinkers, beginning in Ionian Miletus with Thales, Anaximander, and Anaximenes (*29*). The Miletian monists were followed in the fifth century B.C. by a pluralistic

SPECIAL CIRCULATIONS

reaction at Croton, in southern Italy, where Pythagoras and his followers, Alcmeon and Philalaus, saw in numbers and numerical relations the "principles of all things" and founded what may have been the first scientific medical school. Their views were developed further in a new center established in Sicily. It seems likely that the ideas worked out there by Empedocles, and later by Philistion, exerted a determining influence upon the biologic thought of the Hippocratic school in Cos, although the speculations of Heracleitos of Ephesus and of the Atomists (Leucippos and Democritos) undoubtedly figured importantly (*154, 155*). Through its successes in the Persian Wars, Athens gained pre-eminence for a period in the fifth and fourth centuries B.C., during which a succession of brilliant men, including Anaxagoras, Plato, and Aristotle, left an indelible mark. Plato and Aristotle founded schools that were to endure for centuries. Learning and the arts found enthusiastic support also in the courts of the Hellenistic world community established after 350 B.C. by Alexander and his successors. In Alexandria, the Ptolemies set up an institute for advanced study dedicated to the Muses under the guidance of men trained with Aristotle. In the Museum and its Library, anatomy and physiology moved forward during the third century B.C. under Herophylos and Erasistratos, both of whom had come to Alexandria from coastal cities of Asiatic Greece. But thereafter the intellectual impetus slackened, and in the centuries that followed the new ideas were petrified as the dicta of a dozen conflicting sects devoted rather to a polemical support of accepted "principles" than to an unimpassioned search for the truth. Throughout the Greco-Roman period physiology and medicine were dominated by Greeks trained in the Ionic city-states. Thus it is fitting that the physiologic thought of the period should have found its ultimate formulation at the end of the second century A.D. in the encyclopedic writings of Galen, who was reared in Pergamon, was taught in the schools of Alexandria and Athens, and was supported by a lucrative practice in Rome. The intellectual centers in Ionia continued to be active under the protection of the Byzantines as the Empire crumbled in the West and contracted in the East. Though their light burned fitfully, they produced such men as Oribasios of Pergamon, Alexander of Tralles, and Paul of Aegina, who played a vital role in transmitting the Hellenic contribution through the Arabs to the West.

In following the course of ideas during a period so remote from our own, the greatest obstacle we meet is the inadequacy of the sources available. During the break-up of the Roman Empire most of the written record vanished irretrievably. The manuscripts that survive are all too often incomplete, blotted, or misarranged by careless and ignorant copyists. The contributions of many extremely important figures can be made out solely from references in the writings of others. Additional uncertainties arise in connection with the use of words, either as a result of intentional obscurity or through changes in meaning. Although Galen and Hippocrates were separated by a period as long as that which lies between us and Chaucer, one tends to think of them as contemporaries, using the same terms in precisely the same way. As a matter of fact, however, connotations varied markedly, and Galen's interpretations of earlier views may be as far from the mark as our interpretation of his. Furthermore, it should be stressed that any effort to work out a continuous conceptual evolution is to impose a certain artificiality, a regularity that does not accord with the facts, for one of the most confusing aspects of ancient thought lies in its apparent inconsistency. In the absence of an intelligible standard rooted in experimental verification, a Bellman's logic tended to prevail, with general acceptance of the validity of any notion that found sufficiently vigorous support. Thus, an intricate convolution of ideas resulted in a large variety of schemes, each containing a hodgepodge of concepts, some new, some old, some proved, some clearly disproved. Indeed, one gains the impression that in suppressing originality by an overabundance of detail the fertility of the early workers actually contributed to the decline in invention after the first century B.C. The picture of conceptualization during the Greco-Roman period thus resembles much more closely a tapestry in which the same threads recur in different combinations than it does an organic growth from seed. This warning is necessary because in the discussion that follows certain concepts relevant to an understanding of splanchnic vascular physiology are considered rather arbitrarily as separate and distinct developments.

CONCEPTS OF SPLANCHNIC VASCULAR STRUCTURES

Gross Anatomy: The vasculature was probably recognized as a discrete arrangement of cylindrical structures within the body at a very

SPECIAL CIRCULATIONS

early time. However, no clear distinction seems to have been made between arteries and veins, between bronchi and blood vessels, or between hollow vessels and solid structures such as nerves and tendons. These confusions are evident in the oldest surviving descriptions of the splanchnic vessels as an organized and interrelated system. An enumeration of the blood vessels of the body in the earliest Egyptian medical texts—The Papyrus Ebers and The Papyrus Edwin Smith (*27, 133, 164*)—from the period prior to 1600 B.C. includes the ureters, the seminal ducts, and the bile ducts. What is perhaps the first explicit written description of the hepatic and splenic vasculature also contains inferences regarding function that were to have a decisive influence upon conceptualization of splanchnic vascular dynamics. According to the Egyptian physicians (*164*), "There are four vessels to the liver; it is they which give it humor and air, which afterward cause all disease to arise in it by overfilling with blood. There are four vessels to the lung and to the spleen; it is they which give humor and air to it likewise." These ideas reappeared in Greek speculations on bodily composition and persisted in various guises down to modern times. It is surprising and rather humbling to see how slowly anatomical knowledge advanced beyond this beginning.

In a much later description (*6, 77*) attributed to an Asiatic Greek, Diogenes of Apollonia, who is believed to have lived in the latter half of the fifth century B.C., the vessels in man were set forth as follows:

"There are two main blood vessels; these extend from the abdomen along the spinal column, one to the right, one to the left, going down to each of the legs correspondingly, and up to the head past the collar bone through the throat. From these, blood-vessels extend throughout the whole body: from the right-hand one to the right side, from the left-hand one to the left side; the two biggest to the heart along the spine, and others a little higher through the chest below the arm pit to each of the corresponding arms. And the one is called splenetic (after the spleen), the other (after the liver) hepatic. The extreme end of each of them divides, one branch going to the thumb, the other to the rest of the hand and fingers. Two other finer blood-vessels lead from the original (main) blood-vessels on the right to the liver and on the left to the spleen and the kidneys."

Diogenes went on to discuss vessels going to the head and extremities.

He stated that finer vessels appear in the arms in addition to the splenetic and hepatic vessels. "These are opened when there is any pain under the skin, but if the pain is in the abdomen the hepatic and splenetic vessels are bled." In this view (which was to be widely accepted, at least by the laity, for more than two thousand years) the veins in the arms extended directly to the liver and spleen, providing in this manner a direct method of removing local excesses of blood and evil humors in the spleen or liver by phlebotomy. Note that the splanchnic circulation was the focus of interest, the center from which the whole vasculature was presumed to extend.

THE SPLANCHNIC CIRCULATION

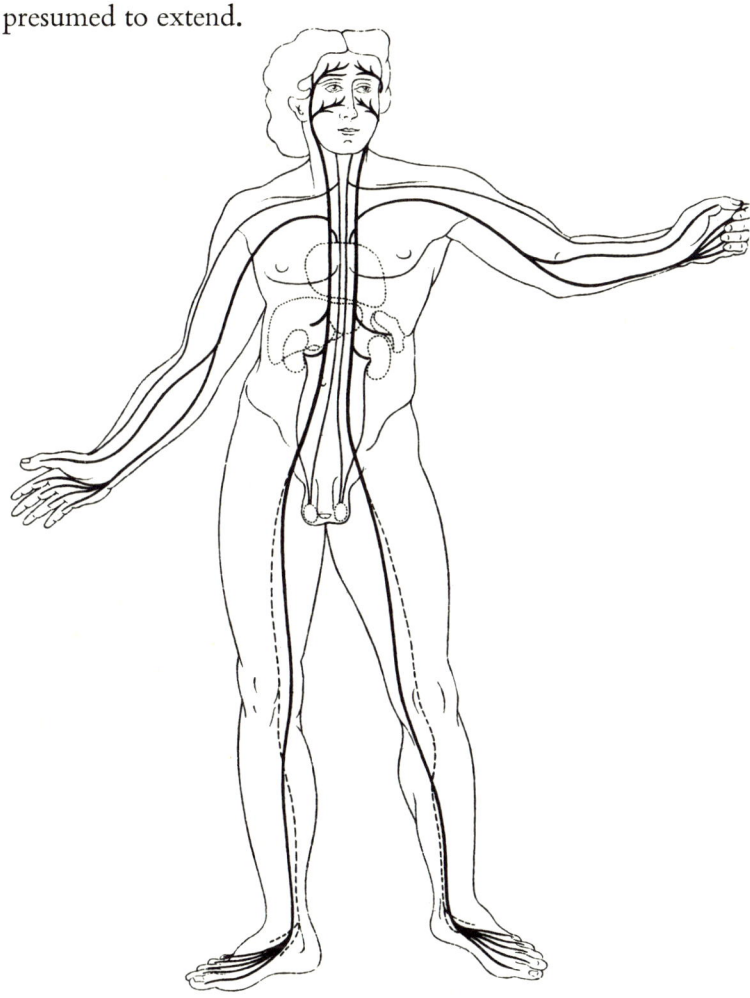

Figure 9. The circulatory system according to Diogenes of Apollonia.

A similar but even more confused scheme is found in the Hippocratic treatise, *Nature of Man*, Chapter XI (*98*).

SPECIAL
CIRCULATIONS

"The thickest of the veins have the following nature. There are four pairs in the body. [The first two mentioned extend from the head along the spine to the genitalia and the lower extremities.] The third pair of veins passes from the temples through the neck under the shoulder-blades, then they meet in the lungs and reach, the one on the right the left side, and the one on the left the right. The right one reaches from the lungs under the breast both to the spleen and to the kidneys, and the left one to the right from the lungs under the breast both to the liver and to the kidneys, both of them ending in the anus. The fourth pair begin at the front of the head and eyes, under the neck and collar-bones, passing on the upper part of the arms to the elbows, then through the forearms to the wrists and fingers, then back from the fingers they go through the ball of the hand and the forearm upwards to the elbow, and through the upper arm on the underside to the armpit, and from the ribs above one reaches to the spleen and the other to the liver."

Here the writer regarded the head as the starting place, but he agreed with Diogenes in providing a direct vascular communication between the veins of the forearms and the splanchnic viscera, for the same purpose of providing a means of phlebotomy to treat abdominal complaints.

Although Aristotle lived a full generation later than these writers and engaged actively in anatomical studies, he quoted their descriptions approvingly in *Historia animalium* (*6*). In another treatise, *De partibus animalium* (*7*), he mentioned a part of the portal system as "the blood vessels which begin at the bottom of the mesentery, and extend throughout the length of it right up to the stomach" (*line 650 a 30*). Aristotle believed that "the blood vessels are a sort of container for the blood," all having "their source in the heart and beginning there" (*line 666 a 21*). In his view,

"The viscera which are below the diaphragm are all of them present for the sake of the blood vessels, in order that the latter may have freedom of carriage and at the same time be attached to the body by means of the viscera, which act as a bond. Indeed, these are, as it were, anchor-lines thrown out to the body through the extended parts; e.g. from the Great Blood-vessel to the liver and to the spleen, for these viscera act, as it were, like rivets and fasten it to the body;

that is to say, the liver and spleen fasten the Great-vessels to the sides of the body (since blood-vessels pass to them from it alone) while the kidneys fasten it to the rear parts" (lines 670 a 7 to 670 a 19).

Although the earlier writings and etymology seem to imply a knowledge of the gastrointestinal tract as a continuous tubular system composed of distinguishable sections extending from the mouth to the anus, the earliest surviving descriptions appear to be those included by Aristotle in *De partibus animalium*. His collaborators, who are believed to have furnished the raw data upon which the biological writings are based, investigated a large number of animal species and thus provided the means for meaningful comparisons. Anatomical divisions are clearly defined, but the local vascular bed goes almost unmentioned.

THE SPLANCHNIC CIRCULATION

Some fifty years after Aristotle, Herophylos, working in the Museum at Alexandria, wrote an account of hepatic anatomy which survives because Galen quoted it approvingly in his work *On anatomical procedures* (*82, 170*).

"In man, the liver is of a good size, big in comparison with that in certain other animals of equal bulk. Where it is applied to the diaphragm it is arched and smooth. Below toward the abdominal cavity and the vena cava it is concave and irregular. Here it may be likened to the fissure through which the vein in embryos enters into it from the navel. The liver is not alike in all, but differs in different animals in breadth, length, thickness, height and number of lobes, and also in the irregularity of the front part at which it is thickest, and the arched top parts where it is thinnest. In some the liver does not have lobes at all but is round and undifferentiated. In some, however, it has two, in some more, and in many four and in some more lobes."

Like Aristotle, Herophylos appears to have been in some doubt about the source of the veins (*159*), but for most of his contemporaries and successors, including Galen, almost 600 years later, there was little doubt that the liver was the "fons venarum." Herophylos seems to have described the gut in some detail. His observation that the "portion continued from the pylorus . . . is twelve fingers' breadth long" was mentioned by Galen (*82, p. 164*). This observation gave the duodenum its name. A younger contemporary at the Museum, Erasistratos, called attention to the heavy muscular coats of the stomach and intestines. To judge from a comment made by Galen, Erasistratos may have de-

SPECIAL CIRCULATIONS

scribed the mesenteric lacteals, for he found that "when the mesentery is exposed the arteries appear full of air—later they seem full of milk" (*82, p. 200*).

The confused record of the next few centuries yields little evidence of major anatomical discoveries, although it seems certain that work continued in the medical schools. It is probable that the full account made available through the writings of Galen is traceable in large part to investigations carried out prior to his time. Galen's enumeration (*82, p. 165*) of a variety of dissecting instruments, "lancets, flat broad probes, two-edged lancets, specilla, oricularia, etc.," bespeaks an ancient craft. The extent of the information which had accumulated is difficult to make out. Galen was undoubtedly verbose, but his works do leave the impression that much remains unsaid as obvious and common knowledge. Thus his description of the vascular system is reasonably exact but quite incomplete. The aorta and venae cavae are clearly differentiated. The mesenteric and celiac arteries were probably recognized. The sources of the splanchnic arterial system and the mesenteric and splenic vessels are described as follows:

"The arteries and veins of the mesentery extend down, like roots, into the concavities of the (intestinal) curves, there meeting one another. Like the roots of trees, these can be traced to a single origin. You will easily find the veins gathered into a single stem, namely, that by the fissure (pylae, or gates) of the liver. The arteries you will not trace so readily, for they are more bloodless and thicker coated and they are in contact with a bloodless organ (mesenteric root glands) which they call the 'mesenteric link' of ligamentous nature by which the mesentery holds the intestines. This extends upward with the arteries lying by it into that part of the spine which lies between diaphragm and kidneys. Here is the starting-point of the arteries in the mesentery, sometimes in one root immediately dividing, sometimes twofold from the start (82, p. 161). . . . The spleen lies on the left, having its concavity towards the right. From the liver there goes to it a vein, a branch of which goes on to the stomach. After sending branches to all the parts of the spleen, part of the vein continues to the convex part of the stomach and the rest to the left region of the omentum" (*82, p. 164*).

The splenic artery is mentioned and the omental vasculature presented in some detail.

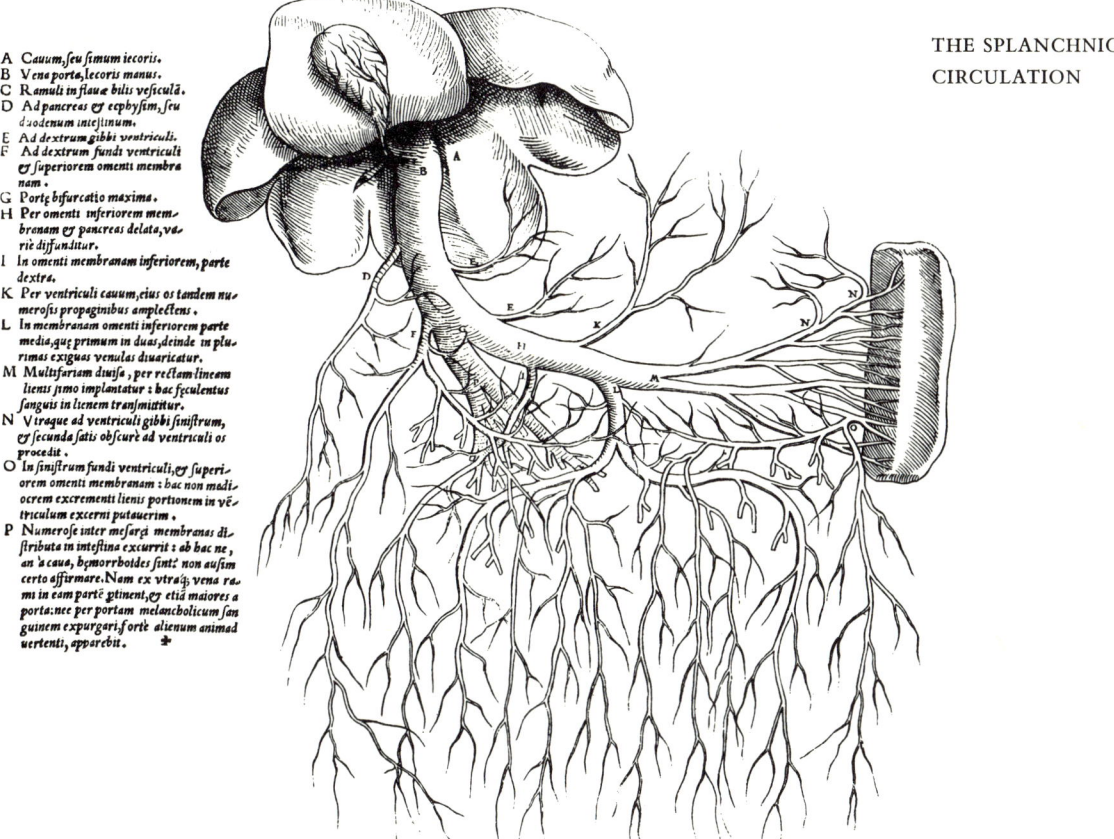

Figure 10. The splanchnic circulation according to Galen as set forth by Vesalius in the *Tabulae Sex*, Venice, 1538. The legends of the figure, as translated by Singer, appear in Notes and Acknowledgments.

Of special interest is Galen's account of the dissection of the vessels of the liver.

"*Into the most concave part run veins from the mesentery. They call this region in which they are all concentrated the 'pyle' (porta) of the liver. There, in all red-blooded animals you will find a large mouth of a vein. Have several*

SPECIAL CIRCULATIONS

instruments ready, some narrower, some broader, so as to use the most suitable. Push one of these into each lobe, pressing it gently forward, and cut down on it with a lancet until you reach the vein in which it is, for the instrument is clearly visible under the thin coat. . . . When bared, without cutting it, remove the surrounding substance of the organ between the vessels. You will thus display one large vein entering each lobe. This divides into many small veins, like the trunk of a tree into branches. These again divide into twigs and end in delicate shoots. . . . If the animal is of considerable size you can preserve the biliary ducts and the arteries belonging to it along with the veins . . . the artery and biliary vessels are clearly seen beside the portal vein."

The extrahepatic biliary tract is then accurately followed out to the duodenum and gallbladder.

"Having examined carefully all these things, proceed to the convex part of the liver, cutting up that lobe the veins of which you laid bare in the concave part. You will see the veins dividing progressively in the convexity but not the arteries. Far less are the biliary ducts here visible."

Perhaps the absence of detail is attributable to the limitations placed upon dissection by the lack of preservatives and a warm climate. Whatever the reason, a false concept of vascular distribution within the hepatic tissues resulted, since Galen seems to have believed that the vessels entering the "concave part" of the liver did not intermingle with the hepatic venous arborizations in the "convex part." This notion was to persist until the work of Glisson, 1400 years later. In other respects Galen's concepts of the gross anatomy of the splanchnic vasculature did not differ greatly from those we accept today.

Finer Structure: Although finer structures could not be made out distinctly, the peculiar texture of the tissues and the obvious lack of homogeneity in any part pointed clearly to a fundamental differentiation. The nature of this differentiation could not be made out by the naked eye, but still it called for an explanation. The oldest and most widely acceptable theory held that the tissues were derived from blood, long considered the substance of life itself. "The natural order," according to Plato (*138*), "is that flesh and sinews should be made of blood, the sinews out of the fibers to which they are akin and the flesh out of the clots which are found when the fibers are separated." Aristotle (*7*) said that the viscera are also composed of blood, "*because they are situated upon the channels of the blood vessels and on the points of ramification. All (including the heart) may be compared to the mud which a running stream deposits, they are as it were deposits left by the current of blood in the blood vessels. . . . (line 647 b 1). Thus just as in the irrigation system the biggest channels persist whereas the smallest ones quickly get obliterated by the mud, though when the mud abates they reappear; so in the body the largest blood vessels persist while the smallest ones become flesh in actuality, though potentially they are blood vessels as much as ever before*" (line 668 a 25).

THE SPLANCHNIC CIRCULATION

In the years following Aristotle, the differences between arteries, veins, and nerves were more sharply defined by the physicians of the medical school at Cos, who had also rediscovered arterial pulsation, a phenomenon familiarly referred to much earlier in the Egyptian medical writings (154, 155). The functions of arteries, veins, and nerves were not understood, but their ubiquity in the body led Erasistratos to conclude that most tissues are formed basically of a varied and intimate commingling of all three. However, Erasistratos believed that the "flesh of the liver" is formed from blood passing into the tissue spaces through the vessel walls and he applied to it the term "parenchyma," from *parencheim*, "to pour in beside" (82).

Of much greater importance to the history of ideas is Erasistratos' concept of an intrahepatic capillary bed.

"*There is a common space into which the veins from the gateway of the liver conduct the unpurified blood, and from which in the first place the biliary passages take over the bile and secondly the branches of the vena cava take over the purified blood. [Thus] there are two kinds of vessels anastomosing at the same place, the one kind extending to the gallbladder and the other to the vena cava, the result is that of the nutriment carried up from the alimentary canal, that part which fits [the diameters of both] is received into both kinds of vessels, some being carried to the gallbladder and the rest passing over into the vena cava*" (81, p. 147).

These ideas are far more explicit in explaining the movement of nutriment from the bowel to the rest of the body by the vascular system than the older, rather vague, notions of seepage and percolation. More than three centuries later Galen was to set out the views of Erasistratos in the only form in which they survive today. It should be stressed that

SPECIAL CIRCULATIONS

Galen was bitterly critical of the Alexandrian scientist, attacking him savagely for his materialism and for his reliance upon morphology as the sole guide to function. Nevertheless he agreed that a system of tiny "labyrinthine" channels must connect the portal vein with the vena cava, thus perpetuating a concept which later proved essential to Harvey's theory of the circulation. Indeed, Galen tended to agree with the old Alexandrian school on most anatomical questions, although he disagreed sharply regarding the composition of the tissue and the character of biologic activity. The first he attributed to appropriate combinations of the body humors, the second to the operation of "natural faculties." He was outraged by Erasistratos' calm dismissal of both hypotheses.

The "doctrine of humors" had a long and involved history which is exceedingly difficult to disentangle. Two lines of thought appear to be discernible. On the one hand, bile, phlegm, and other humors were considered as detrimental by-products or residues, probably instrumental in causing disease, and on the other, bile and phlegm were regarded, like blood, as an integral part of the body fabric. Both opinions have a long pedigree. The first is perhaps the older, seeming to stem from the rational-empirical phase of Egyptian medical thought in which much emphasis was laid upon *wekhedu* (*wḫdw*), a noxious humor absorbed from the gut as a residue of digestion, a principle responsible for post-mortem putrefaction and for a change in the blood during life which found issue in fever and purulent discharges (*133, 164*). Possibly, as some suggest (*164*), this view was taken up and elaborated in the medical school on the isle of Cnidus, an arch-rival of the school on Cos. Certain books in the Hippocratic Corpus (*Ancient Medicine* (*97*) in particular) call attention to the variety and number of humors in the body, some "acid and unmixed," others "pungent and acrid," some produced by the primary disorder, others producing harmful effects by excesses or defects, "all diseases arising from the internal cause of bile and phlegm." Bile was marked out by the Pythagorean and Empedoclean schools also as the root cause of disease, and in view of Plato's intellectual debt to Philistion of Locroi it is not surprising to find bile and phlegm referred to in the *Timaeus* (*138*) as "unwholesome morbid secretions" (*line 82a*). Aristotle's thought (*7*) was even closer to the Egyptian, for he called bile and phlegm "residues" which served no purpose and were "like the sediment produced in the bowel and intestine" (*line 677 a 15*). The second, and opposing, view is more difficult to trace. According to the Homeric poems bile was involved somehow in the expression of grief, anger, and deep emotion (*130*). Bile was thus an essential secretion and was properly considered a basic ingredient of body composition. This idea was apparently cultivated by the school on Cos (possibly as a reaction to Cnidus), and in the Hippocratean treatise, *Nature of Man*, written by Polybus, a son-in-law of Hippocrates, it was given its definitive expression (*98*):

THE SPLANCHNIC CIRCULATION

"*The body of man has itself blood, phlegm, yellow bile, and black bile; these make up the stuff of his body and through these he feels pain and enjoys health. Now he enjoys the most perfect health when these elements are duly proportioned to one another in respect of compounding, power and bulk, that is, when they are perfectly mingled*" (Chap. IV., lines 1–5).

Over the centuries that followed philosophers and scientists like Aristotle and Erasistratos generally favored the first view, laying stress rather upon the elements of Air, Fire, Water, and Earth as the basic constituents of all things than upon the humors (*5*). In contrast, physicians tended to emphasize the Hippocratean thesis, and Galen's enthusiastic support ultimately made the four humors an accepted doctrine of Arabic and medieval medicine.

Possibly the fact that Aristotle and Hippocrates agreed on the importance of the four Elements may account for Galen's curious belief (*81*) that they also agreed on the doctrine of humors. One of the most striking evidences of Greek originality and independence of thought lies in the persistent effort to find an ultimate unity in some quintessence behind the basic Elements—Air, Fire, Water, and Earth; whether it be one of these (Thales, Anaximenes, Heracleitos), an undefinable stuff (Anaximander), atoms differing only in size, shape, and position (Leucippos, Democritos), or an infinite variety of atomized substances (Anaxagoras) (*29*). All these speculations left their mark upon medical thinking and were reflected in conceptualizations of structure and function. Certainly all four Elements were clearly evident in the splanchnic bed and the tissues it supplies; in intestinal gases, in the body heat, in the abundance of fluids, and in the earthy fecal matter.

Air was considered particularly important. The obvious relationship

SPECIAL CIRCULATIONS

between breathing and life, the confusion of mist, wind, flatus, breath, vapor, and other gaseous substances as identities, and the observation of steam rising from freshly shed blood, all conspired to endow "air" with the mysterious trappings of the "soul." Much thought was given to this concept in the Italian and Sicilian medical schools. To the old Egyptian idea of a system of vessels conducting air Empedocles added the hypothesis that air enters the body both by the lungs and by pores in the skin (*77*). Philalaus of Croton suggested at about the same time that the "soul" might be tripartite, divided between the head, heart, and navel —the last apparently derived at the outset from the mother by way of the umbilical cord and correspondingly impulsive and childlike (*77*). These ideas were further elaborated by Plato (*138*), who divided the rational, spiritual, and appetitive aspects of the soul between the brain, heart, and liver. He was rather vague about the route by which the air is dispersed in the body once it entered, although he seems to have suggested that it may be in the vessels. Aristotle (*7*) was similarly vague about distribution but quite assured in his belief that the brain was merely a cooling device that adjusted the temperature of the blood which had been heated in the heart. The centrally placed heart was to Aristotle's mind the obvious seat of the soul, where intellect and emotion were centered and whence "pneuma," or "spirit" was sent forth to animate the rest of the body. Development and differentiation seems to have been contingent, in Aristotle's thought, upon a hereditable "connate pneuma" (*135*). Even more elaborate "pneumatic" theories were worked out by his successors, among them Erasistratos, to account for the pulse and for the absence of blood in the arteries after death. Galen disproved Erasistratos' claim that the arteries contained nothing but air in life by an experimental demonstration of intra-arterial blood in living animals, but he, too, believed that air entered the arteries through the skin and the lungs (*60, 81, 82*). He also thought that the liver elaborated a "natural spirit" or a principle involved in the maintenance of vegetative or nonintellectual function, that the heart produced, possibly from the air, a refined essence necessary for life, a "vital spirit," and that the brain disseminated an essence of the soul (*spiritus animalis* or "animal spirit") necessary in sensory perception and rational activity (*79, 80*). These concepts, evidently parallel to Plato's division of the soul, thus made "air" an extremely important, though not by any means a precisely defined, constituent of the tissues.

"Fire" was another essential element, more rarefied and hotter than air. Heracleitos of Ephesus (*fl.* 500 B.C.) believed that the basis of reality lay in "fire" and constant change stabilized by an "attunement" of opposing forces (77). His writings were influential particularly in determining the thought of the Pythagoreans and, ultimately, the concepts of the Hippocratic school. According to the former, (notably Philalaus of Croton) "man's body is composed of heat" (5, *Chap.* XVIII, *line 20*) and respiration was simply a means of cooling the blood. Aristotle suggested that the "innate heat" was produced in the heart and that the heated blood, after cooling in the lungs and brain, was distributed to the tissues by the arteries. The idea of "innate heat" remained embedded for centuries in biological thought. The proximity of the liver and spleen to the diaphragm and heart accounted for their relatively poor arterial supply, according to Galen, for "they are warmed directly and do not require the heat supplied by the arteries." Far more important from the standpoint of conceptual evolution was the Heracleitean doctrine of "attunement." The Pythagorean teaching of balanced dualities promulgated by Alcmeon of Croton ("Health is the harmonious mixture of the qualities" of the Elements—Dry, Wet, Cold, and Hot) undoubtedly played a part in stimulating Empedocles to return to the traditional four Elements and to postulate coordination between them by opposing forces of attraction and repulsion (77). These ideas proved widely acceptable—to Plato, to Aristotle, to the physicians of the Hippocratic school, and finally to Galen, in whose works they were passed to the West.

CONCEPTS OF SPLANCHNIC VASCULAR FUNCTION

The formulation of meaningful concepts of the function of the splanchnic circulation in the absence of reliable physiologic data depends as much upon an understanding of the ends it serves as upon a knowledge of its anatomy. The Greek physiologists found in the close association of the liver, spleen, and gastrointestinal tract a disarmingly "obvious" role for the splanchnic bed in "sanguification," or the formation of blood from food. Given information or theory on the use of a structure, it is possible to construct a bewildering variety of reasonable

SPECIAL CIRCULATIONS

physiological hypotheses. Indeed, the danger is that an intellectually satisfying hypothesis may result in self-deception and in illusory "discoveries" of nonexistent structures or activities that are required by theory. The attractive concept of sanguification proved to be just such a will o' the wisp in tempting the unwary into ill-grounded speculations on the splanchnic blood flow. Unfortunately, comprehension of the hemodynamic implications of structure necessitates a basis in physical theory and technology which the Greek and Roman thinkers lacked. The laws of fluid flow were but dimly recognized and usually misinterpreted; the source and character of movement were misjudged. Actually, all physical and biologic motion was attributed to the channeling of an activity that was considered an inherent property of Water, Air, and Fire. This idea was developed by Empedocles and taken up by the philosophers that followed him (77). Aristotle (7) certainly stressed the observable qualities rather than the theoretical entities underlying them. "Perhaps," he said, "it is better to say *dynameis* instead of Elements for it is just these four, the fluid substance, the solid, the hot, and the cold, which are the matter of composite bodies." *Dynameis* is a very difficult technical term employed repeatedly throughout the classical medical literature to refer to "powers," "natural faculties," or "properties," which are demonstrable as effects. In the Hippocratic treatise on *Ancient Medicine* (97), for example, *dynameis* are defined as "intensity or strength of the humors," in Galen's writings, as the "cause of activity." Galen (81) marked out the three major faculties of genesis, growth, and nutrition, but since for every observable effect there was a corresponding *dynamis*, the potential number of "powers" was actually infinite. In this instance terminologic distinctions were misconstrued as advances in understanding with a resulting tendency to put a brake upon further analysis. Factual inaccuracy, insufficiency, and indeterminacy all combined to check and distort concept formation. Nevertheless, a driving curiosity coupled with a profound respect for reason and a courageous determination to exclude the supernatural frequently led to concepts that were remarkably perceptive and often startling in their accuracy.

Sanguification: The ancient belief that blood is manufactured in the liver undoubtedly had its origin in the obvious engorgement of the liver with blood. Since food enters the gastrointestinal system and since it must be converted to blood, it is an almost self-evident conclusion that the process of sanguification takes place in the liver, transport from bowel to liver being provided in some manner by the local vascular system. Such was the general theory set out in the earliest medical writings, although the association of the liver with emotion and with divination was not easy at first to exorcise or, alternatively, to incorporate in the theoretical scheme. In a general way, the hypothesis of local sanguification held the field throughout classical times, gaining in detail and sophistication perhaps, but nonetheless remaining fundamentally unchanged over the 500 years from Aristotle to Galen.

In Plato's *Timaeus* (*138*) we find a transitional account in which the liver is described as the organ of prophecy and the processes of digestion and sanguification vaguely ascribed to the stomach and neighboring blood vessels.

"Knowing that . . . the part of the soul which desires meats and drink . . . would not comprehend reason . . . God combined with it the liver, and placed it in the house of the lower nature, contriving that it should be solid and smooth, and bright and sweet, and should also have a bitter quality in order that the power of thought which proceeds from the mind might be reflected as in a mirror . . . and so strike terror into the desires . . . such is the nature of the liver which is placed as we have described in order that it may give prophetic intimations. . . . The spleen is situated on the left-hand side and is constructed with a view of keeping the liver bright and pure—like a napkin, always ready prepared and at hand to clear the mirror. And hence when any impurities arise in the region of the liver by reason of disorders of the body, the loose nature of the spleen, which is composed of a hollow and bloodless tissue, receives them all and clears them all away. . . . When the respiration is going in and out, and the fire, which is fast within, follows it, and ever advances moving to and fro, enters through the belly and reaches the meat and drink, it dissolves them, and dividing them into small portions and guiding them through the passages when it goes, pumps them as from a fountain in the channels of the veins."

Plato attributed the red color of the blood to the burning effects of "Fire," an idea suggesting that transformation of the food to blood resembled the changes produced by heat during cooking and ripening.

The physicians called this process "coction" (*pepsis*) and believed that it operated also in correcting disturbances in the perfect balance (*crasis*) of the humors: "A man is in the best possible condition," according to

SPECIAL CIRCULATIONS

the Hippocratic book on *Ancient Medicine* (*97*, *Chap*. XIX), "when there is complete coction and rest with no particular power (*dynamis*) displayed." Aristotle (*7*) also considered coction and digestion akin to baking, with rearrangement of the Elements by "the agency of heat." After the food is broken up by mastication and swallowed, according to his view, "the natural heat comes into play and effects the concoction of the food." From the stomach the partially concocted food was then taken up by the veins ["like roots"] in the mesentery and the residues were left in the gut. "The blood [or its counterpart] is the final form of the food" after concoction was completed in the liver, with the help of the spleen which "draws off the residual humors from the stomach and by virtue of its blood-like nature can assist in the concoction of them." Bile, a residue formed during concoction in the liver, was eliminated by way of the gallbladder and bile ducts. Evidently Aristotle had accepted many of the ideas set out by Plato, although he elaborated and expanded them with greater care to correlate structure and function. For both, the Empedoclean Elements were essential, the spleen was an excretory organ (though they differed on its nature), and the "innate heat" generated in the heart was the agent of change. Just how this change occurred is not apparent. Aristotle made it clear in his review of other opinions that these questions had been argued at great length for a long time. The debate continued throughout the classical period.

One of the chief sources of disagreement lay in the basic assumptions regarding the composition of matter. According to the theory proposed by Anaxagoras, digestion and concoction consisted in separation of tiny particles (homeomeries) of bile, blood, and other ingredients, as needs required (*77*). Democritos of Abdera, on the other hand, suggested that atoms differing only in shape, size, and arrangement made up all substances and that transmutation could therefore be accomplished simply by an appropriate reorganization (*29*). Erasistratos would have none of these speculations; he insisted only upon the importance of anatomical arrangements and demonstrable physical principles in determining function. According to Galen (*81*), Erasistratos emphasized the role of gastric trituration in "softening of the food, removal of waste within, and absorption when chylified (emulsified)" (*Book* III, *Chap*. IV). Innate heat was unimportant, he claimed, because "it is inconceivable that digestion involving as it does such trifling warmth, should be related to the boiling process" (*Book* III, *Chap.* IV). He refused to speculate on coction other than to agree that it might take place in the veins.

According to Galen, digestion consisted not in chylification but in alteration or a transmutation into the "quality proper to that which is receiving nourishment." The stomach contracted down upon the food in such a way as to avoid breaking it up, in order to promote absorption. And since the "adjacent viscera [were] like a lot of burning hearths around a great cauldron—to the right the liver, to the left the spleen, the heart above, and along with it the diaphragm (suspended and in a state of constant movement), and the omentum sheltering them all" (*Book* III, *Chap.* VII)—there was ample innate heat to assist in coction. From the stomach and intestine, in Galen's view, the nutriment entered the portal veins where it continued to undergo alteration since "things are done slowly in the body and by degrees."

"[In order] that the nutriment may be carried from the liver into the whole body, pure and with no waste product, Nature has contrived organs; some to clear away the thin and light part of it, some the earthy and heavy part, some the intermediate which is watery and serous. The organs that draw away the first are called . . . bile-ducts . . . those . . . which deal with the earthy and heavy part are the spleen, and of the intestines, the lower parts as far as the rectum. The organs of the third or intermediary kind are the ureters, kidney and urinary bladder" (*81, p. 15*).

The spleen was thus "the emunctory of the liver" (*79, 80, On the Use of Parts, Book* IV, *Chap.* XII) drawing the black bile, by way of the splenic vein, away from the liver and, after processing it, ultimately discharging it into the stomach by way of special vessels (possibly the short gastric veins) (*79, 80, Book* IV, *Chap.* XV). The process of coction within the liver was enhanced by the rich vascular network which delayed perfusion and prolonged contact during which alteration and the removal of peccant humors occurred. The yellow bile was separated from the nutriment and returned to the gut via the bile ducts. The chyme thus "submitted to complete coction by the innate heat mounts red and pure to the convex part of the liver, showing by its color that it has received and assimilated a portion of the divine fire"; i.e. the natural spirits (*82, p. 283*). Although his knowledge was no more exact than Aristotle's, Galen belabored at length the similarities between coction and baking or wine-making. The liver was for Galen—and after him for the Western World—primarily the "seat of sanguification and the source of the veins" (*79, 80,* Book IV, Chap. XII).

SPECIAL CIRCULATIONS

Dynamics of Splanchnic Vascular Flow: The supposed function of the splanchnic vasculature in digestion, absorption, and sanguification required it to serve as a route for the movement of chyle and blood from gut to liver and thence to the remainder of the body. The dynamics of this process were never clearly delineated. Empedocles seems to have

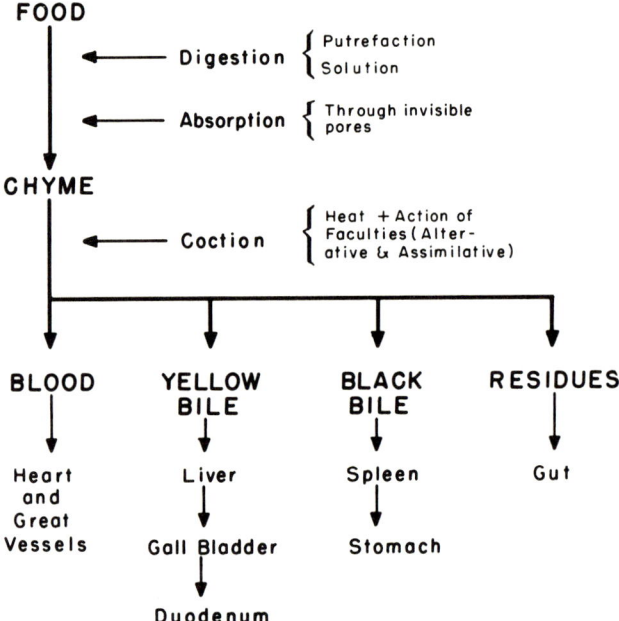

Figure 11. Physiology of sanguification according to Galen. Digested food is absorbed from the stomach and the gastrointestinal tract, enters the portal vessels as chyle, and passes upward to the liver. In the process it undergoes coction which is completed within the liver and the excrement is excreted as yellow bile by way of the gallbladder and bile duct and as black bile after passage in a retrograde manner through the portal vein, splenic vein, and to the spleen by way of a hypothetical splenic duct into the stomach. The heavy earthy material which remains within the gut after digestion is excreted as feces mixed with black and yellow bile.

been the first to attempt to work out the mechanisms by which the inherent mobility of the Elements, so obvious in the tides, in running brooks, in storms, in wind and in flames, might be controlled in living bodies. He called attention to the manner in which fluid may be held suspended in an open tube when the upper end is stopped by the finger because "the air outside, striving to get in, checks the water" (*77*). This phenomenon served as the basis for the hypothesis that blood flows to and fro in the vessels with a kind of tidal movement under the influence of movements of air in and out through skin and lungs. Plato (*138*) accepted this notion with open approval and postulated in addition the interaction of Fire and Air to promote the movement of fluid upward from the belly. Somewhat greater detail was brought to this description by Aristotle (*7*), who attributed control of motion to an unmoving Prime Mover (or Soul) centered in the heart, and who apparently believed the blood to move unidirectionally into the tissues since he likened blood flow to irrigation. The movement of blood was thus assigned to external causes as well as to the innate energies of the fluid itself. Unfortunately, understanding of the operation of surface forces, air pressure, and gravity was obscured by teleology and theology to such an extent as to nullify the actual gain.

THE SPLANCHNIC CIRCULATION

Within Aristotle's school in the Lyceum, men like Theophrastos and Strato struggled with these concepts, first attacking the "teleological principle" itself and then proceeding to the development of a realistic experimental empiricism (*64*). Theophrastos undertook a re-evaluation of the Elements and succeeded in showing that they were susceptible to further analysis and that their qualities were simply attributes, not in themselves material principles. This revision set the stage for the work of Strato who followed Theophrastos as head master of the Lyceum, after a decade in Alexandria where he had tutored the young Ptolemy and where he must have known and influenced Erasistratos. Farrington (*64*) has found in Strato's writings abundant evidence of a well-organized and practical theory of experimental investigation which proved particularly useful in his work on *Pneumatics*. In their earlier work in this field Plato and Aristotle had emphatically denied the existence of a vacuum, whereas the proponents of the Atomic Theory postulated a "continuous void" within which atoms endlessly whirled. Both groups took their positions on the basis of logical deduc-

SPECIAL CIRCULATIONS

tion. Strato, however, reached the conclusion that a "discontinuous void" exists between particles of matter but that a "continuous void" is contrary to nature, adducing as experimental evidence the suction of medical cupping glasses and the compressibility of air. Erasistratos seems to have been deeply impressed by these ideas.

According to Galen (*81*), Erasistratos made the "horror vacui," or suction, an important factor in causing blood flow. He believed that the arteries are normally filled with air, and that when an artery is severed the air escapes, creating a vacuum into which blood in the veins is attracted through connecting capillaries. Erasistratos attributed the pulse to cardiac contraction, believing that the "pneuma" is drawn out of the lung into the left ventricle at each diastole of the heart; "by its passage the pulse is produced in all the arteries throughout the body" (*82, p. 176*). Although Galen proved that the pulse is produced in a blood-filled artery, he did not reject the "horror vacui" principle and agreed with Erasistratos in believing that it operated at least in part to transfer chyme from the intestines into the portal vein, thence to the liver, and finally, after sanguification, to the heart (*81, pp. 99 and 119*). Erasistratos did not accept intrinsic arterial contraction as a cause for the pulse as many others did, but he did think that portal venous peristalsis might promote flow. In addition, he observed that the movements of the stomach and intestines compress the mesenteric veins and he suggested that the vascular contents might be propelled toward the liver in this manner (*81, p. 167*). An appreciation of the importance of a *vis a tergo* apparently led to the realization that vascular resistance might be a determinant. Indeed, Galen reported that Erasistratos attempted to explain the development of ascites by "supposing that blood is prevented from going forward owing to the narrowness of the passages." Erasistratos was obviously on the verge of a correct formulation of hemodynamic principles, but the inadequacies of technology and physical theory robbed him of his opportunity. The fragments of his work that survive in the writings of others are embued with an almost modern scientific temper. Unfortunately, his attitude did not suit the spirit of the age. Empirical and "practical" motives proved more compelling, and his writings perished from neglect.

During the long interval between Erasistratos and Galen there seems to have been little interest in splanchnic circulatory dynamics, although it is hard to be certain that important studies have not been lost in the wreckage of the classical literature. The fragments of Asclepiades and the surviving books of Rufus, Aretaeus, Celsus, and Soranus are much more deeply concerned with clinical problems of diagnosis and management. Nevertheless, the interest in anatomy and physiology that characterized Galen's thinking must have had its origin in his schooling in the scientific centers of the East. Galen disagreed wholeheartedly with what he considered the materialistic teachings of Erasistratos and Asclepiades; he emphasized rather the potentialities and vital forces peculiar to living things. Perhaps this emphasis did much to prevent the destruction of his works during centuries of ecclesiastical dominance, but it also served to retard the development of rigorous critique. Galen (*79–81*) returned to the various *dynameis* and abandoned the search for physical principles as a means of explaining hemodynamics. He accepted many of Erasistratos' suggestions but put more reliance upon "attractive or assimilative faculties" that brought about the absorption of chyme from the intestine for separation of the yellow bile and black bile and that finally promoted the transfer of blood from the concave to the convex part of the liver. The conversion of chyme to blood, chiefly in the veins and liver, was mediated by an "alterative faculty." Galen acknowledged the influence of the "width of the vessels and their mouths" upon flow and distribution, and he believed that movement through the liver was slowed by the tortuosity and length of the intrahepatic vessels in order to prolong contact with the parenchyma during alteration. Erasistratos' suggestion that venous narrowing might obstruct flow was treated with contempt, however, since it seemed obvious to Galen that the "attractive faculty" could overcome any such obstacle. Indeed, he saw no reason why portal venous flow should always move from the gastrointestinal tract to the liver and not on occasion in the opposite direction.

THE SPLANCHNIC CIRCULATION

"*Thus when there is an abundance of nutriment contained in the food-canal it is carried up to the liver by the veins, and when the canal is empty and in need of nutriment this is again attracted from the liver by the same veins. Thus the stronger draws and the weaker is evacuated. So purgative drugs draw their appropriate humors from all over the body by the same stomata* [*in the intestinal wall*] *through which absorption previously took place. One and the same stoma*

SPECIAL CIRCULATIONS

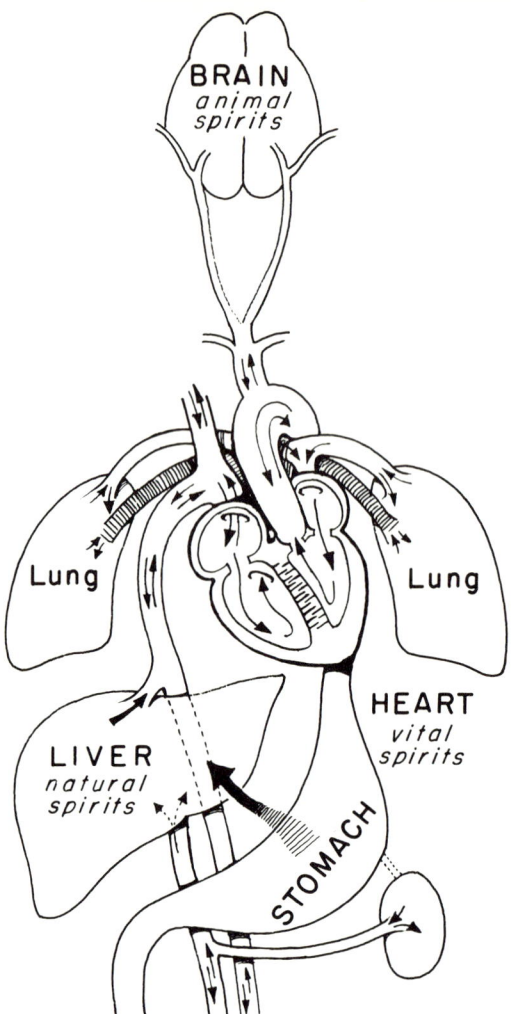

Figure 12. Relationship between the splanchnic and systemic vasculatures according to Galen. The partially digested food enters the portal veins and passes to the liver (heavy arrow) under the influence of the "attractive faculty." Movement to the liver is aided by compression of the veins by gastrointestinal movements and by the suction (or tendency to a vacuum) produced by the attraction of the chyle to the liver. The partially manufactured blood ebbs and flows in the portal veins, carrying chyle to the liver, black bile to the spleen whence it is discharged into the stomach (via a hypothetical duct—dotted lines), and residues to the gut. In the liver sanguification is completed and "natural spirits" added. The blood is then discharged into the large veins where it ebbs and flows, some entering the heart to be endowed with the "vital spirits" and to pass out to the lungs. The blood in the arteries mixed with air coming from the lungs also ebbs and flows, some reaching the brain to be further refined by the addition of the "animal spirits."

subserves two distinct faculties and these exercise their pull at different times in opposite directions—first it subserves the pull of the liver, and during catharsis, that of the drug" (*81, Book* III, *Chap*. XIII).

The success of this idea obviously militates against the development of a more accurate concept of circulatory dynamics and gives full rein to the unpredictable forces exerted by the *dynameis*. The role of the arteries was similarly obfuscated. In addition to the small amount of heat needed in coction, Galen claimed that the arteries of the splanchnic bed carried "pneuma, vapor, and that part of the blood which has been accurately elaborated and refined" (*81, Book* III, *Chap*. XIV). At the skin surface they drew in air during diastolic dilatation,

THE SPLANCHNIC CIRCULATION

"*while those which anastomose at any point with the veins attract the thinnest and most vaporous part of the blood which these contain, and as for the arteries which are near the heart, it is on the heart itself that they exert their traction. . . . So also the traction exerted by the diastole of arteries which go to the stomach and intestines takes place at the expense of the heart itself and the numerous veins in its neighborhood, for these arteries cannot get anything worth speaking of from the thick heavy nutriment contained in the intestines and stomach, since they first become filled with lighter elements.*"

There is not the slightest evidence in any of these comments that Galen saw the possibility of a circulation of blood from the arteries to the veins, but his support for the ideas that anastomoses between the two systems do exist and that blood moves from the portal vein through the liver into the vena cava via vascular connections was ultimately to provide a basis for the new epoch opened by Harvey.

CONTRIBUTION TO CONCEPTUALIZATION

The most important element in the development of concepts during the Greco-Roman period is surely to be found in the escape from the bonds of superstition. The realization that physiological data could be used alone as a basis for thought without need to allow for the caprices of an ineluctable divinity made possible a new search for understanding. The radical shift in the significance attributed to physical form at last gave real meaning to the study of anatomy and to the deduction of its functional implications. Throughout the whole period, the popular acceptance of the old gods and all their powers was actively opposed to

SPECIAL
CIRCULATIONS

the new insights; nowhere more obviously than in the conflict of ideas regarding the splanchnic vasculature. In the beginning haruspicy and all it stood for undoubtedly informed the views even of such independent spirits as Plato and Aristotle; later its influence waned, although it undoubtedly played a role in determining the central position of the liver in the conceptual scheme. As far as we can judge from the record that remains, the knowledge of splanchnic vascular morphology was developed to a point consistent with the technology of the time; the growth of splanchnic vascular physiology was retarded by misinformation and a lack of critique. Perhaps the tendency to regard vigorously expounded ideas as self-validating reflected to some extent a persistent belief in magic. In any case, the failure to establish a rigorous critical canon ultimately resulted in a welter of conflicting and confusing claims in which the truth was hard to follow. It remained the task of the moderns to cope with this difficulty.

The Modern View

During the 1400 years between Galen and Harvey the classical knowledge of anatomy and physiology died out in the West and lingered on in the East, in the Roman universities of Byzantium and in the newer Moslem schools of Egypt, Persia, and Spain. It is true that throughout the far-flung organization of the Western Church—even within temporarily isolated segments like the Irish ecclesiastical community—many manuscripts were carefully guarded, copied, and recopied. Secular thought and speculation, though limited, did not lapse altogether. Throughout the Middle Ages Aristotelian logic occupied a supreme place in the Trivium of professional teaching, and it is not surprising that diagrams of vascular anatomy in monastic leech books (*168*) were patterned upon the Aristotelian accounts. Curiously enough, the biological treatises were not accessible to the West until the thirteenth century, when Arabic translations of Aristotle's and Galen's works came into the hands of translators in Spain and Sicily. The manuscript diagrams suggest an older tradition (*168*), presumably transmitted and perpetuated as a result of the survival of a garbled doctrine of humors and the use of phlebotomy to remove noxious or excessive humors directly from the liver or spleen. The antecubital veins and their supposed direct connections with spleen and liver continued to appear in

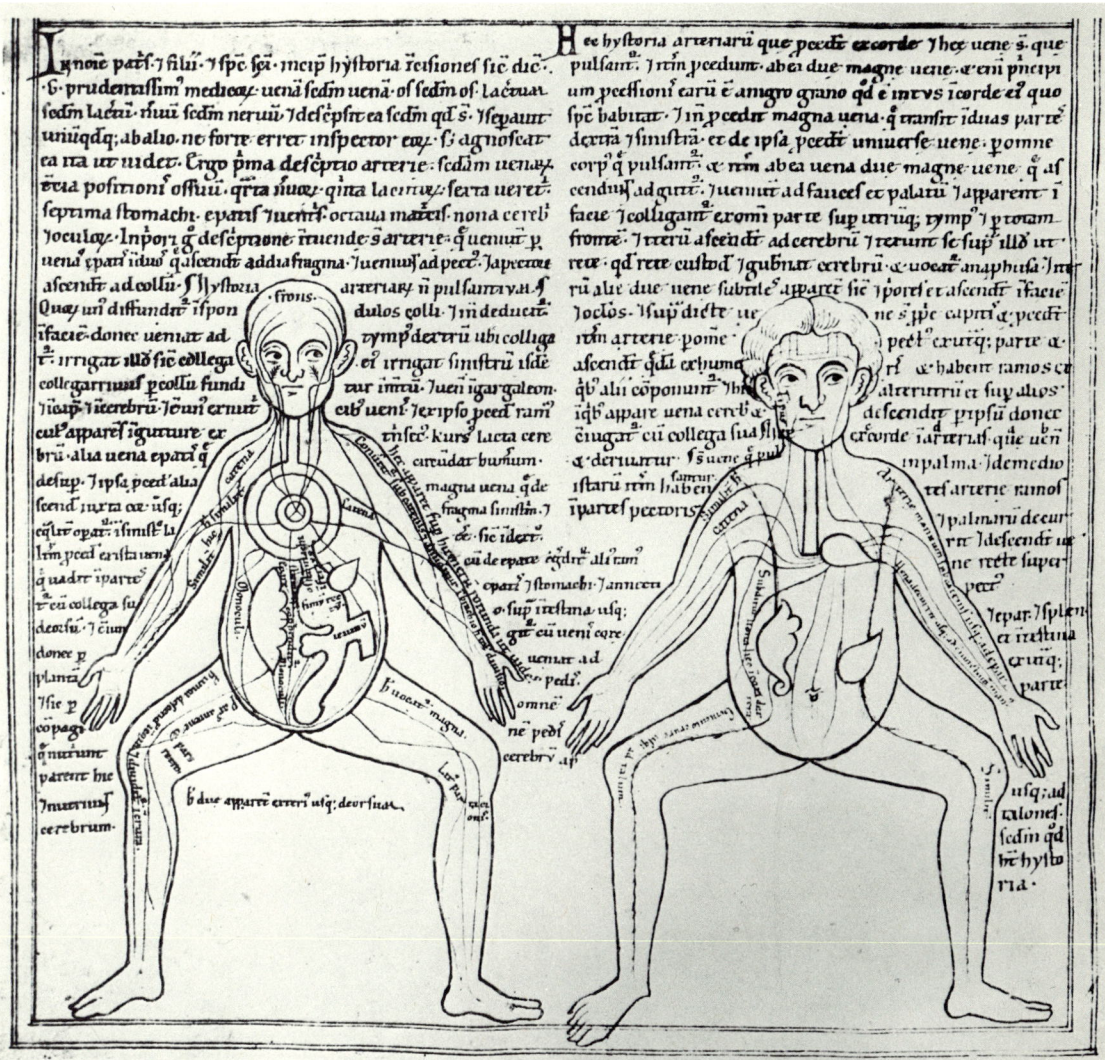

Figure 13. Medieval concept of the splanchnic circulation. Figures taken from a monastic manuscript show distribution of vessels to a multilobed liver on the left and to the stomach and a spleen on the right in a manner reminiscent of the plan outlined by Diogenes of Apollonia and the other authorities quoted in detail by Aristotle. The figure on the left shows the distribution of the arterial system, that on the right the distribution of the veins.

[649]

SPECIAL CIRCULATIONS

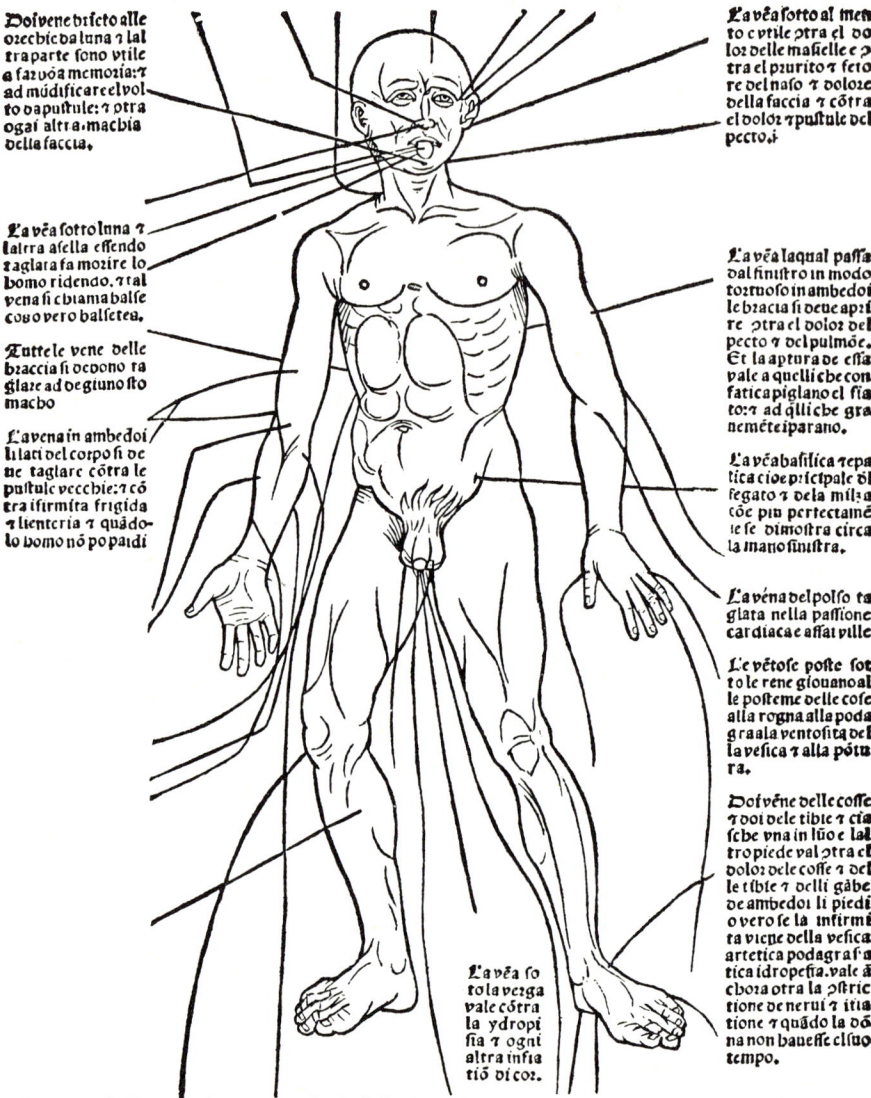

the anatomical atlases (*161*) that began to emerge from the new universities that grew up in Italy, France, Germany, and England during the thirteenth and fourteenth centuries. The revival of the ancient learning within these centers was marked both by a slavishly enthusiastic acceptance of classical authorities and by an increasingly sceptical attitude that grew out of the effort to make sense of the incoherent remnants of the literature. Time and political turbulence had not only destroyed much good but also eliminated a great deal of nonsense and, in doing so, set the stage for the development of the scientific method.

THE SPLANCHNIC CIRCULATION

Anatomical and physiological concepts of the splanchnic circulation improved progressively as the older ideas taken from Aristotle were replaced by those of Galen, during the ascendency of the Humanists. In the anatomical figures the liver was usually portrayed as a five-lobed organ, possibly because pigs or dogs were used in dissections, but human dissection began quite early, certainly in the fourteenth and probably in the thirteenth century, and it seems probable that the figures were not taken too literally. The differentiation of liver into two sections, the upper gibbous and the lower concave, each with its own vasculature—portal and hepatic veins, respectively—was obviously a legacy from Galen, but nevertheless it was a great improvement upon the older ideas of the phlebotomists. The Galenic scheme of the splanchnic circulation persisted down to the time of Harvey. Even anatomists of genius, like Leonardo da Vinci (*113*) and Andreas Vesalius (*48, 176*) in the fifteenth and sixteenth centuries, were so greatly influenced by Galen that their drawings clearly reflect Galen's ideas of the splanchnic circulation rather than their own observations. The information contained in these figures had become more accurate, however, indicating an understanding of the circulatory system far in advance of Galen's.

Figure 14. "Vein man" from Mondino. The Anathomia of Mondino, written in 1316, is considered to be the first modern anatomical work. This figure, taken from that text, shows the points at which bloodletting should be undertaken for various diseases. It can be seen that the Aristotelian concept of the circulation persists, since the splenic and hepatic veins in the antecubital spaces on the right and left, respectively, are clearly indicated. The use of Arabic nomenclature reveals the source of most of his authorities.

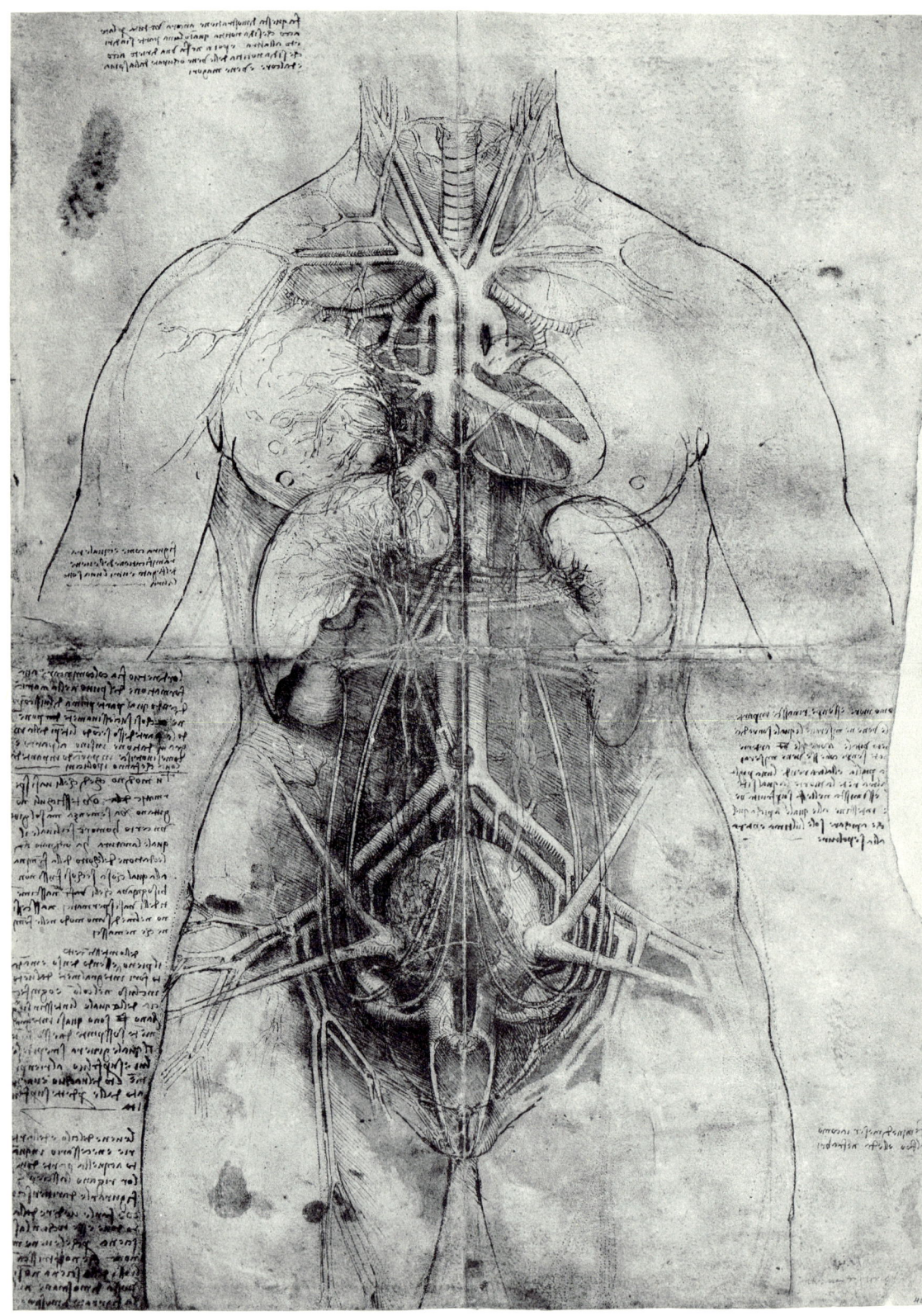

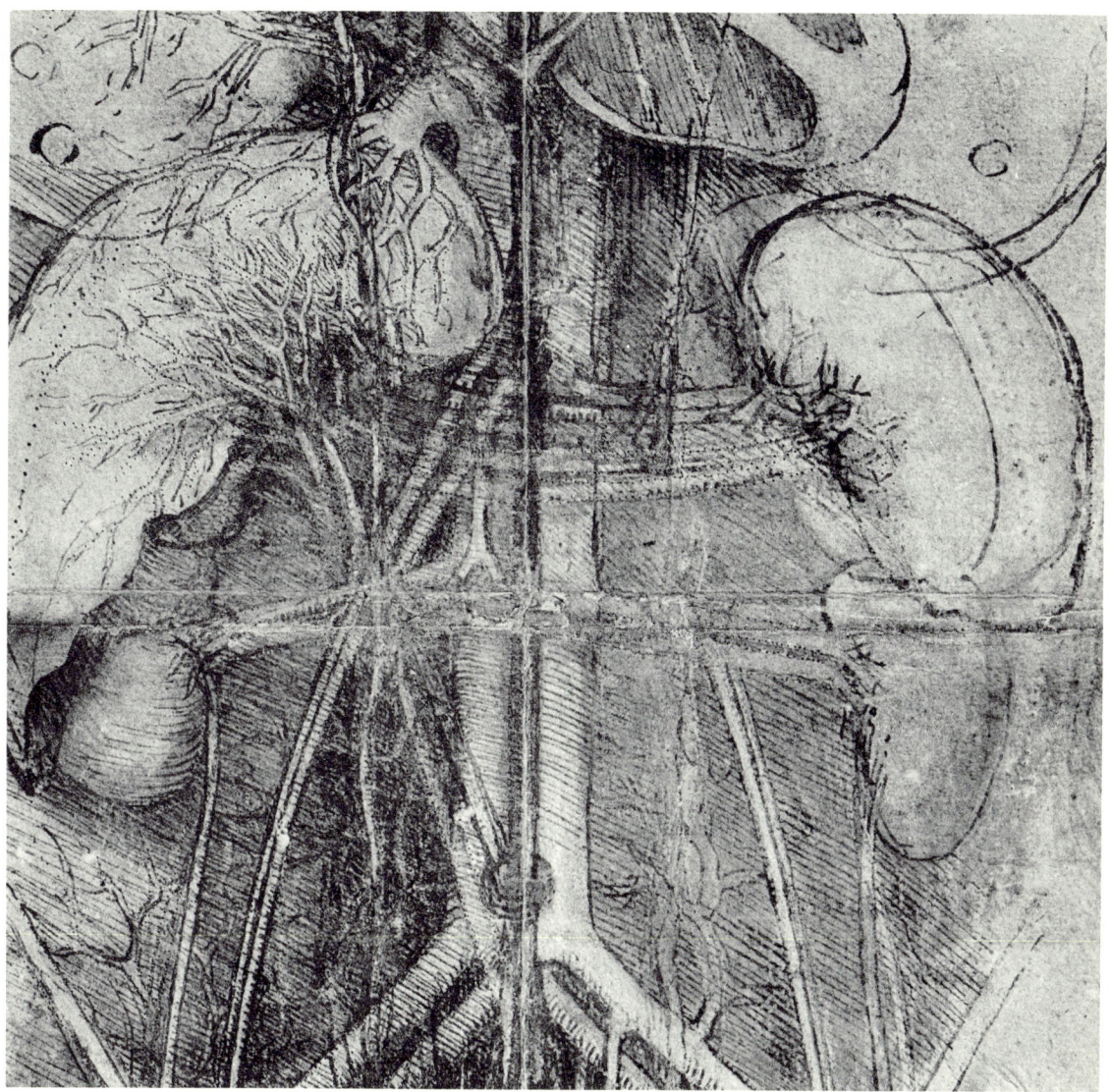

Figure 15. *Opposite page:* Leonardo da Vinci's representation of the female situs viscerum. *Above:* Enlargement of the mid-portion, showing Leonardo's view of the distribution of the blood vessels in the liver and spleen. The gibbous and caval portions of the liver are supplied by vessels that communicate directly and do not interdigitate to any extent. The distribution of the remainder of the portal system is obviously inexact, showing the influence of Galenic ideas. The configuration of the liver, however, is quite accurate.

SPECIAL CIRCULATIONS

PRIMA.

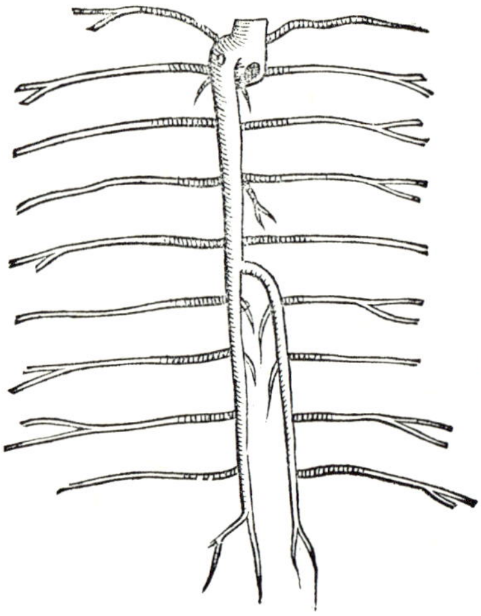

TERTIA.

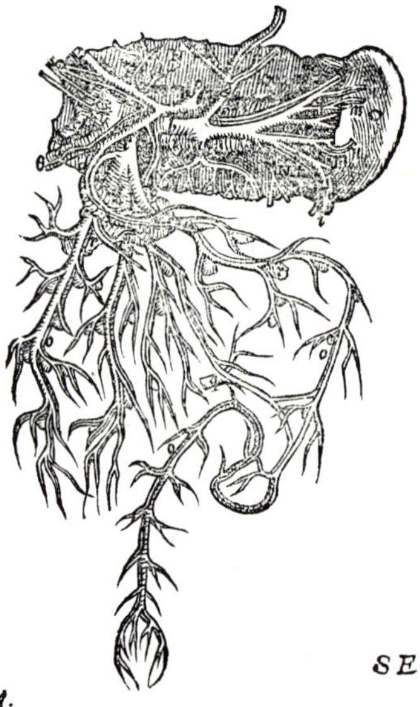

SEXTA.

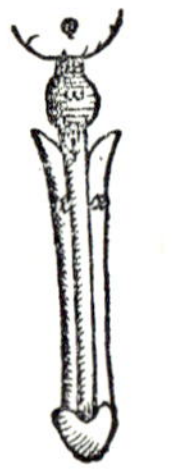

SECVNDA.

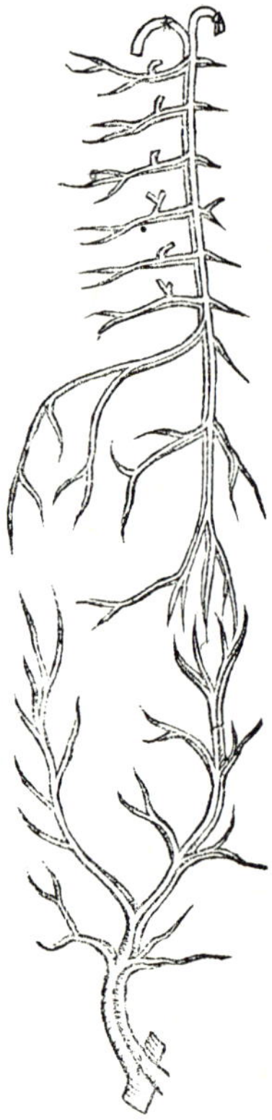

QVARTA.

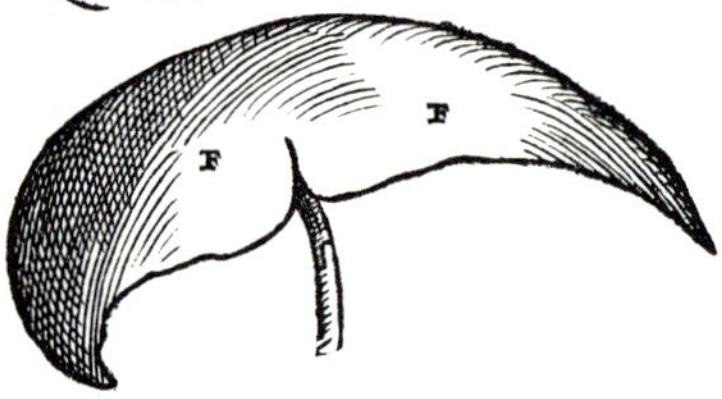

QVINTA.

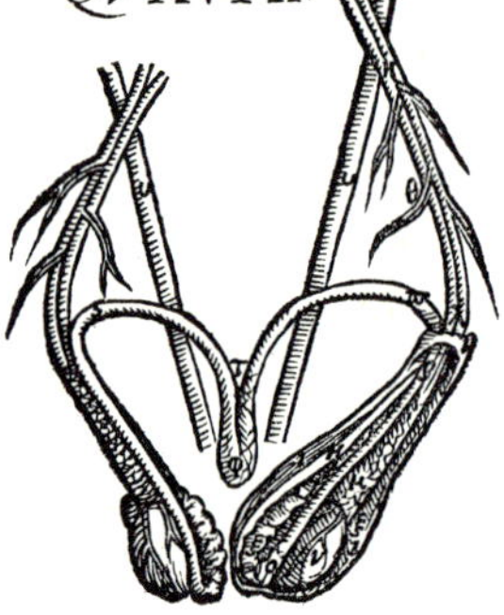

SEPTIMA.

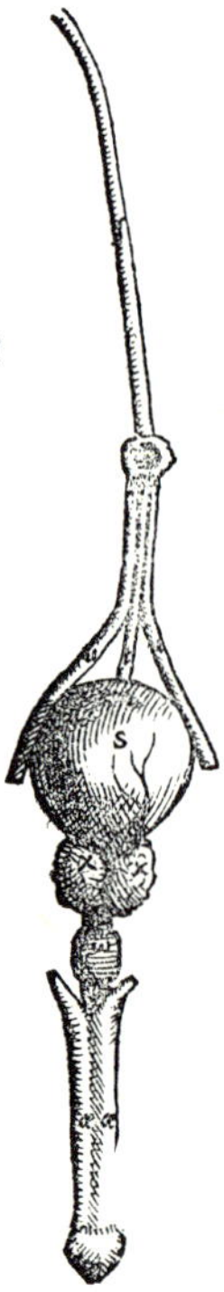

OCTAVA

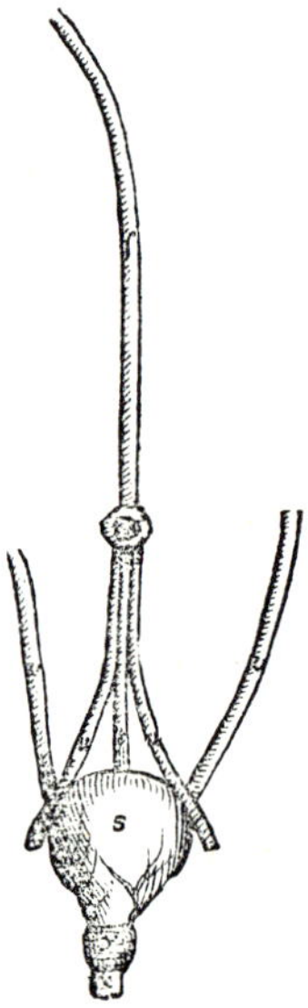

The figure of the liver drawn by Andreas Vesalius in the Tabula Sex (Fig. 10) appears to be porcine, while that in the Fabrica is a much more accurate portrayal of the human organ. Both contain a wealth of detail regarding the character and distribution of lesser vessels. The drawings and their legends indicate a continued belief in the older ideas of circulation within the liver.

THE NEW METHOD—HARVEY AND GLISSON

The remarkable change in outlook that made possible the advances so evident in Vesalian anatomy led ultimately to the development of scientific method. The barren legalities of Aristotelianism and the literary preoccupations of Humanism did not fully satisfy the need for a means of seeking knowledge by a direct appeal to Nature, a need long felt and long debated in the Italian medical schools.

During his years in Pisa and Padua, Galileo succeeded in formulating what he called a "geometrical method" (*83, 144*) which combined (1) analysis of a phenomenon to determine the principle involved, (2) deduction of its consequences, and (3) test by further experiment. William Harvey (1578–1657) studied medicine at Padua during Galileo's time, and it is no accident that he applied the Galilean method in making his discovery of the circulation of the blood. For the Harvey trained in Galenic medicine the liver and the splanchnic bed was the source of the veins (*fons venarum*) and the "factory of the blood" (*sanguificationis officina*), but for the Harvey tempered in the scientific schools of Padua the accepted impermeability of the lungs to the blood was plainly at variance with the belief that blood moved easily through the liver by the channels described by Erasistratos (*92*):

"*The parenchyma of the liver is denser by far [whereas] that of the lungs is of much fairer texture, and spongy by comparison. . . . In the liver there is no inthrust, no driving force; in the lung the blood is pushed in by the pulsation of*

Figure 16. The splanchnic bed according to Vesalius. Blood vessel systems shown here were to be cut out and pasted upon a master chart in order to show the proper relations. *Tertia* refers to the splanchnic bed and is remarkably complete in detail. There is no evidence, however, that Vesalius was in any way aware of the actual distribution of the finer branches of the portal vein in the liver or in the gastrointestinal tract. This figure is taken from the *Fabrica*.

SPECIAL CIRCULATIONS

the right ventricle of the heart and by this inthrust the vessels and porosities of the lungs must be distended. . . . The liver, on the other hand, remains quiescent and has not been seen to dilate and constrict in this way. . . . Everyone agrees that the whole of the juice of the ingesta can pass through the liver into the vena cava in man as in the ox or in very large animals, and people have had to admit exactly this if nutriment is somehow to get through the liver to the veins for the purpose of nutrition and no other way is available."

Just as there are valves in the heart and the great veins in order to maintain flow of blood in one direction, so there are valves for the same purpose "in the mesenteric branches facing towards the vena cava and the porta hepatis."

Harvey calculated that the quantity of blood put out by the heart must be at the very least greatly in excess of the ingesta, and he concluded

"that in animals the blood is driven round a circuit with an unceasing circular sort of movement. In the mesentery the blood enters through the coeliac and superior and inferior mesenteric arteries and proceeds to the intestines; from these together with the chyle which has been drawn into the veins, it returns through the very numerous branches of those veins into the porta hepatis, and through the liver itself into the vena cava. For this reason, the blood in these veins is of the same color and consistence as that in the rest of the veins (though this is a minority view—and one not in accord with Galen as noted above), and it is unnecessary to subscribe to the improbable suggestion that in every capillary offshoot there be a two-fold movement, of chyle upwards and of blood downwards. Is the effect not rather due to the extreme ingenuity of Nature? For if raw chyle were mixed in equal portions with mature blood, the result would not be a maturation, transmutation, and sanguification, but rather (as they are respectively active and passive) an intermediary product deriving from the union of the two substances, like sour wine mixture produced by adding water to wine. When, however, a small portion of chyle is mixed with a large amount of passing blood in this way, and it constitutes only a small portion of the total mass, the change (as Aristotle says) is effected with comparative ease . . . since, when a drop of water is added to a large jar of wine or vice versa, the whole is not a mixture, but is essentially wine or water still. So in opened up mesenteric veins what is found is not chyme, not chyle or blood, either separate or blended, but sensibly, in respect of color and consistence, the same blood as in the re-

mainder of veins. As, however, it contains a modicum, even if an imperceptible one, of chyle that has not undergone concoction, Nature interposed the tortuous hepatic channels to delay the blood and to assure its more complete transmutation, so that it should not reach the heart prematurely in imperfect condition, and thereby overwhelm the vital principle. . . .

"*From the upper part of the splenic venous branch which comes off in the pancreas there arise the posterior, coronary, gastric and gastro-epiploic veins, all of which together with their very numerous twigs and ramifications, are distributed to the stomach in just the same way as the mesenteric veins are distributed to the intestines. Similarly from the lower part of that splenic venous branch, the hemorrhoidal vein passes off downwards to the colon and rectum. The blood returning through these two venous systems carries both with it, on the one hand from the stomach a relatively immature juice—watery, thin, and with its chylification not yet perfected, on the other hand a thicker, more earthy juice which can be regarded as deriving from the feces. In the splenic venous branch there is a thorough mixing of opposites and the blood is suitably tempered. Nature thus deals with the two juices which are resistant, through their respective abnormalities, to coction by mixing them thoroughly and adding to them large amounts of relatively warm blood, supplied in great profusion by the spleen through its multiplicity of arteries. She thus brings the juices to the porta hepatis in a better state of preparation and, thanks to the arrangement of the venous system that I have mentioned, supplements and compensates for what is lacking in both extremes.*"

In his revision and reformulation of the old splanchnic circulatory scheme it is evident that Harvey did not reject the Galenic concepts of coction, of innate heat produced by the heart, and pneuma—animal, vital, and natural. Indeed, Galen's voice is heard repeatedly in Harvey's pages. But the old ideas were moribund. The liver could no longer be considered the center of the vascular system and the source of the blood. "Just as the king has the first and highest authority in the state, so the heart governs the whole body," Harvey said. "It is, one might say, the source and root from which in the animal all power derives, and one upon which all power depends."

The reaction to Harvey's theory consisted at first of a shocked and violent opposition, which was soon submerged under the swelling tide of confirmatory publication (52). Exception was taken in particular

SPECIAL CIRCULATIONS

to the dethronement of the liver from its place of importance in the Galenic system. For a time Gasparo Aselli's lacteals, reported in the year after the publication of *De motu cordis*, appeared to provide a means by which chyle could be conducted directly from the stomach and intestine to the liver for sanguification, but this explanation was soon disproved. Little more than twenty years later, Jean Pecquet (1622–74), then at Montpellier, described the thoracic duct, its entry into the subclavian veins, and the receptaculum chyli in *Experimenta nova anatomica*, published in Paris, in 1651 (*52*). Pecquet attributed the movement of the lymph to respiratory movement, to transmitted pulsation from neighboring arteries and to compression by contracting muscle outside the ducts. Pecquet's findings were confirmed and extended with the description of the entire lymphatic system by Olaf Rudbeck (1630–1702) and Thomas Bartholin (1616–81) during the next few years. These two men argued bitterly over the distribution of credit for the discovery of the lymphatic system and the clear differentiation of lacteals and lymph vessels. Moderns believe that Rudbeck's claim is stronger, but in contemporary writing Bartholin was given first place (*52, 162*). Perhaps the more telling argument against a central role for the liver, accredited to Bartholin by both Glisson and Malpighi, was

SISTE . VIATOR. CLAVDITUR . HOC . TUMULO . QVI . TUMULAVIT. PLURIMOS. PRINCEPS . CORPORIS . TUI . COCUS . ET. ARBITER. HEPAR . NOTUM . SECULIS. SED. IGNOTUM . NATURÆ. QVOD. NOMINIS . MAJESTATEM . ET . DIGNITATIS. FAMA . FIRMAVIT. OPINIONE . CONSERVAVIT. TAMDIU . COXIT. DONEC . CUM . CRUENTO . IMPERIO . SEIPSUM. DECOXERIT. ABI . SINE . IECORE . VIATOR. BILEMQ . HEPATI . CONCEDE. UT . SINE . BILE . BENE. TIBI . COQVAS . ILLI . PRECERIS.	PAUSE TRAVELLER ENCLOSED IN THIS TOMB IS ONE WHO HATH ENTOMBED VERY MANY, PRINCE OF THE BODY, DIGESTER AND ARBITER; THE LIVER, KNOWN TO THE AGES BUT UNKNOWN TO NATURE BECAUSE THE MAJESTY OF HIS NAME AND DIGNITY BY REPORT HE STRENGTHENED BY OPINION HE PRESERVED SO LONG HE DIGESTED UNTIL WITH HIS BLOODY TYRANNY HIMSELF HE DIGESTED AWAY. DEPART WITHOUT LIVER, TRAVELLER AND CONCEDE BILE TO THE LIVER THAT WITHOUT BILE WELL THOU MAY DIGEST FOR THYSELF. PRAY FOR HIM.

Figure 17. Epitaph for the deposed liver composed by Thomas Bartholin, 1643.

found in the engorgement of the hepatic lymphatics on the hepatic side of a peripherally placed ligature, indicating lymphatic flow out of the liver. The lymphatic valves also suggested lymphatic flow away from the liver. Thus even the lymphatic vessels failed to provide for the movement of chyle to the liver. Harvey's claim that the "heart governs the whole body" was then accepted and the concept of the liver as the source of the veins and the factory of the blood relegated to the dust heap. Bartholin (*10*) consequently in 1653 decided "to sing the De Profundis" over the liver, solemnly assigning it to the grave and placing upon its tomb an epitaph which paid tribute to its departed glory and long reign as "*princips corporis,*" "*cocus et arbiter.*" The international character of the seventeenth century advances in medical science appear most clearly in these developments, made by a Frenchman, an Italian, a Swede, and a Dane. The English were equally productive, and among those whose contributions are important Francis Glisson (1597–1677) stands first.

Glisson's work on the liver, *Anatomia hepatis*, published in 1654, is a landmark in the history of ideas of splanchnic vascular physiology. Fellow, Lecturer in Greek, and Dean at Caius College, Cambridge, Glisson embarked upon his medical studies the year after Harvey's great book appeared, and received his degree in 1634, at the age of thirty-seven (*184*). He was appointed Regius Professor of Physic at Cambridge in 1637. Although he held this position as long as he lived, he spent very little time in Cambridge and apparently never discharged the duties for which he was paid. Most of the work for which he is remembered was done in London, where he undoubtedly knew Harvey. He participated actively with his friend, Thomas Wharton (1614-73), in founding the Royal Society and in the affairs of the Royal College of Physicians of which he became president in 1667–69. In view of his learning it is not surprising to find that Glisson was deeply influenced by Aristotelian logic and the ancient writers. His preoccupation with formal, material, efficient, and final causes, with explanations that sought in biologic phenomena an anthropocentric vitalism, and with the whole apparatus of Galenic humors, spirits, and faculties was typical of the period. Nevertheless, Glisson's careful description of the liver far outstrips anything previously published. He described hepatic lobation but stressed the underlying integrity of the liver and actually attributed

SPECIAL CIRCULATIONS

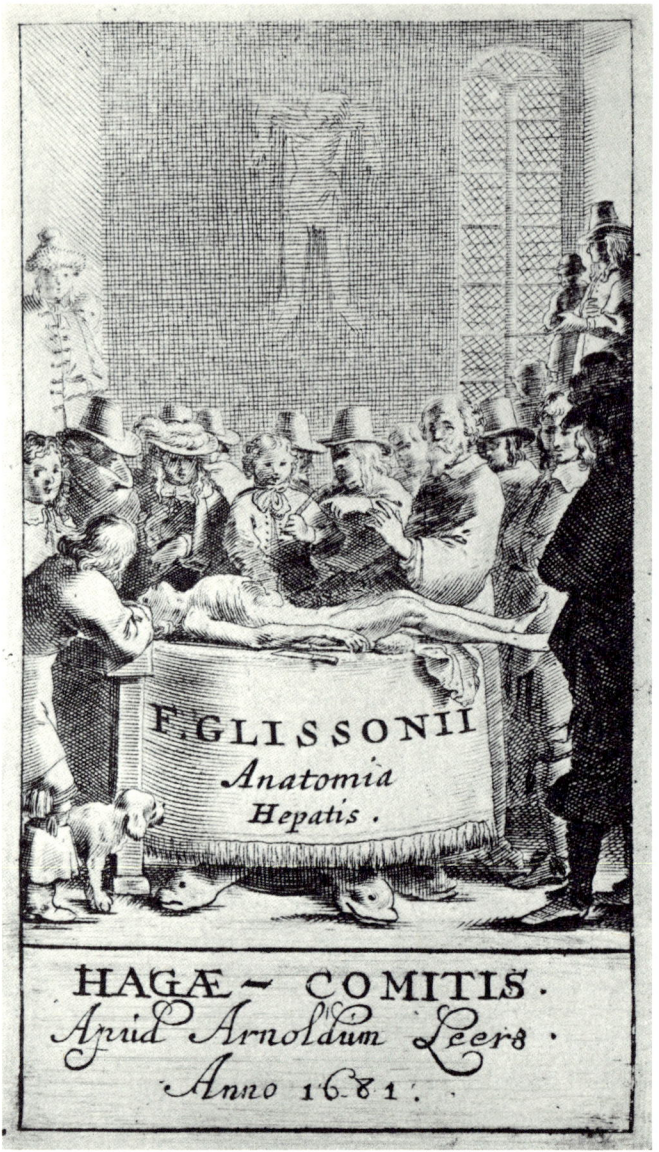

Figure 18. Glisson working in the anatomical theatre in London. This figure is taken from the title page of the 1681 edition of his book on the anatomy of the liver. It shows him, presumably the bearded man, standing at the foot of the cadaver directing the assistant in his dissection and surrounded by interested spectators and students.

the fissures to breaks in continuity produced by bending and twisting of the body upon the relatively unyielding tissue! (*85, Chap.* x). Close examination disclosed a continuous tunic supporting and protecting the liver, closely attached to the parenchyma and vessels (*85, Chap.* IX), following the latter into the substance of the organ and enfolding vein, artery, nerves, and bile ducts (*85, Chap.* xx). This investing membrane, still known today as Glisson's capsule, was to figure prominently in contemporary thinking about the splanchnic circulation.

THE SPLANCHNIC CIRCULATION

Harvey's claim (and Erasistratos' earlier one) that blood must flow from intestine through the liver to the heart was conclusively proved by Glisson. Using a bull's bladder and a cannula as a kind of syringe (*85, Chap.* XXI) he injected "warm water, slightly coloured with milk" into the portal vein of a human cadaver and found that the liver became pale and no longer sanguinous in appearance when all the blood had been washed out of it. Hence, he was led to believe that the liver might be a gland like the pancreas or the parotid which his colleague Wharton had studied. Careful removal of the hepatic parenchyma by cooking the liver in warm water and scrubbing the softened tissue away allowed Glisson to make out the more fibrous framework of vessels, ducts, and nerves. From these preparations he was able to make the first drawings of the distribution of veins and bile ducts in the liver and to show their relationship to one another. Obviously both hepatic and portal venous and biliary ductal (*porus biliaris*) systems were uniformly distributed and regularly related to one another throughout the whole organ, without any obvious distinction between the gibbous and caval portions. Glisson was well aware of the difficulties encountered in trying to make out connections of such fine structures, and he was careful to point out possible errors and to deny anastomoses other than capillary between the three systems. The arteries seemed to go only to the capsule and bile ducts, but not to the parenchyma, and ultimately ending in a capillary bed that he proved by experiment to drain into the hepatic veins. He found that the hepatic duct was always full of bile whereas the gallbladder might be empty, indicating the primacy of the hepatic ducts in the formation of bile. The connection between the biliary tracts and the vascular system could not be made out, but filtration through pores was proposed as one possibility. In this extremity, Glisson fell back upon the ancient "assimilative force"

[661]

SPECIAL CIRCULATIONS

exerted between "similitudes" to explain the movement of bile from the blood with which it is commingled into the bile ducts. The demonstration that all three kinds of vessels spread together throughout the entire structure of the liver and that there is no solid part, as Spigelius had claimed, or limitation of the input and outflow systems to the inferior (caval) and superior (gibbous) moieties, gave further support to the Harveian concept, and evoked new ideas regarding the organization of the vasculature.

The distribution of the abundant supply of nerves was of special interest to Glisson. He accepted the old idea that they are vascular in character and serve to carry a subtle liquid from the brain and spinal "marrow" to the tissues. Curiously enough, a nerve supply could be detected going only to the vessels, bile ducts, and capsular elements within the liver; none entered the parenchyma. Consequently Galen's

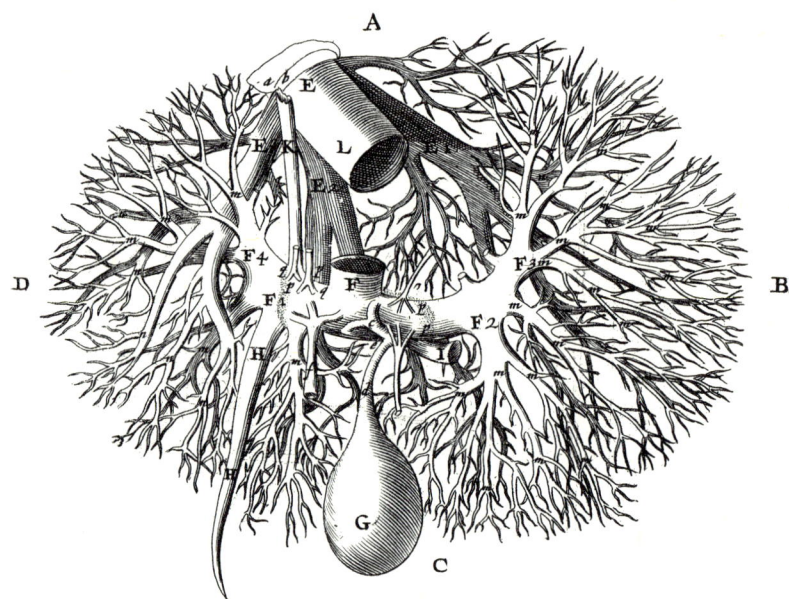

Figure 19. The hepatic vasculature according to Glisson. Drawing made from injected preparations of the vasculature of the liver. The view is from the ventral surface. The interdigitation of the hepatic venous and portal systems is readily seen. It is also evident that Glisson appreciated the close relationship between the biliary tract and the vasculature of the liver.

belief that the innervation of the total splanchnic bed accounts for pain and visceral sensory sensations seemed acceptable, but not quite complete. Glisson sought to make up for the deficiency by suggesting that the nerves might not only conduct animal spirit peripherally but might also act as absorbents conveying lymphoid chyle from the intestines to the spleen and ganglia for elaboration into a "spermatic" fluid necessary for the nourishment of "spermatic" tissues such as brain, bone, connective tissue, skin, and intestine. In the same way, blood might be considered the nutrient for "sanguinous" tissues—fatty reddish parenchymal structures—heart, lungs, kidney, liver, and spleen. In the course of this involved and poorly founded speculation, Glisson developed a most important concept (and its corresponding term) to explain the movement of bile in the *porus biliari*. Blood moves through the veins, he said, in part as a result of transmitted pulsations from the arterial vessels in the capsule and in part by diaphragmatic and abdominal wall contraction, but in the biliary vessels movement must depend upon "irritation" by bile of the tissues which react to rid themselves of the "irritant." Glisson developed this notion more fully in another work, but it was not then generally accepted. More than a century passed before it became one of the basic concepts in neurophysiology. The suggestion seemed to include a role of the capsular tissue as a muscular coat in promoting the flow of bile—and possibly also of blood through the vessels contained within it. Finally Glisson concluded that the liver could not be the center of sanguification in view of its vascular connections and the character of local blood and lymph flow. He suggested that "vital spirit" in the heart and elsewhere in the vasculature was active in the elaboration of blood since "like always produces like." Among the arguments for this view was the observation mentioned by Aristotle that blood first appears in the heart in the chick embryo. The "*usus nobilis ac publicus hepati*" was to purify the blood (*sanguinis depurationeum*); bile was not a nutritive humor but plainly an excrement removed from the blood which underwent coction by the "vital heat," an idea not so very different from that set forth by Galen. Indeed, it is obvious that many of Glisson's ideas were based upon the ancient theories, which is by no means remarkable.

Harvey and Glisson stand at the end of the old and at the beginning of a new intellectual dispensation, in which scientific method is more

THE SPLANCHNIC CIRCULATION

SPECIAL
CIRCULATIONS

clearly formulated and applied and in which critical evaluation of new ideas becomes increasingly more effective not only because of the improvements in instrumentation and communication but also because of the growing realization of the need for conscientious self-discipline. Both men are stressed at this point because they contributed outstandingly to the fund of ideas of function and structure, and especially because they applied the new methodology effectively. Neither could be wholly free of the influence of the ancient beliefs. Indeed, both accepted the older views almost in their entirety and only put forward new formulations that seemed to apply to relatively minute and limited areas. Once questioned and found wanting in one respect, however, ancient theory everywhere broke down as rapidly as a chain reaction. Both men affected and were in turn affected by the thinking of their contemporaries. The new ideas were very much in the air, and neither can be considered an isolated genius far in advance of his time. The rampant speculation so typical of the fifteenth and sixteenth centuries, much of it baseless and ridiculous but some of it seminal, cannot therefore be put in proper perspective by dwelling upon the thought of but two contributors. The ideas of their contemporaries, such as Sanctorius, Borelli, van Helmont, Sylvius, and Willis, in Italy, Holland, and England, respectively, cannot be discussed here in any detail, although their persistent experimental efforts to find mechanical causes, mathematical relationships, and measurable manifestations undoubtedly laid the foundation for the development of quantitative physiology. At the same time their speculations regarding "occult qualities," "fermentation," "ebullition," "archei," and "vital force" perpetuated in various forms the old ideas of "pneuma," "humors," "faculties," and "elementary composition." Certainly these conjectures impinged upon the thought of both Harvey and Glisson.

Another factor that must be borne in mind in considering the formation of concepts in the mid seventeenth century is the status of technology. Technical improvements and inventions are of the utmost importance in the history of physiologic concepts, both because they provided new mechanisms that were relevant to an understanding of function and because they provided new tools that permitted more precise measurement and investigation. The scientists in the Alexandrian Museum failed to see that the heart is a pump because they worked nearly two centuries before the double-action valved pump was invented (Ctesibus, A.D. 5) (*84*). Even then it was used chiefly as a toy, and it seems to have attracted little attention. By Harvey's day pumps and pumping machinery were very much to the fore as a result of developments in mining that were essential to meet the demands imposed by the improved metallurgy and the needs of the expanding populations at the close of the Middle Ages. The invention of the microscope by Galileo undoubtedly advanced the discovery of structure, but progress in defining histology was delayed for more than a century simply because the technology of the period could not provide homogeneous glass, achromatic lenses, or the machined parts necessary for fine adjustments. In many respects the development of modern concepts of the splanchnic circulation since Harvey and Glisson has gone hand in hand with the advance of technology.

THE SPLANCHNIC CIRCULATION

THE NEW ANATOMY—HAND LENS TO ELECTRON MICROSCOPE

Although early microscopists were forced to work with extremely crude instruments, often of their own manufacture, they quickly made an amazing number of discoveries that completely revolutionized the generally accepted conceptual scheme. Marcello Malpighi (1629–94), founder of the anatomical school in the University of Bologna, succeeded in extending the ideas of Harvey and Glisson and in formulating a new understanding of splanchnic vascular structures, despite repeated attacks and interference by the local Galenist opposition. His best known contribution, perhaps, was the first description of blood flow through capillaries studied microscopically in the lung and mesentery, which provided the final structural evidence for Harvey's theory. Moreover, in the course of careful studies of a remarkable variety of animal species, Malpighi (*122*) substantiated, by direct observation, Glisson's belief that the portal and hepatic veins are connected by a capillary system rather than by anastomoses between large branches. He differed in stressing the lobular divisions of the liver, calling attention rather to its intrinsic granularity than to the homogeneity in which Glisson had found evidence of a divinely ordained "perfection." Indeed, Malpighi was able to separate the hepatic parenchyma by maceration and dissection under the microscope into small particulate masses, or "lobules," resembling bunches of grapes and composed in turn of

SPECIAL CIRCULATIONS

"tiny conglobate bodies like grape-seeds" connected by means of central vessels. Unlike Wepfer, who had noted these bodies two years earlier in the pig's liver, Malpighi pursued his discovery through every class of vertebrates and reached the conclusion that the lobule is the fundamental hepatic unit. He thought he could make out a circumscribed "knotted" vascular structure surrounding the lobules, which structure appeared to become more prominent following injection, possibly as a result of distention. Hence it seemed reasonable to conclude that a follicular or cystic structure lay between the vessels and the bile ducts. The latter were therefore believed to take origin in tiny secretory (or "secerning") acini. In this concept the liver was regarded as a compound of blood vessels, bile ducts, and secretory tissue. Malpighi seems to have found the idea so attractive that he returned to it again and again in interpreting the microstructure of other organs such as the spleen, kidney, parotid, and pancreas. However, investigators using new techniques soon put the acinar hypothesis to the test and found it wanting. Although their counterclaims were really no more valid, the character of the arguments and the circumstances under which they were put forward told heavily against Malpighi's views.

The medical schools and the universities had provided the setting and the opportunity for the work of Galileo, Malpighi, and many others, but new sources of support, untrammeled by academic tradition, contributed to the success of Harvey and his successors. The seventeenth century saw a remarkable spread of interest in scientific studies that resulted in the appearance of learned societies, some independent, some supported by national and local governments, for the purpose of promoting research and providing a forum from which new discoveries could be promulgated (24). The members of these academies—the so-called experimental philosophers or *Virtuosi*—concerned themselves with every aspect of knowledge, not infrequently with trivia and the exotic, but more often with useful and "improving" ideas. Collections of various kinds were soon started, and every society had to have its own cabinet, or thesaurus, of curiosities, thus creating a demand for better methods of preservation. In the medical schools, too, a premium was put upon permanent anatomical preparations. A number of men, for the most part in Holland, became remarkably skilled in this art and added measurably to knowledge of the circulation. Perhaps the

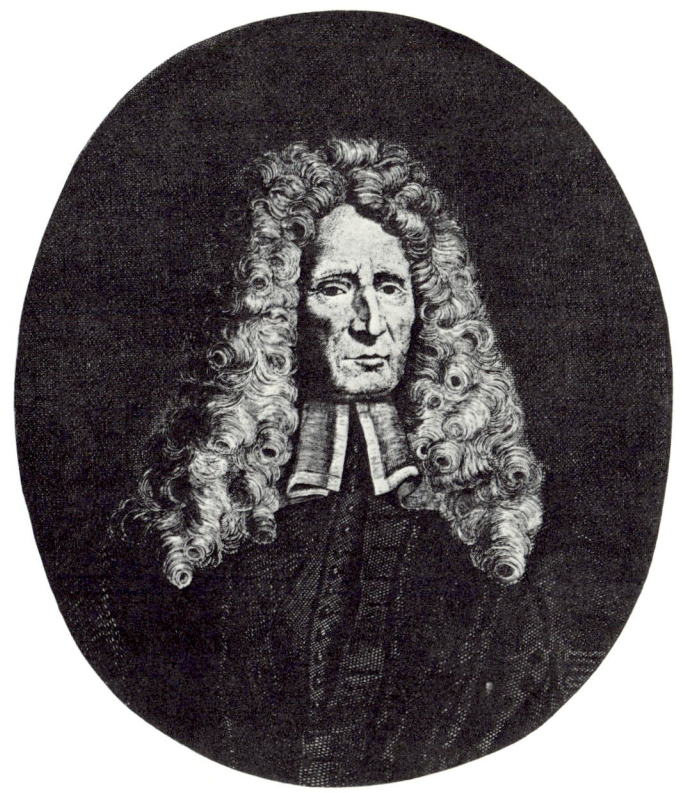

Figure 20. Frederick Ruysch (1638–1731).

best known in his time was Frederick Ruysch (1638–1731), professor of anatomy at Amsterdam. According to one biographer (56), writing in 1825,

"he brought the art of injection to such a pitch of perfection that no one has been able to equal it. He succeeded in making beautiful anatomical preparations, preserving them in the most perfect state of integrity, the injected parts maintaining their consistency, plasticity, and flexibility, even improving with time because the color of the injected material rendered them more life-like. The noise of such an important discovery spread and attracted the curious from all over Europe to his laboratory. The story goes that Peter the Great tenderly kissed the embalmed body of an infant who seemed to smile at him. . . . In 1717 he purchased Ruysch's cabinet and took it to St. Petersburg."

SPECIAL
CIRCULATIONS

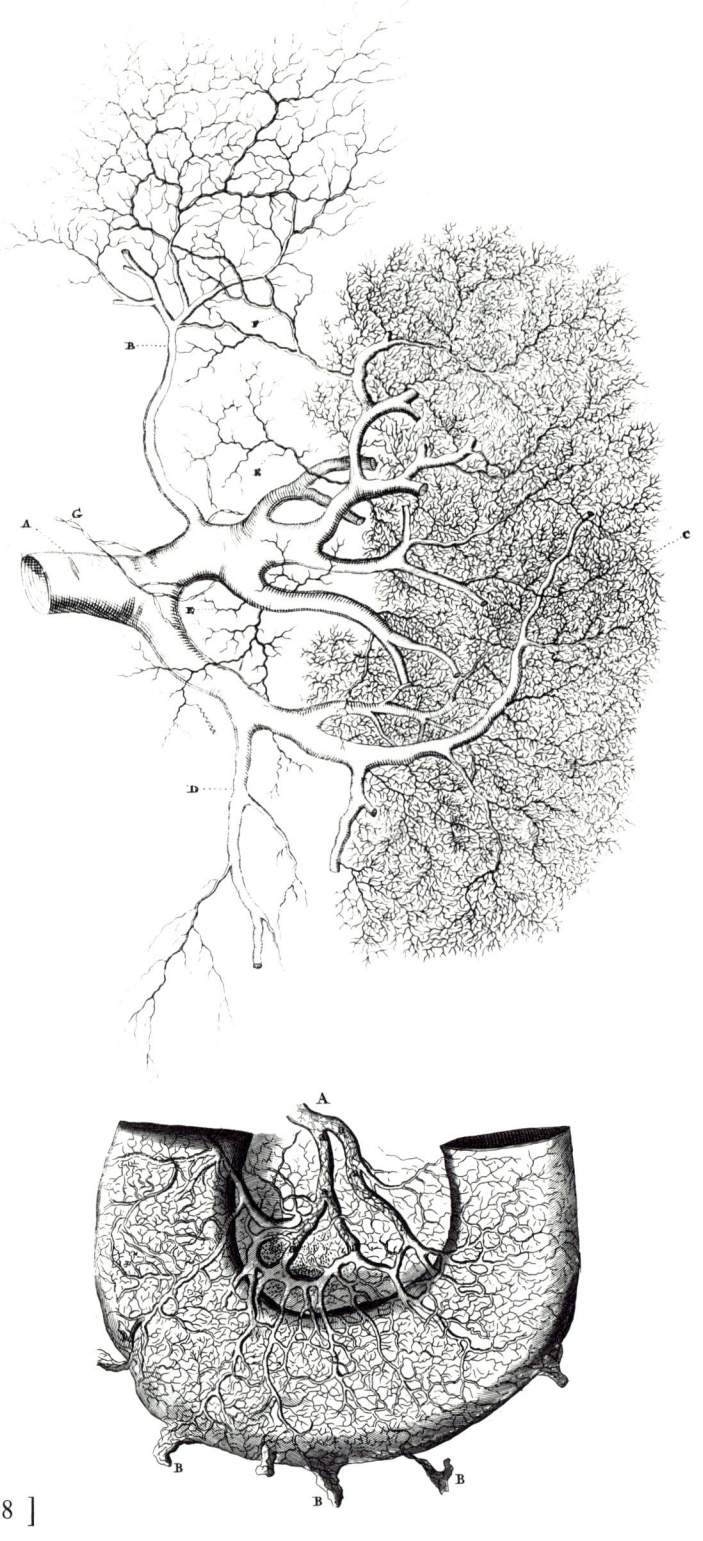

Numerous drawings (*151*) of the preparations of hepatic, splenic, and mesenteric vessels in Ruysch's collection attest to his skill in the use of injection masses composed of suet, wax, and other plastic materials.

When wax was injected under pressure into the portal vein Ruysch found that it flowed directly into the bile ducts as a "continuous thread." Hence he concluded that Malpighi's "acini" were simply points at which the biliary and vascular systems intercommunicate without interruption by a secreting parenchyma (*149*). Since this observation could be tested and easily verified it proved very convincing and was generally accepted. The resulting concept of the hepatic vasculature that found currency during the eighteenth century was set forth in 1737 by Wainewright (*178*):

THE SPLANCHNIC CIRCULATION

"The Liver being supposed to be wholly vascular, its Glands are to be considered as so many innumerable little Grape-like Convolutions of Vessels, which like so many ty'd Bottoms of Thread wound up carefully and conveniently together, have all along in their Passages and Channels, an infinite number of biliary Vessels opening with their little Mouths into them, there to imbibe the Bile in the Circulation of the Blood, which by a Similitude of Parts, and Configuration of Pores they are enabled by Nature to do."

Ruysch's casts of the splenic vasculature afforded equally persuasive support for the belief that the spleen also is "composed altogether of arteries and veins." Albrecht von Haller (1708–77), who occupied a position of extraordinary prestige at the mid-century, espoused Ruysch's view (*89*). The splenic arteries, he said, divide repeatedly into a great number of small branches and finally into very soft brush-like branches very difficult to fill by injection. They terminate in "circles" by which there is a "ready passage for liquor into the corresponding veins. These circles with their parallel branches form . . . bunches—like a pencil-brush but of a shorter rounder kind whence many have mistaken them for glands." Before such an authority, opposing voices received little attention. One of these was Antoine Ferrein of Montpellier (1693–1769),

---

Figure 21. Sample drawings of the splanchnic vasculature taken from Ruysch. In the upper picture, the finer vasculature of the spleen is clearly delineated. The lower picture shows the arrangement of the mesenteric vessels supplying a loop of colon.

SPECIAL CIRCULATIONS

whose work long remained obscure because it was recorded only in brief and uninformative abstracts (*66, 67*). However, Ferrein's work was recognized and much debated before the end of the century. On careful dissection Ferrein had found that the lobule appeared to be composed of two kinds of tissue; one he called "*cortical* that is external, friable and of a reddish hue verging upon yellow, the other *medullary* or central, red, soft and pulpy." He believed the medullary tissue made up the pulpy end of the biliary ducts, thus returning to Malpighi's concept but modifying it by the substitution of a solid structure for a hollow acinus. As time passed, this view in one form or another continued to gain adherents, but uncertainty regarding the character of extravascular parenchyma could not be resolved until after the advent of the compound microscope. Meanwhile, remarkable progress in the delineation of the splanchnic vasculature was made by the use of the hand lens and injection techniques alone.

The appearance of two monographs on the anatomy of the liver, one in Latin by Johannes Müller (*125*) in 1830, the other in English by Francis Kiernan (*102*) in 1833, marked the beginning of a new era in anatomical description. Both presented substantially the same material, although Kiernan's work was much more detailed and exact. Both depended almost solely upon careful dissections aided by the hand lens and vascular injections of colored "size" or quicksilver. They confirmed the earlier work of Malpighi and Ruysch on the general disposition of hepatic venous and arterial systems, as well as Ferrein's discovery that the portal vein enters the lobules both directly and by way of the arterial capillary networks supplying the bile ducts and portal spaces. Kiernan focused special attention upon the relationship of the lobules to the vasculature. He noted the arrangement of the lobule about a central vein that drained into a larger vessel, which he referred to as the *sub-lobular hepatic vein* since the lobule always abutted upon it. Such an organization seemed to differ radically from that of other glands, where the essential feature is the duct rather than the draining vessel. Despite this evidence of the peculiar importance of the blood supply to the bile-forming tissues, neither Müller nor Kiernan could find evidence of a direct communication between the two systems. They agreed that injection of wax under pressure probably results in rupture of some of the fine vessels in the bile duct mucosa, so that wax in the duct is not evidence of a direct communication between bile ducts and blood vessels. Neither worker could make out the finer branches of the biliary ductules, though Kiernan published a figure of a "reticulated plexus" within the lobule, which he admitted was largely imaginary. The sinusoids were seen, but with considerable difficulty, to converge from their origin at the periphery of the lobule to enter the central vein; they appeared to communicate freely by "transverse branches." Kiernan championed the idea that the arterial flow is distributed only to the bile ducts and the portal spaces, ultimately draining as venous blood by way of portal venous branches into the intra-lobular network. He found by experiment that the cortico-medullary appearance reported by Ferrein could be wholly accounted

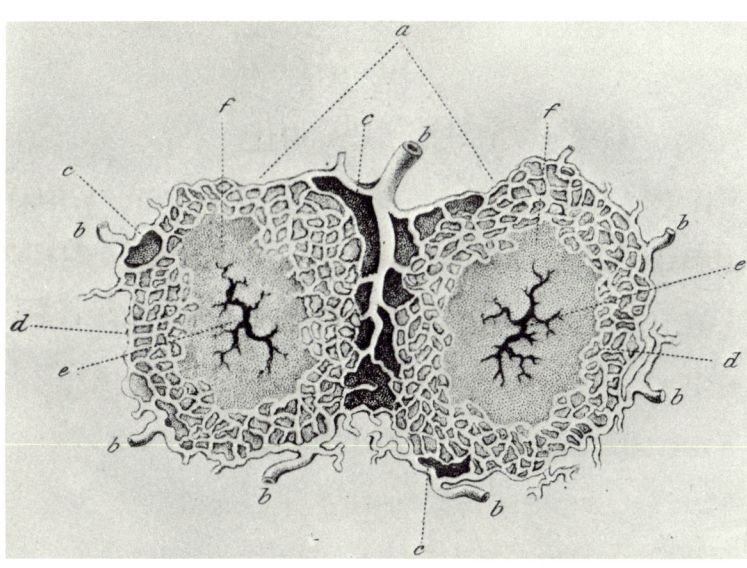

Figure 22. The biliary ductule system within the hepatic parenchyma according to Kiernan. This reticulated plexus which begins midway between the central vein and the portal triads was admittedly an imaginary extrapolation of what Kiernan could see using a hand lens and injected preparations. It is evident that his preconceptions regarding the role of the parenchymal tissue in the formation of bile have played a large role in determining the disposition of the cannuliculi. His legend is presented in full in Notes and Acknowledgments.

SPECIAL CIRCULATIONS

for by vascular congestion without need to postulate a difference in the character of the tissue. Although hollow acini could be eliminated, the bulk of the lobule appeared to be secretory tissue. Further definition of the tissue elements came from technical progress in microscopy. Three major but little recognized advances in technology (4) ushered in a new era of anatomical discovery: the correction of achromatic aberration (which Newton had thought impossible), by combining two types of glass into a single lens [Chester Moor Hall (1703–71), John Dolland (1706–61)]; the manufacture of optical glass by Pierre Louis Guinand (1748–1824) in 1805; and the development of precision screw-cutting lathes in the last quarter of the eighteenth century.

A sound theoretical basis for a histology of the body tissues including the abdominal viscera and their vascular systems had already been established by the work of Marie-François-Xavier Bichat (1771–1802),

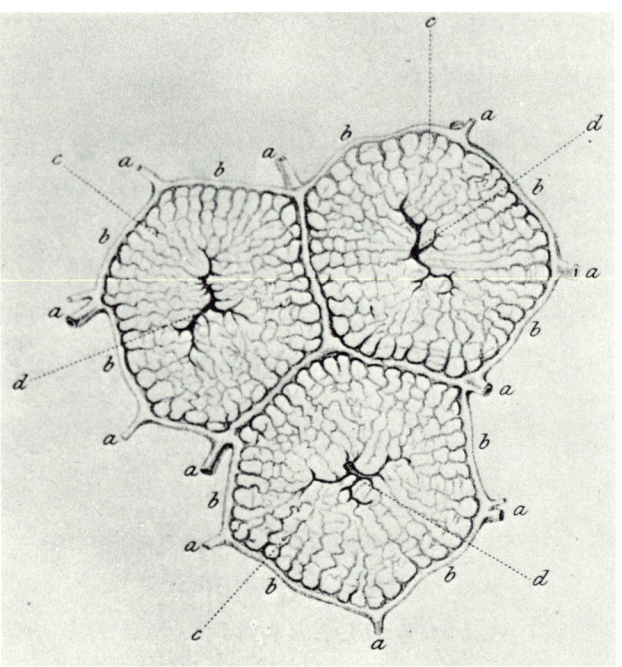

Figure 23. The intralobular distribution of the sinusoids according to Kiernan. For Kiernan's full description see Notes and Acknowledgments.

premier medécin de l'Hôtel Dieu in Paris. Bichat (*20*) sought to define similarities in terms of tissue systems rather than gross structure or function. In his *Anatomie Générale* (1801), for example, he considered the abdominal vascular system a subunit of the "Système vasculaire à sang noir," discussed its parts in relation to one another, and showed that the system consists for the most part of tissues fundamentally like those elsewhere in the body. That is to say, epithelium, connective tissues, vessels, nerves, muscle, etc., do not differ materially from the same units occurring in other parts of the body. Although Bichat introduced—or re-introduced—erroneous physiological ideas that were difficult to eradicate, his concept of cellular organization was a brilliant advance that hastened the formulation of a still more important simplifying generalization—the cell theory. Although Schleiden and Schwann (*158*) deserve credit for this concept, it should not be forgotten that the work was done in the laboratory of Johannes Müller in Coblentz. Müller had contributed importantly to the development of concepts of splanchnic vascular structure. Moreover, from 1830 to 1857, he trained a generation of investigators who laid the groundwork of histology, neurophysiology, and hemodynamics—a contribution that cannot be overrated. Among these men, von Kölliker, J. Henle, and E. H. Weber made important studies of splanchnic cellular structures. The parenchymal cells, their arrangement into columns lying between the hepatic capillaries, and the finer structures of the small bile ducts and blood vessels were soon described. By mid-century the human hepatic cells (11–36μ in diameter) were recognized as a tessellated epithelium containing a "vesicular nucleolated nucleus" (7–9μ in diameter), many fat droplets, and pigment granules. The intralobular capillaries were described as tubular and were pictured as threading their way among the parenchymal cells with numerous anastomoses (*95, 104*). The character of the sinusoidal epithelium, the intrahepatic communications between arteries and portal venous system, vascular innervation, the interhepatic lymphatic system, and the biliary capillary network remained obscure. Von Kölliker (*104*) and others had discovered muscular tissue in the trabeculae of the spleen, and most workers favored the view that an intercapillary network joined the penicillar arterioles and the venous radicles without direct communication with the intertrabecular interstices. A more precise picture of the distribution of connective tissue

SPECIAL CIRCULATIONS

throughout the organ was emerging, which failed to confirm Malpighi's belief that the follicles are encapsulated (*125*). The vasculature of the gastrointestinal tract and the pancreas had been accurately delineated, although certain minute structures—the capillary wall, the arteriovenous communications, and the neural pathways—were poorly understood.

From 1850 to 1950 there was remarkable progress in filling in the anatomical details—an advance that could be attributed to refinements in microscopy and the use of new tools and better techniques of injection, dissection, and three-dimensional reconstruction. Striking improvement in resolving power and magnification came first from improvements in the manufacture of precision tools and optical instruments and later from development of photography, quantum optics, and electronics. Chemical and biochemical discoveries not only made it possible to visualize vascular elements more precisely with various dyestuffs or plastics but also to work more confidently in the living animal under adequate anesthesia and physiological control. Thus a clearer definition of splanchnic capillary anatomy has come from light microscopy of prepared sections by Kupffer (*108*) and of living material through the quartz rod transillumination of sinusoids in liver, spleen, and mesenteries by Knisely (*103*), Wakim (*179*), Seneviratne (*159*), and MacKenzie, et al. (*118*). In addition, ultraviolet microscopy with fluorescent dyes by Ellinger and Hirt (*63*), radiomicrography by Barclay and Daniel (*51*), measurement and reconstruction of capillaries by the injection of various contrast media by many workers, including Beale (*14*), Brissaud and Sabourin (*28*), Hyrtl (*100*), MacGillavry (*117*), Disse (*57*), Chrzonszczewsky (*42*), Mall (*120*), and Deysach (*55*), have contributed importantly. The electron microscope has also yielded information regarding the nature of the capillary epithelial lining and its relationship to the underlying cells (*65*). Finally, certain new plastics appear to yield a more faithful reproduction of the vasculature when used for the injection mass, and study of the casts has provided information regarding vascular distribution throughout the splanchnic bed. The relationship between the biliary system and the vasculature was first accurately defined in 1866 by Chrzonszczewsky (*42*), who used the hepato-cellular excretion of indigo carmine just before death of the animal to mark out the bile capillaries for light microscopy. His findings, though long disputed, have been confirmed by reconstruction methods (Elias, et al.) (*62*) and electron microscopy. Definition of molecular structure of the vascular coats is still in its infancy. Nevertheless much remains to be done with the older methods in working out structural interrelationships and the anatomical basis for functional integration of the various components of the splanchnic vasculature.

By and large, the last century has not been a period in which new concepts of anatomy have developed. It has been marked, rather, by growing investigative skill in the clarification and testing of concepts laid down in the seventeenth, eighteenth, and early nineteenth centuries. The major new conceptual developments have emerged in the course of studies of splanchnic vascular physiology, in many respects as an outgrowth of the new anatomy.

CONCEPTS OF SPLANCHNIC CIRCULATORY PHYSIOLOGY AFTER GLISSON

Local Determinants of Flow in the Splanchnic Bed: Harvey and Glisson differed diametrically in their conceptions of the forces involved in promoting complete circulation. The energy imparted to the blood during each systolic contraction appeared sufficient in Harvey's mind to assure movement to the periphery, through the arterioles and capillary bed, and back to the heart. Glisson, in contrast, could not believe that venous flow depended solely upon the heart. He was particularly impressed by the relatively sluggish and nonpulsatile flow through the portal veins prior to passage through the liver. The extension of the capsule about the vessels into the depth of the liver, the concept of "irritabilia," and the rich neural network terminating in capsular tissue persuaded Glisson that the capsule might contribute actively in the propulsion of venous blood. He also called attention to the possible influence of transmitted arterial pulsation, respiratory activity, and extrinsic muscular contraction. Throughout the following century Glisson's views in this matter were generally accepted by physiologists (*136*). J. G. DuVerney (1648–1730), anatomist of the Academie Royale des Sciences and the Jardin du Roi, said, for example, that "the use of the capsule is to facilitate the course of the blood and bile which would be too slow if it were not acted upon by the intrinsic movement of this membrane," and it was said by Pétrequin (*136*) to have been referred to as an "abdominal heart" designed to force the blood through the liver.

SPECIAL CIRCULATIONS

However, W. Cowper (1666–1710), G. B. Morgagni (1682–1771), and G. D. Santorini (1681–1737) were unable to satisfy themselves that the capsule is muscular, and G. Fantoni (1675–c. 1745) failed, in 1711, to observe any movement in it (*136*). Hence, by mid-century, workers like Haller viewed Glisson's capsule as a supportive structure and the veins as simple elastic conduits. Indeed, Haller (*89*) pointed out the tendency for blood to stagnate in the portal system since the "section of any branch of the vena portarium is always less than the trunk from whence it is derived; where the lights of all the branches together greatly exceed that of the trunk: from whence it follows a great friction or resistance, and a retarded motion." He suggested that such a tendency might be "diminished by motion of the adjacent muscles, and by the respiration, as it is increased by inactivity with sour and viscid aliments."

Numerous observers from Glisson onward had claimed that the arteries could contract actively, but the question of transmitted motion and simple elastic recoil as a possible explanation remained unresolved. Since it was impossible to differentiate fibrous connective tissue from muscle using the methods then available, a variety of elaborate hypotheses developed during the eighteenth century regarding the function and activity of "membranes" (such as those making up the blood vessels), which Haller's anatomical studies proved to be ubiquitous in the body. Although he did not completely agree with those who attributed "vital powers" or contractibility to the arterial membranes, Haller brought forward much evidence to prove that contraction of the arteries might be an important agent in the circulation. This view had already had other more ardent supporters, among them Stephen Hales (*88*). Among his numerous ingenious experiments was the following. Tying a brass tube into the aorta of a dog and employing a level of pressure equal to the normal aortic tension, he injected water and measured the outflow, per minute, from the divided vessels of the intestines. He found that cold water decreased and hot water increased the flow. Further, from studies of the actions of such drugs as alcohol and infusion of cinchona bark he concluded that while one set of agents by constricting the vessels lessens the outflow, another set widens the vessels and increases outflow. In 1722, William Cullen, professor of medicine at Glasgow, extended the idea by suggesting that "the muscular fibres of the arteries become more irritable as the arteries are more distant from the heart" (*47*). This concept became popular not only because the facts seemed to favor it but also because it provided support for the "solidists," who emphasized destruction of the solid elements in the body fabric as the basis for disease, and who had been active in demolishing the last strongholds of the humoral doctrine since the time of Baglivi (1668–1706).

For fifty years after Cullen, contractile activity of the arterial capillaries was accepted as the major factor in the promotion of blood flow. Bichat (*20*) laid special emphasis upon the role of the capillaries in making possible the movement of the blood through the splanchnic bed, and other investigators reported observations that seemed to give the idea confirmation. However, in 1832, Poiseuille (*140, 141*) reported a series of elegant experiments in which the flow through the mesenteric capillaries of frogs, mice, and horses was shown to depend exclusively upon arterial inflow and pressure. The pressure in a mesenteric vein of a horse, isolated with its artery of supply and intervening capillary bed, rose and fell with arterial pressure in the absence of any maintenance of independent venous pressure. This work and that of Magendie (*119*) also served to sustain Haller's impression that respiration and movements of the abdominal wall aided return, for it was found that portal venous pressure varied during the respiratory cycle. Magendie added convincing confirmatory evidence that the driving force of the left ventricle is sufficient to return the blood to the right heart. However, the conclusive demonstration of muscle in the coats of the small arteries and veins by Henle (*94*) in 1840 seemed at first to nullify the findings of Poiseuille and Magendie. In 1859, Claude Bernard (*16*) called attention to the heavy musculature of the hepatic veins and claimed that blood entering the liver by the portal vein reaches "the center of the lobules where it would stagnate because the feeble impulse by which it has been driven thus far would be powerless to move it further. But the hepatic veins in contracting down, squeeze the liver, as it were, like a sponge and the blood, finding an outlet in the direction of the inferior vena cava, is expelled into this vessel which carries it to the heart." During the next fifty years, however, advances in instrumentation and experimental technique were to prove conclusively that vascular smooth muscle plays a major role in determining the distribution of flow and blood volume within the splanchnic bed, rather than the movement of blood through it. The concept of the vasculature itself as an active agent in circulatory dynamics was to survive, but in a modified form.

SPECIAL CIRCULATIONS

Splanchnic Circulatory Dynamics: Although it was recognized in Harvey's day that the principles of hydraulics could be applied in the analysis of cardiovascular dynamics, relatively little progress was made in this direction until Poiseuille. The basic laws governing the distribution of pressures in fluid had been worked out by Simon Stevinus (1548–1620) and Evangelista Torricelli (1608–47) in the sixteenth and seventeenth centuries, but the dynamics of flow in tubular systems defied analysis until after the discovery of the binomial theorem, the "method of fluxions," and the laws of motion by Newton. The major initial contributions in modern hydraulics were made by physiologists interested chiefly in the circulation—Stephen Hales, Daniel Bernouilli (1700–1783), and Poiseuille. Poiseuille not only formulated the relationships between the volume of flow, viscosity of fluid, dimensions of the conduit, pressure gradient, and the resistance to flow in the principle that bears his name, but also invented an instrument, the mercury manometer, by means of which pressure could be measured in quantitative terms (*139, 142, 143*). As noted above, he was the first to measure pressure in the mesenteric veins. Although Poiseuille's contribution was recognized for the advance it was, bringing to him a modest *succès d'estime*, the fundamental implications of his ideas were not fully grasped for almost a century. The measurement of blood pressure directly, in terms of the length of a column of mercury or saline solution (Poiseuille used sodium carbonate) supported at equilibrium, was accepted at once. Instrumentation improved quickly; Ludwig and his students applied the methods of graphic registration that had been developed first in studies of wind velocity by Thomas Young and later by the French school concerned with ballistics (*111*). The use of a closed elastic recording system was introduced in 1861 by Chauveau and Marey (*39*), and increasingly sensitive manometers were developed thereafter (*182*) by Fick (1864), Roy (1887), von Basch (1887), Hürthle (1888), and P. Frederiq (1888). Mean portal venous pressures and simultaneous intra-arterial pressures were reported before the end of the century (*11, 13*), by von Basch in 1875 and by Bayliss and Starling in

1894. Both studies noted the major pressure gradient between the aorta and the portal vein, across the splenic and mesenteric beds (portal venous pressure in the dog is approximately 7 mm. Hg), but neither attempted to explore the distribution of flows and resistances within the system.

Understandably, the inaccessibility of the splanchnic vasculature and the inadequacy of anesthesia and surgical manipulation made it difficult to study splanchnic hemodynamics quantitatively. Moreover, an accurate method of measuring blood flow was not available until 1868, when Dogiel (*61*), working in Ludwig's laboratory, described the "stromuhr." Flows within the splanchnic bed were first measured with the stromuhr by Burton-Opitz (*30–35*) at the beginning of the twentieth century and were reported in a series of papers from 1908 to 1914. The average values for hepatic arterial and portal venous inflows in the dogs studied by Burton-Opitz were, respectively, 25 and 50 ml. per minute per 100

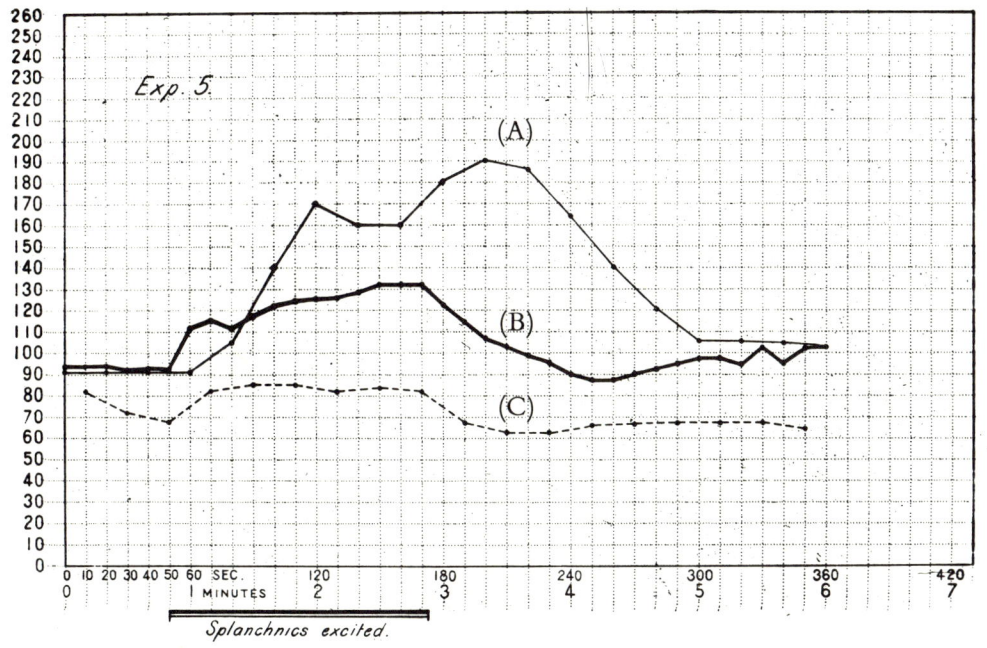

Figure 24. Graph showing the femoral arterial and portal venous pressures in the dog obtained by Bayliss and Starling, 1894. Stimulation of the splanchnic nerve resulted in an elevation of portal venous pressure (A), femoral arterial pressure (B), and inferior caval pressure (C). (Arterial pressure in mm. Hg; venous pressure in mm. $MgSO_4$.)

SPECIAL CIRCULATIONS

grams of tissue. These values were but slightly lower than those which seem to be generally acceptable today after nearly half a century of remarkable technical advances (37). Venous catheterization has made it possible to estimate splanchnic outflow indirectly by clearance procedures and by wedging the catheter deep in a hepatic vein to measure an intrahepatic pressure approximating sinusoidal pressure (25, 169). An approximate value for flow may also be derived from the rate of disappearance of various colloidal substances from the blood (58).

Poiseuille had observed "lamination" early in his work on flow through capillaries, and it was suggested by Sérégé and Soulé (160) in 1905 that this phenomenon causes a more rapid movement of blood from the portal vein through the right lobe than through the left lobe of the liver. The feasibility of direct observation of the flow through the capillaries of the various components of the splanchnic bed—spleen, intestines, mesenteries, and liver—in living animals with electrical illumination was noted by Tigerstedt (175) in 1922. This observation was made possible by the introduction of quartz rod illumination in Krogh's laboratory by Knisely (103) as early as 1934. Streamlining was observed directly by this means, and attention was called to the possibility that the activity of sinusoidal "sphincters" might also result in nonuniform distribution of blood within the liver and spleen. However, roentgenographic visualization of the movement of radiopaque materials through the splanchnic bed (1) and the use of isotopes in evaluating splanchnic circulation time (181) have yielded results suggesting that turbulence induced by respiratory or body movements minimizes the importance of portal venous lamination under most circumstances in intact animals or man. These methods have also failed to show the presence of the valve-like structure between the hepatic arteriolar and portal venous inflows that was postulated by Gad (78) as a means of providing for equalization of inflow pressures. Indeed, numerous studies have made it evident that control of splanchnic perfusion must be vested in the arterioles of the liver, spleen, and gastrointestinal tract, with distribution of flow depending in the main upon the relative distribution of arteriolar resistances, as Mall's anatomical studies (121) had suggested earlier. The role of intrinsic sinusoidal activity remains disputed, but there is little doubt that the heavy musculature of the hepatic veins and their radicles in most species indicates a contractibility that may influence flow and that can certainly alter the volume of blood held in the splanchnic bed.

During the course of the early studies of the splanchnic vasomotor innervation, it was gradually realized that splanchnic venous activity might bring about engorgement and swelling of the liver and the other abdominal viscera. Two new methods, plethysmography and artificial perfusion, both destined for extensive exploitation, were employed to characterize the reactions quantitatively. According to Marey (*123*), the idea of measuring change of organ volume with change in blood flow originated in arguments regarding the character of the arterial pulse. To test the hypothesis that arteries actually dilated with each pulse and did not simply transmit a pressure "shock," Spallanzani fitted rings of fixed diameters around the aorta of an experimental animal in order to detect expansion, Flourens used a watch spring, and Poiseuille passed a segment of the artery through a water-filled jacket connected to capillary tube into which fluid was displaced by dilatation. This apparatus was adapted by Piegu in 1846 for the measurement of the volume changes in an extremity. It was rapidly improved thereafter by Chelius, Fick, Bruisson, Mosso, and others. The initial work on the measurement of changes in the volume of the liver seems to have been carried out in Ludwig's laboratory, where various types of plethysmography were devised to provide a continuous record of the quantity of blood retained or released under different circumstances from the kidney and liver (*93*). Perfusion of the isolated liver at a constant pressure with serum, by Mosso (*124*) in 1875, or with warm saline solution, by Cavazzani and Manca (*38*) in 1895, permitted a more precise evaluation of changes in blood flow and content. So little was known at first, however, about the chemistry and handling of body fluids and tissues that the results obtained were usually erratic and unreliable. With time both methods became extremely important in the clarification of splanchnic hemodynamics. The first records of splenic volume *in situ* were obtained by Roy (*146*) with the help of a hinged metal box, or "oncometer," in which the spleen was enclosed while its circulation was kept intact. This apparatus was modified by Schäfer and Moore (*156*) and by François-Franck and Hallion (*71–75, 90*) to determine changes in the volume of the liver, pancreas, gastrointestinal tract, and spleen during circulatory reactions *in situ*.

SPECIAL
CIRCULATIONS

All these studies showed large changes in volume that were attributed initially to alteration in blood flow alone. From 1915 to 1932, however, studies were reported from Vienna, Berlin, and London in which improved methods of perfusion of the isolated organ yielded evidence of a mechanism (*Lebersperre*) controlling the outflow of blood from the hepatic veins (*8, 12, 110*). First clearly described by Mautner and Pick in Vienna, the "sperre" or "sluice" mechanism, located in the larger hepatic veins, was demonstrated conclusively by Bauer, Dale, Poulsson, and Richards (*12*) in the isolated perfused liver of the dog. Histamine, "peptone," and anaphylaxis constricted this sluice, whereas epinephrine or stimulation of the sympathetic nerve supply released it. The mechanism was not demonstrable in the liver of the cat and only inconstantly in that of the goat.

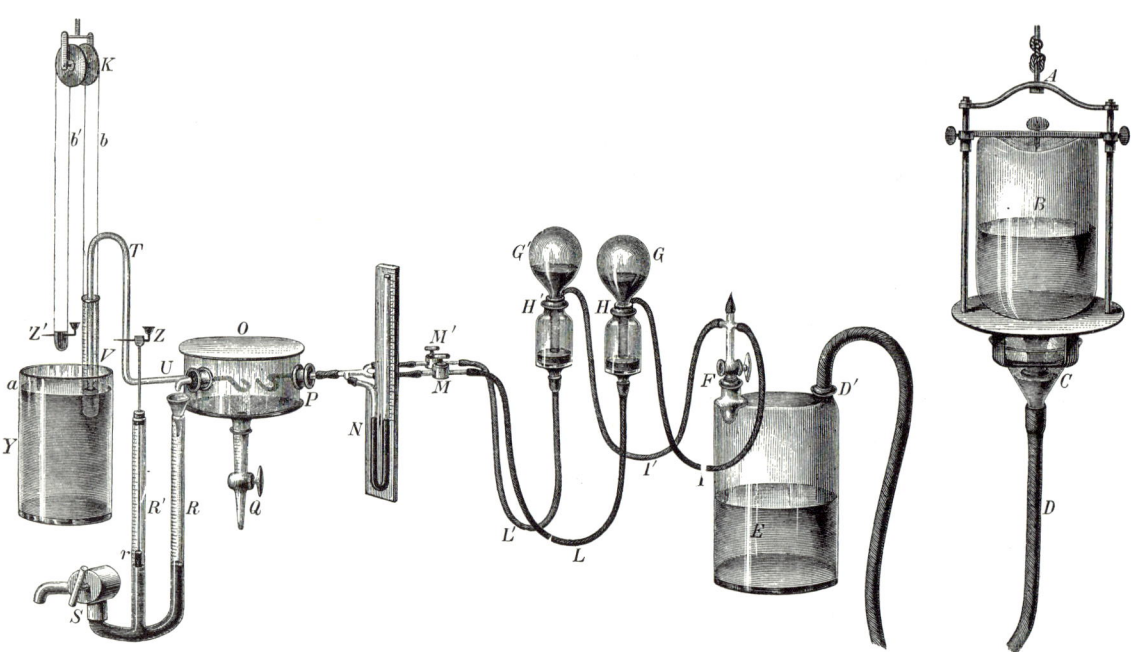

Figure 25. Apparatus used by Angelo Mosso to study the explanted liver. This apparatus was devised in 1876 and used to perfuse the liver of the rat under controlled conditions of perfusion pressure, venous drainage pressure, and external environment. The organ was perfused throughout by defibrinated serum.

Changes in splenic volume also received intensive study by a number of investigators and were attributed variously to altered filling pressure, to constriction or dilatation of trabecular muscle, or to a combination of both factors (9, 53). Engorgement of the portal venous bed was found to depend in the main upon the relationship between inflow and outflow resistances. Recent work on portal venous tone and on the quantity of blood held in the splanchnic bed of the intact animal and man (measured by regional dilution of isotopically labeled human serum albumin) suggests that reflex adjustment in venous smooth muscle may also contribute significantly to the maintenance of portal capacity (26, 44). Vascular muscle may contribute transiently in promoting blood flow but only to the extent to which it brings about a reduction in capacity. Its major contribution lies in the manner in which it determines the loss and distribution of the energy imparted to the blood by myocardial contraction. The new concepts of hemodynamic interrelationships have not only deepened our understanding of the mechanisms of the splanchnic circulation but have also fostered the growth of ideas regarding its role in the body economy both in serving vital tissues and as a part of cardiovascular dynamics.

Splanchnic Circulatory Integrations: Although the liver was no longer generally regarded after Glisson as the "Bowel of Sanguification" nor the spleen as the "emunctory" of the liver, both organs were widely believed to be essential to the purification of the blood coming from the gastrointestinal tract. However, Steno had found that blood drawn from the portal vein resembled in color and coagulability that taken from the vena cava (122). Since malnutrition often complicates the course of jaundice, Malpighi (122) suggested that bile might actually be useful, perhaps in digestion. In support of this view he had proved experimentally that bile comes from the liver alone and that the gallbladder is designed as a receptacle from which the bile may be introduced into the intestine on need. Malpighi believed that the impurities of the blood were removed in the process of bile formation and the blood improved by a "new dissolution and preparation of the nutritive juice." Although he had discovered that splenectomy had no ill effect in the dog, he suggested that the spleen also cooperated by producing a subtle "juice" which promotes hepatic function. Bile continued to be regarded by most physicians, however, as exclusively an "excrementous

SPECIAL CIRCULATIONS

fluid" separated from the blood by a more or less physical process somewhat like filtration. Haller (*89*) believed that the omentum supplied an oily material for bile formation (the dried residue of bile was known to be greasy and inflammable), that another constituent came from the mesenteric and mesocolic veins as a voluminous "subalcaline watery humour," and that a "more putrid water absorbed from the large intestines" constitutes the "acrid alcaline quality in bile." The spleen, according to Haller, is composed solely of arteries and veins in which the blood moves slowly and is "fomented with heat, attenuated and in a manner dissolved by the putrid faeces of the adjacent colon," entering "thus upon a benign putrefaction." This hypothetical reaction prepares the blood so "that it may supply a sort of watery juice to the bile but such as is probably of a subalcaline nature, and rendered somewhat sharp, or lixivial by the remora of the blood." By the end of the eighteenth century, however, it was well established that splenectomy does not alter the appearance or composition of the bile. Even as late as 1830, Kiernan (*102*) concluded on the available evidence that bile was

"a purely excrementitious fluid, stimulating the intestinal canal, but having no influence on the formation of the chyle. The lungs separate from venous blood an excrementitious matter in a gaseous form; the liver extracting from venous blood an excrementitious fluid, may be considered as the abdominal lung."

In general, it had been believed until this time that bile is formed exclusively from portal venous blood, the artery serving solely a nutritive function like the bronchial artery. This conclusion was supported by Haller's observation that bile formation continued in experimental animals even when the hepatic artery was ligated. However, in 1802 Bichat (*20*) set forth an opposing argument, that since the biliary tract is in closer approximation to the hepatic arterial tree than to the portal venous network, bile must be formed from arterial blood. His claim seemed to find support in a *lusus naturae* reported by Abernethy (*2*) in 1793, a one-year-old child with a congenital atresia of the portal vein and a large portal caval anastomosis, in whom bile excretion had not been impaired. A careful examination of Abernethy's specimen indicated a marked increase in arterial vascularization. Eventually, Kiernan's conclusion that bile is derived from blood coming both from the portal vein and from the hepatic arterial capillary net was gradually accepted. The surgical advances of the nineteenth century soon made it possible to show conclusively that the liver is also capable of bile formation when it is perfused by the hepatic artery alone (*165*). (Eck's successful construction of an effective anastomosis between the portal vein and the inferior vena cava in the dog (1877) proved in addition that portal venous perfusion of the liver is not essential to life (*40*). Death shortly after ligation of the portal vein in experimental animals was finally recognized as the result of trapping a large fraction of the blood volume in the mesenteric veins.)

The importance of bile in fat absorption was recognized by Brodie, according to Magendie (*119*), but it was not put upon a firm quantitative basis until the effect of biliary fistula had been investigated in dogs by Bidder and Schmidt (*21*), Bernard, Flint, and others from 1852 to 1867 (*49, 68*). These studies indicated that bile serves a digestive as well as an excretory function. An understanding of bilirubin elimination and bile acid secretion began to emerge from the pioneering research in the chemistry of pigments and steroids by a series of brilliant students who worked on the composition of the bile [Tiedemann and Gmelin (*174*)], the source, path of degradation, and structure of bilirubin [Hoppe-Seyler, Heintz, Berzelius, and Jaffé (*112*)], and the characterization of the bile acids [Strecker (*166, 167*)]. Of even greater importance was the discovery by Claude Bernard (1848) of what he called the "internal secretion" of the liver, its "sugar-producing office" (*17*). Bernard found that the hepatic venous blood contains a much larger quantity of sugar than portal venous or arterial blood, in the absence of detectable sugar in the liver. By 1857 he had isolated glycogen and shown that it is converted in the liver to sugar by a ferment, in proportion to body need (*18*). This work conclusively demonstrated a vital activity of the liver in the regulation of the chemical composition of the blood, a function essential to the integrity of all tissues and dependent in turn upon splanchnic blood flow both for its maintenance and for its impact upon the body as a whole.

During the course of his studies of hepatic glucose production, Bernard was led to examine the effect of the nervous system upon glucose production in dogs and rabbits. In doing so he found that puncture of

SPECIAL CIRCULATIONS

the medulla oblongata in the floor of the fourth ventricle was followed by glycosuria in association with striking changes in the splanchnic circulation. Exploration of the hemodynamic response resulted in the discovery of the splanchnic vasomotor mechanism by which the splanchnic circulation may be integrated in systemic circulatory responses (*19, 153*). By 1850, the concept of vasomotor control had attracted a large following by reason of the advances in instrumentation and the enunciation of more sophisticated concepts of energy-flow relationships, vascular contractibility, and functional coordination. Bernard's finding was quickly confirmed and extended by Brown-Séquard, Waller, and Schiff (*153*). Vulpian produced an obvious ischemia in the dog by stimulation of the splanchnic trunks (*177*), and Pavy found that section was followed by dilatation (*153*). A theory of balanced vasoconstriction-vasodilation was soon elaborated. Indeed, Ludwig (*116*) suggested that "the splanchnic area is the most important regulator of the arterial pressure." Direct effects of splanchnic stimulation upon hepatic, splenic, and mesenteric blood flow and upon portal

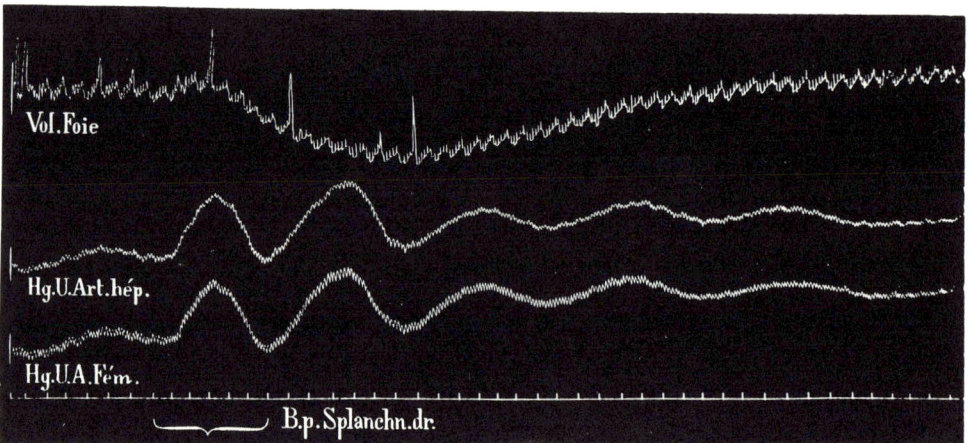

Figure 26. Tracing of femoral and hepatic arterial pressures and liver volume obtained by François-Franck and Hallion in 1896 before and after stimulation of the right splanchnic nerve. It can be seen that the liver volume (Vol. Foie) decreased in association with a rise in both hepatic (Hg. U. Art. Hép.) and femoral (Hg. U. Art. Fém.) arterial pressures. This is one of the earliest tracings giving quantitative expression to change in liver volume.

venous pressure and capacity were observed in experimental animals by von Basch (*11*), Pal (*131*), Mall (*120*), Bayliss and Starling (*13*), Cavazzani and Manca (*38*), François-Franck and Hallion (*71–75, 90*), Burton-Opitz (*30–35*), and many others. It became increasingly obvious during the course of these studies that the responses reported were erratic, inconsistent, and dependent upon species, the kind and extent of surgical manipulation, preparation, anesthesia, and a host of other indeterminate variables. Oliver and Schäfer's discovery (*129*) of epinephrine in 1894 provided a clue to at least one of these factors, making it evident that integration may be mediated by humoral as well as neural intercommunication. However, exploration of the splanchnic vascular responses to epinephrine by Schmid (*157*), Burton-Opitz (*30–35*), Bernard (*16*) Baer and Rössler (*8*), Bauer, Dale, Poulsson, and Richards (*12*) and many others also encountered difficulties of interpretation as a result of variability in response. An outline of the development of these discoveries lies beyond our purview, but it may be said that much remains obscure. Norepinephrine, acetylcholine, serotonin, and histamine have been added as naturally occurring vasoactive materials that profoundly influence the splanchnic circulation in various ways, and others are undoubtedly in prospect. A complete inventory with adequate control of all the elements involved is not yet at hand. Nevertheless, patterns of integration within the splanchnic vasculature, between the visceral and systemic circuits, and between the tissues served by the splanchnic inflow and the remainder of the body have emerged from studies of mechanisms of drug responses.

It seems more and more likely that splanchnic circulatory integrations subserve a goal-seeking activity, aimed, as Bernard (*16*) pointed out, at fixing the composition of the "milieu intérieur," or, as Walter Cannon (*36*) saw it, at the "homeostasis" of vital functions. These important simplifying concepts have proved exceedingly fruitful, although it is not yet clear upon which of the many internal environments within the body priority is placed, nor upon which of numerous essential activities homeostatic responses are geared.

As it happens, splanchnic vascular reactions have been found to serve both the larger goal of systemic circulatory homeostasis and the more immediate need of maintaining the hepatic, pancreatic, and gastrointestinal blood supply. Early in the seventeenth century, Borelli (*23*)

SPECIAL CIRCULATIONS

made computations of the distribution of blood flow through the body and concluded that approximately one twenty-fifth of the aortic flow must enter the splanchnic bed because the summed cross sections of the mesenteric arteries and coeliac axis make up this proportion of the maximal aortic cross section at its origin from the heart. Borelli was far in advance of his time in making a quantitative approach to a physiologic question. Nearly two centuries were to pass before it became evident that local resistances and hydrostatic levels might have a greater influence than arterial dimensions alone, and it was still longer before accurate measurements of cardiac output and hepatic blood flow proved that the splanchnic inflow at rest in man amounts to approximately 25 per cent of the total flow (25). This figure, more than six times larger than Borelli's estimate, indicates a contribution to total peripheral resistance so large that splanchnic vasomotor activity could have a controlling influence upon blood pressure, as Ludwig suggested. Thus, arterial hypertension induced by norepinephrine has been found to be associated with somewhat more constriction in the splanchnic bed than elsewhere in the body, so that the splanchnic fraction of total flow is reduced (15). Also, with assumption of the upright position, an increase in splanchnic vascular resistance contributes importantly in supporting arterial pressure (46). In general, however, splanchnic resistances appear to be determined chiefly by local tissue needs for blood. In hemorrhagic shock, for example, vasoconstriction does not occur in dogs, and, after a short period, vasodilation actually develops, despite persistent hypotension (145).

Local adjustments in vascular capacity also appear to figure prominently in the maintenance of venous return. Malpighi (122) explicitly indicated the role of the spleen as a "lake or special reservoir" in which blood could be pooled or disgorged as needs required. The notion persisted after his time and was frequently mentioned, but it could not be developed in the absence of adequate hemodynamic theory. The elaboration of these principles during the nineteenth century resulted, as noted above, in a better understanding of the distribution of energy within the arteries and across the resistances. Consequently, interest first centered upon intravascular pressures and flows, but since *Windkessel Theorie* also necessarily implied that the quantity of blood in any portion of the vascular bed must depend upon a balance between mean filling pressure and the elastic recoil of the vessel wall, attention was ultimately drawn to the problem of the blood volume and its distribution in the cardiovascular system (*76*). The potential role of the veins, and especially of the splanchnic venous reservoir, in assuring return of blood to the heart was clearly outlined by August Krogh (*107*) in 1912. The volume of blood held in the spleen, liver, pancreas, and gastrointestinal vessels had been shown (see above) to be greatly affected by denervation (dilation), stimulation of the splanchnic nerves (reduction), and the administration of various pressor agents (reduction). Barcroft (*9*) and others found that shrinkage of the spleen occurs in the dog during exercise, after hemorrhage, and in a variety of conditions conducive to arterial hypotension. These findings have been confirmed by modern methods and give strong support to the concept of the splanchnic bed as a compensatory reservoir, integrated in systemic circulatory responses. Since the splanchnic reservoir may contain as much as 20 per cent of the total blood volume in normal man at rest, redistribution involves a quantity large enough to affect systemic adjustment profoundly, with little or no significant change in splanchnic blood flows. The intimate mechanisms of regulatory shifts in blood volumes, flows, and pressures remain obscure. If the past is a reliable guide, elucidation of the humoral and neuromuscular factors involved will almost certainly point the way to new and surprising concepts of splanchnic circulatory physiology.

CONCEPTUAL EVOLUTION IN THE MODERN PERIOD

The rapidity with which concepts today are constructed or demolished, expanded or reformed, can be traced, in large part, to an escape from dogmatism. A critical attitude toward alleged "facts" and interpretations developed slowly during the centuries of uncertainty and disillusion after the fall of Rome to reach full maturity in the modern era. The search for a "Method" during the fifteenth century was, in essence, an attempt to express the changed outlook, in formal terms, to frame a law of scientific critique. Divine authority was rejected by the Greco-Roman philosophers; secular authority was rejected by the moderns. Moreover, in the Renaissance, a remarkable zest for innovation appeared that combined with an advanced technology to yield a rich harvest of new biological information for critical analysis. For the first time, technical devices were made to measure functions as well as dimen-

SPECIAL CIRCULATIONS

sions. From the concept of the circulation we owe to Harvey, there emerged a completely revised view of splanchnic vascular dynamics that the new tools made it possible to evaluate and, at last, to understand in terms of physical principles. It is noteworthy and characteristic that a constant interchange of ideas between every branch of knowledge has accelerated the pace of progress. Hydrodynamics derives as surely from physiologic studies as from engineering investigations; splanchnic hemodynamics leans as heavily upon Newton as upon Poiseuille. Similarly, an understanding of splanchnic vascular reactions has been enlarged by an appreciation of social organizations and of communications theory. Perhaps, also, nuclear physics and biochemistry will join hands some day to clarify the problems of splanchnic vascular tonus and responsivity. So long as concepts can evolve freely, whatever the final answer, the danger of stultification in the grip of authority can be avoided—although it is possible, of course, that other equally embarrassing fallacies may continue to encumber our thought simply because they are unrecognized.

BIBLIOGRAPHY

1. ABEATICI, S., and L. CAMPI. La visualizzazione radiologica della porta per via splenica. Minerva Med., 42:593, 1951.
2. ABERNETHY, J. Account of two instances of uncommon formation in the Viscera of the human body. Phil. Trans., 83:(part I) 59, 1793.
3. AESCHYLUS. The Seven Plays in English Verse by L. Campbell. *Prometheus Bound*, lines 493-496. London, Oxford University Press, 1930.
4. ANGUS-BUTTERWORTH, L. M. Glass. In C. Singer, E. J. Holmyard, and A. R. Hall, Eds. A History of Technology, Vol. IV. Oxford, Clarendon Press, 1958, pp. 358-378.
5. ANONYMUS LONDINENSIS. The Medical Writings. Tr. by W. H. S. Jones, Ed. Cambridge, Cambridge University Press, 1947.
6. ARISTOTLE. The Works. Vol. IV, Historia animalium. Tr. by D'A. W. Thompson. Oxford, Clarendon Press, 1910.
7. ARISTOTLE. Parts of Animals. Tr. by A. L. Peck. Movement of Animals, Progression of Animals. Tr. by E. J. Forster. (Loeb Classical Library). Cambridge, Harvard University Press, 1945.

8. BAER, R., and R. RÖSSLER. Beiträge zur Pharmakologie der Lebergefässe. I. Mitteilung: Über die Abhängigkeit der Histaminwirkung von der Durchströmungsrichtung. (Versuche an isoliert durchströmter Hundeleber). Naunyn-Schmiedeberg's Arch. exp. Path. Pharmak., 119:204, 1927.
9. BARCROFT, J., H. A. HARRIS, D. ORAHOVATS, and R. WEISS. A contribution to the physiology of the spleen. J. Physiol. (Lond.), 60:443, 1925.
10. BARTHOLIN, T. Vasa lymphatica, nuper hafniae in animantibus inventa, et hepatis exequiae. Paris, Du Puis, 1653.
11. BASCH, S. VON. Ueber den Einfluss des gereizten n. splanchnicus auf den Blutstrom innerhalb und ausserhalb seines Verbreitungsbezirkes. Ludwig's Arb. physiol. Anst. Leipzig, 10:229, 1876.
12. BAUER, W., H. H. DALE, L. T. POULSSON, and D. W. RICHARDS. The control of circulation through the liver. J. Physiol. (Lond.), 74:343, 1932.
13. BAYLISS, W. M., and E. H. STARLING. Observations on venous pressures and their relationship to capillary pressures. J. Physiol. (Lond.), 16:159, 1894.
14. BEALE, L. S. Lectures on the Principles and Practice of Medicine. The Liver. London, Churchill, 1889.
15. BEARN, A. G., B. BILLING, and S. SHERLOCK. The effect of adrenaline and noradrenaline on hepatic blood flow and splanchnic carbohydrate metabolism in man. J. Physiol. (Lond.), 115:430, 1951.
16. BERNARD, C. Leçons sur les propriétés physiologiques et les altérations pathologiques des liquides de l'organisme, Vol. 2. Paris, Baillière, 1859, Huitième et Neuvième Leçons, pp. 192–223.
17. BERNARD, C. Leçons sur le diabète et la glycogenèse animale. Paris, Baillière, 1877.
18. BERNARD, C. Leçons de physiologie expérimentale appliquée à la médecine. 2 Vol. Paris, Baillière, 1855–56.
19. BERNARD, C. Leçons sur la physiologie et la pathologie du système nerveux. 2 Vol. Paris, Baillière, 1858.
20. BICHAT, X. Anatomie générale, appliquée à la physiologie et à la médecine. 2 Vols. Paris, Brosson, 1801.
21. BIDDER, F. H., and C. SCHMIDT. Die Verdauungssaefte und der Stoffwechsel. Mitau, G. A. Reyher, 1852.
22. BOISSIER, A. Mantique Babylonienne et mantique Hittite. Paris, Geuthner, 1935.
23. BORELLI, G. A. De motu animalium.... Part I and II. Neapoli, Typis Felicis Mosca, 1734.
24. BRADLEY, S. E. The tradition of scientific critique. J. clin. Invest., 36:866, 1957.

25. BRADLEY, S. E., F. J. INGELFINGER, G. P. BRADLEY, and J. J. CURRY. The estimation of hepatic blood flow in man. J. clin. Invest., 24:890, 1945.
26. BRADLEY, S. E., P. A. MARKS, P. C. REYNELL, and J. MELTZER. The circulating splanchnic blood volume in dog and man. Trans. Ass. Amer. Physns. 66:294, 1953.
27. BREASTED, J. H. The Edwin Smith Surgical Papyrus, Published in Facsimile and Hieroglyphic Transliteration with Translation and Commentary in Two Volumes. Vol. I. Chicago, University of Chicago Press, 1930.
28. BRISSAUD, E., and C. SABOURIN. Sur la lobulaire du foie et les voies de la circulation sanguine intra-hépatique. C.R. Soc. Biol. (Paris), 40: 757, 1888.
29. BURNET, J. Early Greek Philosophy. 4th Ed. London, Macmillan, 1930.
30. BURTON-OPITZ, R. Über die Strömung des Blutes in dem Gebiete der Pfortader. I. Das Stromvolum der Vena Mesenterica. Pflüg. Arch. ges. Physiol., 124:469, 1908.
31. BURTON-OPITZ, R. Über die Strömung des Blutes in dem Gebiete der Pfortader. I. Das Stromvolumen der Vena lienalis. Pflüg. Arch. ges. Physiol., 129:189, 1909.
32. BURTON-OPITZ, R. The vascularity of the liver. III. The effect of stimulation of single nerves of the hepatic plexus upon the flow in the hepatic artery. Quart. J. exp. Physiol., 4:103, 1911.
33. BURTON-OPITZ, R. The vascularity of the liver. IV. The magnitude of the portal inflow. Quart. J. exp. Physiol., 4:113, 1911.
34. BURTON-OPITZ, R. The vascularity of the liver. VI. The influence of the greater splanchnic nerves upon the venous inflow. Quart. J. exp. Physiol., 5:189, 1912.
35. BURTON-OPITZ, R. The vasomotor nerves of the portal vein. Amer. J. Physiol., 36:325, 1915.
36. CANNON, W. B. The autonomic nervous system: an interpretation. Lancet, I:1109, 1930.
37. CATTON, W. T. Physical Methods in Physiology. London, Pitman, 1957.
38. CAVAZZANI, E., and G. MANCA. Contribution à l'étude de l'innervation du foie: Les nerfs vaso-moteurs des ramifications portes hépatiques. Arch. ital. Biol., 24:33, 1895.
39. CHAUVEAU, A., and J. MAREY. Appareils et expériences cardiographiques: Démonstration nouvelle du mécanisme des mouvements du coeur par l'emploi des instruments enregistreurs à indications continues. Mém. Acad. Méd. (Paris), 26:268, 1863.
40. CHILD, C. G., III. Eck's fistula. Surg. Gynec. Obstet., 96:375, 1953.

41. CHILDE, V. G. The Dawn of European Civilization. 6th Ed. London, Routledge and Kegan Paul, 1957.
42. CHRZONSZCZEWSKY, N. Zur Anatomie und Physiologie der Leber. Virchows Arch. path. Anat. 35:153, 1866.
43. CICERO. De divinatione. Tr. by W. A. Falconer. (Loeb Classical Library). Cambridge, Harvard University Press, 1953, pp. 214–539.
44. COMBES, B., J. R. K. PREEDY, H. O. WHEELER, R. M. HAYS, and S. E. BRADLEY. The hemodynamic effects of hexamethonium bromide in the dog, with special reference to "splanchnic pooling." J. clin. Invest., 36:860, 1957.
45. COON, C. S. The History of Man. London, Cape, 1955.
46. CULBERTSON, J. W., R. W. WILKINS, F. J. INGELFINGER, and S. E. BRADLEY. The effect of the upright posture upon hepatic blood flow in normotensive and hypertensive subjects. J. clin. Invest., 30:305, 1951.
47. CULLEN, W. Institutions of Medicine, Part I. Physiology. 3rd Ed. Edinburgh, Elliot, 1785.
48. CUSHING, H. W. A Bio-bibliography of Andreas Vesalius. New York, Schuman's, 1943.
49. DALTON, J. C. A Treatise on Human Physiology. 7th Ed. Philadelphia, Lea, 1882.
50. DANIEL, G. Lascaux and Carnac. London, Lutterworth Press, 1955.
51. DANIEL, P. M., and M. M. L. PRICHARD. Variations in the circulation of the portal venous blood within the liver. J. Physiol. (Lond.), 114:521, 1951.
52. DAREMBERG, C. Histoire des sciences médicales.... Vol. 1. Depuis les temps historiques jusqu'à Harvey. Vol. 2. Depuis Harvey jusqu'au XIXe Siècle. Paris, Baillière, 1870.
53. DEBOER, S., and D. C. CARROLL. The mechanism of the splenic reaction to general CO poisoning. J. Physiol. (Lond.), 59:312, 1924.
54. DERRY, D. E. Mummification. II. Methods practised at different periods. Ann. Égypt. Serv. Antiquités, 41:240, 1942.
55. DEYSACH, L. J. The nature and location of the "sphincter mechanism" in the liver as determined by drug actions and vascular injections. Amer. J. Physiol., 132:713, 1941.
56. DICTIONAIRE DES SCIENCES MÉDICALES. Biographie médicale. Vol. 7. A. J. L. Jourdan, Ed. Paris, Panckoucke, 1825.
57. DISSE, J. Ueber die Lymphbahnen der Säugethierleber. Arch. mikr. Anat., 36:203, 1890.
58. DOBSON, E. L., and H. B. JONES. The behavior of intravenously injected particulate material. Acta med. scand., Suppl. 273, 1, 1952.
59. DOBSON, J. F. Herophilus of Alexandria. Proc. roy. Soc. Med. (Sect. Hist. Med.), 18:19, 1925.

SPECIAL CIRCULATIONS

60. DOBSON, J. F. Erasistratus. Proc. roy. Soc. Med. (Sect. Hist. Med.), 20:825, 1927.
61. DOGIEL, J. Die Ausmessung der strömenden Blutvolumina. Ber. Sächs. Ges. d. Wiss. Leipzig, 19:200, 1867.
62. ELIAS, H. The liver cord concept after one hundred years. Science, 110:470, 1949.
63. ELLINGER, P., and A. HIRT. Mikroskopische Untersuchung an lebenden Organen. 1. Mitteilung. Methodik; Intravitalmikroskopie. Z. Anat. Entwickl. Gesch., (Part 1) 90:791, 1929.
64. FARRINGTON, B. Greek Science, Its Meaning for Us. Vol. I. Thales to Aristotle. Vol. II. Theophrastus to Galen. Harmondsworth, Penguin, 1949.
65. FAWCETT, D. W. Observations on the cytology and electron microscopy of hepatic cells. J. nat. Cancer Inst., 15:1475, 1955.
66. FERREIN. A. Un mémoire sur la structure et les vaisseaux du foye. Hist. Acad. roy. Sci., 57:51, 1733.
67. FERREIN. A. Sur la structure des visceres nommés glanduleux, et particulierement sur celle des reins et du foie. Mém. Acad. roy. Sci., 94:709, 1749.
68. FLINT, A. Handbook of Physiology, for Students and Practitioners of Medicine. New York, Macmillan, 1905.
69. FORBES, R. J. Chemical, culinary, and cosmetic arts. In C. Singer, E. J. Holmyard, and A. R. Hall, Eds. A History of Technology, Vol. I. New York, Oxford University Press, 1954, pp. 238–298.
70. FOWLER, W. W. Roman essays and interpretations. In his Ancient Italy and Modern Borneo: A Study in Comparative Culture. Oxford, Clarendon Press, 1920, pp. 146–165.
71. FRANÇOIS-FRANCK, C. É., and L. HALLION. Recherches expérimentales sur l'innervation vaso-constrictive du foie (1er mémoire: Historique et technique). Arch. physiol. norm. path., ser. 5, 8:908, 1896.
72. FRANÇOIS-FRANCK, C. É., and L. HALLION. Recherches expérimentales sur l'innervation vaso-constrictive du foie (2e mémoire: Topographie). Arch. physiol. norm. path., ser. 5, 8:923, 1896.
73. FRANÇOIS-FRANCK, C. É., and L. HALLION. Recherches expérimentales sur l'innervation vaso-motrice du foie (3e mémoire: Réflexes vasoconstricteurs). Arch. physiol. norm. path., ser. 5, 9:434, 1897.
74. FRANÇOIS-FRANCK, C. É., and L. HALLION. Recherches expérimentales sur l'innervation vaso-motrice du foie (4e mémoire: Répartition des réflexes vaso-constricteurs; leur effets mécaniques; leur intervention en présence des poisons traversant le foie). Arch. physiol. norm. path., ser. 5, 9:448, 1897.
75. FRANÇOIS-FRANCK, C. É., and L. HALLION. Circulation et innervation vasomotrice du pancreas. Arch. physiol. norm. path., ser. 5, 9:661, 1897.

76. FRANK, O. Die Grundform des arteriellen Pulses. Erste Abhandlung. Mathematische Analyse. Z. Biol., 37:483, 1899.
77. FREEMAN, K. Ancilla to the Pre-Socratic Philosophers. A complete translation of the Fragments in Diels, Fragmente der Vorsokratiker. Cambridge, Harvard University Press, 1957.
78. GAD, J. Studien über Beziehungen des Blutstroms in der Pfortader zum Blutstrom in der Leberarterie. Dissertation. Berlin, G. Schade, 1873.
79. GALEN. De l'utilité des parties du corps humain. In his Oeuvres anatomiques, physiologiques et médicales. Tr. by C. Daremberg. Paris, Baillière, 1854, Vol. I, pp. 111–706.
80. GALEN. De l'utilité des parties du corps humain. In his Oeuvres anatomiques, physiologiques et médicales. Tr. by C. Daremberg. Paris, Baillière, 1856, Vol. II, pp. 1–211.
81. GALEN. On the Natural Faculties. Tr. by A. J. Brock. (Loeb Classical Library). New York, Putnam, 1916.
82. GALEN. On anatomical Procedures.... (De anatomicis Administrationibus). Tr. by C. Singer. Publication of the Wellcome Historical Medical Museum, N.S., No. 7. London, Oxford University Press, 1956.
83. GALILEI, GALILEO. Dialogues Concerning Two New Sciences. Tr. by H. Crew and A. de Salvio. New York, Macmillan, 1914.
84. GILLE, G. Machines. In C. Singer, E. J. Holmyard, and A. R. Hall, Eds. A History of Technology, Vol. II. New York, Oxford University Press, 1956, pp. 628–658.
85. GLISSON, F. Anatomia hepatis.... Hagae, Arnoldum Leers, 1681.
86. GOETZE, A. Old Babylonian Omen Texts. (Yale Oriental Series, Babylonian Texts, Vol. 10). New Haven, Yale University Press, 1947.
87. GUTHRIE, W. K. C. The Greeks and their Gods. Boston, Beacon, 1955.
88. HALES, S. Statical Essays. 2nd Ed. corrected. 2 Vol. London, Innys, 1740.
89. HALLER, A. VON. Physiology—Course of Lectures upon the Visceral Anatomy and Vital Œconomy of Human Bodies—compiled for the use of the University of Göttingen. Vol. I—in English by S. Mihles. London, Innys and Richardson, 1754.
90. HALLION, L., and C. É. FRANÇOIS-FRANCK. Recherches expérimentales exécutées à l'aide d'un nouvel appareil volumétrique sur l'innervation vaso-motrice de l'intestin. Arch. physiol. norm. path., ser. 5, 8:478, 1896.
91. HARRISON, J. E. Prolegomena to the Study of the Greek Religion. 3rd Ed. Cambridge, Cambridge University Press, 1922.
92. HARVEY, W. Movement of the Heart and Blood in Animals. An Anatomical Essay. Tr. by K. J. Franklin. Oxford, Blackwell, 1957.

SPECIAL CIRCULATIONS

93. Héger, P. Expériences sur la circulation du sang dans des organes isolés. Bruxelles, H. Marceau, 1873.
94. Henle, J. Ueber die Contractilität der Gefässe. Wschr. ges. Heilk., p. 329, 1840.
95. Hering, E. The liver. In S. Stricker's Manual of Human and Comparative Histology. Tr. by H. Powers. Vol. 2. New York, New Sydenham Society, 1872, pp. 1–33.
96. Herodotus. The Histories. Tr. by H. Cary. New York, Appleton, 1899. Book IX, Calliope, 61.
97. Hippocrates. Vol. I. Tr. by W. H. S. Jones. (Loeb Classical Library). London, Heinemann, 1923.
98. Hippocrates. Vol. IV. Tr. by W. H. S. Jones. (Loeb Classical Library). Cambridge, Harvard University Press, 1953.
99. Hussey, M. I. Anatomical nomenclature in an Akkadian omen text. J. Cuneiform Stud., 2:21, 1948.
100. Hyrtl, J. Lehrbuch der Anatomie des Menschen. 16th Ed. Wien, Braumüller, 1882.
101. Kemp-Welch, A. The emblem of St. Ansano. Burlington Mag., 18:337, 1911.
102. Kiernan, F. The anatomy and physiology of the liver. Phil. Trans., 123:711, 1833.
103. Knisely, M. H., E. H. Bloch, and L. Warner. Selective phagocytosis. I. K. danske vidensk. Selsk. biol. Skft., 4:(#7) 1, 1948.
104. Kölliker, A. Manual of Human Microscopical Anatomy. Tr. by G. Busk and T. Huxley. J. De Costa, Ed. Philadelphia, Lippincott, Grambo, 1854.
105. Körte, G. Bronzeleber von Piacenza. Mitt. dtsch. archeol. Inst. Rom., 20:348, 1905.
106. Krause, E. Diogenes von Apollonia. Erster Teil. Janus, 14:228, 1909.
107. Krogh, A. The regulation of the supply of blood to the right heart (with a description of a new circulation model). Skand. Arch. Physiol., 27:227, 1912.
108. Kupffer, C. Ueber Sternzellen der Leber. Briefliche Mittheilung an Prof. Waldeyer. Arch. mikr. Anat., 12:353, 1876.
109. Lacaille, A. D. Personal communication. The Wellcome Historical Medical Museum, London, N.W.1, England.
110. Lampe, W., and J. Méhes. Gefässstudien an der überlebenden Warmblüterleber. III. Mitteilung: Die Wirkung von Hormonen auf die Lebergefässe. Naunyn-Schmiedeberg's Arch. exp. Path. Pharmak., 119:66, 1926.
111. Langendorff, O. Physiologische Graphik. Ein Leitfaden der in der Physiologie gebräuchlichen Registrirmethoden. Leipzig, Deuticke, 1891.

112. LEMBERG, R., and J. W. LEGGE. Hematin Compounds and Bile Pigments; Their Constitution, Metabolism, and Function. New York, Interscience, 1949.
113. LEONARDO DA VINCI. Quaderni d'Anatomia. Vol. I. Tredici Fogli della Royal Library di Windsor: Respirazione, Cuore, Visceri addominali. Christiania, Dybwad, 1911.
114. LINTON, R. The Tree of Culture. New York, Knopf, 1955.
115. LOUD, G. News from Armageddon. Illus. Lond. News, 188:1108, 1936.
116. LUDWIG, C., and L. THIRY. Über den Einfluss des Halsmarkes auf den Blutstrom. S.-B. Akad. Wiss. Wien, math.-nat. Kl. (1. Abteilung), 49:421, 1864.
117. MACGILLAVRY, T. H. Zur Anatomie der Leber. S.-B. Akad. Wiss. Wien, math.-nat. Kl. (2. Abteilung), 50:207, 1865.
118. MACKENZIE, D. W., JR., A. O. WHIPPLE, and M. P. WINTERSTEINER. Studies on the microscopic anatomy and physiology of living trans-illuminated mammalian spleens. Amer. J. Anat., 68:397, 1941.
119. MAGENDIE, F. Précis élémentaire de physiologie. 2 Vol. Paris, Méquignon-Marvis, 1816–17.
120. MALL, F. P. The contraction of the vena portae and its influence upon the circulation. Johns Hopk. Hosp. Rep., 1:111, 1896.
121. MALL, F. P. A study of the structural unit of the liver. Amer. J. Anat., 5:227, 1906.
122. MALPIGHI, M. Discours anatomiques sur la structure des visceres sçavoir du foye, du cerveau, des reins, de la ratte, du polype du coeur, et de poulmons. 2nd Ed. Paris, d'Houry, 1687.
123. MAREY, E. J. La Circulation du sang à l'état physiologique et dans les maladies. Paris, Masson, 1881.
124. MOSSO, A. Von einigen neuen Eigenschaften der Gefässwand. Ludwig's Arb. physiol. Anst. Leipzig, 9:156, 1875.
125. MÜLLER, J. De glandularum secernentium structura penitiori earumque prima formatione in homine atque in animalibus. Lipsiae, Vossii, 1830, pp. 82–84.
126. MÜLLER, J. Ueber die Structur der eigenthümlichen Körperchen in der Milz einiger pflanzenfressenden Säugethiere. Arch. Anat. Physiol., Leipzig, 1:80, 1834.
127. NOUGAYROL, J. Textes hépatoscopiques d'époque ancienne conservés au Musée du Louvre. Rev. Assyriologie et Archéologie Orientale, 38:67, 1941.
128. NOUGAYROL, J. Textes hépatoscopiques d'époque ancienne conserves au Musée du Louvre (III). Rev. Assyriologie et Archéologie Orientale, 44:1, 1950.

SPECIAL CIRCULATIONS

129. Oliver, G., and E. A. Schäfer. On the physiological action of extract of the suprarenal capsules. J. Physiol. (Lond.), 16:I, 1894.
130. Onians, R. B. The Origins of European Thought about the Body, the Mind, the Soul, The World, Time and Fate. 2nd Ed. Cambridge, Cambridge University Press, 1954.
131. Pal, J. Ueber die Innervation der Leber. Med. Jb., Wien, n.F. 3:67, 1888.
132. Pallottino, M. The Etruscans. Tr. by J. Cremonan. Harmondsworth, Penguin, 1955.
133. Papyrus Ebers, The Greatest Egyptian Medical Document. Tr. by B. Ebbell. Copenhagen, Levin and Munksgaard, 1937.
134. Pease, A. S. M. Tulli Ciceronis de divinatione liber primus. Part I, with commentary. University of Illinois Studies in Language and Literature, Vol. 6, No. 12, 1920.
135. Peck, H. L. The connate pneuma: an essential factor in Aristotle's solutions to the problems of reproduction and sensation. In Science, Medicine and History; Essays on the Evolution of Scientific Thought and Medical Practice, written in Honour of Charles Singer, E. A. Underwood, Ed. London, Oxford University Press, 1953, Vol. I, pp. 111-121.
136. Pétrequin, J. E. Recherches sur les usages de la capsule dite de Glisson, pour servir à l'histoire de la circulation hépatique; mémoire présenté à la société de médecine de Gand. Gaz. méd. Paris, Ser. 2, 6:449, 1838.
137. Piggott, S. Prehistoric India to 1000 B.C. Harmondsworth, Penguin, 1950.
138. Plato. Timaeus. In the Dialogues of Plato. Tr. by B. Jowett. New York, Random, 1937, Vol. II, pp. 3-68.
139. Poiseuille, J. L. M. Recherches sur la force du coeur aortique. Paris, Didot, 1828.
140. Poiseuille, J. L. M. Recherches sur les causes du mouvement du sang dans les veines. J. univ. hebd. méd. chir. prat., 1:289, 1830.
141. Poiseuille, J. L. M. Recherches sur les causes du mouvement du sang dans les veines. 2e partie. J. univ. hebd. méd. chir. prat., 3:97, 1831.
142. Poiseuille, J. L. M. Recherches sur les causes du mouvement du sang dans les vaisseaux capillaires. Ann. Sci. nat. (Zoologie), 5:111, 1836.
143. Poiseuille, J. L. M. Recherches expérimentales sur le mouvement des liquides de nature différente dans les tubes de très petits diamètres. Ann. Chim. (Phys.), 21:76, 1847.
144. Randall, J. H., Jr. The development of scientific method in the school of Padua. J. Hist. Ideas, 1:177, 1940.

145. REYNELL, P. C., P. A. MARKS, C. CHIDSEY, and S. E. BRADLEY. Changes in splanchnic blood volume and splanchnic blood flow in dogs after haemorrhage. Clin. Sci., 14:407, 1955.
146. ROY, C. S. The physiology and pathology of the spleen. J. Physiol. (Lond.), 3:203, 1880–82.
147. RUTTEN, M. Trente-deux modèles de foies en argile inscrits provenant de Tell-Hariri (Mari). Rev. Assyriologie et Archéologie Orientale, 35:36, 1938.
148. RUYSCH, F. Museum anatomicum Ruyschianum; sive catalogus rariorum, quae in authoris aedibus asservantur; adornatus ab eodem. Amstelodami, apud H. et viduam T. Boom, 1691.
149. RUYSCH, F. Opusculum anatomicum de fabrica glandularum in corpore humano, continens binas epistolas: quarum prior est Hermanni Boerhaave ad Fredericum Ruyschium; alter Frederici Ruyschii ad Hermannum Boerhaave. In his Opera omnia anatomico-medico-chirurgica, Vol. IV. Amstelodami, apud Janssonio-Waesbergios, 1737.
150. RUYSCH, F. Epistola anatomica, problematica quarta, ad F. Ruyschium auctore J. J. Campdomerco. De glandulis, fibris, cellulisque lienalibus, etc. In his Opera omnia anatomico-medico-chirurgica, Vol. II. Amstelodami, apud Janssonio-Waesbergios, 1737.
151. RUYSCH, F. Epistola anatomica, problematica quinta, ad F. Ruyschium auctore G. Frentz. De vasis sanguiferis perisottii tibiae, ut et viis, per quas vesicula fellea sarcinam acquirit. In his Opera omnia anatomico-medico-chirurgica, Vol. II. Amstelodami, apud Janssonio-Waesbergios, 1737.
152. RUYSCH, F. Opera omnia anatomico-medico-chirurgica, Vol. I. Amstelodami, apud Janssonio-Waesbergios, 1737.
153. SAMUEL, S. S. Principes fondamentaux de l'histoire du système nerveux nutritif. J. Physiol. (Paris), 3:572, 1860.
154. SARTON, G. A History of Science. Vol. I. Ancient Science through the Golden Age of Greece. Cambridge, Harvard University Press, 1952.
155. SARTON, G. A History of Science. Vol. II. Hellenistic Science and Culture in the Last Three Centuries B.C. Cambridge, Harvard University Press, 1959.
156. SCHÄFER, E. A., and B. MOORE. On the contractility and innervation of the spleen. J. Physiol. (Lond.), 20:1, 1896.
157. SCHMID, J. Beeinflussung von Druck und Stromvolumen in der Pfortader durch die Atmung und durch experimentelle Eingriffe. Pflüg. Arch. ges. Physiol., 126:165, 1909.
158. SCHWANN, T. Mikroskopische Untersuchungen über die Uebereinstimmung in der Struktur und dem Wachsthum der Thiere und Pflanzen. Berlin, Sander, 1839.

SPECIAL CIRCULATIONS

159. SENEVIRATNE, R. D. Physiological and pathological responses in the blood-vessels of the liver. Quart. J. exp. Physiol., 35:77, 1949.
160. SÉRÉGÉ, H., and E. SOULÉ. Sur la vitesse de circulation du sang dans le foie droit et dans le foie gauche chez le chien. C.R. Soc. Biol. (Paris), 58:519, 1905.
161. SINGER, C. The Fasciculo de Medicina, Venice 1493, Part I. In Monumenta Medica, Vol. II, H. E. Sigerist, Ed. Florence, Lier, 1925.
162. SKAVLEM, J. H. The scientific life of Thomas Bartholin. Ann. med. Hist., 3:67, 1921.
163. SNELL, B. The Discovery of the Mind. The Greek Origins of European Thought. Tr. by T. G. Rosenmeyer. Cambridge, Harvard University Press, 1953.
164. STEUER, R. O., and J. B. DE C. M. SAUNDERS. Ancient Egyptian and Cnidian Medicine: The Relationship of their Aetiological Concepts of Disease. Berkeley, University of California Press, 1959.
165. STOLNIKOW. Die Stelle vv. hepaticarum im Leber und gesammten Kreislaufe. Pflüg. Arch. ges. Physiol., 28:255, 1882.
166. STRECKER, A. Untersuchung der Ochsengalle. Erste Abhandlung. Justus Liebigs Ann. Chem., 65:1, 1848.
167. STRECKER, A. Untersuchung der Ochsengalle. Zweite Abhandlung. Justus Liebigs Ann. Chem., 67:1, 1848.
168. SUDHOFF, K. Tradition und Naturbeobachtung in den Illustrationen medizinischer Handschriften und Frühdrucke vornehmlich des 15. Jahrhunderts. Stud. Gesch. Med., Leipzig, 1:1, 1907.
169. TAYLOR, W. J., and J. D. MYERS. Occlusive hepatic venous catheterization in the study of the normal liver, cirrhosis of the liver and noncirrhotic portal hypertension. Circulation, 13:368, 1956.
170. TEMKIN, O., and W. L. STRAUS, JR. Galen's dissection of the liver and of the muscles moving the forearm; translated from the "Anatomical Procedures." Bull. Hist. Med., 19:167, 1946.
171. THULIN, C. O. Die Etruskische Disciplin. I. Die Blitzlehre. Göteborg Högsk. Arskr., 11:(pt. 5), 1906.
172. THULIN, C. O. Die Etruskische Disciplin. II. Die Haruspicin. Göteborg Högsk. Arskr., 12:(pt. 1), 1906.
173. THULIN, C. O. Die Etruskische Disciplin. III. Die Ritualbücher und zur Geschichte und Organisation der Haruspices. Göteborg Högsk. Arskr., 15:(pt. 1), 1909.
174. TIEDEMANN, F., and L. GMELIN. Die Verdauung nach Versuchen. Heidelberg, Groos, 1826, Vol. 1, p. 80.
175. TIGERSTEDT, R. Die Physiologie des Kreislaufes. 2nd Ed. Berlin, Gruyter, 1922.
176. VESALIUS, A. De humani corporis fabrica libri septem. Basileae, Oporini, 1543.

177. VULPIAN. Sur les effets des excitations produites directement sur le foie et les reins. C.R. Soc. Biol. (Paris), ser. 2, 10:5, 1858.
178. WAINEWRIGHT, J. An Anatomical Treatise of the Liver, with the Diseases Incident to It. London, Clarke, 1737.
179. WAKIM, K. G., and F. C. MANN. The intrahepatic circulation of blood. Anat. Rec., 82:233, 1942.
180. WEBSTER, T. B. L. From Mycenae to Homer. London, Methuen, 1958.
181. WHEELER, H. O., B. COMBES, A. W. CHILDS, and O. L. WADE. The splanchnic circulation time. Trans. Ass. Amer. Physns., 68:177, 1955.
182. WIGGERS, C. J. The Pressure Pulses in the Cardiovascular System. New York, Longmans, Green, 1928.
183. WOOLLEY, C. L. A Forgotten Kingdom. Harmondsworth, Penguin, 1953.
184. YOUNG, J. Glisson and Wharton. N.Z. med. J., 22:24, 1923.

XI

The Cerebral Circulation

THE heart and the brain were undoubtedly recognized by primitive man as the most vital of the organs, even though it was not until three hundred years ago that the relationship between them began to be clarified. The pulsations of the brain during life are mentioned in the Smith Papyrus, one of the earliest of medical texts, which was written around the seventeenth century B.C. (56), although this may have been a copy of a much older text dating back to the thirtieth century B.C. The ancient Egyptians and the early Greeks apparently did not distinguish between tendons, nerves, and blood vessels; the Ebers papyrus uses the same word (*met*) to describe them indiscriminately (73), and our words neuron and neurology come from the Greek νεῦρον, which originally meant "tendon."

By the sixth century B.C., Pythagoras had characterized the brain as the organ of reasoning, a concept which, though obvious to us, was nevertheless denied by Aristotle two hundred years later. One pupil of Pythagoras, Alcmeon of Croton (*c.* 500 B.C.), was the first anatomist

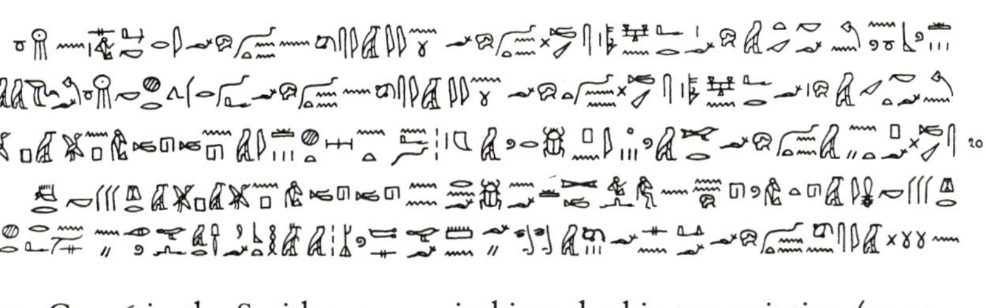

Figure 1. Case 6 in the Smith papyrus, in hieroglyphic transcription (seventeenth century B.C.). It outlines the examination of a gaping cranial wound, describes the convolutions of the brain and notes the cerebral pulsations, "... and something therein throbbing and fluttering under thy fingers, like the weak place of an infant's crown before it becomes whole...."

SPECIAL CIRCULATIONS

and physiologist whose writings, though fragmentary, have come down to us. He recognized an ebb and flow of blood in the veins and the importance of blood for mental function. He taught that sleep was caused by the retreat of blood from the brain into the great veins; death occurred when this retreat was permanent (73). Empedocles (c. 480 B.C.), and later Diogenes of Apollonia (c. 400 B.C.), emphasized the importance of air, or Pneuma, to the proper functioning of the brain (66). This material was distributed by the heart through the vascular system. Pleasure, sensation, and intellect, and their pathological alterations, could be traced to the proportion of air and blood which were available to the brain and other organs. Democritos (470–380 B.C.) developed this further in conjunction with his atomic theory of the world, in which the molecules of the spirit of life, like those of fire, were smooth, round, and mobile, and were present in the air, to which they returned at death (73).

Hippocrates of Cos (c. 460–370 B.C.) and the physicians of the school which he developed wrote extensively on the brain, as well as on many other organs. The treatise *On the sacred disease* (21), a study of epilepsy written by one of the Hippocratic physicians about 400 B.C., gives one of the earliest accounts of the anatomy of the veins of the neck:

"and veins run toward it [the brain] from all parts of the body, many of which are small, but two are thick—the one from the liver and the other from the spleen. . . . The remaining part of it [the vein from the liver] rises upward across the clavicle to the right side of the neck, and is superficial so as to be seen, near the ear it is concealed, and there it divides; its thickest, largest, and most hollow part ends in the brain; another . . . to the ear, another to the eye, and another to the nostril."

Superficial vessels of the brain were described without much accuracy, and the interior of the brain itself was thought by these physicians and by Aristotle to be bloodless. They believed the brain to be a large gland, whose function, among others, was to cool and purify the blood, releasing excess fluids and other material by way of the nasal discharge. Mental disturbances were attributed to the retention of humors in the brain:

"And by the same organ [the brain] we become mad and delirious, and fears and terrors assail us, some by night and some by day, and dreams and untimely

wanderings, and cares that are not suitable, and ignorance of present circumstances, desuetude and unskillfulness. All those things we endure from the brain, when it is not healthy, but is more hot, more cold, more moist or more dry than natural" (21).

THE CEREBRAL CIRCULATION

Although cerebral physiology was not to become more precise for many centuries, knowledge of the anatomy of the brain, its coverings, and its blood vessels showed steady progress from that time forward.

After the death of Aristotle in 322 B.C., the scientific center of the world moved from Athens to Alexandria. There Herophylos of Chalcedon (*c.* 300 B.C.) carried on his studies and teachings of anatomy (66). He described the meninges, the confluence of the cerebral sinuses which bears his name, and the *rete mirabile*, or "marvelous network," of anastomotic vessels between the arterial systems of the head and brain which, although well developed in lower animals, such as the dog, cat, and ox, does not exist in man. The contributions of Herophylos to other areas of anatomy and physiology were many. He re-established the brain as the seat of intelligence and consciousness, differentiated between sensory and motor nerves, clearly distinguished veins from arteries, and recognized pulsation as an active process in the arteries.

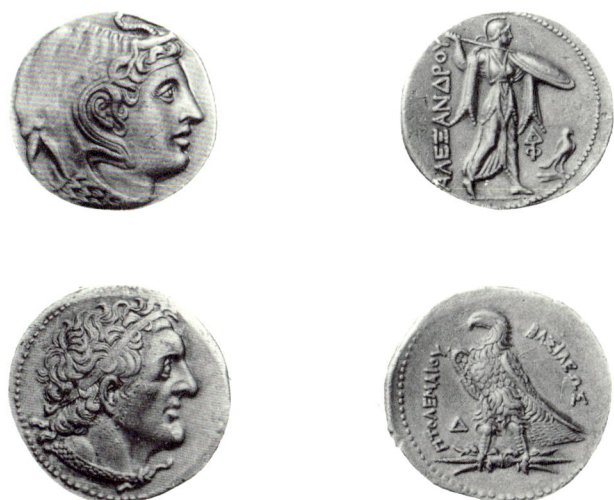

Figure 2. Early coins of Alexandria showing (above) Alexander and the goddess Athena, (below) Ptolemy Soter and the eagle of Zeus.

Galen: Rete Mirabile and Animal Spirit

SPECIAL CIRCULATIONS

Nearly five hundred years intervened between Herophylos and the next significant contributor to cerebral anatomy and physiology. Galen of Pergamon (A.D. 129–199), whose impact on circulatory physiology is detailed elsewhere in this volume, constructed from the theories of the Greeks who had preceded him a doctrine of cerebral nutrition and function, which, like his other concepts, dominated physiology for nearly 1500 years (66).

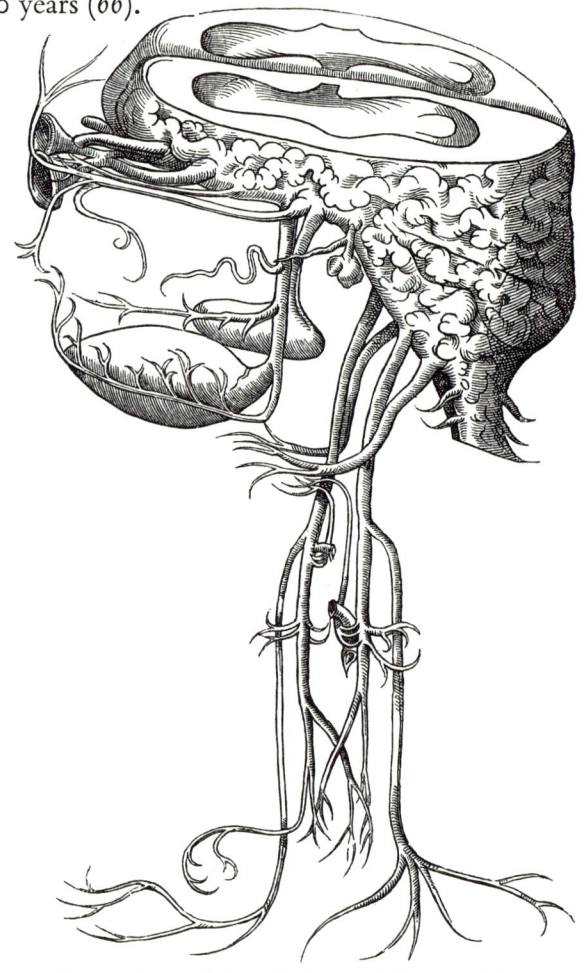

Figure 3. The Galenic view of the relations of the cranial nerves to the base of the brain and to the cerebral ventricles. From an early sketch by Vesalius which was published without his permission in 1539.

Galen was the first of the ancients to demonstrate that arteries contain blood. In his scheme the brain was nourished both by arterial and venous blood. The latter, originating in the liver and intestines, brought food and *natural spirit* to all the organs, including the brain (cf. Alcmeon). By way of the arteries came a considerably smaller quantity of blood, but this had been enriched in the left ventricle by *vital spirit* brought in from the outside air through the trachea, lung, and pulmonary vein (cf. Diogenes and Democritos). In the *rete mirabile* at the base of the brain there was formed a third principle, the *animal spirit*, which was distributed to all the muscles by way of the nerves, which were supposedly hollow. The *animal spirit* resulted in distension of muscles; its absence caused contraction. In this, he borrowed freely from still another Greek, Erasistratos of Chios (66), a younger contemporary of Herophylos.

THE CEREBRAL CIRCULATION

Galen's concept, though largely derivative, was systematic, based upon some experimental evidence, and fairly logical. In a remarkable way it recognized, long before the origin of chemistry, the requirements of the brain as well as other organs for some substrate, and its ability to create from these a third and different principle—call it animal spirit or the nerve impulse—responsible for cerebral function. Although Harvey overthrew the Galenic theory of the circulation, he and his successors for many years accepted and developed Galen's concept insofar as it concerned the functions of the brain and nervous system.

Following Galen there was no further development of the physiology and little progress even in the anatomy of the cerebral circulation until the Renaissance. Mondino de' Luzzi (1270–1326), who restored the science of anatomy, paid relatively little attention to the brain. He did, however, describe the choroid plexus lying between the ventricles and postulated that opening or closing this communication controlled mental processes (66, 54). Berengario da Carpi (c. 1520) gave a more detailed description of the choroid plexus and recognized its arterial and venous components (66). More important, perhaps, he was the first to deny the existence of the *rete mirabile* in man, thus destroying the source of Galen's *animal spirit* and contradicting a host of anatomists who believed they had demonstrated it in the human brain.

The state of anatomy and physiology in the Renaissance just before

SPECIAL
CIRCULATIONS

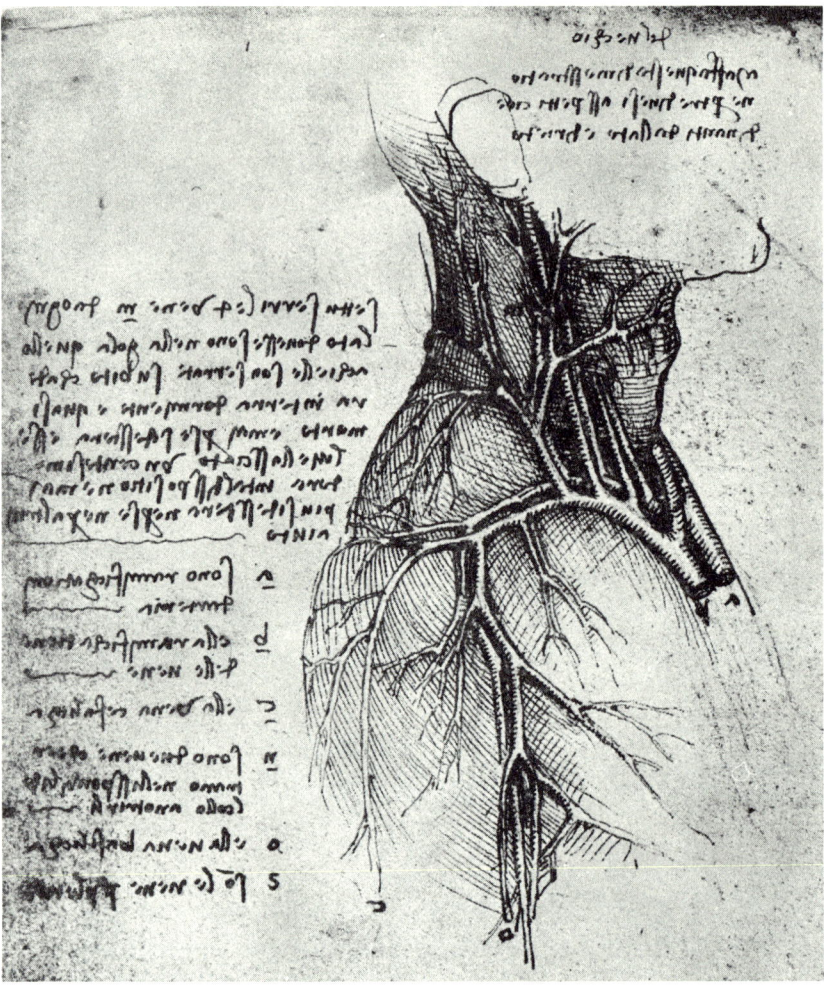

Figure 4. The vessels of the neck, from a drawing by Leonardo da Vinci.

Vesalius's revival and reorganization of it may be appreciated, perhaps, from the anatomical notebooks (*43*) and drawings of Leonardo da Vinci (1452–1519). He described with some accuracy the vessels of the neck, and recognized that cervical compression could produce unconsciousness. He suggested that little over half a minute ("the hundredth part of an hour") need elapse before irreversible damage and death might occur —something of an underestimate but in the right order of magnitude. He referred on several occasions to a *rete mirabile* in the human head, suggesting that he had not performed such dissections himself. It is interesting that da Vinci's concepts of circulatory physiology, especially in reference to the brain, were considerably more primitive than those of Galen. He considered the factors responsible for bringing blood to the head against the force of gravity, proposed and dismissed respiratory movement as the propelling force, and settled on a highly vitalistic explanation in terms of spiritual heat, which he presumed could cause blood to ascend as mercury rises in a heated retort. He recognized that the mental effects of wine result from the action of certain of its ingredients on the brain, but offered no explanation of the mechanism of transport between the gastrointestinal tract and the brain other than a rising "as though towards the sky" (43).

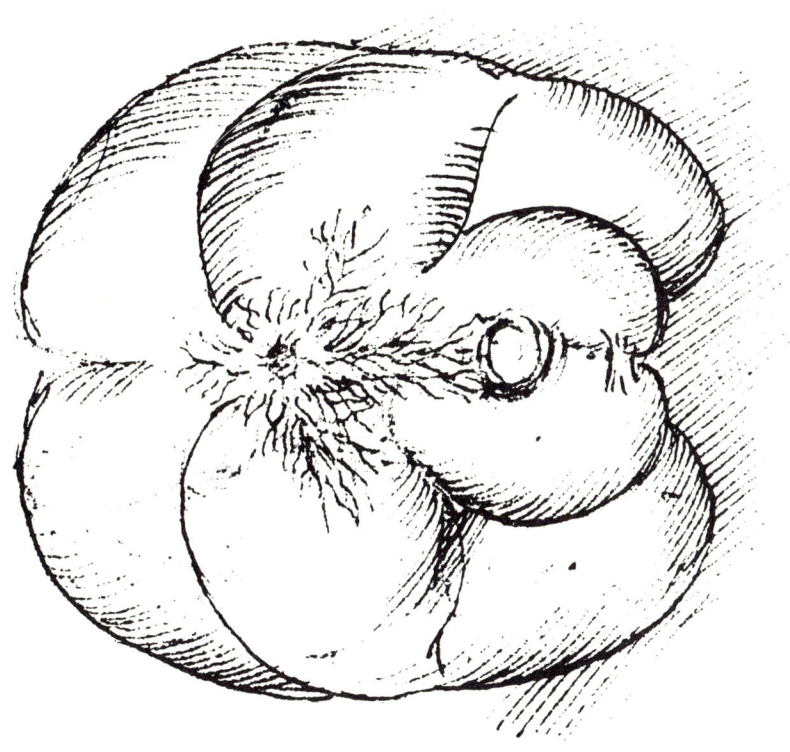

Figure 5. The *rete mirabile*, from a drawing by Leonardo da Vinci.

Vesalius: Galen Refuted

SPECIAL CIRCULATIONS

With Vesalius (1514–64) the anatomical sciences took a great forward leap, and, although his treatment of the vascular system of the brain did not compare in accuracy and beauty of detail with his descriptions of bones and muscles, or of the brain itself, he corrected a number of errors propounded by Galen that had been perpetuated for more than a thousand years. His discussion of the course of the soporal (internal carotid) artery and the absence of the plexus reticularis (*rete mirabile*) in man is especially interesting.

"How much has been attributed to Galen, easily leader of the professors of dissection, by those physicians and anatomists who have followed him, and often against reason! In confirmation, there is that blessed and wonderful plexus reticularis which that man everywhere inculcates in his books.

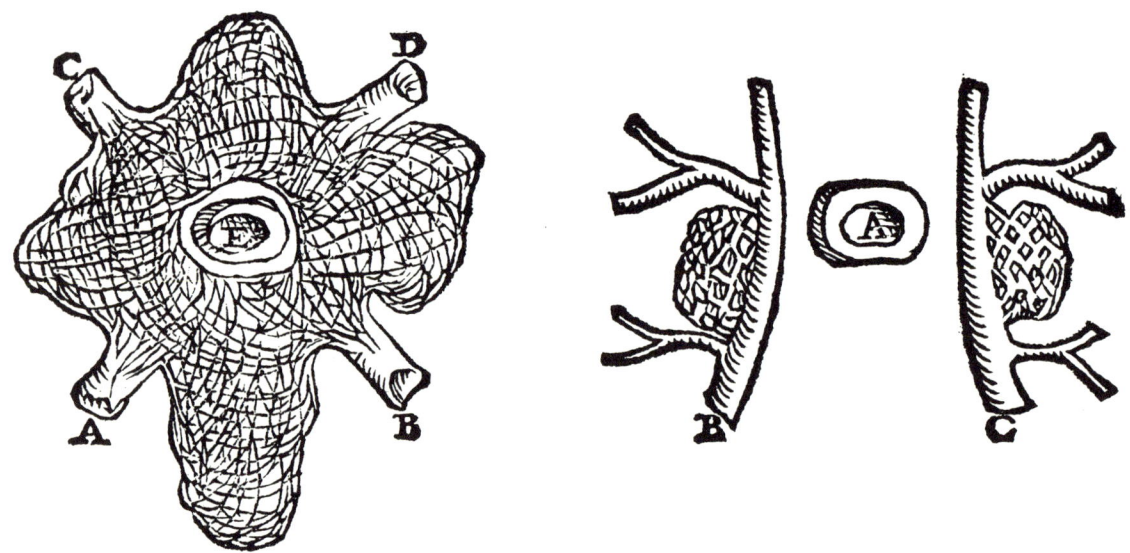

Figure 6. Vesalius's representation of Galen's description of the *rete mirabile*.
Left: A and B indicate the arteries entering the skull to form the plexus. C and D represent the vessels into which the subdivisions of the plexus are reunited. E is the pituitary gland. *Right:* The arrangement of the arteries on either side of the pituitary gland in cattle and in sheep but not in man.

There is nothing of which physicians speak more often. They have never seen it (for it is almost non-existent in the human body), yet they describe it from Galen's teaching. Indeed, I myself cannot wonder enough at my own stupidity and too great trust in the writings of Galen and other anatomists; indeed, I who so much labored in my love for Galen that I never undertook to dissect a human head in public without that of a lamb or ox at hand, so as to supply what I could in no way find in that of man and to impress it on the spectators, lest I be charged with failure to find that plexus so universally familiar by name. For the soporal arteries quite fail to produce such a 'plexus reticularis' as that which Galen recounts" (74).

It is no small matter to question established authority when questioning is heresy, and it required many years of subservience to a concept which he knew was wrong before even Vesalius could openly repudiate it. But his break with Galenic tradition was purely in terms of anatomical detail; he used his discoveries to strengthen the teleological and vitalistic notions of orthodox physiology:

"*... but the Maker of the Universe has used far greater ingenuity than Galen imagined. For He has contrived for the great soporal artery a tortuous channel with a long passage* [carotid canal] *in the bone, and He has willed for this passage the very thing for which Galen imagined that the plexus had been built, to wit, that the vital spirit be thoroughly concocted in the many turnings and twistings of the artery and its matter be so prepared for producing animal spirit. Galen said that the artery, when it had entered the cranial cavity, was divided into innumerable branches which were so interwoven and intermixed that they formed a plexus comparable to a bunched-up fisherman's net, or heap of nets ...*

"*How far these things are from the truth and how much they demonstrate indifference to nature will be seen by him who has learned the actual course of that branch of the soporal artery*" (74).

In Book III of De humani corporis fabrica, Vesalius described the vascular system and included a detailed drawing of the vessels of the brain. Although it was the most complete description up to that time and for many years beyond, it contains many inaccuracies, the most glaring, perhaps, being the description of a large communication between the carotid artery and the transverse sinus.

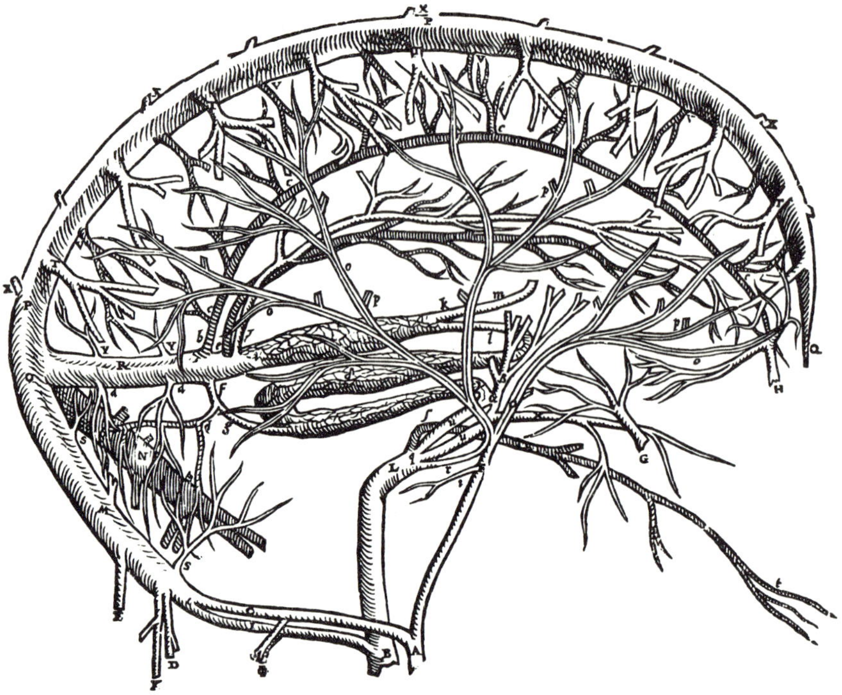

SPECIAL CIRCULATIONS

Figure 7. The vessels of the brain, from the *Fabrica* of Vesalius.

Realdus Columbus (1516–59), who had been an assistant to Vesalius, learned through vivisection that the pulsations of the brain were synchronous with those of the heart and arteries (66), which, with his demonstration of the lesser circulation, paved the way for Harvey's revolutionary discovery two generations later.

In *De motu cordis* (19), Harvey did not refer to the cerebral circulation, although he assumed it to be large. In fact, at the end of the seventh chapter of that great work, he used this assumption to argue against the prevalent idea that the function of the right ventricle was merely the nutrition of the lung.

"It is altogether incongruous to suppose that the lungs need for their nourishment so large a supply of food, so pulsatorily delivered, and also so much purer and spiritous (as being supplied directly from the ventricles of the heart). For they cannot need such more than does the extremely pure substance of the brain, . . ." (19).

While Harvey was revolutionizing the physiological concepts of the circulation, some of his contemporaries were making more modest contributions to the anatomy and function of the brain and its vessels. François de la Boe Sylvius (1614–72) published one of the most complete descriptions of the dural sinuses up to that time and, more important, established the science of pathological anatomy (54). Nyman (1594–1638) of Wittenberg, an outstanding clinician who used necropsy for study of the mechanisms of disease, concluded on anatomical grounds that apoplexy was caused by obstruction of the torcular Herophili (54). The greatest of these scientists was Thomas Willis, an active London physician, whose work, *Cerebri anatome nervorumque*, was a landmark in neuroanatomy (78). He gave, perhaps not the first, but the most extensive description of the anastomotic circle of arteries at the base of the brain which bears his name. Following the tradition of his day, his description was extremely literary but hardly succinct:

"For in as much as the carotidick arteries do communicate between themselves in various places, and are mutually ingrafted; from thence a double benefit results, though of a contrary effect: because by this one and the same means care is taken, both lest the brain should be defrauded of its due watring of the blood, and also lest it should be overwhelmed by the too impetuous flowing of the swelling stream or torrent. As to the first, lest that should happen, one of the Carotids perhaps being obstructed, the other might supply the provision of both; then, lest the blood rushing with too full a torrent should drown the channels and little Ponds of the brain, the flood is chastised or hindered by an opposite emissary, as it were a Flood-gate, and so is commanded to return its flood, and haste backwards by the same ways, and to run back with an ebbing Tide" (79).

In addition, Willis corrected the misconception that the anterior spinal artery was a nerve and made important contributions to functional cerebral anatomy. He established the presence of fine vessels throughout the brain substance by injecting dye into the great vessels and demonstrating an abundance of dark spots on the cut surface of the brain. Willis accepted the Galenic concept of animal spirits and regarded their storage to be one of the functions of the autonomic ganglia. In this he was merely reflecting the scientific opinion of his time. No less a scientist than René Descartes (1596–1650) had written, "that part of

SPECIAL
CIRCULATIONS

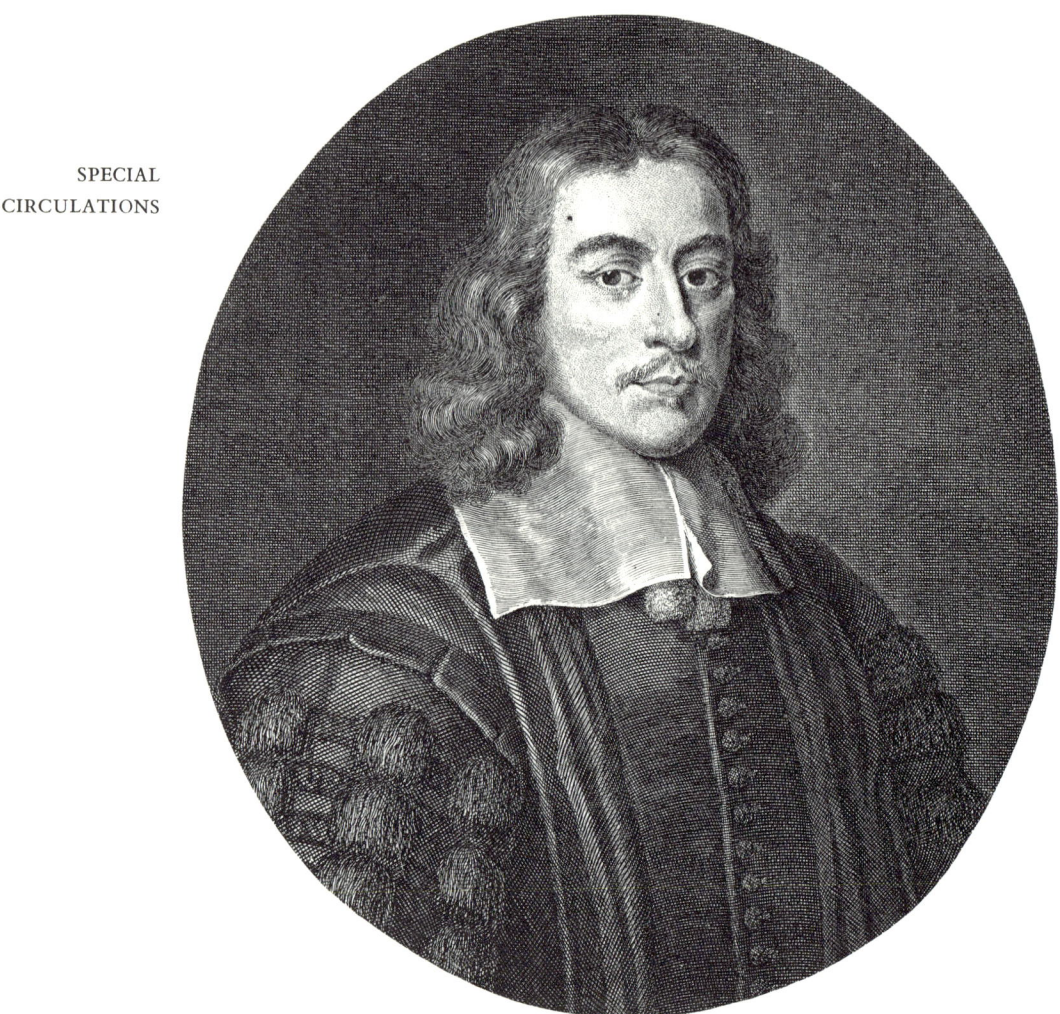

Figure 8. Thomas Willis (1621–75).

the blood which penetrates as far as the brain serves not only to nourish and maintain its substance but also principally to produce there a certain very subtle spirit—the animal spirit" (73). Not until ten years before his death did Harvey break with this tradition which he had implicitly accepted in *De motu cordis*. In 1649, he wrote in the second disquisition to Riolan,

THE CEREBRAL CIRCULATION

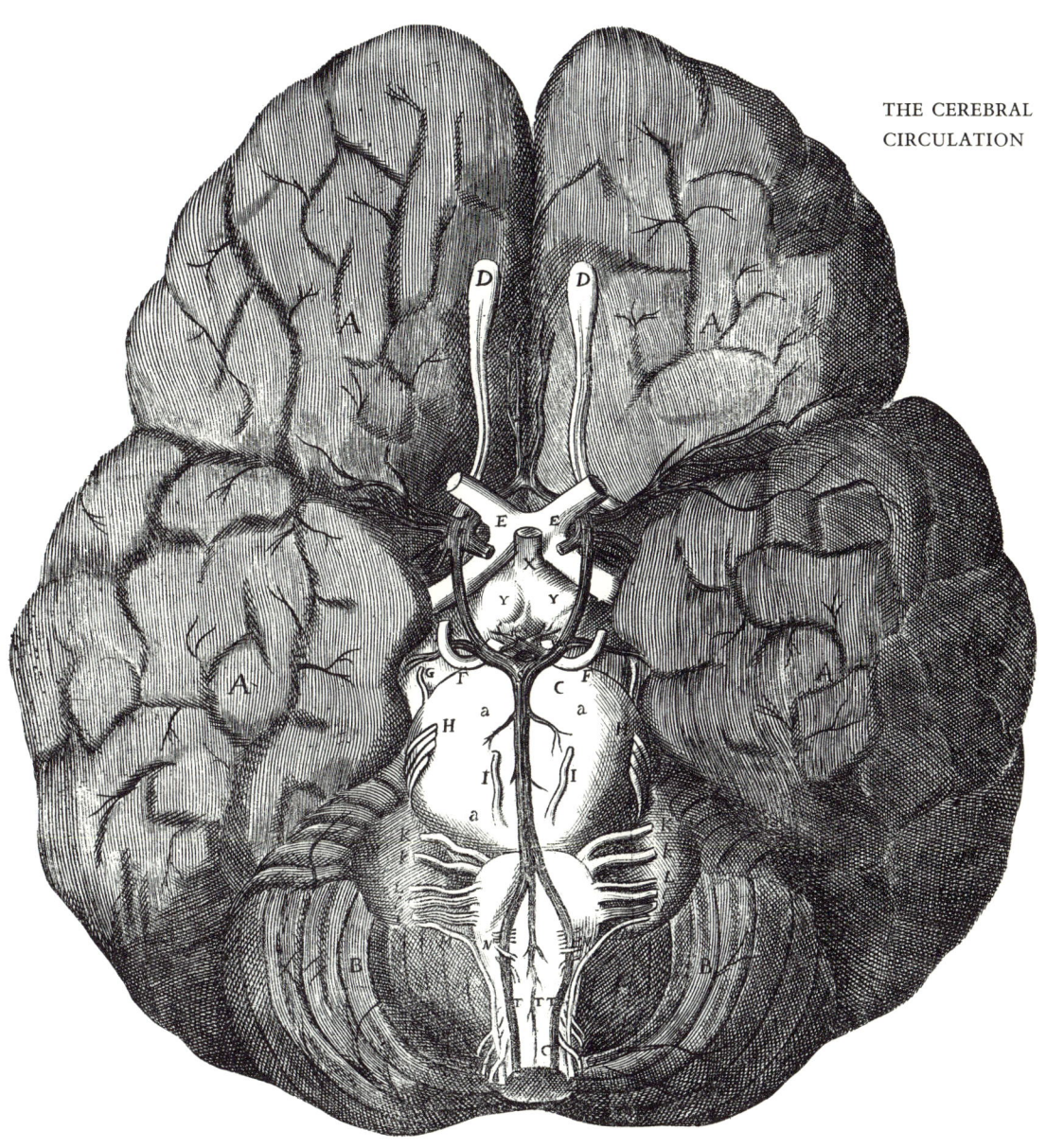

Figure 9. The Circle of Willis and the cranial nerves. This plate was drawn by Willis's friend, Christopher Wren.

SPECIAL CIRCULATIONS

"Persons of limited information, when they are at a loss to assign a cause for anything, very commonly reply that it is done by the spirits. . . . Some speak of corporeal, others of incorporeal spirits; and they who advocate the corporeal spirits will have the blood, or the thinner portion of the blood, to be the bond of union with the soul, the spirit being contained in the blood as the flame is in the smoke of a lamp or candle, and held admixed by the incessant motion of the fluid. . . . There is nothing more uncertain and questionable, then, than the doctrine of the spirits . . ." (76).

It is perhaps fitting that Harvey, who had put the mysteries of the circulatory system on a simple mechanical basis, should have dealt so severely with vitalistic and supernatural concepts in other areas. Thirty years later the "animal spirits" became the subject of some very interesting scientific speculation. John Mayow, in 1681, wrote,

"The animal spirit is 'spiritus nitroaeriens' [*the oxygen of Lavoisier*] *. . . the blood returning from the brain to the heart is for the greater part deprived of* [*oxygen*] *which it has left in the brain for the production of animal spirit"* (73).

These statements of Harvey and Mayow seem to be proper preludes to what we shall call the Modern Era.

Cerebral Blood Flow: Early Experiments and Conflicting Ideas

The important characteristic of the modern physiology which began with Harvey is its dependence on the inductive approach. Experimental methods have played a determining role in the development of knowledge concerning the cerebral circulation. When satisfactory methods have been used by critical observers, significant progress has been made. Even poor techniques, in the hands of those who recognized their limitations, have led to the development of important concepts. But where inadequate methods have been coupled with an uncritical and dogmatic approach, earlier and more valid observations have been negated and neglected and errors have become established for several generations.

The modern chapter on the circulatory physiology of the brain begins with an impressive bit of deductive reasoning. In 1783, Alexander Monro the younger put forward this view:

THE CEREBRAL CIRCULATION

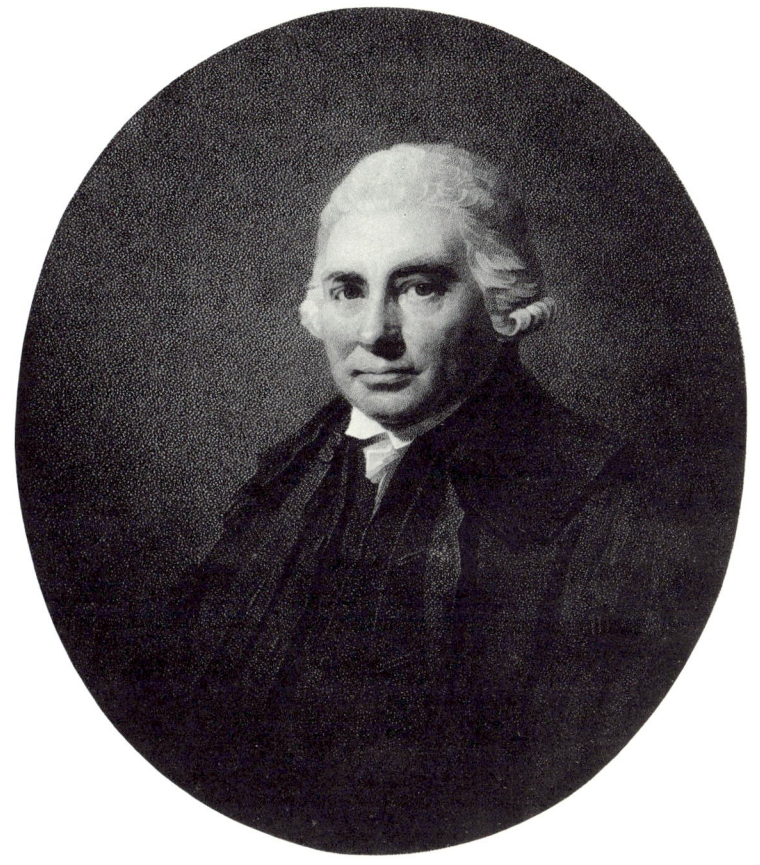

Figure 10. Alexander Monro (1733–1817).

"*For being enclosed in a case of bone, the blood must be continually flowing out of the veins that room may be given to the blood which is entering by the arteries. For, as the substance of the brain, like that of the other solids of our body is nearly incompressible, the quantity of blood within the head must be the same, or nearly the same at all times whether in health or disease, in life, or after death . . .*" (47).

Abercrombie supported this thesis forty years later by deduction again and with the same arguments, but Kellie (1824) confirmed their postulates in actual experiments (23). He found that the brains of animals killed by exsanguination still contained blood, except where he had broken the integrity of the skull by trephining before death.

SPECIAL CIRCULATIONS

The Monro-Kellie doctrine pertained only to the constancy of the blood volume of the brain, and although Burrows (1846) pointed out that cerebrospinal fluid represented a volume which was by no means fixed (4), production or absorption of this fluid would be sufficiently slow under ordinary circumstances as not to argue against the general validity of the doctrine in the adult with an intact skull over relatively short periods of time. The doctrine does not, however, apply to blood flow, which may still vary widely within the confines of a constant total blood volume.

Perhaps the oldest method for studying the cerebral circulation in the living state was that employed by Donders, who in 1851 reported his observations of pial vessels in animals in the calvarium of which he had fixed and sealed a glass window (9). He observed variations in the size of those vessels in different states and especially during asphyxia, in which they were significantly dilated. Since Donders, a large number of investigators including Ackermann (1), in 1858, Nothnagel (51), in 1867, and more recently, Forbes (13), Cobb (7), and Wolff (80), have employed various modifications of the technique, which although impossible to quantify in terms of blood flow, permits observation under relatively normal conditions.

In searching for more quantitative methods for studying the cerebral circulation, investigators soon decided to put the Monro-Kellie principle to good use by converting the cranio-vertebral cavity into an oncometer. Salathé (1876), von Schulten (1884), Knoll (1886), Falkenheim and Naunyn (1887), and Dean (1892) measured changes in cerebrospinal fluid pressure (20), which they interpreted as alterations in intracranial volume concomitant with changes in blood flow. It is, of course, apparent that such an approach could measure at best only directional changes, while the technique of Roy and Sherrington (1890), which measured changes in the vertical diameter of the brain in the open cranium, was subject to an even greater variety of serious errors. Yet the observations of Roy and Sherrington (55) were closer to the truth than many before and since, and their deductions were so brilliant and perceptive that they should have dominated the field, had they not been rudely and erroneously brushed aside only a few years after their conception. They found that under many of their experimental con-

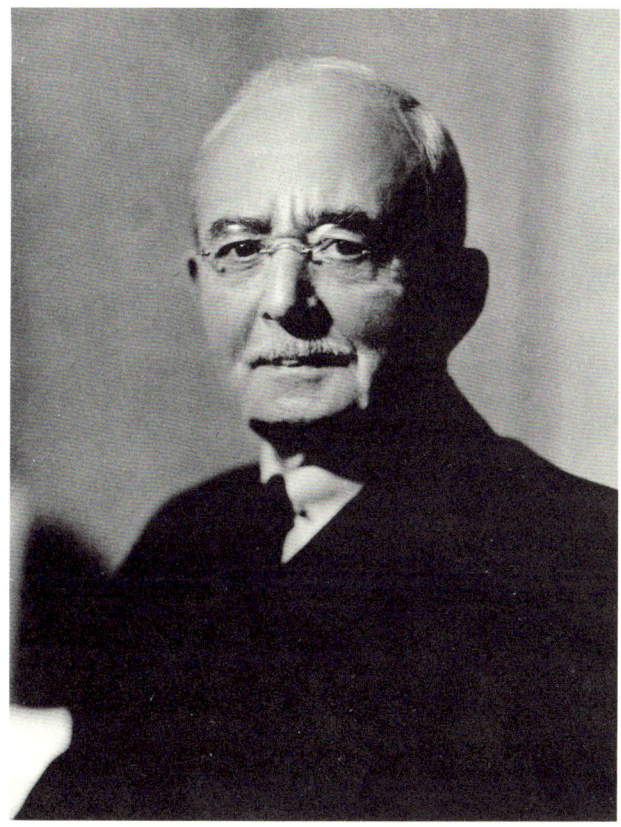

Figure 11. Charles S. Sherrington (1861–1952).

THE CEREBRAL
CIRCULATION

ditions, "the blood supply of the brain varies directly with the blood pressure in the systemic arteries," from which they deduced:

"*In whatever way produced, anaemia of the central nervous system excites the vasoconstrictor nerves with the result that owing to constriction of the vessels of the digestive, urinary and other systems, the arterial blood pressure rises, causing an increased flow of blood through the cerebrospinal blood vessels.*"

Although they sought for and found no evidence of intrinsic control by way of vasomotor nerves, they observed, during asphyxia and following the intravenous infusion of strong acids, a marked expansion of the brain which was independent of arterial blood pressure.

SPECIAL
CIRCULATIONS

From these observations and others they derived the following conclusion, remarkable for its clarity, originality, and prescience:

"*We conclude then, that the chemical products of cerebral metabolism contained in the lymph which bathes the walls of the arterioles of the brain can cause variations of the calibre of the cerebral vessels: that in this reaction the brain possesses an intrinsic mechanism by which its vascular supply can be varied locally in correspondence with local variations of functional activity*" (55).

Six years later, Leonard Hill published his book, *The Physiology and Pathology of the Cerebral Circulation; An Experimental Research* (20), which was to dominate the field for nearly two generations. Rejecting all previous work as being based upon fallacious methods, he proceeded to develop and extol an approach of his own.

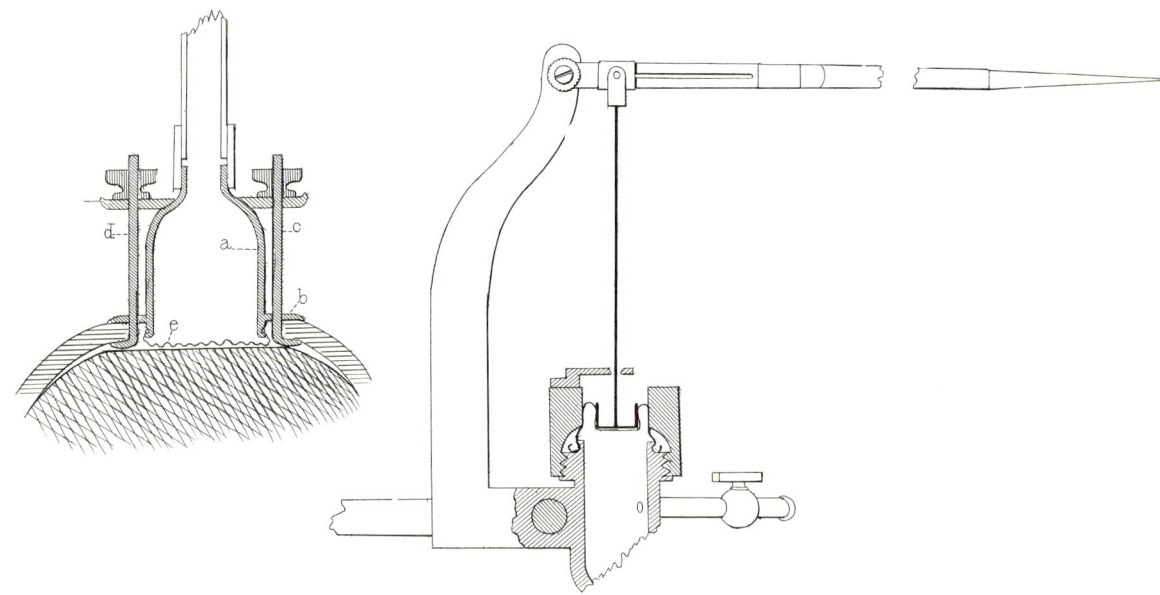

Figure 12. Illustration from Roy and Sherrington of method for recording changes in intracranial volume as a measure of cerebral circulation. *Left:* Metal capsule fixed over aperture in skull. The lower end of the bell-shaped capsule is sealed by a flexible, delicate animal membrane (e). The upper opening of the capsule leads to the recording apparatus. *Right:* Recording apparatus. A light piston conveys to the recording lever any changes in the volume of the brain.

"The exact method of experiment by which I have arrived at these important results is simultaneous record of — (1) arterial pressure in the central carotid, (2) general venous pressure in the right auricle, (3) cerebral venous pressure in the torcular Herophili, (4) cerebro-spinal fluid pressure taken by trephining the atlas and screwing a tube into the hole and connecting this with a manometer; or, intracranial pressure taken by means of the cerebral pressure gauge."

THE CEREBRAL CIRCULATION

The modern student of hemodynamics may find it difficult to understand just how four such pressure measurements could possibly yield information on blood flow, but Hill never critically evaluated his own method, or for that matter ever clearly indicated how he drew conclusions regarding blood flow from cerebral venous pressure. Since there are only large channels of very low resistance between the torcu-

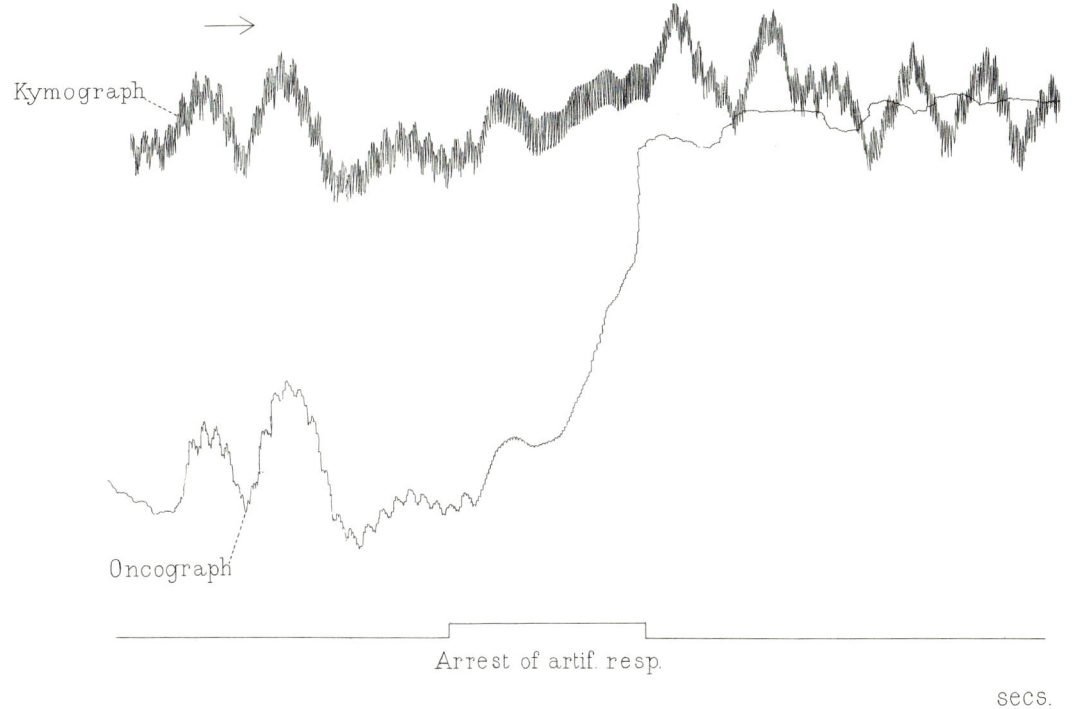

Figure 13. Pressure tracings from Roy and Sherrington showing effect of asphyxia on intracranial volume (oncograph) and systemic arterial blood pressure (kymograph). This was one of the earliest demonstrations that asphyxia was associated with dilatation of cerebral vessels.

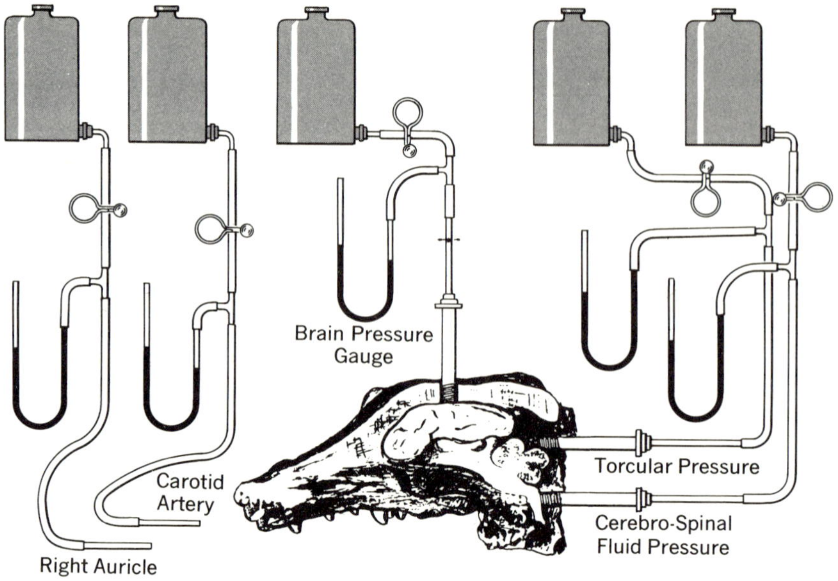

SPECIAL
CIRCULATIONS

Figure 14. Illustration from Hill showing his method of studying the cerebral circulation of the dog. From left to right, the five manometers are arranged to record pressure from the right auricle, the carotid artery, the subdural space, the torcular Herophili, and the spinal canal, respectively.

lar and the right atrium, pressure in one would reflect that in the other quite faithfully under all conditions; even in states of extreme cerebral vasodilation, venous pressure at the torcular could rise only imperceptibly. Armed with this technique, peculiarly unsuited to discovering evidence for intrinsic circulatory control of the brain, Hill found none, insisted that none existed, and rebuked those who, with better methods or more sagacious reasoning, found evidence for its presence. Stimulation of the cervical sympathetics, asphyxia, amyl nitrite, acids, convulsions, injections of lethal doses of suprarenal extract, which others had shown to affect cerebral vessels, appeared to Hill to have no effect on these vessels at all. In his experiments they behaved as if they were lead pipes:

"*We have been entirely unable to confirm the results that Roy and Sherrington obtained with acids, and have not found the slightest evidence of active dilatation of the cerebral vessels.* . . .

"In every experimental condition the cerebral circulation passively follows the changes in the general arterial and venous pressures. The intracranial or cerebral venous pressure varies directly and absolutely with general venous pressure, but only proportionally with general arterial pressure. . . . It is by means of the splanchnic area that the blood supply to the brain is controlled. . . . The brain has no direct vasomotor mechanism, but its blood supply can be controlled indirectly by the vasomotor centre acting on the splanchnic area. The vasomotor centre is part of the central nervous system, and feels the same needs and is stimulated by the same centripetal impulses as affect the rest of that system, and thus it maintains a supply of blood to the central nervous system which corresponds to its functional activity."

THE CEREBRAL CIRCULATION

The first signs of revolt against Hill's conclusions appeared after the first quarter of the twentieth century. Using refined adaptations of oncometric techniques or direct observation of pial vessels, investigators were reaffirming the observations of Donders and of Roy and Sherrington with respect to local effects of carbon dioxide and other agents on the cerebral circulation and of stimulation of certain constrictor or dilator nerves (*80*). By the use of a cooled thermocouple, Schmidt was able to obtain qualitative information with respect to blood flow in various regions of the brain (*59, 61*) and to compare the characteristics of cerebral circulation with that of muscle. None of these methods, however, measured cerebral blood flow directly and quantitatively. As early as 1887, Gärtner and Wagner (*15*) had attempted a direct approach by estimating the outflow from the lateral sinus in laboratory animals. They made no claim, however, to measuring total cerebral blood flow. It was not until 1943, in fact, that the first reliable quantitative measurements of cerebral blood flow were made by Dumke and Schmidt in the macacque monkey (*10*).

Measurement of Cerebral Blood Flow

During the fifty years following the first attempts by Gärtner and Wagner, there were numerous efforts to make such measurements, but these ran afoul either of instrumental deficiencies or the *rete mirabile*, which, having ceased to be a problem for anatomists some three hundred years before, now troubled the physiologist by so confounding the cerebral circulation with that of the rest of the head as to make it

SPECIAL CIRCULATIONS

practically impossible to isolate the two in animals where this rich anastomosis occurred. The earliest attempt at measurement of the cerebral blood flow was probably that of Jensen, in 1904, who arrived at a value of 125 ml. per 100 gm. per minute in the dog and rabbit (*22*). Activity appears to have lagged until, thirty years later, three other values appeared in the literature, ranging from 60 to 130 ml. per 100 gm. per minute in the same species (*80*). In his exhaustive review of 1936, Wolff questioned the reliability of these values, on the basis of the free anastomoses which Bouckaert and Heymans had shown to exist between the intra- and extra-cranial circulation in the species studied. Recognizing that such anastomoses are relatively minor in the primate, Dumke and Schmidt (*10*) used the monkey, in which it was possible to isolate the arterial inflow to the brain and to direct it through a simple and ingenious "bubble flowmeter" which they had adapted from Soskin's laboratory. In animals anesthetized with pentobarbital they arrived at a mean value of 86 ml. per 100 gm. of brain per minute, found a correlation between blood flow and arterial blood pressure, and demonstrated an intrinsic response of cerebral vessels to a number of drugs. Even before these quantitative values were available, however, a reappraisal of Hill's conclusions had been going on, and, based upon the work of such men as Cobb, Forbes, Wolff, Schmidt, and a number of others throughout the world, a new concept of the control of the cerebral circulation was emerging, which was remarkably similar to that of Roy and Sherrington, but considerably better documented. This concept, as stated by Forbes and Cobb (*14*), who were most instrumental in its formulation, acknowledged the over-riding importance of the arterial blood pressure: "This factor appears to dominate all others. The arterial pressure, in turn, depends on complex reflexes from the cardiovascular centers of the central nervous system, the carotid sinuses, and other reflex mechanisms. These reflexes, therefore, play a vital part in controlling the supply of blood to the brain." Their concept also includes the important thesis that intrinsic factors may modify the effect of blood pressure:

"Active changes in caliber of cerebral arteries . . . may overcome moderate or gradual fluctuations in arterial pressure . . . [they] result from the following conditions: Direct trauma to vessels' walls. Changes in chemical composition

of the arterial blood. . . . Asphyxia of the tissues due to slow blood flow. . . . Regional activity of the brain. There is evidence that active areas of gray matter have a local vasodilation. This may be due to a local increase in CO_2 or other products of active cellular metabolism. Activity of cerebral vasoconstrictor nerves (sympathetic). Activity of cerebral vasodilator nerves (parasympathetic). These last two conditions have less effect on cerebral blood flow than the chemical conditions mentioned. . . ."

Many problems remained unsettled, and there was much new information to be acquired in this field. These studies had been made almost exclusively in animals, and the effects of species differences, anatomical peculiarities, anesthesia, and sometimes drastic surgery combined to produce inconsistent results. Experiments on the effects of drugs yielded information of limited practical value since these depended largely on the species used, dosage, and route of administration. Finally, information on the state of the cerebral circulation in human disease was to a large extent lacking. In 1944, Schmidt (*60*) summarized the state and needs of the field at that time:

"It is unfortunate indeed that now, when data concerning the behavior of the human cerebral circulation are urgently desired, the only thing that can be said is that a considerable amount of fundamental research will have to be done before such data become available. Yet in the past the first step toward real advances in clinical experimentation has often been dissatisfaction with the methods previously utilized, and it is to be hoped that history will repeat itself here."

Because Schmidt communicated to those about him his long-standing interest in the cerebral circulation and his "dissatisfaction with the methods previously utilized," it was not by chance that, at that time, a method which appeared to be capable of measuring the human cerebral circulation (*34*) was being developed in his laboratory (*61*).

Studies on the Human Cerebral Circulation

One of the earliest series of observations on the human cerebral circulation was that of Mosso (*48*), in 1881, who recorded changes in the volume of intracranial contents by sealing a tambour system to the scalps of patients with cranial defects. He made continuous recordings

SPECIAL CIRCULATIONS

in a number of physiological states, including sleep, and inferred changes in cerebral blood flow from his measurements, often quite correctly. In 1927, the Boston psychiatrist, Abraham Myerson, in collaboration with Halloran and Hirsch (*50*), made possible most of the recent advances in the field by showing that cerebral venous blood could be obtained readily and safely in man through a needle inserted into the superior bulb of the internal jugular vein. Later workers have shown that such blood is, in fact, representative of cerebral venous blood (*36*) not significantly contaminated by blood of extracerebral origin (*65*). This permitted estimation of the arteriovenous difference for oxygen across the human brain for the first time. The Fick Principle, described elsewhere in this volume, can be used for measuring blood flow not only for the body as a whole but for any organ, providing its oxygen consumption and arteriovenous oxygen difference are known. Although the oxygen consumption of the brain was not known, if it could be assumed to be constant, then the cerebral arteriovenous oxygen difference would be an inverse measure of the cerebral blood flow. On the basis of this assumption, W. G. Lennox and E. L. Gibbs used changes in the arteriovenous oxygen difference to infer changes in cerebral blood flow in a variety of physiological and pathological states (*41*, *77*). In many of these studies, where consciousness was unimpaired, this assumption and the conclusions based upon it are now known to have been valid; in other conditions, especially of intracranial disease and coma (*77*), the inferences were misleading. In 1933, F. A. Gibbs (*16*) devised an ingenious technique based upon a heated thermocouple which could be inserted into the internal jugular in the form of a needle and by means of which it was possible to measure directional changes in flow through that vessel.

Using the Monro-Kellie Principle, Ferris (*12*), in 1941, made measurements of the displacement of cerebrospinal fluid following occlusion of both internal jugular veins as an index of cerebral arterial inflow. The values obtained were quite low since it was not possible to occlude all of the venous return from the brain nor to prevent some of it from flowing into the rather distensible veins of the face and scalp.

The nitrous oxide technique was based upon the Fick Principle, but employed, instead of oxygen, an inert gas, the uptake of which by the brain would be less affected by functional state or disease and capable of estimation from simple physical principles:

"Unfortunately, the brain, unlike the kidney, does not specifically and selectively remove foreign substances from the blood and excrete them for accurate measurement. Furthermore, although it does consume large quantities of oxygen, that consumption cannot independently be measured or even assumed to be constant since it would be expected to vary with activity and disease. The brain does, however, absorb by physical solution an inert gas such as nitrous oxide, which reaches it by way of the arterial blood. It was hoped that the quantity of this gas absorbed by the brain would be independent of the state of mental activity and susceptible of measurement on the basis of physical solubility alone. If this were found to be the case, then the numerator of a Fick equation applied to the brain could be derived" (25).

That concept arose quite naturally. While serving as a research fellow in the laboratory of Joseph Aub, I participated in studies on experimental shock which employed the Fick Principle for measurement of cardiac output. During that period I had attended a symposium in which André Cournand and Dickinson Richards described the remarkable studies which they were making in clinical shock. I was impressed that these studies were more accurate, more relevant, and, because of the rigorous restrictions of clinical investigation, far more physiological than any which had been made in lower animals. When, two years later, I learned from Carl Schmidt the importance of the cerebral circulation and was given the opportunity to participate in some of the critical studies in the monkey, it was natural that there should have been a motivation to attempt measurements in man and that the Fick Principle should have been chosen as the first point of departure.

Preliminary studies in the dog confirmed the hope that nitrous oxide would be taken up rapidly and in appreciable quantities by the brain with the attainment of satisfactory equilibrium between it and cerebral venous blood in a reasonable time, and experiments in the monkey demonstrated a satisfactory agreement between values calculated from the theory and those directly measured (34).

In July of 1944, the first studies of cerebral blood flow using the newly developed technique were performed in man (34), and after some of the assumptions had been validated (65) and the solubility con-

SPECIAL CIRCULATIONS

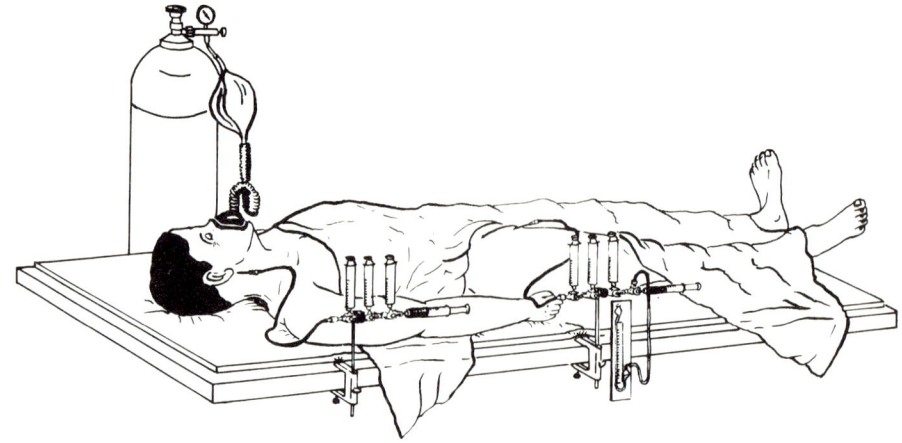

Figure 15. Measurement of cerebral blood flow in man by nitrous oxide technique.

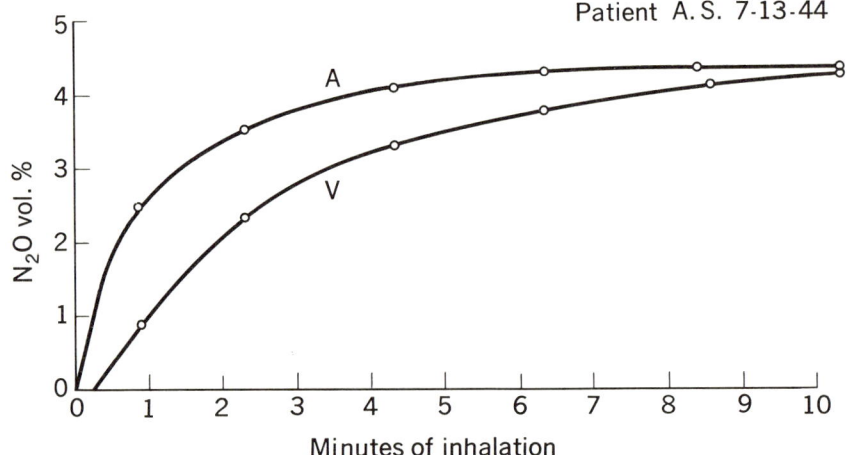

Figure 16. Curves obtained in the first study with the nitrous oxide method in man, July 13, 1944, in a patient with hypertension. The value for cerebral blood flow is 57.5 ml./100 gm./min.

stant of the gas in brain more precisely evaluated (*31*), a more definitive description of the technique appeared in 1948 (*36*). The nitrous oxide technique, or some modification of it (*58*, *39*), was quickly adopted by a number of investigators throughout the world and employed for the study of the human cerebral circulation under physiological conditions and in disease (*29*, *38*), and for the evaluation of the effects of a large number of drugs (*68*).

In 1947, F. A. Gibbs and his associates applied the Stewart Principle of dye dilution to measurement of total intracranial blood flow (*17*), and some years later Nylin (*52*) used a similar principle, but adapted it to obtain greater precision. Methods based upon dye injection have not been employed extensively, perhaps because of the technical problems of making injections into the internal carotid arteries.

The nitrous oxide technique has two important limitations. Since it requires a period of at least ten minutes for each determination, it may be used only in steady states and not for the measurement of a rapidly changing blood flow. However, Lewis and his associates (*44*) have adapted the technique to continuous measurement by substituting the gamma-ray-emitting inert gas krypton, Kr^{79}. The second limitation is its ability to measure only the over-all circulation of the brain, rather than that of particular regions within it. Recently, by employing the same theory of inert gas exchange (*27*) which is the basis of the nitrous oxide technique, it has been possible to arrive at quantitative estimates of the circulation in as many as forty different regions of the brain of the unanesthetized cat (*33*).

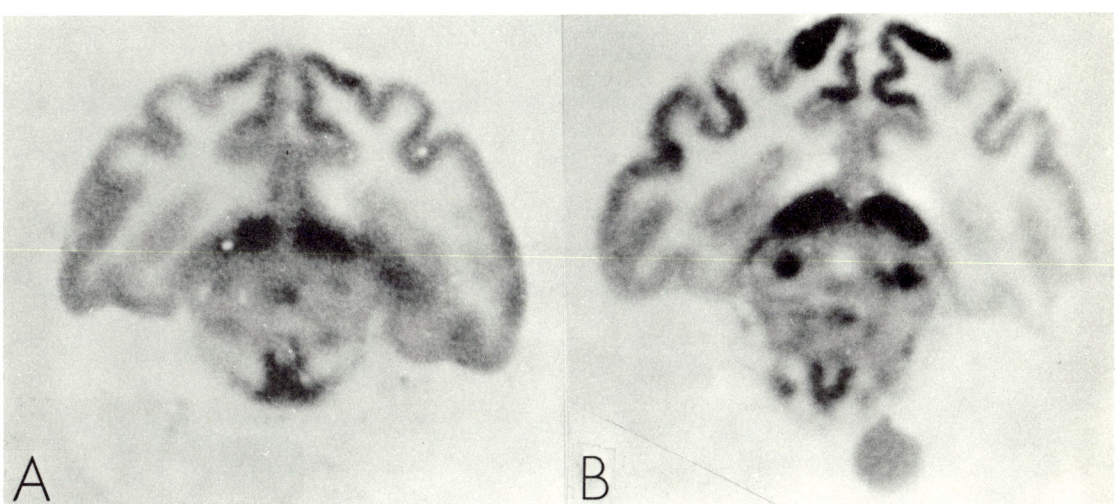

Figure 17. Autoradiogram showing the distribution of the gas $CF_3\ I^{131}$ in the cat brain used in measurement of local cerebral blood flow. Experiment A was performed in the dark, and Experiment B during photic stimulation; the effect of optical activity on the blood flow in the lateral geniculate and visual cortex is clearly evident.

SPECIAL CIRCULATIONS

Much of the information obtained from measurement of the cerebral circulation in man was new and unique, especially that obtained by studies on a large variety of clinical disorders, or on the effects of therapeutic doses of a large number of drugs (*68*). In the latter field especially, a number of older ideas had to be revised: substances like alcohol, nicotinic acid, histamine, aminophylline, and caffeine, which were formerly regarded as vasodilators in the cerebral circulation, were now found to have either no effect, or a complex and ambiguous one, or actually to exert an appreciable cerebral vasoconstrictor action in clinical studies.

Variations in Disease

The cerebral circulation was measured in a large number of clinical disorders (*26*), in many of which it was found to be a factor relevant to the disease process. It was found to be reduced in patients with increased intracranial pressure, in polycythemia, and in cerebral arteriosclerosis, and elevated in patients with severe anemia, thus confirming theories based upon post mortem findings or upon physical concepts. In essential hypertension, cerebral blood flow was found to be normal (*30*), so that a generalized cerebral ischemia, one of the theories invoked to explain the hypertension, was discounted. The value of efforts to reduce the blood pressure in this disorder was substantiated by demonstration (*32*) that the increased cerebrovascular tone could and would relax in response to a wide variety of surgical and pharmacological (*68*) therapies, and the cerebral circulation would be thus maintained in the face of a reduction in blood pressure to more nearly normal levels. Sleep was found to be associated with no reduction, and in fact a slight increase, in cerebral blood flow (*46*). This definitively invalidated the ischemic theory of sleep, which had had many proponents from the time of Alcmeon.

With respect to the regulation of the cerebral circulation, the studies in man further supported the importance of intrinsic factors, but in addition, because anesthesia and surgical interference no longer obscured the results, they permitted a new interpretation of the role of the blood pressure to emerge:

"*Studies in intact human beings have strengthened the concept that a normal arterial blood pressure is zealously maintained by numerous homeostatic mechanisms such as the carotid sinus reflex and central control of peripheral vascular tone; and that as long as the mean arterial blood pressure remains above a critical minimal level, cerebral blood flow is actually regulated intrinsically by changes in cerebrovascular resistance"* (*26*).

Just a few years before this information had become available, the importance of extracerebral mechanisms in the regulation of the cerebral circulation had been emphasized and it had been concluded that they were of greater significance than the cerebral vasomotor influences (*75*).

The more quantitative studies in man have also further characterized the factors responsible for this intrinsic control. Intracranial pressure, viscosity of the blood, and physical changes in the vessels themselves have been shown to be of some importance (*26*). One factor which remains unclear in its import is that of neurogenic control of cerebral vessels.

Neurogenic Control

As early as 1830, Brachet had demonstrated an engorgement of the superficial cerebral vessels following section of the cervical sympathetic chain (*45*), which was confirmed later by Nothnagel (*51*) and by Ackermann (*1*). Claude Bernard (*45*) described an increase in cortical temperature resulting from the same procedure, while, conversely, Donders (*9*) observed a constriction on pial vessels following stimulation of the sympathetic innervation of the head. Roy and Sherrington (*55*) obtained inconstant effects from section or stimulation of the vagus in the rabbit or the vagosympathetic trunk in the dog, which appeared to follow changes in arterial or central venous pressure, and concluded that there was no reason for believing that vasomotor nerves for the brain were to be found in the nerves of the neck. Hill (*20*) also concluded that there was "no evidence whatever of . . . the existence of any vasomotor nerves supplying the brain."

In 1938, Forbes and Cobb (*14*) summarized the work of the intervening fifty years:

"During the past few years, however, workers in different laboratories, using different experimental methods, have obtained convincing evidence that in animals cerebral vasoconstrictor nerves do exist, but that they exert slight influence on arterial caliber or on cerebral blood flow compared with the effect

SPECIAL CIRCULATIONS

of constrictor nerves in other organs. . . . A vasodilator mechanism has also been described. Furthermore, improved histological methods have demonstrated beyond question the presence of nerve fibres—myelinated and nonmyelinated—on the cerebral vessels and meninges both in animals and in man."

In formulating this concept they referred to work in their own laboratory which employed direct visualization (14), Schmidt's thermoelectric measurements in various parts of the brain (59, 61, 62), and those of Bouckaert and Jourdan with the perfused, isolated brain (14), all of which confirmed the occurrence of a slight cerebral vasoconstriction following stimulation of the cervical sympathetics. Evidence for a vasodilator innervation was obtained jointly by Cobb, Finesinger, Chorobski, and Penfield, and was traced by the latter two from the facial nerve through the geniculate ganglion and the greater superficial petrosal nerve to the carotid plexus (5). Penfield, in 1932, had demonstrated unmyelinated nerve fibers on intracerebral blood vessels in the cat, dog, monkey, and man (14).

It is one thing to establish the existence of intracranial vascular nerves, capable of constricting or dilating cerebral vessels, but quite another to demonstrate their physiological function. Studies in man have failed to reveal any generalized tonic effect exerted by the cervical sympathetics on cerebral vascular tone (18) except, possibly, in pathological states (45), and the role of neurogenic influences on the normal cerebral vessels remains obscure.

Carbon dioxide, on the other hand, and oxygen, perhaps to a lesser extent, have been shown by studies in man (35, 41) to occupy the prominent place which many previous workers, beginning with Roy and Sherrington, had assigned to them. These studies have given further support to the theory that the concentration of one or both of these metabolic gases is the mechanism whereby blood flow was adapted to metabolic and functional demand locally and generally in the brain (68).

Cerebral Metabolism

One very important advantage derived from quantitative measurement of cerebral blood flow was the opportunity it provided for calculation of the rate of oxygen utilization and energy exchange in the brain.

This function has had a long and interesting history in philosophical and physiological speculation. After Lavoisier's demonstration that living organisms did not contradict the law of the conservation of matter, physiology became considerably more materialistic and mechanistic. Debates between vitalists and mechanists marked this period, with names like Magendie, Helmholtz, and Claude Bernard on the side of mechanism. The last fortress of vitalism was the brain and the mental processes which took place there. This became the final battleground. Some appreciation of the feelings of that time may be gleaned from the lectures of Professor Lawrence, published in London in 1823 (*40*).

"... *sensation, perception, memory, judgment, reasoning, thought, in a word all the manifestations called mental or intellectual are the animal functions of their appropriate organic apparatus, the central organ of the nervous system.... In opposition to these views it has been contended that thought is not an act of the brain, but of an immaterial substance residing in or connected with it. This large and curious structure*, which in the human subject receives one-fifth of all the blood sent out from the heart, *which is so peculiarly and delicately organized, nicely enveloped in successive membranes and securely lodged in a solid bony case, is left almost without an office, being barely allowed to be capable of sensation. It has indeed the easiest lot in the animal economy; it is better fed, clothed and lodged than any other part and has less to do.*" [Emphasis added.]

The similarity to the Hippocratic discourse (p. 704) on the same theme is striking, but even more striking is the flat and quite accurate statement of the magnitude of the human cerebral circulation more than a hundred years before it is presumed to have been measured. Although the mechanists might postulate, as indeed they did, that thought was a chemical process which like all others conforms to the doctrine of the conservation of matter and energy, they were far from proving it, and a search for the "energy equivalent of thought" was vigorously pursued. Lombard, in 1866, and in the next twenty years, Schiff, Paul Bert, Corso, and Tanzi (*73*) measured the temperature of the head in man and demonstrated in an unconvincing manner that this temperature rose with mental work and heightened emotions, attributing this to an increased chemical activity of the brain. In 1892, Angelo Mosso (*49*)

SPECIAL CIRCULATIONS

reported more exact studies of the temperature of the brain itself in animals and man, measured by mercurial thermometers sensitive to 0.002°C. He found the cerebral temperature, which he interpreted as an index of cerebral metabolism, to fall in sleep and in narcosis and to rise considerably during convulsions or following the injection of stimulant drugs. In a conscious animal "great psychical activity" produced only a slight rise in temperature. He characterized the brain as the seat of great chemical activity:

"Observations made while an animal is awake tend to show that the development of heat due to cerebral metabolism may be very considerable even in the absence of all intense psychical activity. The mere maintenance of consciousness belonging to the wakeful state involves very considerable chemical action" (49).

Leonard Hill took issue with those conclusions and disproved them to his satisfaction by demonstrating that the arteriovenous difference for oxygen and carbon dioxide was smaller for cerebral venous blood than it was for blood from the femoral vein: "The results of a long series of experiments showed us that the brain is not a seat of active combustion. The combustion of muscles is vastly greater than that of the brain, both in rest and in spasm" (20). Although he was careful to point out that the error involved in the gas analyses was of the order of 1 per cent, he neglected to measure the blood flow, which, of course, explains his erroneous conclusion.

Twenty years after Mosso predicted a high metabolic activity in the brain on the basis of its temperature, the first measurement of its oxygen utilization in vivo was attempted. Alexander and Cserna obtained a value of 13 ml. for the cerebral oxygen consumption (per 100 gm. of brain per minute) in the dog. Succeeding investigators reported similar values: 11 ml. by Handley, 10 ml. by Gayda and by Rein, 7.5 ml. by Schmidt, and 6.6 ml. by Hou, in the same species (63). Since the necessary precautions to prevent the inclusion of extracerebral circulation in the measurement of the cerebral blood flow were not always taken, these values are erroneously high.

In 1945, using the monkey in order to avoid that difficulty, Schmidt and his associates (63) obtained a value of 3.7 ml. per 100 gm. per minute for cerebral oxygen consumption in lightly anesthetized animals.

This value fell in deeper anesthesia and doubled during convulsions.

The nitrous oxide method made possible the calculation of the oxygen consumption of the human brain in various states of functional activity and, more than a century after the question was first posed, a measure of the energy equivalent of the thought process, whatever meaning might be attached to it. The normal, conscious human brain was found to consume oxygen at a rate of approximately 3.5 ml. per 100 gm. per minute, equivalent to an energy utilization of 20 watts (*28*), and approximately one-fifth of the resting oxygen utilization of the whole body. One very interesting finding of two independent groups (*72, 57*) was that the brain does not participate in the generalized increase in oxygen consumption which is characteristic of hyperthyroidism. On the basis of this finding, Sokoloff developed his important concept of the physiological action of thyroxin on protein synthesis (*69*).

When consciousness was impaired by some generalized metabolic disturbance, such as insulin hypoglycemia or diabetic acidosis, cerebral oxygen utilization fell, and in deep anesthesia or coma of various types it remained at approximately half of the normal value (*28*). It appeared that in these states, at least, the new findings on the brain supported Barcroft's conclusion: "There is no instance in which it can be proved that an organ increases its activity under physiological conditions without also increasing its call for oxygen" (*3*).

An interdependence between functional activity, metabolism, and blood flow had been postulated for the brain since the time of Roy and Sherrington, although it was many years before any experimental evidence was adduced to support it. Alexander and Révész (*2*), in 1912, found some evidence for increased metabolism in response to optical stimulation, and in 1927, Cobb and Talbott (*8*) reported an increase in the vascularity of the olfactory bulbs of cats exposed to ammonia. Schmidt and Hendrix (*62*), and later Serota and Gerard (*64*), using thermoelectric probes inserted into the brain, found evidence for increased blood flow or metabolism in appropriate areas after stimulation of various sensory pathways. Quite recently, Sokoloff and his associates (*67*) obtained quantitative evidence for an increase in blood flow in the visual cortex and lateral geniculate body in unanesthetized cats after prolonged photic stimulation. In man, Penfield and his associates (*53*) found evidence of localized increase in circulation following electrical stimulation of the cerebral cortex.

Relation to Mental Function

SPECIAL CIRCULATIONS

With the application of more quantitative studies in man, however, it soon became evident that the complexities of mental function were not always correlated with the over-all energy exchange of the brain. Neither hyperventilation nor moderate hypoxia produced a detectable decrease in cerebral oxygen utilization, even though both were accompanied by definite mental changes. This led to the conclusion that "the higher psychic functions are associated with biochemical changes so subtle and complex as to render any attempt to describe them in terms of mere oxygen utilization no more adequate than to predict the fidelity of a radio by its power requirements" (*35*). Many examples were found in the next few years to reinforce the truth of that statement.

In 1948, it was found that the cerebral circulation and oxygen consumption in schizophrenia (*37*) was not different from normal and that barbiturate semi-narcosis, which produced marked mental and behavioral change in such patients, was associated with no change in those functions. A few years later, Mangold and his associates (*46*) demonstrated that sleep, as opposed to anesthesia, was accompanied by no measurable decline in cerebral utilization of oxygen, and thus made untenable those theories attributing sleep to the action of some endogenous narcotic substance. In 1955, Sokoloff, et al. (*70*) found that the performance of mental arithmetic did not increase the energy exchange of the brain, and two years later (*71*), found that this function was also unaltered during the action of a psychotomimetic drug.

Although it is reasonable to postulate that such mental alterations as are listed above are the reflections of highly localized but significant changes in oxygen metabolism within the brain, it is also useful to reflect upon the concept of the early mechanisms of the "energy equivalent of thought," and whether a relationship which may be expected to exist between energy expenditures and the mechanical or osmotic work of other organs has any meaning with respect to the higher functions of the brain, where "important defects ... may surely lie beyond oxidation, or, indeed, beyond biochemistry. For the brain is neither a pump nor a motor; its current counterparts seem to be instruments of computation and communication. In such an instrument, although a defective power supply will produce dysfunction, meaningfulness of content and accuracy are by no means always correlated with the power used" (*28*).

The concepts regarding the cerebral circulation are today, as they were two thousand years ago, inextricably bound up with the functions of the brain and the mysteries of the mind. In that time, much has been learned about the vessels of the brain—their anatomical disposition, their nerve supply, and their ability to react to a large number of stimuli. That ability forms the basis for the intrinsic regulation of the cerebral circulation, first postulated in 1890, then vigorously denied, and now held to be its most important determinant. The physiological and pharmacological aspects of the cerebral circulation have been considerably clarified in the past decade by studies in man; in fact, it may be said that more basic information has been obtained in this field by means of clinical studies than was ever possible with experiments in lower animals. Knowledge of the cerebral circulation in human disease and in relation to states of consciousness and mental activity has in some cases led to a better understanding of fundamental mechanisms; in many instances, however, this knowledge has led to a greater awareness of the complexities of the brain.

BIBLIOGRAPHY

1. ACKERMANN, T. Untersuchungen über den Einfluss der Erstickung auf die Menge des Blutes im Gehirn und in den Lungen. Virchow's Arch. path. Anat., 15:401, 1858.
2. ALEXANDER, F. G., and G. RÉVÉSZ. Über den Einfluss optischer Reize auf den Gaswechsel des Gehirns. Biochem. Z., 44:95, 1912.
3. BARCROFT, J. The Respiratory Function of the Blood. Cambridge, Cambridge University Press, 1914.
4. BURROWS, G. On Disorders of the Cerebral Circulation and on the Connection between Affections of the Brain and Diseases of the Heart. London, Longman Brown, Green and Longmans, 1846.

SPECIAL CIRCULATIONS

5. CHOROBSKI, J., and W. PENFIELD. Cerebral vasodilator nerves and their pathway from the medulla oblongata. Arch. Neurol. Psychiat. (Chicago), 28:1257, 1932.
6. CHOULANT, L. Geschichte und Bibliographie der anatomischen Abbildung. Leipzig, Weigel, 1852.
7. COBB, S. Cerebral circulation. A critical discussion of the symposium. Proc. Ass. Res. nerv. ment. Dis., 18:719, 1938.
8. COBB, S., and J. H. TALBOTT. Studies in cerebral circulation. II. A quantitative study of cerebral capillaries. Trans. Ass. Amer. Phys., 42:255, 1927.
9. DONDERS, F. C. Die Bewegung des Gehirns und die Veränderungen der Gefässfüllung der Pia mater, auch bei geschlossenem, unausdehnbarem Schädel unmittelbar beobachtet. Nederl. Lancet, 1850. Abstr. in Schmidts Jb. ges. Med., 69:16, 1851.
10. DUMKE, P. R., and C. F. SCHMIDT. Quantitative measurements of cerebral blood flow in the macacque monkey. Amer. J. Physiol., 138: 421, 1943.
11. EDWIN SMITH SURGICAL PAPYRUS. Tr. by J. H. Breasted. Chicago, University of Chicago Press, 1930.
12. FERRIS, E. B., JR. Objective measurement of relative intracranial blood flow in man. Arch. Neurol. Psychiat. (Chicago), 46:377, 1941.
13. FORBES, H. S. The cerebral circulation. I. Observation and measurement of pial vessels. Arch. Neurol. Psychiat. (Chicago), 19:751, 1928.
14. FORBES, H. S., and S. COBB. Vasomotor control of cerebral vessels. Proc. Ass. Res. nerv. ment. Dis., 18:201–217, 1938.
15. GÄRTNER, G., and J. WAGNER. Ueber den Hirnkreislauf. Wien. med. Wschr., 37:601, 640, 1887.
16. GIBBS, F. A. A thermoelectric blood flow recorder in the form of a needle. Proc. Soc. exp. Biol. (N.Y.), 31:141, 1933.
17. GIBBS, F. A., H. MAXWELL, and E. L. GIBBS. Volume flow of blood through the human brain. Arch. Neurol. Psychiat. (Chicago), 57:137, 1947.
18. HARMEL, M. H., J. H. HAFKENSCHIEL, G. M. AUSTIN, C. W. CRUMPTON, and S. S. KETY. The effect of bilateral stellate ganglion block on the cerebral circulation in normotensive and hypertensive patients. J. clin. Invest., 28:415, 1949.
19. HARVEY, W. Exercitatio anatomica de motu cordis et sanguinis in animalibus. Movement of the Heart and Blood in Animals. An Anatomical Essay. Tr. by K. J. Franklin. Oxford, Blackwell, 1957.
20. HILL, L. The Physiology and Pathology of the Cerebral Circulation; An Experimental Research. London, Churchill, 1896.
21. HIPPOCRATES. On the Sacred Disease. Tr. by F. Adams. In The Genuine Works of Hippocrates, Vol. II. New York, Wood, 1886.

22. JENSEN, P. Über die Blutversorgung des Gehirns. Pflügers Arch. ges. Physiol., 103:171, 1904.
23. KELLIE, G. Transactions of the Med. Chir. Soc., Edinburgh, I, 84 and 123, 1824 (cited by L. Hill, see ref. 20).
24. KETY, S. S. Quantitative determination of cerebral blood flow in man. Methods in Medical Research, 1:201, 1948.
25. KETY, S. S. Blood flow and metabolism of the human brain in health and disease. Trans. Stud. Coll. Phys. Philad., 18:103, 1950.
26. KETY, S. S. Circulation and metabolism of the human brain in health and disease. Amer. J. Med., 8:205, 1950.
27. KETY, S. S. The theory and applications of the exchange of inert gas at the lungs and tissues. Pharmacol. Rev., 3:1-41, 1951.
28. KETY, S. S. General Metabolism of the Brain *in vivo*. In D. Richter, Ed. International Neurochemical Symposium, 2nd. Metabolism of the Nervous System. London, Pergamon, 1957.
29. KETY, S. S. The Physiology of the Cerebral Circulation in Man. In J. McMichael, Ed. Circulation; Proceedings of the Harvey Tercentenary Congress. Oxford, Blackwell, 1958.
30. KETY, S. S., J. H. HAFKENSCHIEL, W. A. JEFFERS, I. H. LEOPOLD, and H. A. SHENKIN. The blood flow, vascular resistance, and oxygen consumption of the brain in essential hypertension. J. clin. Invest., 27:511, 1948.
31. KETY, S. S., M. H. HARMEL, H. T. BROOMELL, and C. B. RHODE. The solubility of nitrous oxide in blood and brain. J. biol. Chem., 173:487, 1948.
32. KETY, S. S., B. D. KING, S. M. HORVATH, W. A. JEFFERS, and J. H. HAFKENSCHIEL. The effects of an acute reduction in blood pressure by means of differential spinal sympathetic block on the cerebral circulation of hypertensive patients. J. clin. Invest., 29:402, 1950.
33. KETY, S. S., W. M. LANDAU, W. H. FREYGANG, JR., L. P. ROWLAND, and L. SOKOLOFF. Estimation of regional circulation in the brain by the uptake of an inert gas. Fed. Proc., 14:85, 1955.
34. KETY, S. S., and C. F. SCHMIDT. The determination of cerebral blood flow in man by the use of nitrous oxide in low concentrations. Amer. J. Physiol., 143:53, 1945.
35. KETY, S. S., and C. F. SCHMIDT. The effects of altered arterial tensions of carbon dioxide and oxygen on cerebral blood flow and cerebral oxygen consumption of normal young men. J. clin. Invest., 27:484, 1948.
36. KETY, S. S., and C. F. SCHMIDT. The nitrous oxide method for the quantitative determination of cerebral blood flow in man: Theory, procedure and normal values. J. clin. Invest., 27:476, 1948.

SPECIAL CIRCULATIONS

37. KETY, S. S., R. B. WOODFORD, M. H. HARMEL, F. A. FREYHAN, K. E. APPEL, and C. F. SCHMIDT. Cerebral blood flow and metabolism in schizophrenia. The effects of barbiturate semi-narcosis, insulin coma and electroshock. Amer. J. Psychiat., 104:765, 1948.
38. LASSEN, N. A. Cerebral blood flow and oxygen consumption in man. Physiol. Rev., 39:183, 1959.
39. LASSEN, N. A., and O. MUNCK. The cerebral blood flow in man determined by the use of radioactive krypton. Acta physiol. scand., 33:30, 1955.
40. LAWRENCE, W. Lectures on Comparative Anatomy, Physiology and Zoology. London, Smith, 1823.
41. LENNOX, W. G., and E. L. GIBBS. The blood flow in the brain and the leg of man, and the changes induced by alteration of blood gases. J. clin. Invest., 11:1155, 1932.
42. LEONARDO DA VINCI. I. Manoscritti di Leonardo da Vinci della Reale Biblioteca di Windsor: Dell'-Anatomia Fogli B. Torino, Roux, 1901.
43. LEONARDO DA VINCI. The Notebooks. Tr. by MacCurdy. New York, Braziller, 1956.
44. LEWIS, B. M., L. SOKOLOFF, R. L. WECHSLER, W. B. WENTZ, and S. S. KETY. A method for the continuous measurement of cerebral blood flow in man by means of radioactive krypton (Kr^{79}). J. clin. Invest., 39:707, 1960.
45. LINDÉN, L. The effect of stellate ganglion block on cerebral circulation in cerebrovascular accidents. Acta med. scand., suppl. 301, 1955.
46. MANGOLD, R., L. SOKOLOFF, E. CONNOR, J. KLEINERMAN, P. O. G. THERMAN, and S. S. KETY. The effects of sleep and lack of sleep on the cerebral circulation and metabolism of normal young men. J. clin. Invest., 34:1092, 1955.
47. MONRO, A. Observations of the Structure and Functions of the Nervous System. Edinburgh, Creech, 1783.
48. MOSSO, A. Ueber den Kreislauf des Blutes im menschlichen Gehirn. Leipzig, Viet, 1881.
49. MOSSO, A. The temperature of the brain, especially in relation to psychical activity. Proc. roy. Soc. (Lond.), 51:83–85, 1892.
50. MYERSON, A., R. D. HALLORAN, and H. L. HIRSCH. Technic for obtaining blood from the internal jugular vein and internal carotid artery. Arch. Neurol. Psychiat. (Chicago), 17:807, 1927.
51. NOTHNAGEL, H. Die vasomotorischen Nerven der Gehirngefässe. Virchows Arch. path. Anat., 40:203, 1867.
52. NYLIN, G., and S. HEDLUND. Blood Flow and Pool in Heart, Lungs and Brain. In J. McMichael, Ed. Circulation; Proceedings of the Harvey Tercentenary Congress. Oxford, Blackwell, 1958.

53. PENFIELD, W., K. v. SANTHA, and A. CIPRIANI. Cerebral blood flow during induced epileptiform seizures in animals and man. J. Neurophysiol., 2:257, 1939.
54. RASMUSSEN, A. T. Some Trends in Neuroanatomy. Dubuque, Iowa, Brown, 1947.
55. ROY, C. S., and C. S. SHERRINGTON. On the regulation of the blood supply of the brain. J. Physiol. (Lond.), 11:85, 1890.
56. SARTON, G. A History of Science; vol. 1, Ancient Science Through the Golden Age of Greece. Cambridge, Mass., Harvard University Press, 1952.
57. SCHEINBERG, P. Cerebral circulation and metabolism in hyperthyroidism. J. clin. Invest., 29:1010, 1950.
58. SCHEINBERG, P., and E. A. STEAD, JR. The cerebral blood flow in male subjects as measured by the nitrous oxide technique. Normal values for blood flow, oxygen utilization, glucose utilization, and peripheral resistance, with observations on the effect of tilting and anxiety. J. clin. Invest., 28:1163, 1949.
59. SCHMIDT, C. F. The intrinsic regulation of the circulation in the hypothalamus of the cat. Amer. J. Physiol., 110:137, 1934.
60. SCHMIDT, C. F. The present status of knowledge concerning the intrinsic control of the cerebral circulation and the effects of functional derangements in it. Fed. Proc., 3:131, 1944.
61. SCHMIDT, C. F. The Cerebral Circulation in Health and Disease. Springfield, Ill., Thomas, 1950.
62. SCHMIDT, C. F., and J. P. HENDRIX. The action of chemical substances on cerebral blood-vessels. Proc. Ass. Res. nerv. ment. Dis., 18:229–276, 1937.
63. SCHMIDT, C. F., S. S. KETY, and H. H. PENNES. The gaseous metabolism of the brain of the monkey. Amer. J. Physiol., 143:33, 1945.
64. SEROTA, H. M., and R. W. GERARD. Localized thermal changes in cat's brain. J. Neurophysiol., 1:115, 1938.
65. SHENKIN, H. A., M. H. HARMEL, and S. S. KETY. Dynamic anatomy of the cerebral circulation. Arch. Neurol. Psychiat. (Chicago), 60:240, 1948.
66. SINGER, C. A Short History of Anatomy from the Greeks to Harvey. 2nd ed. New York, Dover, 1957.
67. SOKOLOFF, L. Local blood flow in neural tissue. In W. F. Windle, Ed. (National Multiple Sclerosis Society) New Research Techniques of Neuroanatomy. Springfield, Ill., Thomas, 1957.
68. SOKOLOFF, L. The action of drugs on the cerebral circulation. Pharmacol. Rev., 11:1, 1959.
69. SOKOLOFF, L., and S. KAUFMAN. Effects of thyroxin on amino acid incorporation into protein. Science, 129:569, 1959.

SPECIAL CIRCULATIONS

70. SOKOLOFF, L., R. MANGOLD, R. L. WECHSLER, C. KENNEDY, and S. S. KETY. The effect of mental arithmetic on cerebral circulation and metabolism. J. clin. Invest., 34:1101, 1955.
71. SOKOLOFF, L., S. PERLIN, C. KORNETSKY, and S. S. KETY. The effects of d-lysergic acid diethylamide on cerebral circulation and over-all metabolism. Ann. N.Y. Acad. Sci., 66:468, 1957.
72. SOKOLOFF, L., R. L. WECHSLER, R. MANGOLD, K. BALLS, and S. S. KETY. Cerebral blood flow and oxygen consumption in hyperthyroidism before and after treatment. J. clin. Invest., 32:202, 1953.
73. SOURY, J. Le Système nerveux central, structure et fonctions. Paris, Carré et Naud, 1899.
74. VESALIUS, A. De humani corporis fabrica, liber VII. Tr. by C. Singer. In Vesalius on the Human Brain. London, Oxford University Press, 1952.
75. WEISS, S. The regulation and disturbance of the cerebral circulation through extracerebral mechanisms. Proc. Ass. Res. nerv. ment. Dis., 18:571, 1938.
76. WHITTERIDGE, G. De motu locali animalium, 1627. In J. McMichael, Ed. Circulation, Proceedings of the Harvey Tercentenary Congress. Oxford, Blackwell, 1958.
77. WILLIAMS, D., and W. G. LENNOX. The cerebral blood-flow in arterial hypertension, arteriosclerosis and high intracranial pressure. Quart. J. Med., N.S. 8:185, 1939.
78. WILLIS, T. Cerebri anatome nervorumque descriptio et usus. Geneva, Samuel de Tournes, 1676.
79. WILLIS, T. Practice of Physik, 1684. Quoted by L. Rogers. The Function of the Circulus Arteriosus of Willis. Brain, 70:172, 1947.
80. WOLFF, H. G. The cerebral circulation. Physiol. Rev., 16:545, 1936.

XII

Physiological Changes in the Circulation after Birth

THE purpose of this essay is to bring together some of the evidence which has accumulated and the theories which have been discussed over the last few centuries as to the nature of the changes in the circulation after birth. The evidence is lopsided, first, because so much of the experimental work is very recent (and therefore probably ill-digested), and second, because, although a good deal is known about the fetal and newborn lamb, little is known about other species. The use of the lamb for such studies is traditional. Fabricius (*91*) wrote that he had provided a precise anatomical description of the fetus of the lamb because the fetal lamb, as well as the fetal ox, had been singled out for description by the ancients; a fetal or newborn lamb was, no doubt, as easily come by in sixteenth century Padua as elsewhere today, and is of a size such that dissection and experiment are not difficult. So far as the relatively few observations on the human infant are concerned, it would appear that the changes in its circulation after birth are not unlike those in the lamb.

The Course of the Circulation in the Fetus

For a proper understanding of the changes in the circulation at birth, we need to know not only the course of the circulation in the mammalian fetus (Fig. 1), but also the magnitude of the volume of blood flow through the fetus and its constituent parts (Fig. 2), and the physiological conditions under which the fetus lives. Until thirty years ago few direct observations had been made upon the living mammalian fetus, either *in utero* or after delivery by Caesarean section. There were, however, several theories as to the course of the circulation in the fetus,

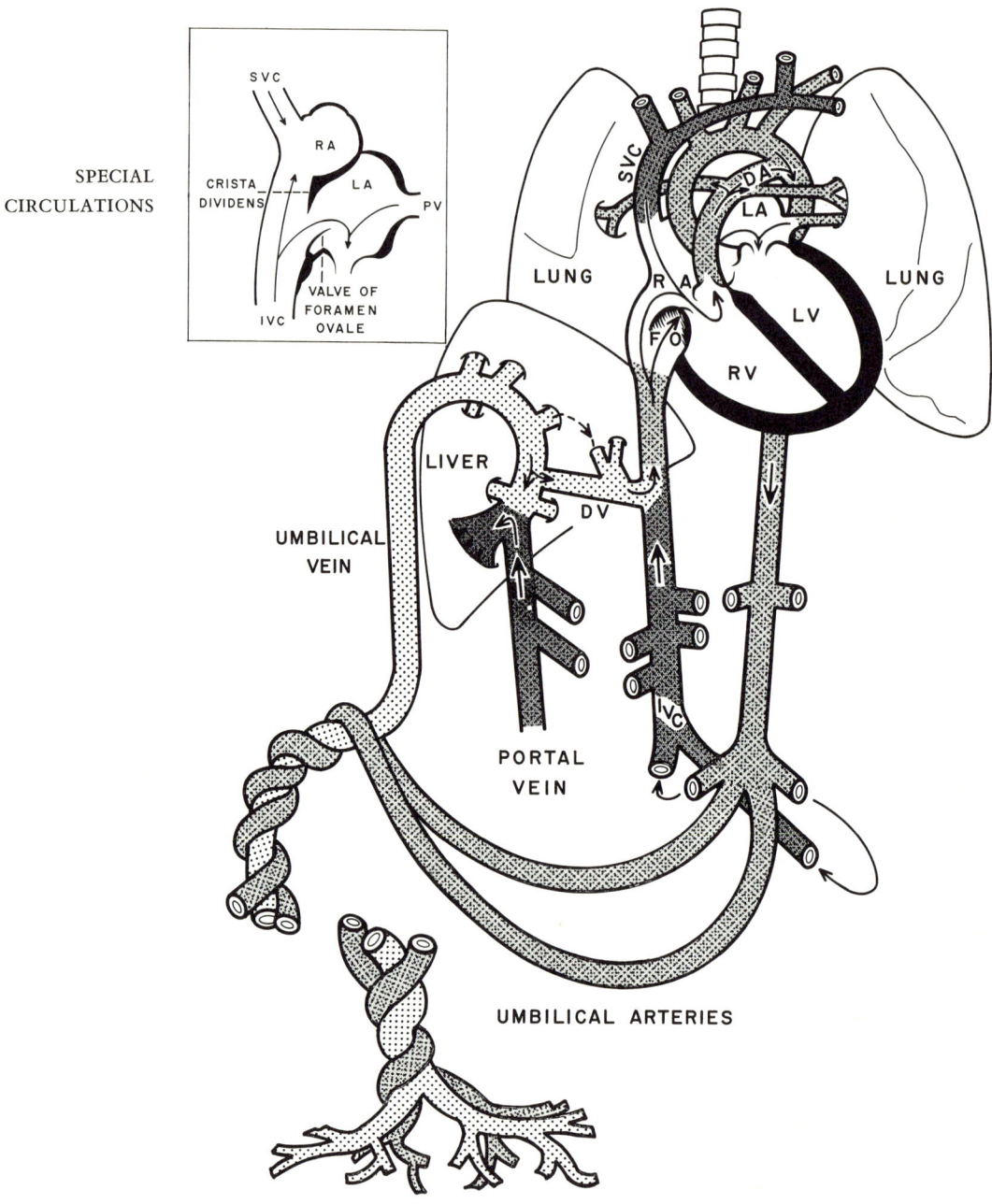

Figure 1. The fetal circulation. The inset shows in greater detail the entry of the great veins into the heart.

based upon anatomical considerations. Both Aranzi (9) and Harvey (114) were aware that the uterine (maternal) and umbilical (fetal) blood vessels were not directly connected with one another in the placenta. Moreover, once Harvey had established the fact that the blood circulated, it became evident that the two great fetal channels, the foramen ovale and the ductus arteriosus, enabled the two ventricles of the heart to work in parallel, pumping the blood from the great veins to the arteries. It was equally evident that some of the arterial blood passed to the fetal tissues and the remainder to the placenta, where it was in some way rejuvenated or refreshed, since once the umbilical cord was tied the fetus could not long survive without breathing. But the details of how the blood circu-

CHANGES IN
CIRCULATION
AFTER BIRTH

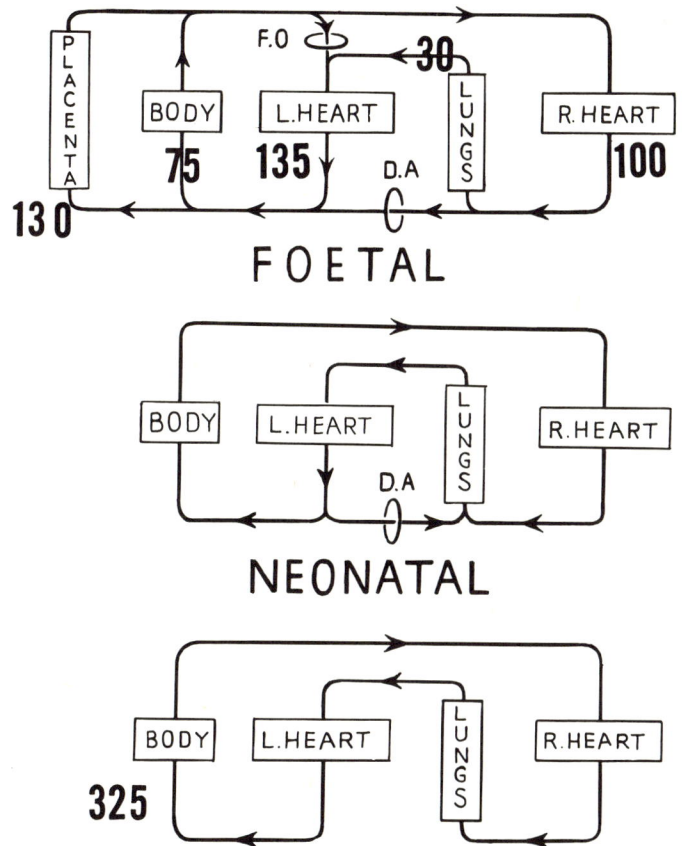

Figure 2. Schematic representation of the principal changes in the circulation at birth. The numerals represent the volume of blood flow, in ml./kg./min., through the great vessels.

SPECIAL
CIRCULATIONS

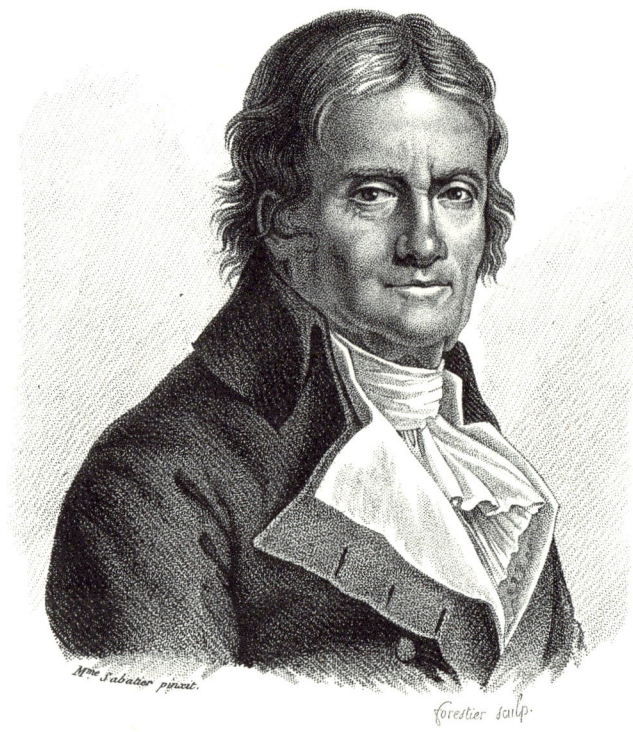

Figure 3. Raphael Bienvenu Sabatier (1732–1811).

lated, of how much mixing of the various blood streams occurred within the heart and great vessels, and of the physiological control of the fetal circulation, were all unknown. Hypotheses there were in abundance, but they varied in repute with the reputation of their protagonists, since no experimental method of testing their validity was available. This is in no wise to diminish the importance of the era of anatomizing, for it was the speculation of this period which prompted the first physiological investigations.

These investigations were designed to illuminate two problems. The first was concerned with how the blood gases crossed the placental barrier, and with measurement of the oxygen and carbon dioxide contents of the fetal blood. The second related to the conflicting hypotheses as to the course of the circulation in the fetus. In 1774 Sabatier (Fig. 3) had presented to the Académie Royale des Sciences in Paris a memoir which was destined to have a powerful influence on subsequent thought (*173*). His view was that all the blood returning from the placenta up the inferior vena cava entered the left atrium by way of the foramen ovale (Fig. 4). Thence it passed into the ascending aorta and the vessels supplying the head and upper limbs. Venous blood returning from the superior vena cava entered the right atrium, and passed through the ductus arteriosus and descending aorta to the placenta. The fetal circulation was thus considered to be a figure-of-eight. "Cette mécanique si simple, et que je crois n'avoir été connue de personne, fait que le sang qui a circulé dans le placenta, ne lui est rapporté que lorsqu'il a parcouru toutes les parties du corps du foetus." This is a classical example of a teleological argument. Sabatier's hypothesis derived from a study of the Eustachian valve, a membranous structure lying at the upper end of the inferior vena cava adjacent to the right atrium. Sabatier believed that the Eustachian valve prevented the blood ascending the inferior vena cava from

CHANGES IN CIRCULATION AFTER BIRTH

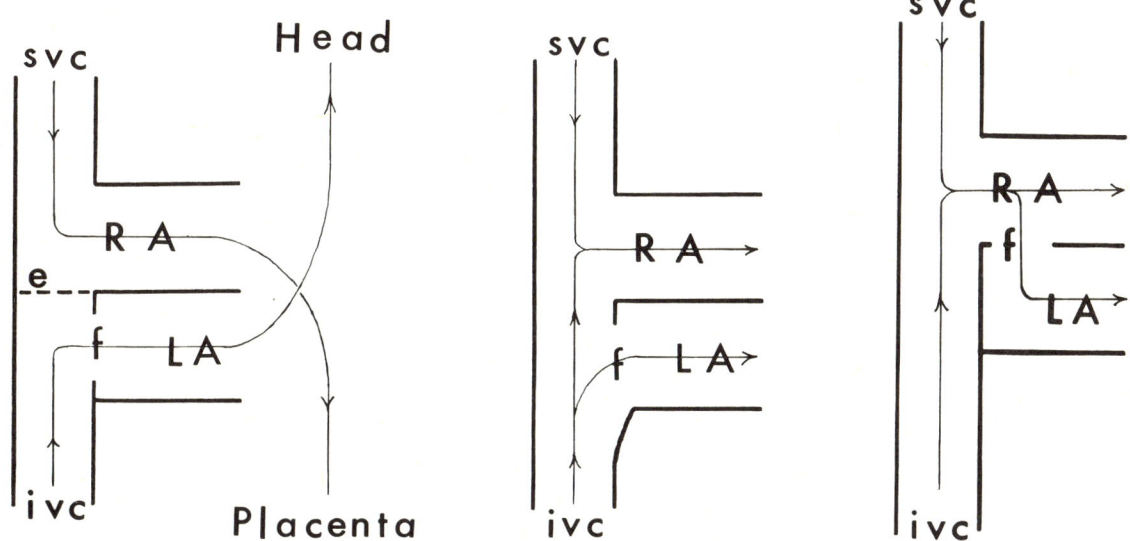

Figure 4. Schematic representations of the entry of the great veins into the heart.

Left: Based on Sabatier, showing the foramen ovale (f) and the Eustachian valve (e). *Middle:* Based on Wolff and Kilian, showing the foramen ovale (f). *Right:* Based on Pohlman, showing the foramen ovale (f) as lying between the two atria.

SPECIAL CIRCULATIONS

entering the right atrium and that it directed this blood into the left atrium through the foramen ovale. Now although the Eustachian valve is prominent in the human fetus, it is absent in many animals, and therefore his argument could not be of universal application. However, it was not the proposed function of the valve which gained such wide acceptance for Sabatier's views, so much as the ingenious and teleological figure-of-eight theory with its implication that the head and heart received purer blood than the rest of the fetus. This scheme was embraced by many subsequent writers. It was not accepted by Kilian (*138*), mainly as the result of a paper by Wolff (*201*). The latter had noted, as did Sabatier, that the two atria were *not* in direct communication with one another in the fetus; the upper part of the inferior vena cava lay between them and had independent openings into each. Wolff supposed that about two-thirds of inferior vena caval blood flow might enter the left atrium through the foramen ovale, the remainder entering the right atrium (Fig. 4). He did not believe that the Eustachian valve was an essential feature of the fetal circulation, and he clearly visualized mixing of two caval blood streams within the right atrium, although only inferior vena caval blood entered the left atrium.

Early in the twentieth century a third hypothesis was presented by Pohlman (*158, 159*). This concept was founded on the view, incorrectly attributed to Harvey and widely current in the early eighteenth century, that the right and left atria were directly joined by the foramen ovale in the fetus. After reviewing the literature, Pohlman wrote of Sabatier's conception of the fetal circulation ("the prevalent one at the time") that it was "physically impossible, morphologically inaccurate and developmentally unnecessary," and he concluded that experimental work must be undertaken. He chose the pig as a subject, and removed the uterus, with the fetuses it contained, from sows killed in the slaughterhouse. The umbilical circulation remained intact and the fetal hearts continued to beat for many hours, although since the uterine circulation was no longer present conditions were far from normal. Pohlman found that the pressures in the two ventricles were equal, and he studied the course of the circulation by injecting "corn-starch granules suspended in normal salt solution." The numbers of granules counted in samples of blood taken simultaneously from the two ventricles were found to be equal, whether the injection was made into the umbilical vein or into the superior vena cava. He concluded that the "blood of the two cavae mixed in the right auricle, and that mixed blood enters the foramen ovale" (Fig. 4).

Thus, by 1920 there were three quite distinct hypotheses as to the course of the circulation from the great veins into the atria of the fetus. None of the original papers was illustrated by diagrams of the course of the circulation, although Wolff published some rather complicated drawings of the fetal heart (Fig. 5) to show the relation of the foramen ovale to the left atrium and inferior vena cava. Even today textbooks of anatomy and physiology reflect the consequent confusion.

CHANGES IN CIRCULATION AFTER BIRTH

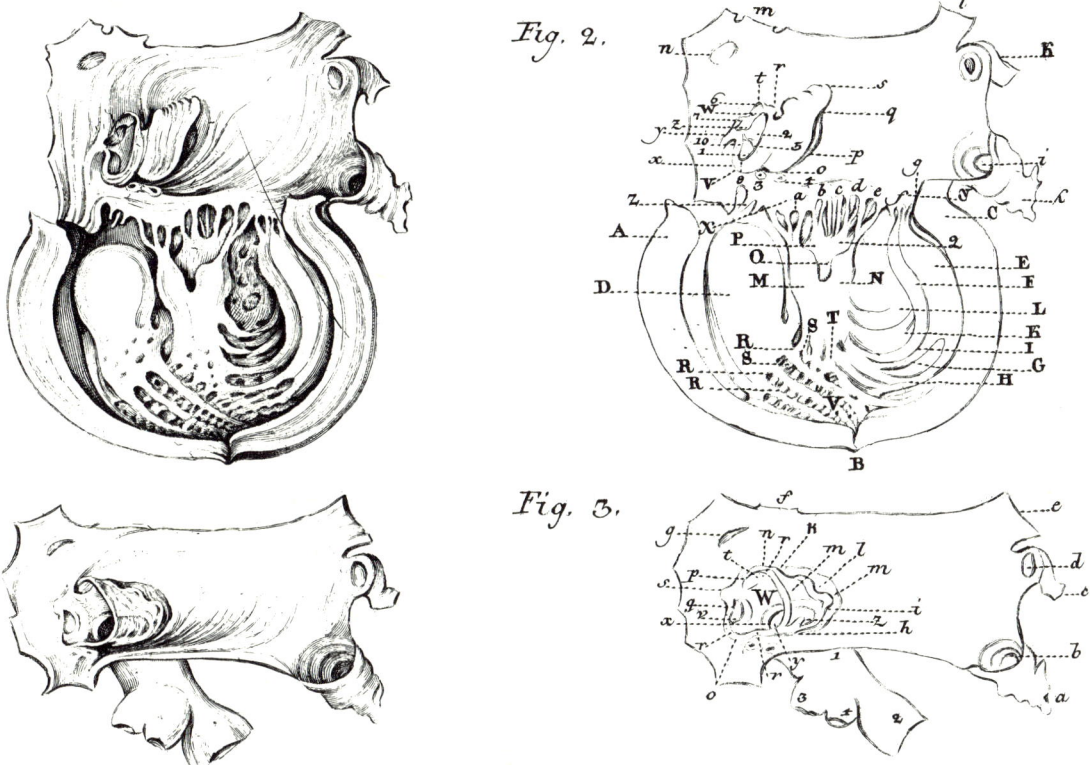

Figure 5. A diagram from Wolff (1776) of a human fetal heart. The upper figure shows the inside of the left atrium (with the valve of the foramen ovale) and ventricle. The lower figure shows the hepatic veins (1, 2, 3, 4) joining the inferior vena cava and the foramen ovale (w) leading thence into the cavity of the left atrium, which has been opened.

SPECIAL CIRCULATIONS

Sabatier's figure-of-eight scheme was thought to lead to a considerably greater oxygen content of the blood in the ascending aorta compared with that in the descending aorta (Fig. 4). Pohlman's scheme would lead to no difference between the two, while Kilian and Wolff's would lead to an intermediate condition.

Pohlman's work bridges the gap between the anatomical and experimental physiological periods. At first sight it belongs to the latter, and yet it really cannot be accepted as a serious attempt to discover what happens *in utero*. For that purpose it is essential to preserve, not only the umbilical circulation intact, but also the mother in as good a physiological condition as possible, so that placental function may be preserved. Since the cat and dog (to take two of the commoner laboratory animals) are rather small at birth, it was an obvious step to use the larger domestic animals. As early as 1884–8, Cohnstein and Zuntz had made some observations on fetal lambs (53, 54). However, it was not until 1927 that Huggett demonstrated that a fetal goat could be kept in reasonable physiological condition, still attached by the umbilical cord to its mother, after delivery by Caesarean section (122). This demonstration marked a great step forward. The essential point was that even after delivery of the fetus, and after rupture of the amniotic membranes, the uterus did not contract to such an extent that placental function was seriously impaired. The technique used by Huggett is of interest and importance, for it was followed closely by workers in this field for the next twenty years. The goat was anesthetized with urethane supplemented with ether and was placed in an old discarded domestic bathtub which had been filled with warm saline. The goat lay nearly supine, with its head just clear of the fluid. The fetus was delivered beneath the surface of the saline to mimic the intra-uterine environment as closely as possible. Huggett took samples of blood from the umbilical artery and vein and from the carotid artery. In six goats the mean O_2 saturation was 45 per cent in the umbilical vein, 33 per cent in the carotid artery, and 17 per cent in the umbilical artery (which is the same as that in the descending aorta). The CO_2 content of the umbilical arterial blood was greater than that of carotid arterial blood. This evidence supported what we may call, for the sake of simplicity, the Sabatier and the Kilian-Wolff hypotheses; it contradicted Pohlman's observations. Huggett also determined the O_2 and CO_2 dissociation curves of fetal blood and maternal blood, and hence calculated the diffusion gradient for these gases across the placenta. Working singlehanded he was at a disadvantage, and although he was aware that fetal blood is "highly active," he took no steps to inhibit metabolic activity during these estimations. Therefore, although he correctly concluded that there was a diffusion gradient across the placenta which is probably adequate to account for oxygen exchange, this conclusion was based on an erroneous fetal dissociation curve which suggested that the blood contained less oxygen than that of the mother at a given partial pressure. Within a few years others repeated these experiments on various species and came to the opposite (and correct) conclusion (*8, 21, 116*). It is now well established that the O_2 dissociation curve of the fetus usually lies substantially to the left of that of the mother. Nevertheless Huggett's work showed what could be done, and began the new era of experimental fetal physiology.

With the new methods it became possible to obtain other evidence on the distribution of blood flow through the fetal heart. Direct observation after opening the chest showed that the blood in the right atrium was darker than that in the left atrium in fetal guinea-pigs and kittens (*16, 200*). Previously, Kellogg had found that the oxygen content of blood samples withdrawn simultaneously from the right and left ventricles in fetal puppies was identical (*135*). These measurements seemed incompatible with the direct observations, but Barcroft pointed out that in Kellogg's experiments the O_2 content was very low (2.4 ml./100 ml., corresponding to an oxygen saturation of only about 10 per cent) (*18*). Kellogg's observations would therefore be consistent with almost complete cessation of umbilical blood flow, and no difference between the O_2 contents of blood from the two ventricles would then be expected. In the fetal lamb, as in the fetal goat (*122*), Barcroft, et al. found that the O_2 saturation of carotid blood was intermediate between that of the umbilical vein and the umbilical artery (*19*). This discovery provided further evidence against Pohlman's concept of blood mixing within the heart, but did not distinguish between the schemes put forward by Sabatier on the one hand and Wolff and Kilian on the other. For this purpose some new technique was necessary.

Even in the 1930's the true anatomical disposition of the two atria and the foramen ovale in the fetus was not generally appreciated, in spite of the beautiful illustrations of some of the earlier anatomists which

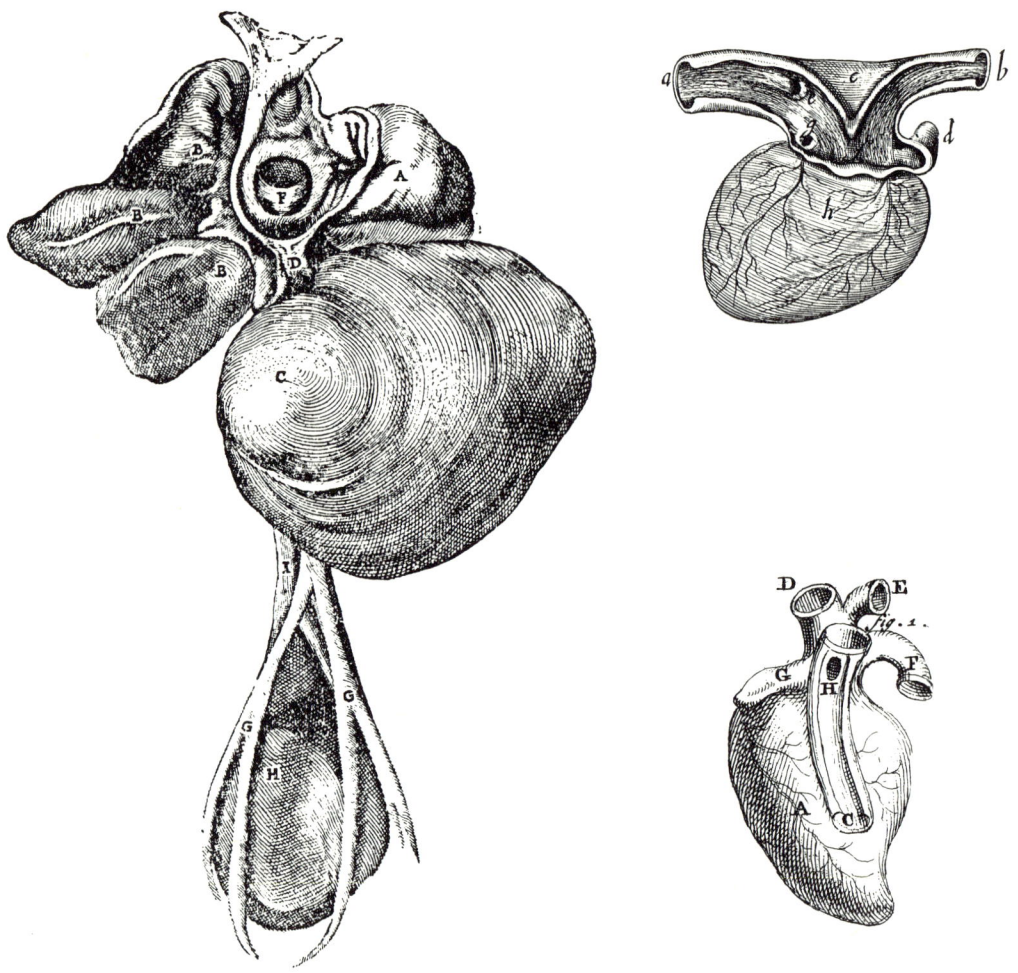

Figure 6. Early illustrations of the foramen ovale.

Left: Human fetus according to Fabricius, showing the heart A, lungs B, liver C, inferior vena cava D, and foramen ovale F, "foramen cum suo ostiolo ad dextrum cordis ventriculum." *Top right:* Lower's representation of the entry of the great veins into the heart of quadrupeds, such as the sheep, dog, horse, or cow, showing the inferior vena cava (a), superior vena cava (b), intervenous tubercle (c), right atrium (d), foramen ovale (e), and coronary sinus (g). *Bottom right:* The foramen ovale in the fetus, according to Drake (1728), *A, the body of the heart. C, the ascending trunk of the vena cava. D, F, the* Arteria Magna. *E, the* Axillary *artery. G, the* right *auricle. H, the* Anastomosis *between the* vena cava, *and the vein of the lungs, called the Foramen Ovale, which is closed with a valve in the adult."*

clearly show the foramen ovale opening off the inferior vena cava (Fig. 6). Many still believed that the foramen ovale joined the two atria (*134, 135, 155, 159*), a notion which presented a difficult conceptual problem. As Barcroft wrote in 1946, "I found it hard to believe that in a single chamber as small as the atrium of the right side of the heart, the entering streams of blood should so completely fail to mix that each should issue retaining its distinctive composition." At a meeting of the Physiological Society in London in 1937, Barcroft and Barron happened to see a cineangiographic film, presented by Barclay and Franklin, of the blood flowing through the veins of an adult animal. They realized that this method could be used to delineate the course of the circulation within the fetus, and so to arrive at a solution of the problem. The two groups of investigators joined forces to carry out experiments on fetal lambs approaching term; the results were clear (*11, 15, 18*). Radiopaque contrast medium injected into the superior vena cava entered the right atrium only. Contrast medium, injected into an umbilical vein or femoral vein, passed to the inferior vena cava, and thence divided into two streams, the greater entering the left atrium directly through the foramen ovale, and the lesser entering the right atrium (Figs. 1 and 7). This

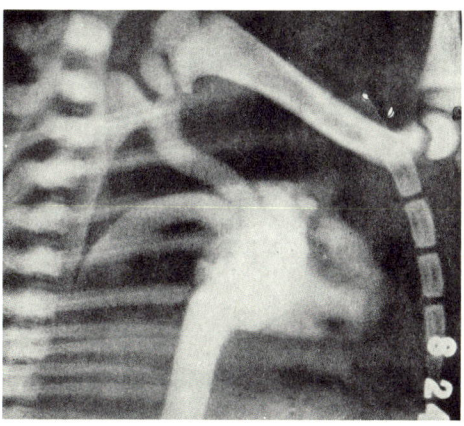 (a)   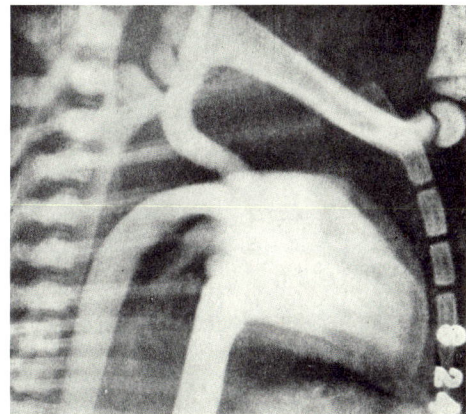 (b)

Figure 7. Contrast medium, injected into an umbilical vein of a lamb fetus, has passed up the inferior vena cava, and the immediate appearance of the shadow in the aortic arch and brachio-cephalic artery shows that much has passed through the foramen ovale into the left heart (a). One second later the pulmonary arteries are beginning to show, indicating a smaller flow through the right heart (b).

SPECIAL CIRCULATIONS

conclusion has been confirmed by subsequent workers using substantially the same method on fetal babies (*143*) and puppies (*112*). Thus, after many years, the conclusions which Wolff and Kilian reached on purely anatomical considerations were confirmed by direct experimental methods.

This satisfactory result does not end the matter, because the answer which has been arrived at is only qualitative in nature. Sabatier, and Nicholls before him, had suggested that the head and upper limbs received blood, if not direct from the placenta, certainly with relatively little venous admixture. This is true, since no superior vena caval blood normally enters the left atrium and since the O_2 content of blood in the carotid artery exceeds that in the descending aorta. The next question is, by how much does mixture within the heart alter the composition of the confluent blood streams? It is indeed remarkable, as Barclay, Franklin, and Prichard have pointed out (*15*), that in the earlier accounts of the fetal circulation some important vascular channels have often been ignored. Barclay, et al. mention the venous drainage of the heart from the coronary sinus and Thebesian veins into the right atrium; there is also the pulmonary venous return into the left atrium. If we are to understand the fetal circulation quantitatively, the contribution of these vessels cannot be disregarded.

These quantitative aspects of the fetal circulation have recently been explored in fetal lambs delivered by Caesarean section under pentobarbitone or dialurethane anesthesia. In these animals, simultaneous blood samples were withdrawn from a number of different vessels, and analyzed for their O_2 content (*73*). The mean results from six lambs are shown in Fig. 8. The oxygen content of pulmonary venous blood was found to be substantially less than that in the pulmonary arteries, and that of coronary sinus blood to be less than that of superior vena caval blood. The problem of mixing of blood streams within the fetal heart is therefore more complicated than at first appears. Nevertheless one general conclusion would seem inescapable. Four streams of blood enter the heart, one from the inferior vena cava 67 per cent saturated with oxygen, one from the superior vena cava 25 per cent saturated, one from the pulmonary veins 42 per cent saturated, and one from the coronary veins and left hemiazygos system (through the coronary sinus) about 15 per cent saturated. Three streams of blood leave the heart; that to the ascending aorta is 62 per cent saturated, that to the descending aorta 58 per cent saturated, and that to the lungs 52 per cent saturated. Leaving aside the details, there is no doubt that under these experimental conditions mixing is very effective, and that it takes place *in both atria* (in the left atrium because of blood entering from the pulmonary veins in a quantity which is far from negligible).

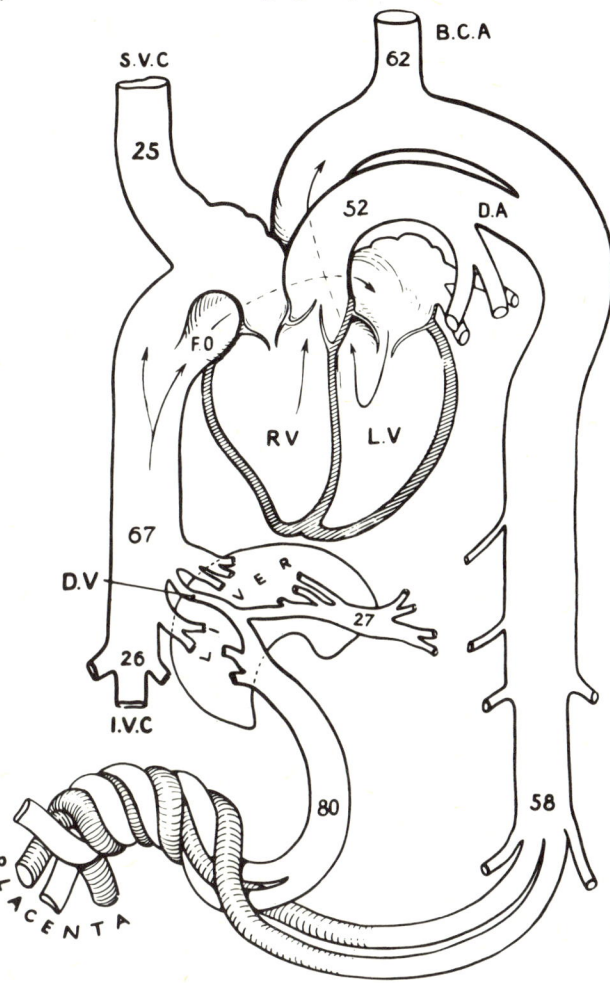

Figure 8. The circulation in the fetal lamb. The figures indicate the percentage O_2 saturation of blood withdrawn simultaneously from the great vessels, and are averages from six lambs. I.V.C., inferior vena cava; S.V.C., superior vena cava; D.V., ductus venosus; F.O., foramen ovale; D.A., ductus arteriosus; B.C.A., brachio-cephalic artery.

SPECIAL CIRCULATIONS

We may now consider once again the proposition first made by Nicholls and Sabatier nearly two centuries ago, that insofar as mixing is incomplete, the brain and the heart are likely to have a supply of blood which is in some respects advantageous. The mean difference in oxygen saturation between the carotid and umbilical arteries was only 6 per cent, with a difference in partial pressure of only 3 to 4 mm. Hg. This is no great advantage, since the mean carotid oxygen saturation was about 62 per cent, with a partial pressure of nearly 25 mm. Hg. Similarly in fetal rhesus monkeys blood samples withdrawn from branches of the ascending aorta (brachial or carotid artery) and descending aorta (femoral artery) with the body of the fetus still *in utero* showed a mean difference of only 9 per cent (*66*). There are other observations in the literature on goats (*122*) and lambs (*19*) which show larger differences between the O_2 saturation of carotid and umbilical arterial blood samples, particularly in premature fetuses, than those described above. But these may have been due either to withdrawal of blood samples from the two vessels at some minutes' interval, or to a departure from good physiological conditions. For a reduction in umbilical blood flow, occasioned by constriction or spasm of the umbilical vein or by hemorrhage, leads to a considerable increase in the difference between the O_2 contents of the carotid and femoral arteries in a fetal lamb (*63*). Certainly the last word has not yet been said on this subject, and we need more quantitative information on various species and under differing physiological conditions.

There is a further point. The oxygen saturation of blood in the descending aorta, which supplies the hinder end of the fetus, is intermediate between that of the pulmonary trunk, which supplies the lungs, and that of the ascending aorta, which supplies the coronary vessels, head, and forequarters (Fig. 8). The umbilical vein supplies the left side of the liver only. Therefore, if we wish to represent the oxygen tension or oxygen content of the blood supplying the fetal tissues by a single figure, that of the descending aorta or one of its radicles (e.g. an umbilical artery) should be used. The use of samples withdrawn from the umbilical vein for this purpose cannot be justified, as will be appreciated from Fig. 1.

We may now try to complete the picture which has been built up of the fetal circulation in the lamb, the one species in which sufficient data are so far available, by calculating the volume of blood flow through the different vessels. This can be estimated in the following way. At four points in the circulation, two bloodstreams, of different oxygen content, mix. In the right atrium a stream containing 67 per cent oxygen from the inferior vena cava mixes with one containing about 25 per cent oxygen from the superior vena cava; the mixture ejected into the pulmonary trunk contains 58 per cent oxygen. It is therefore possible to calculate the contribution from each of the two confluent streams. By an extension of this argument, and by making certain assumptions, the relative volume of blood flow through each of the principal vessels has been calculated as a proportion of the combined output of both ventricles. The results of these calculations are shown in Fig. 9. The placenta is a low

CHANGES IN CIRCULATION AFTER BIRTH

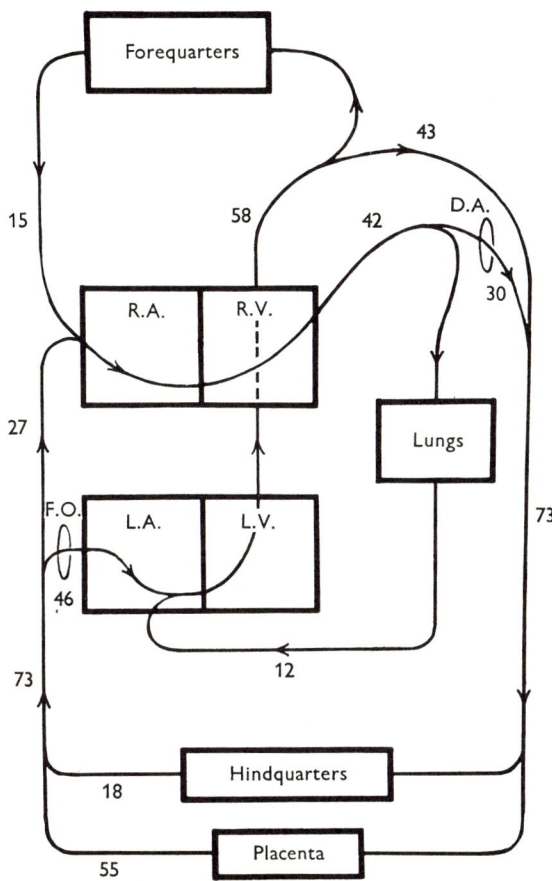

Figure 9. The circulation in the mature fetal lamb. The figures indicate the rate of blood flow as a percentage of the combined output of both ventricles.

[757]

SPECIAL CIRCULATIONS

resistance circuit, in parallel with the fetal tissues (both systemic and pulmonary), through which flows 55 per cent of the combined output of both ventricles. The blood flow through the lungs (12 per cent) is far from negligible. The foramen ovale and ductus arteriosus carry 46 per cent and 30 per cent of the total cardiac output, respectively. As the ventricles work in parallel to drive blood from the great veins to the arteries, there is no need for their output to be equal, and the output of the left ventricle (58 per cent) was found to be significantly greater than that of the right ventricle (42 per cent). It should be emphasized that these are mean figures only, calculated from observations on six lambs which were within a few days of term, and under specified conditions of anesthesia and experiment. They provide us with a model, a mental picture of how the fetal circulation works. It is the only model which we have as yet for this purpose and we ought not to be surprised if it does not prove to be of universal application.

It is possible to replace the figures for the proportion of total cardiac output by actual estimates of blood flow. In 1949, Cooper and Greenfield used an ingenious method for measuring umbilical blood flow (57). They placed a fetal lamb in a plethysmograph, still attached to its mother by the umbilical cord. When the umbilical veins were occluded, the volume of the fetus began to decrease at a rate which gave an estimate of umbilical flow. By this means, and by direct measurements from a flowmeter inserted into the abdominal portion of the umbilical vein, the umbilical blood flow/kg. body weight was estimated to be, on the average, 130 ml./min. at the end of gestation in the lamb (2, 58, 68). Using this figure, we can calculate that the combined output of both ventricles should be $100/55 \times 130$ or 235 ml./kg./min. This agrees with the figure of 240 ml./kg./min. obtained by Barcroft and Torrens (27) from measurements on three mature fetal lambs using a cardiometer. Similarly, pulmonary blood flow is calculated as about 30 ml./kg./min., which is consistent with direct measurements of flow through the left lung. Systemic blood flow through the other tissues of the fetal lamb is therefore 235 (total cardiac output) minus 130 (umbilical flow) minus 30 (pulmonary flow) = 75 ml./kg./min. These estimates of blood flow are shown in Fig. 2, which provides a rough idea of the blood flow in the mature fetal lamb under one particular set of experimental conditions. More recent measurements with an electromagnetic flowmeter

(*64*) have shown that in mature fetal lambs under light chloralose anesthesia umbilical blood flow may range from 132 to 260 ml./kg./min., giving a rather higher calculated flow through the fetal body. We must envisage during the next few years a progressive revision of our ideas as to the volume and distribution of fetal cardiac output as experimental techniques improve and approximate the natural conditions *in utero* more closely.

The Fetal Environment

We also have to consider another aspect of the problem. In order to understand how and why the changes which take place at birth do in fact occur, it is necessary to appreciate the particular physiological circumstances under which both the fetus and the newborn animal or baby live.

The fetus floats in the amniotic fluid within the body of its mother, protected from heat, cold, and many types of sensory stimuli, and supplied through its umbilical cord with the substances necessary for life and growth. Particular attention has been given to the means whereby oxygen is supplied to the fetus. There was a time, at the turn of the century, when physiology was enlivened by a celebrated dispute as to whether oxygen was transferred through the lungs, from the atmosphere to the blood, by a process only of diffusion, or whether this was aided by secretion. It is not surprising, therefore, to find in the literature of the period discussions of these two possibilities in regard to the placenta. However, by the time experimental fetal physiology began, this dispute had been settled, and when, in 1927, Huggett concluded that there was a gradient in the partial pressure of oxygen between the maternal and fetal side of the placenta in goats, sufficient to supply oxygen by diffusion, this conclusion was not contested. The size of the diffusion gradient has been calculated, assuming that the directions of flow of maternal and fetal blood streams within the placenta are wholly countercurrent, and that samples of uterine venous and umbilical venous blood are truly representative of those leaving the area where oxygen transfer takes place. We can be happy about neither of these assumptions (*33*), yet the calculations give a rough idea of the size of the diffusion gradient to be expected, about 40 mm. Hg for the syndesmochorial (*106*)

SPECIAL CIRCULATIONS

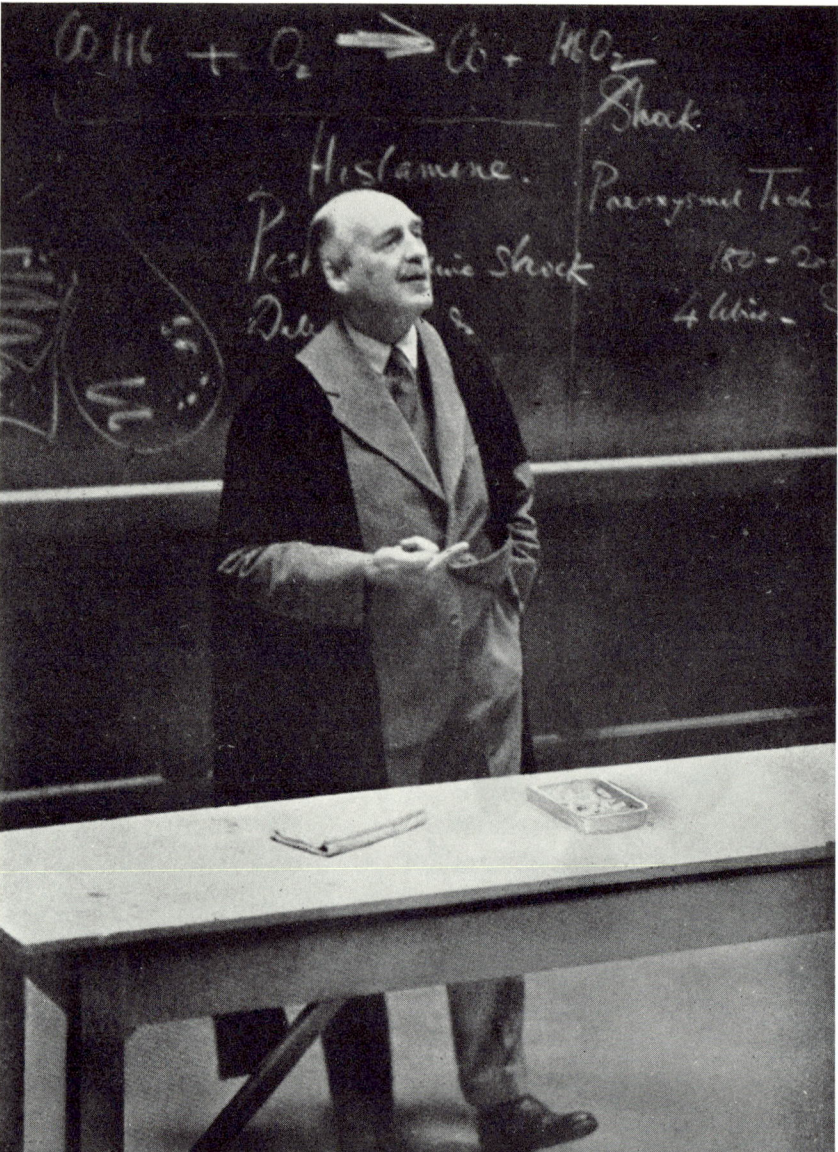

Figure 10. Joseph Barcroft (1872–1947).

placenta of the sheep and about 10 mm. Hg in the hemochorial placenta of the rabbit (*31, 32*). In man it has been calculated as about 20 mm. Hg (*161*). From this, and because the blood in the umbilical vein is diluted with blood containing even less oxygen before it reaches the fetal tissues (Figs. 1 and 8), it follows that the fetus must live in an environment in which the oxygen partial pressure is considerably less than that of the mother. It is this difference which led Barcroft (Fig. 10), who, between the early 1930's and the onset of World War II, laid the foundations of fetal physiology as an experimental science, to use the phrase "Mount Everest *in utero*" as a succinct description of one of the principal problems of fetal existence.

When we turn from generalization to measurements, the difficulties begin. Measurements of arterial oxygen saturations and partial pressures are available from experiments in fetal lambs and from the cord blood of babies after delivery, but the agreement between them is poor. In adults the arterial oxygen partial pressure is about 95 mm. Hg. In lambs near term the umbilical arterial blood has an oxygen saturation of about 58 per cent (Fig. 7), with a partial pressure of a little over 20 mm. Hg. Barcroft's 1946 figures are rather lower, and the 1957 figures of Kaiser and Cummings are lower still (*131*), with a calculated umbilical arterial oxygen tension of only just over 15 mm. Hg. In the human baby the mean oxygen saturation of umbilical arterial blood given by many authors from different countries under a variety of operative conditions (Caesarean or vaginal delivery) varies from 9.8 to 42 per cent, corresponding to an oxygen partial pressure of only 8 to 16 mm. Hg (*35, 52, 85, 116, 170, 182, 194, 202*). The significance of these observations lies in two features; first, the very wide range of values obtained even in the same species, and second, the very low absolute values which have been recorded.

In order to get these figures in perspective we must turn to other considerations. It has been widely believed by mammalian physiologists that, except under very extreme conditions immediately preceding death, the oxygen consumption of an animal is independent of the partial pressure of oxygen in the circulating blood. The reasons for this belief are twofold. First, it has been known for the last forty years or more that the oxygen consumption of minced tissues and of tissue slices does not decrease until the oxygen partial pressure (for example, in a Warburg flask) is reduced to a few mm. Hg. Evidently most mammalian enzyme systems, and particularly the cytochrome oxidase system, are capable of

SPECIAL
CIRCULATIONS

accepting molecular oxygen at a very low partial pressure. Second, observations on adult man at high altitudes and on animals such as dogs (*104, 113*) indicate that oxygen consumption does not decrease until the oxygen partial pressure of the inspired air is very much reduced, equivalent to an oxygen content of less than 6 per cent at sea level, when there is immediate danger of cardiovascular collapse.

In the mammalian fetus, the only available information concerns the anesthetized lamb, in which oxygen consumption is reduced when the umbilical arterial oxygen saturation falls much below 50 per cent (i.e. a partial pressure of about 20 mm. Hg) and yet the circulation is maintained (*68*). When the arterial oxygen partial pressure falls below this level, lactate accumulates in the blood, which suggests that the energy requirements of the animal are then being partly supplied by anaerobic glycolysis. Yet lactate is not readily transferred from the fetal lamb to its mother across the placenta (*28*). The relevance of these observations for our present purpose is that they provide an index by which we may judge whether observations are being made under conditions which approximate physiological normality. It is hard to believe that under normal intra-uterine conditions the supply of oxygen is so deficient that oxygen consumption is reduced, and that lactic acid, and hence hydrogen ions, are likely to accumulate. Using this criterion then, the normal arterial oxygen partial pressure is nearly 25 mm. Hg in the fetal lamb, compared with slightly less than 100 mm. Hg in the newborn. This provides a rough indication of the height of the "Mount Everest *in utero*" at which the fetus lives. For instance, Houston and Riley studied four men acclimatized to an altitude of 20,000 feet in a low pressure chamber, and observed an arterial oxygen saturation of 52 per cent at an oxygen tension of 29 mm. Hg (*121*).

No comparable data are available for the human baby. But it will be noted that the mean umbilical arterial oxygen partial pressure on delivery was only 8 to 16 mm. Hg. It is hard to avoid the conclusion that the majority of human babies are grossly asphyxiated on delivery, and that the mean values obtained for the oxygen content of cord blood are a poor index of normal intra-uterine conditions. This conclusion is supported by the observation that the blood pH and buffer base rises progressively during the twenty-four hours after birth (*127*). The difference between the umbilical arterial oxygen partial pressure observed in lambs and babies should occasion no surprise, for in experiments on lambs a large incision is made in the uterus, which does not contract immediately the fetus is removed, nor does the placenta separate; in human birth the conditions are altogether different.

So much for the fetal circulation and environment. We must now turn to the dramatic events which occur in the circulation at birth.

CHANGES IN CIRCULATION AFTER BIRTH

The Process of Birth, Rupture of the Cord, and the First Breath

It is not possible to give a concise analysis of the events which immediately precede the separation of the baby from its mother, for the process of birth may be rapid or prolonged, it may occupy an hour or two or a day or two. During this process the fetus is subjected to various hazards, including mechanical injury, infection, and hemorrhage, and what is more to our present purpose, asphyxia and depletion of its carbohydrate reserves. The importance of the latter will be discussed toward the end of this chapter. Meanwhile, we must consider the immediate mechanical effects of delivery.

Let us begin with the simplest situation, that in which birth is rapid and the umbilical cord is at once torn or tied. This often occurs naturally. Thus, in one instance, a ewe became more and more restless over a period of half an hour, walking about her pen and stopping to grunt from time to time. Then, standing still, she suddenly delivered her lamb with two strong efforts, the cord tearing as the lamb fell to the ground; the vessels contracted at once so that there was no loss of blood. This sequence of events can be duplicated experimentally in a lamb delivered by Caesarean section under local anesthesia. So long as the placental circulation is intact the lamb lies quietly beside its mother without breathing. When the cord is tied there is an immediate but transient rise in blood pressure; this is attributed to the large increase in peripheral vascular resistance which occurs when umbilical arterial flow is arrested, followed a few seconds later by a fall in cardiac output as the umbilical vein empties. During the next one and a half minutes the heart begins to accelerate and the blood pressure rises as the lamb uses up the oxygen in its blood and becomes asphyxiated (Fig. 11). This second and larger rise in pressure is attributed to reflex mechanisms excited by oxygen lack and carbon dioxide excess. Finally, the lamb

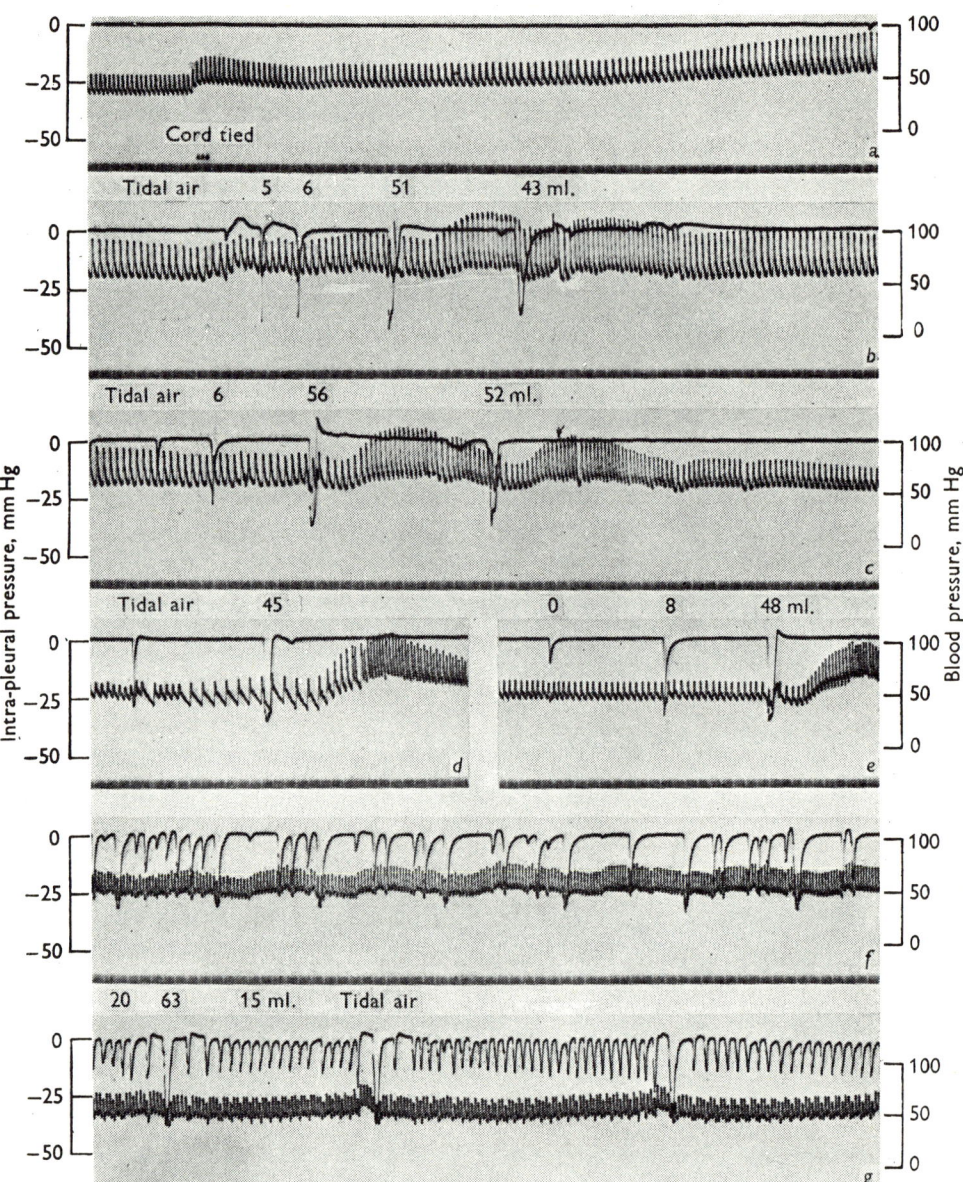

Figure 11. A record of the first breaths in the mature fetal lamb, delivered under local anesthesia. Records show the femoral arterial and intrapleural pressures. The figures above each respiratory effort record the tidal air, in ml. Records a–c are continuous; d was taken 4 min., e 5 min., and g 20 min. after tying the umbilical cord.

begins to make strong respiratory efforts, such that the intra-pleural pressure falls to -40 mm. Hg or less (Fig. 11B), and after a few more minutes regular breathing is established (Fig. 11F, G). The arterial pressure returns toward the initial level, but levels off about 10 mm. Hg above it. This experiment differs from the natural sequence of events in two respects: a newborn lamb is usually already asphyxiated on delivery (because the cord has been compressed during the second stage of labor), and the sensory stimuli are more severe during natural birth. These circumstances no doubt explain why many healthy animals and babies begin to make respiratory efforts when they are still only partly delivered. The experiment described above demonstrates that asphyxia alone is sufficient to start breathing, in the absence of gross sensory stimulation.

CHANGES IN CIRCULATION AFTER BIRTH

The immediate change in systemic blood pressure at birth was first measured by Cohnstein and Zuntz (53, 54). Previously, Schultze (179), in an interesting but purely speculative book, had suggested that an increased vascular capacity of the lungs when pulmonary respiration began might lead to a fall of arterial pressure, a circumstance which he thought would favor contraction of the umbilical arteries. Cohnstein and Zuntz (53, 54) did a few experiments which demonstrated a tendency for the pressure to rise. This result countered Schultze's views, and no further observations appear to have been made on the subject for another fifty years. In 1938, Barcroft, et al. reported that ligation of the cord was followed by a rapid but transient rise of arterial pressure (about 40 mm. Hg) (20). They considered that this rise was initiated by the respiratory movements but believed that some other mechanism was also involved (that this is so is clearly demonstrated in Fig. 11, in which the immediate rise occurs long before respiratory movements begin). In 1940, Windle stated that any *considerable* rise in systemic pressure with the beginning of breathing should be regarded as evidence of *previous* asphyxial depression of the fetus (199). Prolonged asphyxia of the fetus causes a fall in arterial pressure, and relief of this on ventilation restores the pressure to, or above, the initial level; this phenomenon often occurs in newborn rabbits or puppies. And yet Windle's interpretation is not necessarily always correct, as can be seen from Fig. 12. This shows a large rise in arterial pressure in a lamb. The lamb was well oxygenated in the fetal state; the cord was then tied and ventilation was begun, but the minute volume was inadequate and the lamb was somewhat (but

SPECIAL CIRCULATIONS

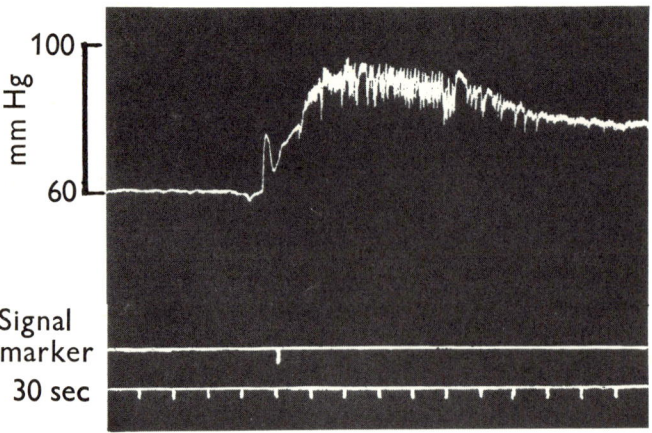

Figure 12. The effect of underventilation after tying the umbilical cord (at the signal mark) in a mature fetal lamb. The blood pressure rose abruptly when the placenta was cut off, fell, and then rose even higher during the consequent anoxemia.

not grossly) asphyxiated. The autonomic nervous system is well developed in the newborn lamb and it is not surprising that the blood pressure should rise on acute asphyxia. It is evident that interpretation of the acute changes in systemic arterial pressure at birth in any particular individual is speculative unless a great many other facts are known. And it is interesting that, in all the discussions as to the nature and sequence of the changes in the circulation at birth, few authors have paid serious attention to the fact that the ductus arteriosus is a wide channel connecting the pulmonary and systemic vascular beds.

The circulation through the lungs. The history of the development of ideas as to the circulation of blood through the lungs of the fetus, and the changes which occur at birth, has some interesting features (*15, 94*). Harvey (*114*) considered that there was no return flow from the lungs to the left atrium in the fetus. Lower believed there was a small pulmonary blood flow during fetal life which increased considerably at birth (*145*) and most authors thereafter accepted this view (*110, 174*). In 1801, Bichat suggested that the ductus arteriosus gradually shut down during gestation, and thereby diverted more and more of the right ventricular blood to the lungs (*38*). In 1826, Kilian went even further and proposed that pulmonary flow in the fetus was as great as, and perhaps even relatively greater than, that to the adult lungs (*138*). He thought it was ridiculous to speak of a slight pulmonary circulation. All of these views were based on anatomical considerations alone, as indeed are the more recent ones of Patten and Toulmin (*157*). The latter suggested, on the basis of measurements of the cross sectional areas of the great vessels at different gestational ages, that pulmonary flow might increase toward term. They thus reached, by different means, the same conclusion as Bichat, though apparently they were unaware of his speculations. According to Bichat, and to Patten and Toulmin, the transition from the fetal to the neonatal condition was gradual, rather than abrupt. Until comparatively recently there was no direct evidence as to whether pulmonary blood flow increased at birth, or, if it did so, how this change was effected.

The first direct measurements on the pulmonary circulation in the fetus and the newborn were made in 1942 by Barclay, et al., using cineangiography in the fetal lamb (*12*). Earlier studies by this method had shown that radiopaque contrast medium, injected into the superior vena cava, passed from the pulmonary trunk through the fetal lungs. The mean pulmonary circulation time in the fetal lamb was now found to be rapid, 2.7 seconds, and since the vessels are wide it was concluded that pulmonary flow must have been considerable. The mean pulmonary circulation time decreased some minutes after breathing had begun, at a time at which (judged by cineangiography) the ductus arteriosus had closed. At this time, then, "the whole flow passes to the pulmonary arteries and adult circulation is established." It is not clear whether this implies that pulmonary blood flow is increased because of closure of the ductus arteriosus, although this conclusion seems to be intended. The only other evidence which was available at the time, and which bore on the point in question, were the measurements of Hamilton, Woodbury, and Woods, who in 1937 recorded the pressures in the right and left ventricles of dog and rabbit fetuses by pushing a needle through the chest wall into the ventricular cavities. They found that before breathing began the pressures in the right and left ventricles were similar. Inspiration lowered the right ventricular pressure more than the left, and this difference was attributed to a fall in pulmonary vascular resistance (*111*). These observations were subsequently criticized by Abel and Windle

SPECIAL CIRCULATIONS

(*1*) and by Barclay, Franklin, and Prichard (*15*) because they disagreed with the interpretation of the changes in pressure observed, and because the method of pressure measurement involved transfixing the heart blindly through the chest wall. On the other hand, Barcroft accepted these findings as indicating that after birth "if the blood traversed the ductus, it would do so from the aorta to the pulmonary trunk, and not in the direction proper to the fetal circulation" (*18*). However, since he believed (erroneously as it will appear later) that the ductus arteriosus closed completely within a few minutes of birth, this possibility was not considered further.

Whatever changes in pulmonary blood flow may occur, it is evident that there must be a change in pulmonary arterial pressure at birth or some time thereafter. In the fetus the blood flows from pulmonary trunk to aorta through the ductus, so that the pulmonary arterial pressure is greater than that in the aorta; in the adult it is considerably less. Direct measurements of pulmonary arterial and aortic pressures in mature fetal lambs whose chests had been opened showed that, when artificial ventilation was begun, pulmonary arterial pressure fell rapidly toward the adult level, while aortic pressure fell transiently and then rose up to, or somewhat above, the initial level (*10*). In 1952–3, using the same preparation, blood flow through the left lung was measured, and was found to increase three- to ten-fold on ventilation (Fig. 13), although pulmonary arterial pressure had fallen and left atrial pressure had risen (*77*). These measurements afforded direct proof of the hypothesis that pulmonary vascular resistance fell abruptly when the lungs were first ventilated.

The precise mechanism by which this change in the lungs is effected is not known. The fact that collapse of a lung in adult man does not necessarily lead to gross cyanosis suggests that the same mechanism may also operate in the adult, and it was tempting to believe that the mechanism had some simple anatomical basis (*146*). Ventilation with 100 per cent nitrogen of the lungs of a fetal lamb, while it was still attached to its mother by the umbilical cord, caused an immediate fall in pulmonary vascular resistance similar to that seen on ventilation with air or oxygen. Distension of the lungs with warm saline, under the same conditions, did not cause a fall in vascular resistance. The increase in pulmonary flow at birth was therefore attributed primarily to distension of the lungs with

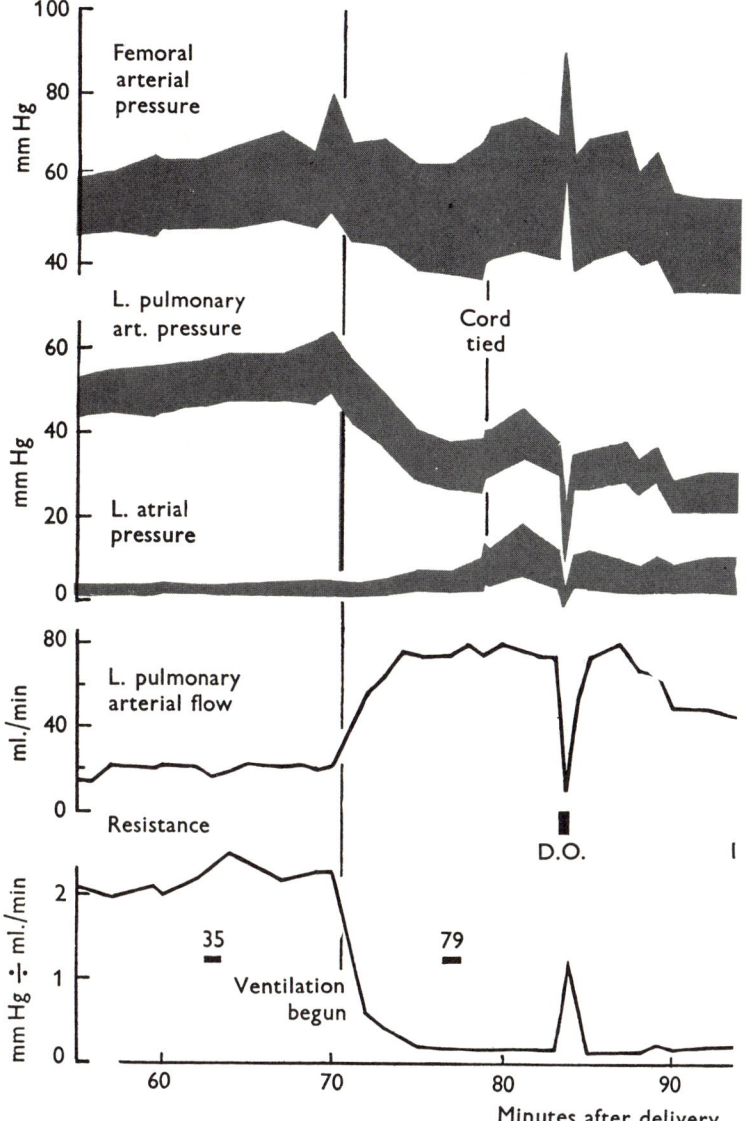

CHANGES IN CIRCULATION AFTER BIRTH

Figure 13. Some of the pulmonary vascular changes on expanding the lungs of a mature fetal lamb. Artificial positive pressure ventilation of the lungs with air caused a great fall in pulmonary vascular resistance, and an increase in pulmonary blood flow. Twelve minutes later temporary occlusion of the ductus arteriosus (D.O.) caused a rise in femoral pressure and a fall in pulmonary pressure and flow, showing that blood had been flowing from the aorta into the pulmonary trunk.

SPECIAL CIRCULATIONS

a gas, and since the same change was seen on ventilation of an isolated perfused fetal lung, it was independent of the integrity of the central nervous system. This suggested that the principal change in vascular resistance was related to some feature of the pulmonary architecture which resulted in compression or convolution of alveolar vessels in the fetal or collapsed condition, as described by Reynolds (167).

The alternative hypothesis, that the high vascular resistance of unexpanded fetal lungs is due to tonic vascular constriction, now seems to be the more likely explanation. Injection of small doses of acetylcholine or histamine (1–3 μgm./kg.) into a fetal pulmonary artery caused profound vasodilatation (69). Indeed, it was not uncommon to observe an increase in blood flow equal to that seen on subsequent ventilation of the lungs. After a short period of ischemia caused by interrupting flow in the unexpanded fetal lung, flow increased considerably above the initial level, and changes in the arterial oxygen saturation of the fetus also caused relatively large alterations in pulmonary blood flow. It is therefore evident that the physiological mechanisms which control pulmonary vascular resistance in the fetal and neonatal period, and particularly those related to the concentrations of the blood and alveolar gases, deserve further study.

Nisell (153) suggested that the decrease in pulmonary vascular resistance at birth might be due to perfusion of the lungs with blood containing less oxygen than under fetal conditions. However, in the newborn lamb the mixed venous blood contains more oxygen than in the fetus. On the other hand, ventilation of the lungs of a newborn lamb with different gas mixtures does undoubtedly alter vascular resistance, a decrease in the oxygen content of the inspired air causing a rise in pulmonary arterial pressure and vascular resistance, as in adult cats (39, 42, 83, 84). Blood flow through those areas of the lungs which are inadequately ventilated will therefore be smaller, so that blood returning from well-ventilated areas should be less diluted with venous blood. It is also possible that the pulmonary blood vessels in the fetus are under reflex control. Daly and Daly (61) have shown in the adult dog that anoxic stimulation of carotid chemoreceptors causes a reflex fall of pulmonary arterial blood pressure, attributed to pulmonary vasodilatation.

There are some mechanical factors of secondary importance. Borst, McGregor, Whittenberger, and Berglund (44) and Carlill, Duke, and

Jones (*49*) found in the adult dog and cat that a rise of left atrial pressure causes a slight fall of pulmonary vascular resistance. The same is true of the isolated lungs of newborn lambs (*64*). In the intact newborn lamb there is a rise of left atrial pressure when ventilation is begun, and this may contribute to the fall of pulmonary vascular resistance which is observed, though it is probably only a small contribution. The pulmonary arterial pressure, and hence pulmonary blood flow, is also directly affected by the patency, or otherwise, of the ductus arteriosus. When the ductus arteriosus is closed in the newborn lamb, pulmonary arterial pressure and flow are reduced (Fig. 13).

The closure of the foramen ovale, and changes in atrial pressure. The foramen ovale was known to Galen, who gave a description of it and of its valve, which lies on the left atrial side of the orifice (Figs. 1, 5). He noted that it might prevent the return of blood from the left atrium to the inferior vena cava, and also that in newborn animals, four or five days old, the membrane over the opening was found to be uniting with it, though such union was not yet complete. Subsequent authors quoted and amplified his account, though naturally it was not until Harvey's discovery of the circulation of the blood that its significance could be properly appreciated. It is possible that it was Harvey who first used the term "foramen ovale" (*94*). Franklin, et al. have pointed out that the foramen is often not oval, and that its valve in some species is quite unlike the other valves of the heart, e.g., in the calf it is tubular in shape and in the horse it is fenestrated, perforated at its further end by a remarkable number of holes which vary in size (*96*). Nevertheless the name "foramen ovale" is now hallowed by tradition and use, and the "valve" seems to function admirably, whatever the variations in shape. Even though the relation of these structures to the left atrium was repeatedly and lucidly described, there were occasional papers even up till the end of the nineteenth century which asserted that blood passed through it from the left atrium to the inferior vena cava. This is yet another illustration of the fact that arguments as to function, which derive from anatomical considerations alone, often carry little conviction in the absence of experimental observations in living animals. However, on purely anatomical grounds it was generally supposed that the valve of the foramen ovale must close by the

SPECIAL CIRCULATIONS

pressure in the left atrium rising above that on the other side of the orifice.

The first experimental observations, in 1938, by Barclay and Franklin (*13*), using cineangiography, suggested that the foramen ovale was functionally patent for some time after birth in lambs delivered by Caesarean section. The next year Barcroft, Kramer, and Millikan found that when a newborn lamb was given oxygen to breathe, the arterial oxygen saturation rose to 95 per cent within five minutes (*26*); this response was clearly "inconsistent with the short-circuiting of any amount of blood through the foramen ovale so great as to be physiologically important." Subsequent cineangiographic observations confirmed this view, and it was concluded that the foramen ovale became closed a few minutes after birth in the lamb (*15, 18*).

Yet this was not the end of the story. Indirect measurements of oxygen content, particularly when breathing pure oxygen, are not necessarily good guides to the presence or absence of small shunts. Thus if inferior caval oxygen saturation is 67 per cent and pulmonary venous saturation 95 per cent, a right-to-left shunt through the foramen ovale, such that one quarter of left atrial blood is derived that way, will only reduce left atrial oxygen saturation to 88 per cent, and this difference may be overlooked. Condorelli, Dagianti, Polosa, and Giuliano used a dye dilution method in unanesthetized lambs, injecting very small volumes of fluid intravenously, and concluded that there was a right-to-left shunt through the foramen ovale up till the fifth day from birth (*56*). Stahlman, Merril, and Le Quire (*186*) have recently confirmed this observation, and Lind and Wegelius also concluded from cineangiograms that there was a similar shunt in some newborn human infants (*143*). There is therefore a conflict of opinion as to when the foramen ovale closes functionally, with the balance favoring the view that it may normally be open for some days from birth. It would be desirable to get some quantitative measure of the size of these shunts when present; the possibility of species differences must also be considered. In the foal, for instance, the fenestrated valve of the foramen ovale has been found collapsed and full of recent clot within a few hours of delivery, but the number of such observations is few.

We must now consider the mechanism of functional closure. In the fetal lamb left atrial pressure was found to be less than inferior vena caval pressure by 1 to 1.5 cm. H₂O (76). Since about two-thirds of inferior vena caval flow passes through the foramen ovale the valve is thus held open during the greater part of the cardiac cycle. But when the umbilical cord is tied, inferior vena caval flow is abruptly reduced and there is a very large fall of inferior vena caval pressure (Fig. 14, C.O.), which is sometimes sufficient in itself to reverse the pressure gradient across the foramen ovale. On ventilation, pulmonary flow increases and left atrial pressure therefore rises. Figure 14 shows an experiment in which left atrial pressure rose above inferior vena caval pressure within 1.5 minutes of beginning ventilation, even though the

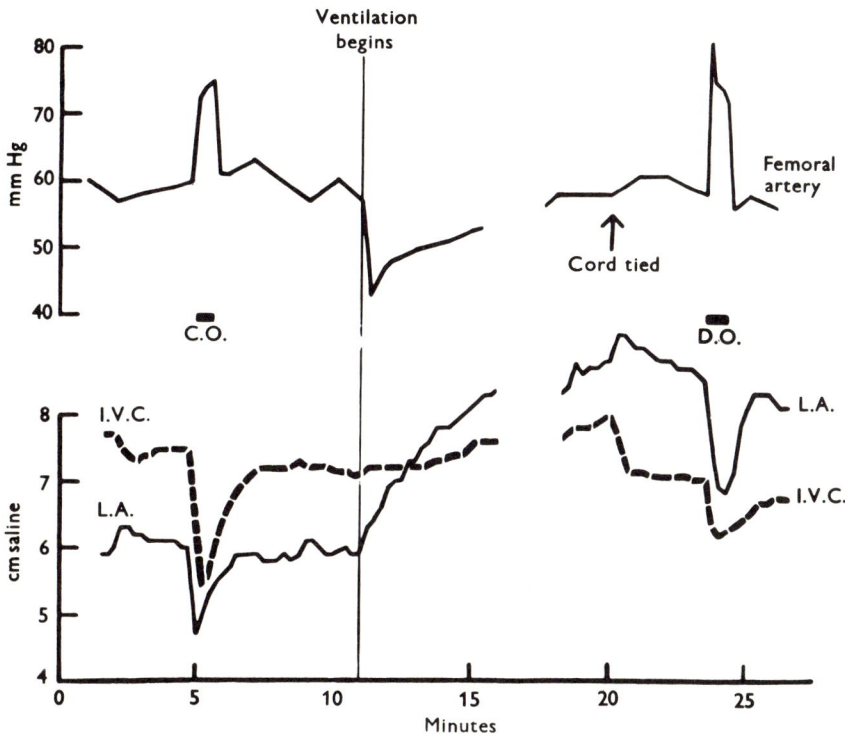

Figure 14. Closure of the foramen ovale in a mature fetal lamb. The figure shows the mean femoral arterial pressure (above) and the pressures recorded by saline manometers in the left atrium (L.A.) and inferior vena cava (I.V.C.). At C.O. the umbilical cord was occluded for a short period, and at D.O. the ductus arteriosus was occluded. Both occlusion of the cord and ventilation of the lungs contribute to the reversal of the pressure gradient across the foramen ovale.

SPECIAL
CIRCULATIONS

cord was not tied and umbilical blood flow therefore continued. When the cord was tied the pressure difference across the foramen ovale became even greater. This suggests that there are two reasons why the valve of the foramen ovale may become functionally shut, a fall in inferior vena caval pressure and a rise in the left atrial pressure. As these experiments were all carried out on anesthetized lambs with open chests, they are not inconsistent with the observations of Condorelli, et al., quoted in the previous paragraph; that is, they were designed to study mechanisms rather than natural history.

Figure 14 also shows the influence of patency of the ductus arteriosus. When the ductus arteriosus was open, blood flowed through it from the aorta to the pulmonary arteries, pulmonary flow was large, and left atrial pressure was high. When the ductus arteriosus was temporarily occluded (D.O.) the pressure difference between the left atrium and the inferior vena cava was much reduced. There are other factors which will almost certainly prove to be of importance. There is evidence, which will be considered later, that cardiac output may increase in the lamb after birth. If cardiac output increases, it is likely that atrial pressures will rise, unless the heart is able to do more work at the same filling pressure (e.g. because of an increase of sympathetic tone). Thus the account given in the preceding paragraph may require modification as we learn more about the control of the circulation in the newborn animal and as investigations are extended to other species.

As Galen observed, within a few days after birth the valve of the foramen ovale becomes adherent to the edges of the opening, and anatomical closure is soon completed, within two days in some foals, within eight days in the lamb, and even longer in the monkey. Patten, from postmortem observations on human infants, concluded that anatomical closure may take some weeks (*156*); observations on healthy infants are naturally not available.

Anatomical closure of the foramen ovale does not necessarily complete the changes in atrial pressure which follow birth. In 1956, Van Harreveld and Russell measured the pressures in the right and left atria of open-chested kittens, from one day to two months of age (*192*). In the adult cat and dog the mean pressure in the left atrium is greater than that in the right atrium; in the kitten within twenty-four hours of birth this difference is present but of questionable statistical significance. Three days later the difference becomes highly significant, and it increases thereafter, until at two months of age the pressure in the left atrium is almost double that in the right atrium. These changes undoubtedly require confirmation in animals with closed chests and normal respiration, but even as they stand they are very interesting, for they suggest a progressive alteration in the cardiovascular system for many weeks after birth. As Van Harreveld and Russell point out, this is roughly paralleled by the development of a large difference between the wall thickness of the two ventricles.

In the fetus the thickness of the two ventricles is approximately the same. Harvey compared them to twin kernels in a double nut and observed that the cone of the right ventricle extended to the tip of the left (*114*). During the three centuries after Harvey, the difference between the relative thickness of the fetal and adult ventricles was mentioned from time to time, but few actual measurements were made or inferences drawn therefrom. In 1955, Keen, using human postmortem material, found that during the first month after birth there was an atrophy of the free wall of the right ventricle by about 20 per cent; at the same time, the left ventricle increased in thickness (*132*). In animals similar changes occur. The atrophy of the right ventricle can be attributed to a reduction in the work of the right heart which, when the ductus arteriosus has closed after birth, has to pump the same volume of blood as the left ventricle, but at a considerably lower pressure. The increase in left ventricular thickness is attributable to the fact that systemic arterial pressure continues to rise after birth, as it does during gestation.

In the adult, left atrial pressure exceeds right atrial pressure. Opdyke, et al. explained this difference by the smaller capacity and elasticity of the left atriovenous system as compared with the right (*154*). But Van Harreveld and Russell suggested that since a ventricle is filled against its own elastic resistance, it is the capacity and elasticity of the ventricle which determines mean atrial pressure (*192*). Obviously both atriovenous and ventricular systems are of importance so long as the atrioventricular valves are open. The rise in left atrial pressure relative to right atrial pressure after birth is thus attributed to the increase in wall thickness of the left ventricle as compared with the right.

SPECIAL CIRCULATIONS

The closure of the ductus arteriosus. The ductus arteriosus was known to Galen and was incorporated by Harvey into a logical scheme of the circulation. In 1564 Leonardo Botallo published a short description of part of the heart, and "through strange turns of events and the carelessness of many writers in checking their references, it carried Botallo's name into anatomical nomenclature through the terms 'trou de Botallo' (foramen ovale) and 'Ductus arteriosus (Botalli)' " (*94*). In fact this appellation was quite undeserved, and there is no evidence that Botallo ever described the ductus arteriosus. Hieronymus Fabricius ab Aquapendente probably published the first accurate drawings of the special blood-channels of the fetus; those showing the ductus arteriosus are reproduced in Fig. 15. Since then there have been many speculations as to the cause of the gross changes which occur in the vessel so soon after birth. In the mid nineteenth century it was suggested that obliteration might be due to "inflammation," intimal proliferation, or thrombosis. But, in 1859, von Rauchfuss found thrombi in the ductus of only four out of 1400 newborn infants at postmortem, and his observations have since been confirmed (*152*, *162*). In 1900, Gérard distinguished two phases, primary functional closure by some mechanical process soon after birth and later secondary anatomical obliteration of the lumen (*100*, *101*). His views were widely accepted (*196*), although as late as 1930 Patten still continued to hold the view that a gradual process of closure, dependent on changes similar to those seen in endarteritis obliterans, might be responsible (*155*). However, attention generally turned to a consideration of the various mechanical hypotheses.

First it was suggested that the vessel might be constricted or compressed by external forces. In 1869, Walkhoff proposed that the change in position of the ductus after birth led to kinking, interruption of blood flow, and hence to clotting (*195*). In 1889, Schanz stated that the aortic end of the ductus was fixed, and that when breathing began the ductus was stretched by the pericardium and its vascular attachments, leading to mechanical obliteration of the lumen (*177*). In 1912, Stienon discussed dilatation of the aortic isthmus (i.e. that part of the aorta which lies between the origin of the vessels to the head and upper limbs and the entry of the ductus arteriosus) or left pulmonary artery, and dislocation of the thoracic viscera as possible factors in closure (*187*).

CHANGES IN CIRCULATION AFTER BIRTH

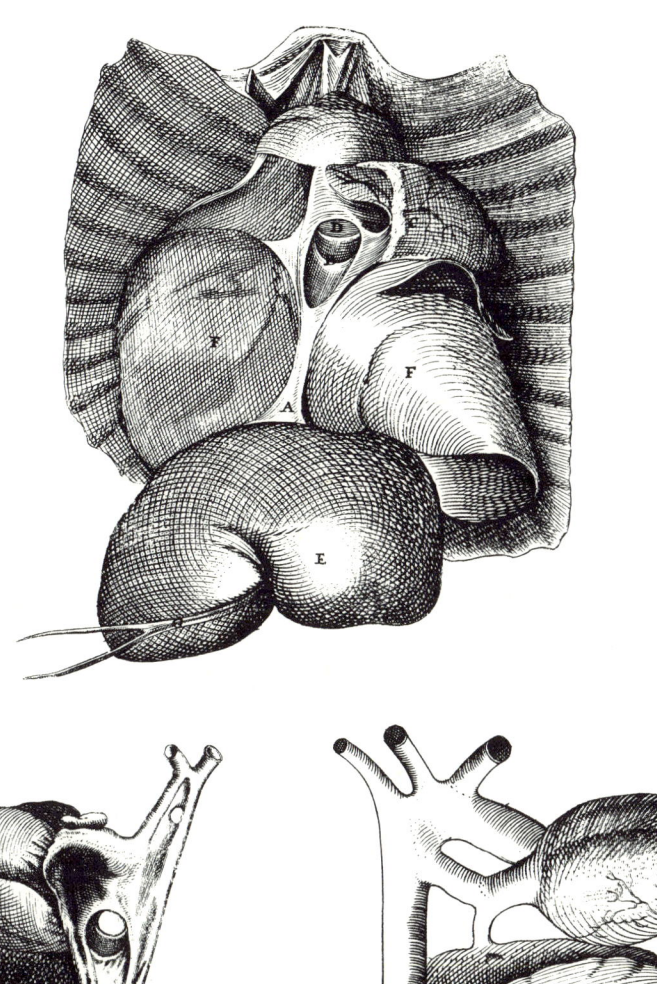

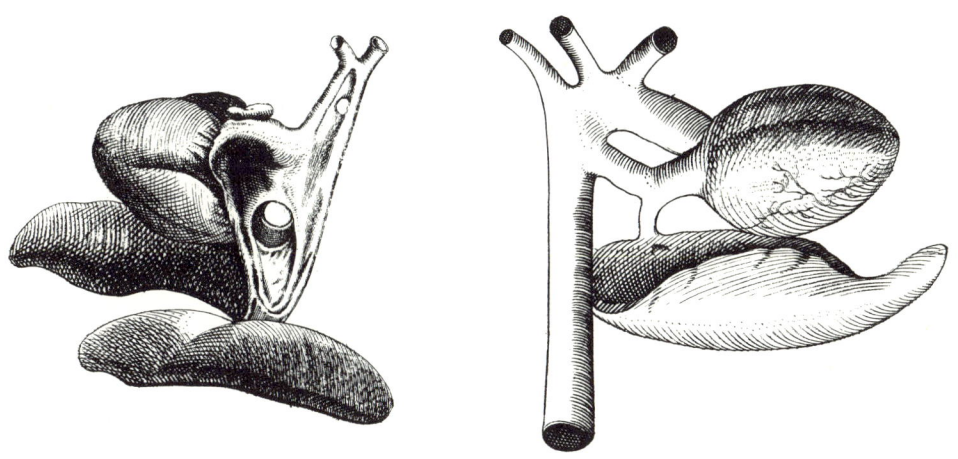

Figure 15. Fetal blood channels according to Fabricius.
Top: Lamb heart. The inferior vena cava (A) is shown as opened and running toward the heart (C) from the liver (E); the foramen ovale is labelled D, and its valve B. *Left:* Human heart, showing the location of the foramen ovale and its valve. *Right:* Human heart, showing the ductus arteriosus.

SPECIAL CIRCULATIONS

In 1926, Melka concluded that the aorta and pulmonary artery compressed the ductus between them, since the ligamentum arteriosum is flattened from side to side (*148*). Some have thought that dilatation of the left bronchus or traction on the left recurrent laryngeal nerve compressed the ductus, while others, such as Linzenmeier, believed that kinking was the principal cause of closure, but added subsidiary factors (*144*). All these speculations were based on postmortem material. It is true that the position and appearance of the ductus alters after birth. Barcroft noted that in the lamb it shortened, and the angles of its junction with the pulmonary artery and aorta became more obtuse (*18*). But no one who has watched this change in the newborn living animal, in the guinea pig (*136, 137*), lamb, or puppy, could believe that traction, compression, or kinking by external forces could possibly play any part in the natural method of closure. The vessel is too wide and too short to be kinked, and it visibly shortens as it constricts.

The second hypothesis was proposed in 1894 by Strassmann, who thought that the tongue of tissue at the acute angle formed by the junction of ductus and aorta could act as a valve (*188*). When breathing began, pressure rose in the left heart and fell in the right heart, the aorta pressed on the ductus, and mechanical closure resulted. Incidentally, Aranzi (*9*) had also supposed that there was a valve at the aortic end of the ductus, so the mistake had been made before. But on this occasion it had far-reaching results, for Strassmann's opinion was supported by others who had studied various species (*97, 111, 139, 169, 199*). It was also vigorously attacked, on the grounds that the piece of tissue in question was too thick to act as a valve and that the experiments which purported to show that blood cannot pass from the aorta through the ductus to the lungs were crude and carried out under unphysiological conditions (*15, 105, 178, 190*). It has now been established, as a result of cineangiographic and other investigations, that in the lamb, the puppy, and the human baby there is no functional valve at the aortic end of the ductus arteriosus (*3, 11, 77, 112, 143, 172*).

The third hypothesis is that primary functional closure of the ductus arteriosus is effected by contraction of the longitudinal and circular muscle in the media of the vessel. This appears to have been suggested first in 1856 by Virchow (*193*). In 1857, Langer recognized that the microscopic structure of the ductus was rather different from that of the pulmonary trunk and aorta (*141*). This finding has been confirmed by many subsequent workers (*45, 62, 101, 105, 117, 120, 124, 136, 176, 190*). The ductus has a looser structure than that of its adjacent vessels, and (in man, at least) less elastic tissue and no external elastic lamina. In the foal these differences are more obvious, in the lamb less so (Fig. 16); however, they do not provide a logical explanation of why the ductus arteriosus should constrict after birth but not the adjacent vessels.

The first systematic experimental studies to determine why the ductus arteriosus constricts at birth were those undertaken by Barcroft, Kennedy, and Mason (*25*) and by Kennedy and Clark (*136, 137*) in fetal guinea pigs. Direct observation showed that functional closure was effected by muscular constriction, a conclusion that has since been confirmed in lambs. A wide variety of procedures were effective, including normal breathing, inflation of the lungs with oxygen, intravenous injection of oxygen gas, mechanical or electrical stimulation of the ductus, injection of epinephrine, hemorrhage, and stimulation of various nerves. From the evidence presented it was impossible to decide what stimuli, alone or in combination, were effective under normal physiological conditions. Nevertheless, Kennedy and Clark's experiments suggested that the level of the arterial oxygen tension was important, and that a rise in it might cause constriction of the ductus even in the absence of the central nervous system. In 1953, Record and McKeown observed in human patients with persistent patency of the ductus arteriosus that there was a higher incidence of a history of fetal distress at birth than in the remainder of the population (*163, 164*). Moreover, the observations of Alzamora, et al. indicated that persistent patency of the ductus was more common in children born at high altitudes (*4*). Therefore, Record and McKeown exposed guinea pigs to a low oxygen environment after birth, and found at postmortem that the ductus arteriosus was wider than in control animals. We thus arrive at the hypothesis that an increase in the oxygen tension of the blood may cause contraction of the ductus arteriosus. This was at first regarded as inherently improbable, so that Barcroft, writing of Kennedy and Clark's work, was prompted to say, "it is known that the coronary vessels will relax in default of oxygen, but the conception of oxygen as a stimulus

CHANGES IN
CIRCULATION
AFTER BIRTH

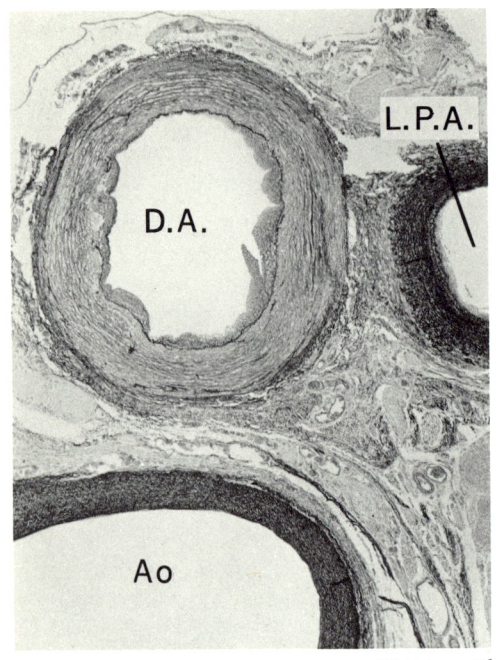

HUMAN STILLBORN   FULL TERM × 16

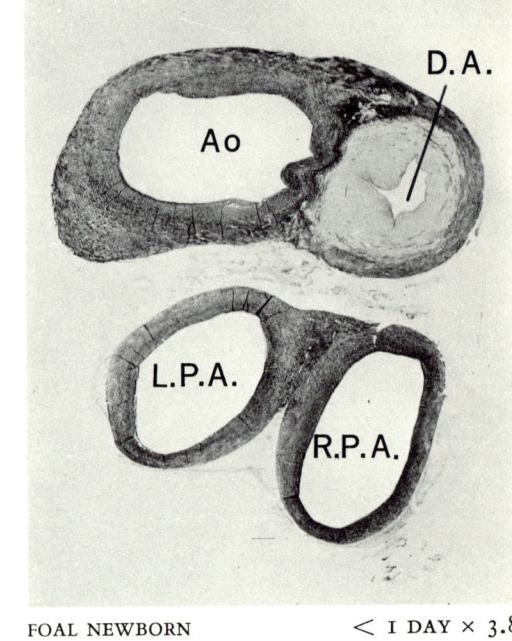

FOAL NEWBORN   < 1 DAY × 3.8

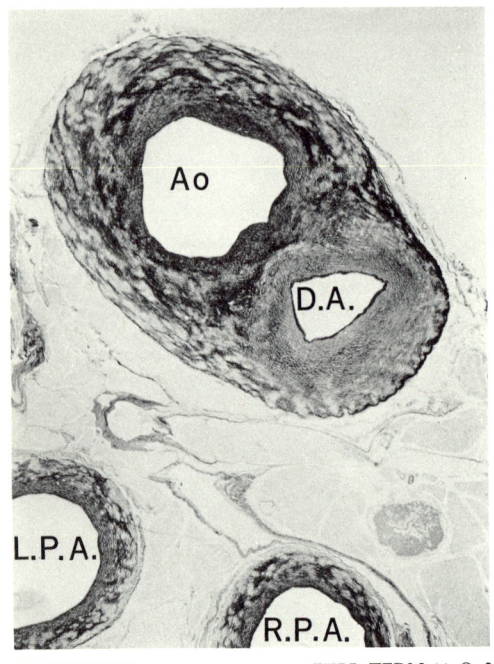

LAMB FETUS   FULL TERM × 9.5

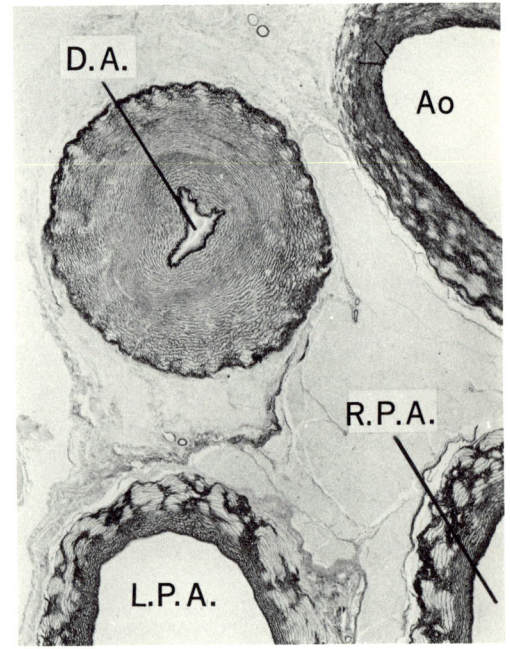

LAMB NEWBORN   1 DAY × 13

to unstriped muscle seems to constitute a challenge, and demands further exploration" (*18*).

In the lamb the ductus arteriosus is such a large vessel that changes in its external diameter can be measured directly with a pair of calipers (*42*). Using this method it was found that the ductus constricted, visibly and measurably, when the oxygen saturation of the arterial blood was raised, in either the fetal or the neonatal condition (Fig. 17). This occurred even though the transmural pressure across the wall of the ductus was maintained, in the absence of the central nervous system and even in an isolated ductus-heart-artificial lung preparation. However, equally good evidence was also adduced that acute asphyxia, or (what is possibly the operative factor) infusion of sympathomimetic amines into the blood of fetal lambs, also causes constriction of the ductus. In the newborn lambs it was quite apparent that, under different circumstances, either asphyxia or a rise in arterial oxygen saturation might be the most important variable in causing immediate contraction of the smooth muscle. Whether it is possible for asphyxia to cause prolonged contraction, for many hours, is not known. Recent experiments (Kovalčík, unpublished) have shown that the ductus arteriosus from the fetal lamb or the guinea pig, suspended in an isolated organ bath, contracts on exposure to oxygen or norepinephrine.

CHANGES IN CIRCULATION AFTER BIRTH

Blood Flow Through the Ductus Arteriosus after Birth

Postmortem evidence from infants dying at varying ages after birth led to the conclusion that the ductus did not completely close for some days or weeks (*50, 100, 101, 124, 142, 175, 198*). Before the seventh day many specimens were easily or widely patent as judged by insertion of a 2 mm. probe (*150*). Yet postmortem material is by its very nature suspect, and that is why Barcroft and others have been unwilling to

---

Figure 16. Sections of the ductus arteriosus (D.A.), aorta (Ao), right and left pulmonary arteries (R.P.A., L.P.A.) of a stillborn human fetus, newborn foal, and fetal and newborn lamb, stained to show the elastic fibers. There are very few of these in the ductus arteriosus of the foal, more in the human, and relatively more in the lamb, as compared with those in the aorta and pulmonary arteries. (Courtesy of Dr. M. M. L. Prichard.)

accept this as convincing evidence of continued patency in healthy babies (*10*).

In the fetus, blood flows through the ductus arteriosus from pulmonary trunk to aorta. In the newborn, if the pulmonary vascular resistance is much decreased after birth, one would expect that blood should flow in the opposite direction so long as the ductus is open. Both Windle (*199*) and Barcroft (*18*) considered this possibility. In 1898 Gibson first described the murmur usually associated with persistent patency of the ductus arteriosus in the child or adult man (*102*). In 1940, Windle argued that if the ductus remained open after birth

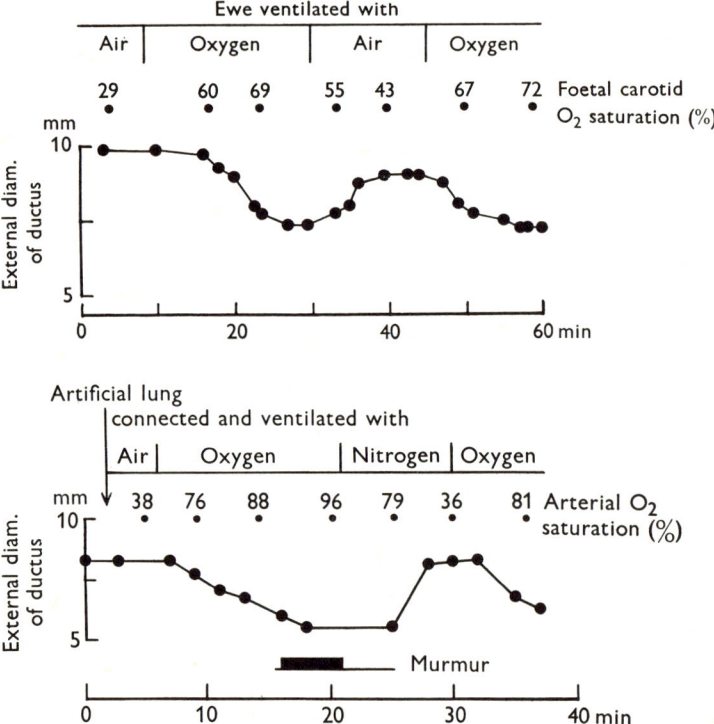

Figure 17. Two experiments to show constriction of the ductus arteriosus when the arterial O_2 saturation is raised. The upper record shows the effect in a fetal lamb when the ewe was ventilated with air or oxygen. The lower record is taken from an experiment using an isolated heart-ductus-artificial lung preparation, which suggests that the phenomenon may be due to a direct action of O_2 on the vessel wall.

"one should expect to hear the characteristic murmur of a patent ductus in every infant, but this is not the case." He therefore concluded that there was some mechanism which rapidly brought about functional closure of the ductus at birth (*199*). Barcroft also inferred from cineangiographic experiments on newborn lambs that the ductus was *completely* closed within a few minutes of birth (*18*). On the evidence which was then available these conclusions were justified, though we now know that neither Windle nor Barcroft was correct.

Experiments of several different kinds have shown that the ductus arteriosus is normally patent for many hours or even days after birth in the lamb, calf, and foal. Perhaps the most striking feature is the very loud and widely conducted murmur (Fig. 18), which is heard over the third or fourth rib in the mid-axillary line (that is, immediately over the junction of the ductus with the pulmonary trunk), and which radiates medially in the direction of flow from the aorta (*5, 43, 74*). This murmur disappears on occlusion of the ductus arteriosus. This evidence has been

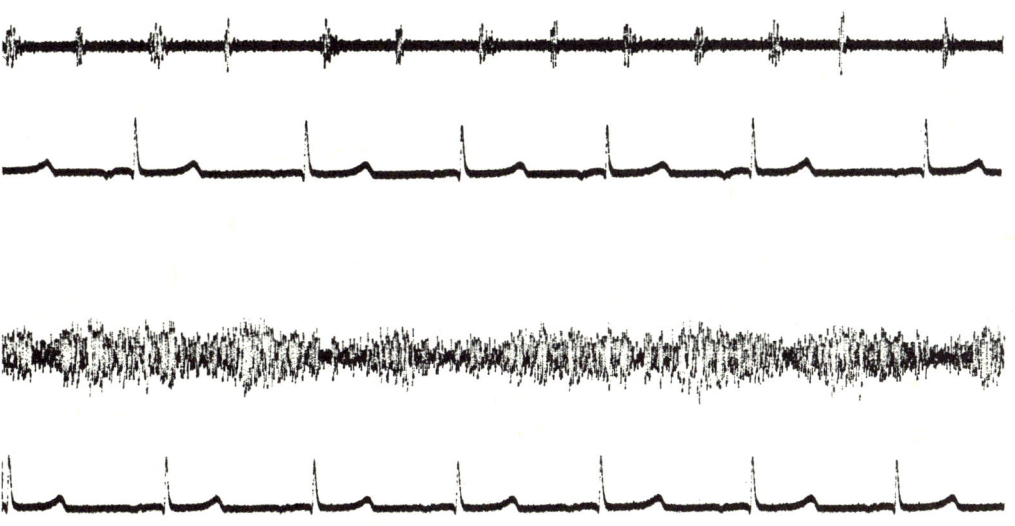

Figure 18. Phonocardiogram and electrocardiogram of an unanesthetized newborn lamb, born naturally. *Above:* heart sounds recorded over the apex beat. *Below:* the murmur recorded over the junction of the ductus arteriosus and pulmonary trunk.

supplemented by cineangiographic observations using improved methods, by measurements of pressure (Fig. 13) and of the oxygen contents of blood samples withdrawn from the great vessels, and by observation of the "thrill" due to turbulent flow in the pulmonary trunk. The volume of blood flow through the ductus can be very large; in some lambs, it comprised as much as half the total pulmonary flow an hour after birth. So long as the ductus was wide open, there was no murmur, even though flow was very large. It was only when the vessel was partly constricted that the velocity of flow exceeded a certain value, critical for any particular vessel diameter and determined by the Reynolds number (a physical constant for a given fluid), and thus gave rise to turbulence. As the vessel constricted still further there came a point when both turbulence and the murmur disappeared. The relationship between the physical variables, the factor $v\rho d/\eta$ (where v is the velocity, ρ the density, and η the viscosity of the blood, and d is the diameter of the ductus) and the comparative intensity of the murmur is shown in Fig. 19. Only when $v\rho d/\eta > 800$ (the Reynolds number for blood) is the murmur apparent. These observations have been described rather fully because an understanding of the physical principles involved makes it clear that there can be a very large flow through the ductus with little or no turbulence. It is only when certain conditions of flow velocity and vessel diameter are satisfied that turbulence occurs and a murmur can be heard. Although the presence of the characteristic murmur inevitably leads to the conclusion that blood is flowing through the ductus, its absence does not mean that blood is *not* flowing through the ductus.

In 1954, Lind and Wegelius concluded, on the basis of cineangiographic examination in six newborn infants, that the ductus was still patent at birth in humans; but at that time they were inclined to think that this condition was abnormal (*143*). The next year Eldridge, Hultgren, and Wigmore observed that, in most infants within three days from birth, the oxygen content of blood withdrawn from the heel was less than that withdrawn from the hand. They attributed this difference to the presence of a *right-to-left* shunt, probably through the ductus (*86*). It has since been suggested that the direction of flow may have been altered by reason of the discomfort involved in obtaining the capillary blood samples, since subsequent observations on simultaneous blood samples from the left atrium and descending aorta show that this right-to-left shunt decreases rapidly in magnitude during the first hour after birth (*125*). In 1955, Prec and Cassels found unusual dye dilution curves after injection into the umbilical veins of newborn infants (*160*); since older infants did not show the same phenomenon, they supposed that the ductus arteriosus must have been open. In 1957, James and

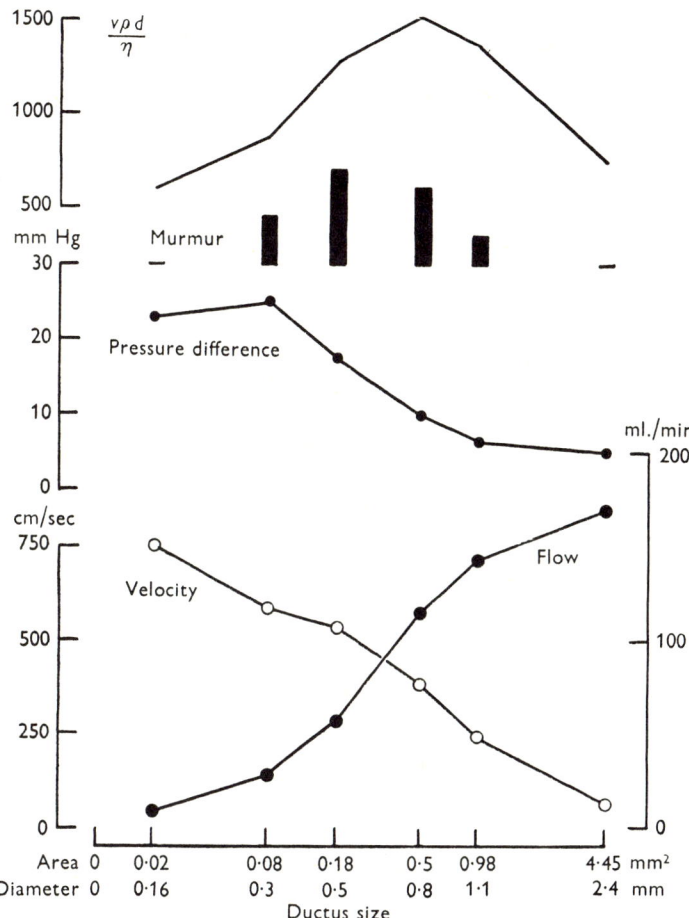

Figure 19. Newborn lamb. The pressure difference between the two ends of the ductus arteriosus, and the volume and velocity of flow through it, have been plotted against its internal diameter and cross sectional area. The comparative intensity of the murmur was measured from phonocardiograph records.

SPECIAL
CIRCULATIONS

Rowe, using mongols (*126*), and Adams and Lind, using normal babies (*3*), observed that the oxygen content of pulmonary arterial blood exceeded that of the right ventricular blood, from samples withdrawn by catheters introduced through a saphenous or umbilical vein. Finally, in 1958, Burnard detected and recorded in about a third of normal babies a faint cardiac murmur, appearing in mid-systole and increasing in volume until it disappeared in the second heart sound (*48*). It was best heard in the fourth and fifth interspace to the left of the sternum, usually appearing within a quarter of an hour of birth and lasting for several hours. It was more common in babies that had been asphyxiated, and was less often heard when the rectal temperature was below average.

All told, these observations strongly suggest that, in the human baby, the ductus arteriosus is normally patent, though partly constricted, for some hours or days after birth. The evidence is less conclusive than in animals, mainly because the murmur is not so easy to hear. The reason for this difference is not yet known, but there are several possibilities arising from the physical factors involved.

The Neonatal Circulation

The fact that the ductus arteriosus normally remains patent for some time after birth gives rise to an intermediate condition of the circulation—intermediate, that is, between the fetal and adult circulation. Figure 2 summarizes what we know of the changes in the great vessels at birth. In the fetus both ventricles work in parallel to drive the blood from the great veins to the arteries. Tying the umbilical cord removes the placenta from the circulation, and the valve of the foramen ovale closes when the left atrial pressure rises above that in the inferior vena cava. These changes take place rapidly, and give rise to the neonatal circulation, in which the ductus arteriosus is still open, left heart output is greater than right heart output, and the thickness of the walls of the two ventricles is still much the same. Pulmonary arterial pressure falls toward the adult level and systemic arterial pressure is somewhat increased over the fetal value. Finally, after a variable period of time, the ductus arteriosus closes to produce the adult type of circulation, in which blood is circulated through the heart and lungs by the two ventricles operating in series.

The neonatal circulation has certain special characteristics which may prove to be of some importance to those who have to deal with newborn infants and animals. Some of these characteristics derive solely from the continued patency of the ductus arteriosus and these will now be considered. First, the output of the left heart is inordinately high and can lead to cardiac failure. Several such cases have been reported in human infants; in one such the ductus was tied at two weeks of age, with subsequent recovery (Burnard, personal communication). Second, continued patency of the ductus could be a temporary advantage during the first hour or two of life when the lungs are not fully expanded and when the arterial blood is not fully saturated. For it enables partly oxygenated blood to recirculate through the lungs and thus to pick up more oxygen from those portions which are well ventilated. Under such conditions artificial occlusion of the ductus causes a fall in the O_2 content of the circulating blood (*41*, *75*). Third, in asphyxia, pulmonary arterial pressure may rise and the direction of blood flow through the ductus arteriosus may then revert to the fetal state, from pulmonary trunk to aorta (*42*, *126*). Under these circumstances the blood supply to the abdominal viscera and the lower limbs will contain less oxygen than that to the heart, head, and upper part of the body. There are two other features of the neonatal circulation which may be mentioned here but will be considered in more detail later in this chapter, *viz.*, the volume of cardiac output and the ability of the fetal cardiovascular system to withstand anoxia.

The Ductus Venosus

The first account of the ductus venosus is probably that published by Vesalius in 1564, the year of his death (*94*). Its discovery has been widely, but incorrectly, attributed to Aranzi (1530–89). The umbilical vein joins the portal vein, and from the trunk which unites these vessels, the portal sinus, there springs the ductus venosus, which runs surrounded, or almost surrounded, by the substance of the liver to the junction of the main hepatic veins with the inferior vena cava (Fig. 1). Vesalius recognized that it was less than half as wide as the umbilical vein. Another distinctive feature of the ductus venosus is that, unlike the hepatic branches of the umbilical and portal veins, it usually gives no

SPECIAL
CIRCULATIONS

branches to the liver substance. Harvey was led to believe from its anatomical situation that all the portal and umbilical venous blood passed through it to the heart, and that the liver therefore had practically no function in the fetus. In 1753, Bertin used wax injections to study the relation of the ductus venosus to the hepatic vessels (Fig. 20) and revived interest in the vessel in a work which Franklin has described as a major contribution to knowledge of the fetal liver (37). Haller (1757) disagreed with Harvey and believed that perhaps as much as six-sevenths of the umbilical venous blood passed through the substance of

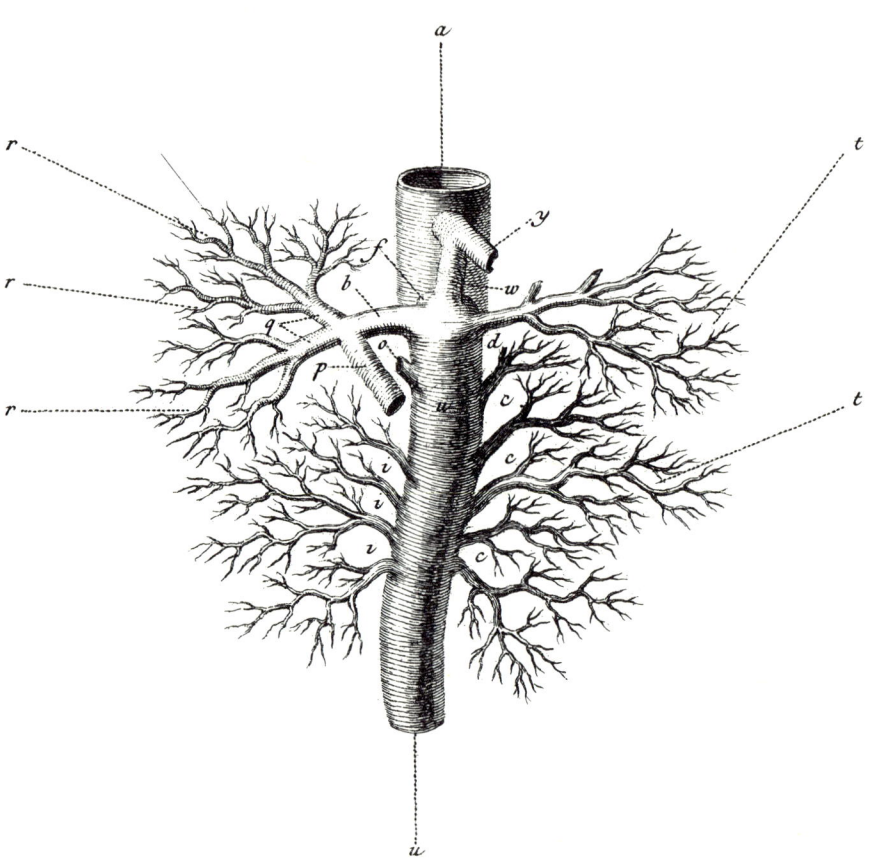

Figure 20. The venous supply to the fetal liver showing the umbilical vein (u), portal vein (p), and the ductus venosus "le canal veineux," (w) running to meet the left hepatic vein (y) as it enters the vena cava (a).

the liver, only one-seventh flowing through the ductus venosus (*110*). In 1801, Bichat mentioned a spur at the origin of the ductus venosus, which he believed might oppose the entry of portal venous blood. He also made direct observations in living guinea pig fetuses, noticing that umbilical venous blood was redder than that in the portal vein (*38*). Once again the inconclusiveness of inferences drawn from anatomical evidence may be observed, for twenty-five years later Kilian believed that the ductus venosus was the direct continuation of the portal vein (*138*). The other anatomical point which must be mentioned is that although the ductus venosus is normally present in the human, lamb, and many other species until birth (*15*), it disappears at an early stage of gestation in the horse (*203*) and pig (*79, 140*). It is not therefore essential to survival in all species, and in those in which it does disappear, *all* of the umbilical and portal venous blood passes through the liver substance.

The first experimental observations were carried out in the 1940's by angiography in the lamb (*14, 15*). In the human fetus very similar appearances have since been found (*143*). Radiopaque contrast medium injected into the umbilical vein passed rapidly through the ductus venosus to appear in the inferior vena cava (Fig. 21). Later investigations showed that the oxygen saturation of blood in the ductus venosus was identical with that in the umbilical vein (*6*). As the oxygen saturation of portal venous blood is much less (Fig. 8) it is unlikely that any portal venous blood normally enters the ductus venosus. In 1944, Barclay, Franklin, and Prichard suggested, on the basis of cineangiograms, that at least a ninth, and probably more, of the umbilical venous blood passes to the inferior vena cava via the ductus venosus (*15*). However, no direct measurements of blood flow have yet been achieved. Occlusion of the ductus venosus in the mature fetal lamb caused no significant change of blood pressure, heart rate, or carotid arterial oxygen saturation, so although a large volume of blood may normally flow through it, this alternative pathway is of questionable significance at the end of gestation.

When contrast medium is injected into the umbilical vein of the fetus, it passes the origin of the ductus venosus to reach the end of the portal sinus; but when injected into the portal vein none enters the portal sinus (*14, 15*). This disparity suggests that some umbilical venous

SPECIAL
CIRCULATIONS

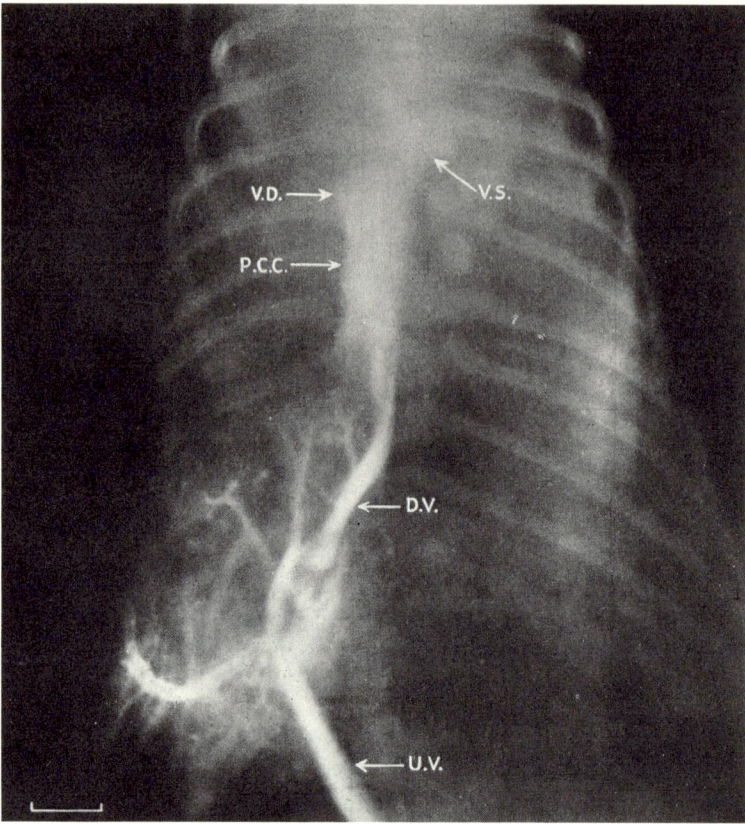

Figure 21. Cineradiograph of an umbilical vein injection into a lamb fetus. U.V., umbilical vein; D.V., ductus venosus. The posterior (inferior vena) caval channel, P.C.C., appears to be bifurcating into its terminal left (V.S.) division through the foramen ovale, and its right (V.D.) division in the right atrium.

blood may normally spill over into the portal vein, although, being diluted with portal venous blood, it might no longer be sufficiently radiopaque to throw a shadow during angiography. This overflow could be of biological interest. Thus, in the fetal lamb, the left side of the liver (about two-thirds of the whole) is supplied with umbilical venous blood which is 80 per cent saturated with oxygen (Fig. 8); the right side is supplied by branches of the portal vein after its junction with the portal sinus. If these right-sided branches contain only portal venous blood, the oxygen saturation will be low, 27 per cent according to Fig. 8; if they contain half portal and half umbilical venous blood the saturation will be 53.5 per cent. There is no experimental evidence yet available to settle this point, and it is difficult to obtain blood samples from the portal supply to the right side of the liver; we are still uncertain about the course of the circulation of the blood to the right side of the liver. The difference between the blood supply of the two sides of the fetal liver is also of interest for two other reasons: first, because it has been reported that there are more hemopoietic foci in the right than in the left side of the liver (*88*), and second, because degenerative changes, macroscopically visible, have been described as being more severe on the right than the left side in babies that are stillborn or die within three days of birth (*107, 108*). Both of these observations would be consistent with the view that the right side is less well supplied with oxygen than is the left.

This seems an appropriate place to digress for a moment, to consider the pressure in the umbilical vein. The first measurements of umbilical venous pressure were made, in 1884, in fetal lambs by Cohnstein and Zuntz; these measurements are illustrated in Fig. 22. The values recorded were high, 16 to 34 mm. Hg, but the high values may

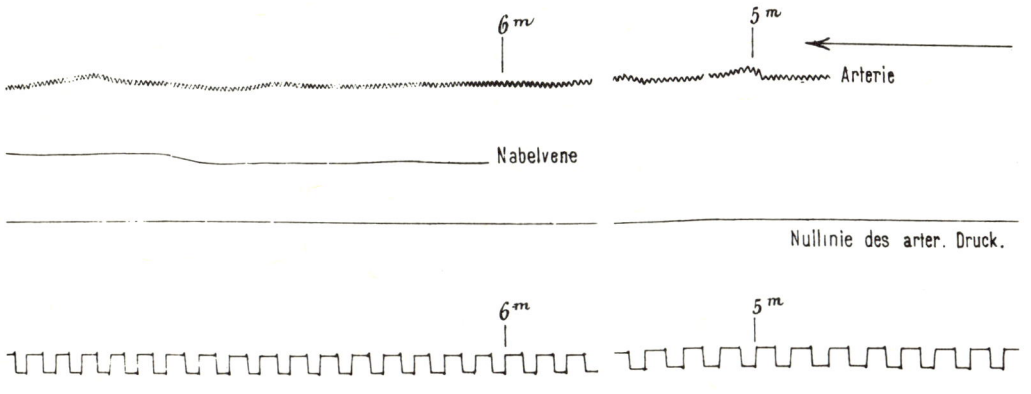

Figure 22. Excerpts from the first published record, by Cohnstein and Zuntz (1884), showing umbilical arterial and venous pressures, measured with a mercury manometer and displayed on a kymograph.

SPECIAL
CIRCULATIONS

have been due to the fact that one whole umbilical vein was obstructed (there are two such veins in sheep). According to Barcroft the pressure in the umbilical veins of the fetal lamb at term is 9 to 18 mm. Hg (*18*). Most subsequent observations agree with these (*64, 166*). The point is an important one, because if we accept a figure of about 65 mm. Hg for the aortic pressure in a fetal lamb near term, about 10 mm. Hg for the abdominal umbilical vein, and zero for the inferior vena cava, it follows that the umbilical circulation offers 85 per cent and the liver and ductus venosus only 15 per cent of the total vascular resistance of the circuit. Most of the vascular resistance lies between the cotyledonary arteries and veins (probably in the fetal villi), and since umbilical blood flow is proportionately so large this vascular bed constitutes one of the most important determinants of fetal blood pressure (*64*). This resistance changes during gestation and may be, to a limited extent, under some degree of physiological control even though the umbilical blood vessels are not innervated. It is also clear that the vascular resistance of the liver and ductus venosus (which are in parallel) are likely to be of comparatively small importance in determining umbilical blood flow. However, changes in umbilical blood flow and in hepatic vascular resistance might alter the distribution of portal and umbilical venous blood to the two sides of the liver.

To return to the ductus venosus, in 1942 Barclay, Franklin, and Prichard observed that the cineangiograms of newborn lambs showed lateral indentations of the ductus venosus at its origin from the portal sinus. "From time to time the indentations vary in degree, and when the ductus venosus shadow disappears, the umbilical vein shadow ends at, or near to, the line joining the indentations." They therefore postulated the existence of a smooth muscle sphincter at this point, whose presence was subsequently confirmed in a variety of species (*15, 29, 30*). A partly contracted bovine specimen is seen in Fig. 23, which shows a view of the ductus venosus from the umbilical vein. This sphincter is innervated by branches of the vagi, which may be post-ganglionic sympathetic fibers. It is thought to contract within a few minutes of birth and thus to effect functional closure of the vessel. This approximately coincides in time with the partial constriction of the ductus arteriosus after birth, but nothing is known about the physiological mechanism responsible. Anatomical closure is not effected for some

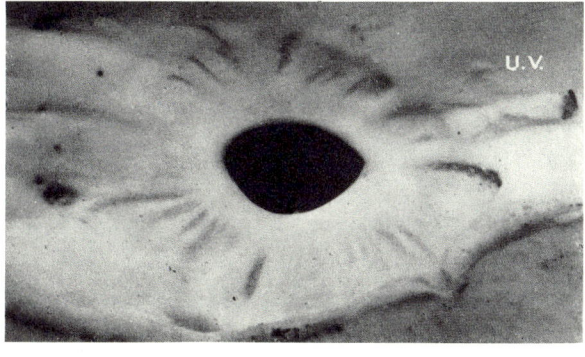

Figure 23. A view of the ductus venosus from the umbilical vein in the bovine fetus, showing the partly contracted sphincter. The scale is in mm.

days or weeks later (*175*). In the human baby a soft catheter may be passed from the umbilical vein through the ductus venosus for a few days after birth (*172*) though a resistance is felt which may be due to the sphincter. It would seem desirable, on physiological grounds, that the sphincter should close rapidly after birth, since otherwise part of the portal venous blood will bypass the liver. Whether temporary or permanent patency of the ductus venosus is common after birth is not known, nor has the effect of asphyxia been studied.

Changes in Blood Volume and Cardiac Output after Birth

The first observations on the distribution of blood between the fetus and the placenta were carried out in 1884 by Cohnstein and Zuntz on rabbits. Although these early experiments were technically rather crude (*18*), the general conclusions drawn from them have been substantially confirmed by later work in goats and lambs (*23, 24, 87*). During the earlier part of gestation most of the blood is in the placenta; toward the end of gestation most of the blood is in the fetus (Fig. 24). In the first two-thirds of gestation about one-sixth of the combined weight of fetus and placenta is blood, whereas only one-twelfth to one-fifteenth of the weight of an adult sheep is blood. Toward term the ratio decreases slightly, but even at birth the blood volume of the fetal lamb (excluding the placenta, about 120 ml./kg.) is proportionately greater than that of an adult sheep (65 ml./kg.).

SPECIAL CIRCULATIONS

When an animal, or a baby, is born, some of the blood which is in the placenta may drain into the fetus. Gunther (*109*) quotes a passage by Erasmus Darwin (1801) as follows:

"Another thing very injurious to the child is the tying and cutting of the navel-string too soon; which should always be left till the child has not only repeatedly breathed but till all pulsation in the cord ceases. As otherwise the child is much weaker than it ought to be, a part of the blood being left in the placenta, which ought to have been in the child."

Estimates of this change in volume have been made since the end of the nineteenth century. In 1876, Budin (*168*) and in 1884, Cohnstein and Zuntz (*54*) reported the amount so transferred in babies to be 60 to 100 grams. Subsequent investigators have confirmed these observations in man (*78, 109, 115, 197*), lambs (*17, 18*), and foals (*171*). Our problem is to decide whether this placental transfusion is important from a circulatory standpoint. As the average baby at the moment of birth

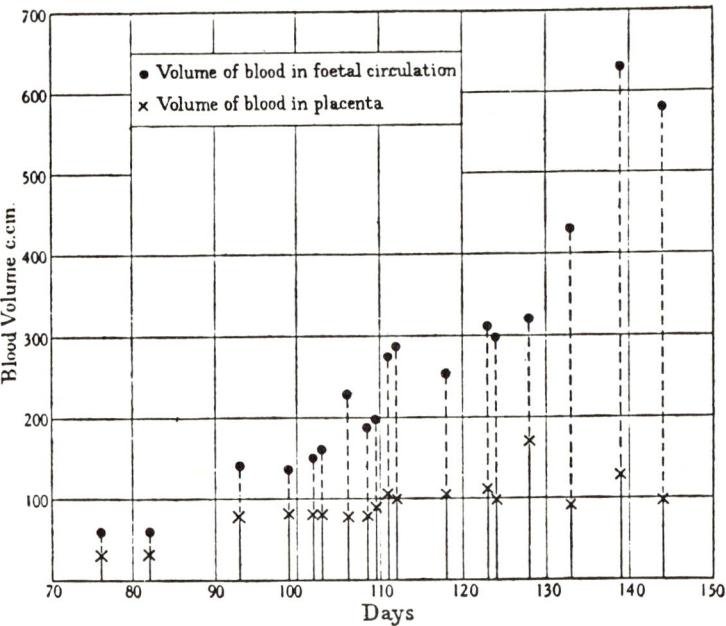

Figure 24. The distribution of blood between the fetus and the placenta in sheep.

probably contains about 370 ml. blood (*98*), placental transfusion may amount to 25 per cent of the fetal blood volume.

It has been suggested that part of the blood derived from the placenta may be used to increase the volume of blood in the lungs. On this question, opinions have differed to the extent that Barclay, Franklin, and Prichard have even proposed that the pulmonary blood volume may decrease after birth (*15*). The first direct measurements in 1939 by Abel and Windle on kittens suggested that there was no change an hour after birth (*1*). These observations were criticized on technical grounds; later experiments on guinea pigs by Sinha (*181*) and particularly by Everett (*89*) and Everett and Simmons (*90*), who administered radioactive iron to the mothers, led to the conclusion that the pulmonary blood volume doubled after sixteen hours. It is apparent in view of these disparate results that more experimental information is needed.

Various authors have noticed that the baby or animal is generally more active after birth than *in utero* (*15, 199*) and it therefore seemed likely that cardiac output might have increased. There is also the possibility that blood flow will increase through the respiratory muscles and the intestines. On the other hand, as Clement Smith has mentioned, the removal of the circulation through the placenta might be expected to reduce cardiac output (*183*). The only direct information available is presented in Fig. 2. It was concluded that the combined output of both ventricles in the fetal lamb at term was about 235 ml./kg./min. The output of the left ventricle was estimated at 135 and that of the right ventricle at 100 ml./kg./min. In sixteen newborn lambs, from less than one day up to sixty days of age, cardiac output measured by the direct Fick method averaged 325 ml./kg./min. (*59*). This value suggests that there may have been an increase in cardiac output after birth. The increase in pulmonary blood flow, from 30 to 325 ml./kg./min., is not far from the range of increase, three- to ten-fold, observed on direct measurement with a flowmeter in the left pulmonary artery after positive pressure ventilation. Systemic blood flow, according to these calculations, increased from 75 to 325 ml./kg./min. It is clearly desirable that the results of these calculations be checked by other methods.

There are physiological considerations which make these calculations appear reasonable. These considerations derive from the fact that, other things being equal, the rate of cooling of a solid body is propor-

SPECIAL
CIRCULATIONS

tional to its surface area. Even in a neutral thermal environment a small newborn animal has a relatively high metabolic rate. In the lamb there is a threefold increase in oxygen consumption shortly after birth (68). In fetal lambs the rate of oxygen consumption is about 5 ml./kg./min., much the same as in adult sheep, but within a few hours from birth it increases to 12 to 15 ml./kg./min. This is necessary if the lamb is to maintain its body temperature. A hint of a similar striking increase in goats was given in an earlier paper by Barcroft, Flexner, and McClurkin (22). Barron and Meschia (32) calculated the maximal possible O_2 consumption of a mature fetal rabbit as 7.7 ml./kg./min., while recent measurements of the O_2 consumption of a newborn rabbit in a neutral thermal environment show that it is more than double this figure. Information in other species is less complete, and suggests that there may be considerable differences in the changes which take place in basal metabolic rate (at a neutral thermal environment) *after* birth. While there is evidence in the puppy (99) and the pig (151) of an increase similar in magnitude to that in the lamb, in the rat the minimal O_2 consumption increases only by about 50 per cent during the first two days after birth (191). In the rhesus monkey it doubles over the first two weeks (66); in the human infant it does not increase much during the first week after birth but does thereafter (47).

The newborn of all mammalian species have to face the problems of maintaining a higher metabolic rate on exposure to cold, which they inevitably suffer to some extent even when provided with a nest, burrow, pouch, or swaddling clothes (93). They all react to cold by an increase in metabolic rate (47, 59, 119, 147, 151, 191). So in different species, at different times from birth and under different physiological conditions, we must expect an increase in either cardiac output or in arteriovenous oxygen difference proportionate to the increase in oxygen consumption.

The Development of Nervous Control of the Circulation

It may well be asked whether in a fetus, which is so well protected from changes in its external environment, and whose capacity for physical exercise is limited, the size or distribution of the cardiac output needs to be regulated or indeed is ever regulated with any nicety. One example may be given, of the response to oxygen lack, which will generally be admitted as a possible hazard to fetal survival. Oxygen lack causes a rise in arterial blood pressure in mature fetal lambs, and hence a passive increase in umbilical blood flow, which thus enables relatively more oxygen to be taken up from the placenta (*40, 64*). Such few measurements as have been made show little evidence of an increase in cardiac output under these circumstances, but there is certainly a redistribution of cardiac output, since pulmonary vascular resistance rises (*69*). It should not be assumed that this can be construed as evidence of nervous regulation of the circulation; the phenomena could be attributed to the local effect of oxygen lack, fall of pH, or perhaps to direct liberation of catecholamines (*55*).

Nevertheless the regulation of the circulation in the fetus and at birth is probably to some extent under nervous control. It is not easy to provide a satisfactory answer to the question "how much?" One of the most striking observations of recent years, made by Jost (*128, 129*), might suggest the answer "not at all." Jost found that rabbit fetuses, decapitated *in utero* on the nineteenth day of gestation, continued to live and grow from a weight of less than 2 grams (headless) to 17 to 25 grams on the twenty-eighth day. However, this is only part of the evidence.

One of the earliest and simplest of experiments was to stimulate the vagus and to see whether the heart slowed. In fetal and newborn puppies (*118, 149*) and in newborn kittens (*7*) it did slow. In newborn rabbits the evidence is conflicting (*133, 184*), possibly because the nerve is fragile and easily damaged (*65*). In fetal lambs early in the second half of gestation stimulation of the vagus slows the heart, and stimulation of the left cardiac nerves accelerates it. In both fetal lambs and babies there is also an adequate supply of sympathomimetic amines in the adrenal glands. The cardiovascular system, in both the fetal and the newborn lamb and rabbit, responds to the injection of epinephrine, norepinephrine, and acetylcholine in the way to be expected from observations on adult animals of the same species, having regard to the special features of the fetal circulation (*65, 70*). These observations suggest that the efferent mechanisms are available which can regulate the circulation toward the end of gestation and at birth.

The next question is whether the vasomotor reflexes are functional at birth. Clark concluded that, in the dog and rat, they did not develop

SPECIAL CIRCULATIONS

until after birth (*51*), and Bauer (*34*) reached the same conclusion about rabbits. Yet partial anoxia or asphyxia of newborn puppies causes an abrupt rise of blood pressure and heart rate. There is also evidence that the baroreceptor (*81*) and chemoreceptor (*67*) mechanisms are functional, even in an animal which is so immature at birth as the rabbit and in which the blood pressure does not rise during *acute* anoxia. It seems possible that some of Clark's difficulties arose from the fact that he recorded the blood pressure of newborn puppies and kittens with a mercury manometer on a kymograph, and he also may not have realized how sensitive some newborn animals are to the effect of anesthetics. The introduction of improved manometers since the last war has certainly made experiments on small animals much easier. In the lamb, which is larger and therefore simpler to handle, there is good evidence that baroreceptor reflexes are present before birth (*60, 80, 123*). At term acute anoxia caused a large rise of blood pressure and heart rate, while injection of hexamethonium (which blocks autonomic ganglia) caused a fall of pressure (*40*); neither response was present halfway through gestation. Comline and Silver (*55*) also showed that anoxia liberated considerable quantities of epinephrine and norepinephrine from the adrenals toward term. Thus some of the normal adult mechanisms for cardiovascular regulation are present at birth, although it is uncertain to what extent they are actively concerned in the regulation of the circulation in early fetal life.

The mean arterial blood pressure, which rises gradually during gestation and after birth, may also give some indication of the development of nervous control of the circulation, although it should not be forgotten that the heart and blood vessels are growing at the same time. At birth the blood pressure is a little over 30 mm. Hg in the rabbit and kitten, about 40 in the puppy, 50 in the human baby, and over 60 in the lamb, calf, and foal. In newborn babies the very striking changes in skin color which occur during anoxia, and the large changes in heart rate which are sometimes observed, strongly suggest that they are not very different from other newborn animals of the same size.

Let us return briefly to Jost's experiments. His headless rabbits lived until near the end of gestation, but they would not have been able to survive birth, for they could not breathe. Whether an animal that is born in a more mature condition, such as a lamb, could survive until term without its brain has still to be discovered. And it is also uncertain whether the transformation of the circulation at birth is a purely mechanical process or whether some degree of nervous control is essential.

The Ability to Withstand Asphyxia

Another profound difference between the fetus and the newborn animal on the one hand, and the adult on the other hand, is in their ability to survive asphyxia or anoxia. Anyone who has tried to drown a puppy or kitten must be aware of this fact. So far as scientific literature is concerned, Paul Bert (1870) is usually credited with the first demonstration that the newborn survives longer in nitrogen than the adult animal (36). But two centuries earlier, Robert Boyle (46), in a series of "new pneumatical experiments about respiration," found that the newborn kitten survived about three times as long without oxygen as an adult animal of the same size. Systematic measurements, which have been made only comparatively recently (92, 103, 130, 165), showed that the tolerance of the newborn to anoxia is related to its maturity at birth. Thus, while adults survived breathing nitrogen for only three minutes or so, newborn rats survived on the average fifty minutes, kittens twenty-five minutes, puppies twenty-three minutes, newborn rabbits seventeen minutes, and guinea pigs (which are more mature at birth) only seven minutes. Lambs and calves are unable to survive oxygen lack for more than a few minutes at birth. As in the adult, the ability to survive prolonged asphyxia or anoxia is increased as the body temperature is reduced. The striking difference between the adult and the newborn can be illustrated by experiments in dogs and puppies (189). In adult dogs circulatory failure occurs and resuscitation is not feasible when the systolic pressure falls below 100 mm. Hg, but newborn puppies were revived when the pressure had fallen to as low as 8/6 mm. Hg. During the period of anoxia, which lasted twenty minutes or more with survival, respiratory efforts were infrequent and gasping, and the carbon dioxide tension of arterial blood rose to 100 to 150 mm. Hg with a very large fall in pH.

The observations of Fazekas, Alexander, and Himwich (92) showed that glycolysis is important for the survival of young animals during anoxia, since their survival time is greatly reduced on administration of iodoacetic acid or fluoride, which inhibit enzymes important in glyco-

CHANGES IN CIRCULATION AFTER BIRTH

SPECIAL CIRCULATIONS

lysis. These observations raised a number of possibilities, that metabolic rate might be higher in older animals, that glycolysis might proceed faster in younger ones, and so on. One of the difficulties in testing these hypotheses was that the newborn of most laboratory animals are too small to provide serial blood samples; however, the fetal lamb is suitable (71). At ninety days gestation age it will survive at least forty minutes of complete asphyxia after tying the cord, whereas at term (147 days) the circulation fails after ten to fifteen minutes. Adult sheep cannot be revived after seven minutes of rebreathing nitrogen from a bag. An interesting feature of these observations is that the decrease in survival time of lambs during asphyxia begins well before birth and therefore cannot be attributed to the better oxygenation of the blood or the changes in the circulation after birth. There is no evidence that glycolysis proceeds faster in younger fetal lambs, nor is the oxygen consumption of older fetal lambs greater per kg. of body tissue. But the carbohydrate reserves of the cardiac ventricles are much greater in the younger lambs, which have a proportionately longer survival time. In all the mammalian species investigated the cardiac glycogen is high (40 mg./gram) early in gestation, and falls towards adult values (less than 5 mg./gram) with increasing age (*180*). In different species and at different ages from birth the survival time was found to bear a roughly linear relation to the initial carbohydrate store of the heart (Fig. 25).

This observation, which has been confirmed by further experiments in the rat (*185*) and monkey (*66*), raises an interesting problem. The direct correlation between initial cardiac glycogen and the time to the last gasp after the onset of asphyxia suggests that the circulation is the limiting factor. So long as its blood supply is sufficient the respiratory center continues to discharge, even in the absence of oxygen. Presumably the cells derive sufficient energy by anaerobic glycolysis, and the continued circulation is needed both to bring glucose to the tissues and, by removing and redistributing acid metabolites, to prevent the tissue pH from falling too rapidly. This theory is supported by the observation that, in premature fetal lambs, intravenous infusion of glucose and alkali prolongs survival during total asphyxia (*72*); both glucose and alkali are required. In mature fetal lambs and monkeys, survival during asphyxia (to the last breath) can be prolonged by the same means, and recovery is facilitated.

These experiments demonstrate the importance of the circulation during birth asphyxia. There can be no doubt that the ability of the newborn of many species to survive prolonged asphyxia is of real value, particularly in man.

Earlier, reference was made to the special characteristics of the neonatal circulation. These include the continued patency of the ductus arteriosus and its possible consequences, the equal thickness of the two ventricles, the volume of cardiac output, and possibly the immaturity of nervous control. The ability of the cardiovascular system to keep on working in the face of complete and prolonged asphyxia is another

CHANGES IN
CIRCULATION
AFTER BIRTH

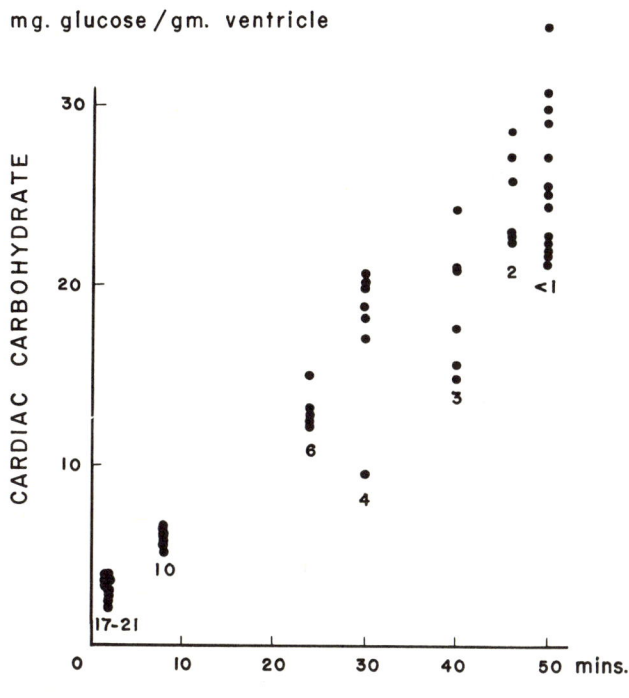

Figure 25. The relation between the carbohydrate content of the ventricles of young rats and the mean survival time in nitrogen. The numeral beneath each group indicates the age in days.

SPECIAL
CIRCULATIONS

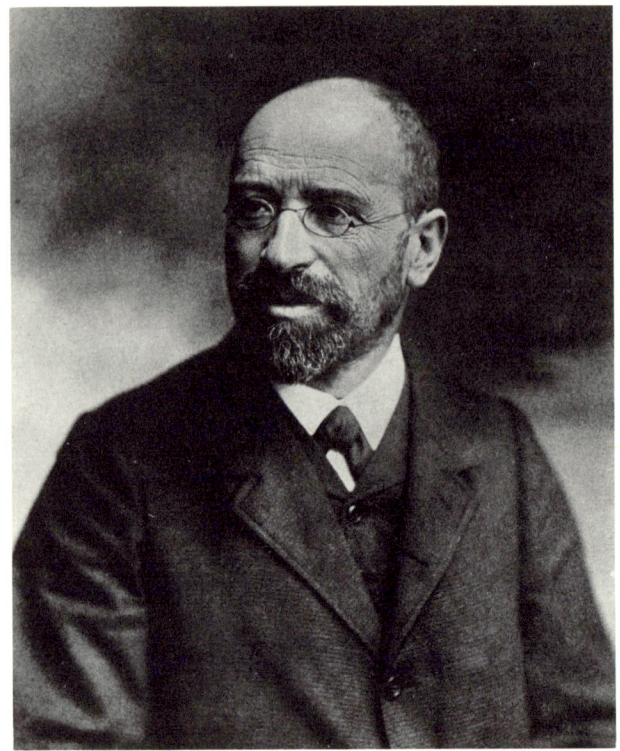

Figure 26. Nathan Zuntz (1847-1920).

remarkable feature, and must be remembered when physiological or pathological changes in the newborn are analyzed.

Conclusion

The development of knowledge of the circulation before and after birth has been slow compared with that of the adult. From the discovery of the circulation of the blood until the end of the nineteenth century, theories were built on the gross anatomical facts, but could not be tested further. Even the introduction of the microscope had little influence. Then in 1884 the brilliant paper by Cohnstein and Zuntz showed what might be done with the simple instruments (like the mercury manometer) which were then available. It is astonishing that their example was not followed until Huggett's experiments in 1927.

The first record of fetal arterial blood pressure was probably made in 1876 and that of umbilical venous pressure in 1884, but the pressure in the pulmonary artery does not seem to have been measured until 1950. This gives some idea of how recent is our knowledge of important parts of the fetal and neonatal circulation. Where, then, do we stand now?

CHANGES IN CIRCULATION AFTER BIRTH

We are in an insecure position, and it is only by accepting much of the evidence published during the last ten years, in many instances still unconfirmed by other workers and different techniques, that it has been possible to put together a connected story. During these ten years there have been considerable advances in our knowledge of fetal and neonatal physiology, not limited to the circulation, but in fields closely related, as in thermoregulation, or more distantly, as in enzyme development. A general misconception about young animals, that they can be regarded as miniature but passive and ineffectual adults, has been replaced by the realization that, because of their immaturity, small size, and rapid growth, their physiology is indeed different, yet they do need and possess mechanisms for regulating their internal environment satisfactorily, in the conditions in which they ordinarily find themselves. Even the existence of this misconception does not explain why so little systematic and critical attention has been given to such problems. There is even one place in the fetal circulation, the junction between portal vein and portal sinus, where there is still some uncertainty as to the direction of blood flow. Quantitative measurements of blood flow have been few, although the methods are available. Much needs to be learned about the nervous control of the fetal and neonatal circulations. Do the carotid chemoreceptors fire continuously in response to the low oxygen tension of fetal arterial blood, and does their rate of discharge therefore decrease abruptly at birth? Do the baroreceptors of the carotid sinus and aortic arch increase their thresholds as the blood pressure rises during gestation and after birth? How is the cardiac output partitioned between the fetus and placenta at different ages and under different physiological conditions? And to what extent, if at all, can circulatory changes in the fetus or placenta limit fetal growth or survival at birth? Every fresh discovery in the adult circulation brings its repercussions, and work upon the living fetus or newborn infant presents special difficulties.

SPECIAL CIRCULATIONS

Finally a word must be said about the integration of physiological mechanisms. For to understand fully the fetal circulation and its changes at birth we also need to understand the nervous and hormonal mechanisms which regulate every aspect of fetal and neonatal physiology. The circulation cannot properly be studied in isolation, nor the infant without its mother. What, for instance, are the factors which determine the growth of the placenta and its vessels, both fetal and maternal? And how is this growth adjusted to fetal development? It is curiosity and speculation which provide the principal driving force for all research, and the broad gap between embryology and the classical physiology of adult mammals seems likely to provide an ample field for both.

BIBLIOGRAPHY

1. ABEL, S., and W. F. WINDLE. Relation of the volume of pulmonary circulation to respiration at birth. Anat. Rec., 75:451, 1939.
2. ACHESON, G. H., G. S. DAWES, and J. C. MOTT. Oxygen consumption and arterial oxygen saturation in foetal and new-born lambs. J. Physiol. (Lond.), 135:623, 1957.
3. ADAMS, F. H., and J. LIND. Physiologic studies on the cardiovascular status of normal newborn infants (with special reference to the ductus arteriosus). Pediatrics, 19:431, 1957.
4. ALZAMORA, V., A. ROTTA, G. BATTILANA, R. ABUGATTAS, C. RUBIO, J. BOURONCLE, C. ZAPATA, E. SANTA-MARIÁ, T. BINDER, R. SUBIRIA, D. PAREDES, B. PANDO, and G. G. GRAHAM. On the possible influence of great altitudes on the determination of certain cardiovascular anomalies. Pediatrics, 12:259, 1953.
5. AMOROSO, E. C., G. S. DAWES, and J. C. MOTT. Patency of the ductus arteriosus in the newborn calf and foal. Brit. Heart J., 20:92, 1958.
6. AMOROSO, E. C., G. S. DAWES, J. C. MOTT, and B. R. RENNICK. Occlusion of the ductus venosus in the mature foetal lamb. J. Physiol. (Lond.), 129:64P, 1955.
7. ANREP, B. v. Ueber die Entwicklung der hemmenden Functionen bei Neugeborenen. Pflügers Arch. ges. Physiol., 21:78, 1880.
8. ANSELMINO, K. J., and F. HOFFMANN. Die Ursachen des Icterus neonatorum. Arch. Gynäk., 143:477, 1930.
9. ARANZI, G. C. De humano foetu libellus. Bononiae, Rubrius, 1564.

10. ARDRAN, G. M., G. S. DAWES, M. M. L. PRICHARD, S. R. M. REYNOLDS, and D. G. WYATT. The effect of ventilation of the foetal lungs upon the pulmonary circulation. J. Physiol. (Lond.), 118:12, 1952.
11. BARCLAY, A. E., J. BARCROFT, D. H. BARRON, and K. J. FRANKLIN. A radiographic demonstration of the circulation through the heart in the adult and in the foetus, and the identification of the ductus arteriosus. Brit. J. Radiol., 12:505, 1939.
12. BARCLAY, A. E., J. BARCROFT, D. H. BARRON, K. J. FRANKLIN, and M. M. L. PRICHARD. Pulmonary circulation times before and after functional closure of the ductus arteriosus. J. Physiol. (Lond.), 101:375, 1942.
13. BARCLAY, A. E., and K. J. FRANKLIN. The time of functional closure of the foramen ovale in the lamb. J. Physiol. (Lond.), 94:256, 1938.
14. BARCLAY, A. E., K. J. FRANKLIN, and M. M. L. PRICHARD. The mechanism of closure of the ductus venosus. Brit. J. Radiol., 15:66, 1942.
15. BARCLAY, A. E., K. J. FRANKLIN, and M. M. L. PRICHARD. The Foetal Circulation and Cardiovascular System, and the Changes that They Undergo at Birth. Oxford, Blackwell Scientific Publications, 1944.
16. BARCROFT, J. Foetal circulation and respiration. Physiol. Rev., 16:103, 1936.
17. BARCROFT, J. Four phases of birth. Lancet, II:91, 1941.
18. BARCROFT, J. Researches on pre-natal life. Oxford, Blackwell Scientific Publications, 1946.
19. BARCROFT, J., D. H. BARRON, A. T. COWIE, and P. H. FORSHAM. The oxygen supply of the foetal brain of the sheep and the effect of asphyxia on foetal respiratory movement. J. Physiol. (Lond.), 97:338, 1940.
20. BARCROFT, J., D. H. BARRON, K. KRAMER, and G. A. MILLIKAN. Factors which influence the oxygen supply of the brain at birth. Fiziol. Z. U.S.S.R., 24:43, 1938.
21. BARCROFT, J., R. H. E. ELLIOTT, L. B. FLEXNER, F. G. HALL, W. HERKEL, E. F. MCCARTHY, T. MCCLURKIN, and M. TALAAT. Conditions of foetal respiration in the goat. J. Physiol. (Lond.), 83:192, 1934.
22. BARCROFT, J., L. B. FLEXNER, and T. MCCLURKIN. The output of the foetal heart in the goat. J. Physiol. (Lond.), 82:498, 1934.
23. BARCROFT, J., and T. GOTSEV. Acquisition of blood by the foetus from the placenta at birth. J. Physiol. (Lond.), 90:27P, 1937.
24. BARCROFT, J., and J. A. KENNEDY. The distribution of blood between the foetus and the placenta in sheep. J. Physiol. (Lond.), 95:173, 1939.
25. BARCROFT, J., J. A. KENNEDY, and M. F. MASON. The relation of

the vagus nerve to the ductus arteriosus in the guinea-pig. J. Physiol. (Lond.), 92:1P, 1938.
26. BARCROFT, J., K. KRAMER, and G. A. MILLIKAN. The oxygen in the carotid blood at birth. J. Physiol. (Lond.), 94:571, 1939.
27. BARCROFT, J., and D. S. TORRENS. The output of the heart of the foetal sheep. J. Physiol. (Lond.), 105:22P, 1946.
28. BARKER, J. N., and H. G. BRITTON. Lactate and pyruvate metabolism in the foetal sheep. J. Physiol. (Lond.), 143:50P, 1958.
29. BARRON, D. H. The "sphincter" of the ductus venosus. Anat. Rec., 82:398, 1958.
30. BARRON, D. H. The changes in the fetal circulation at birth. Physiol. Rev., 24:277, 1944.
31. BARRON, D. H., and F. C. BATTAGLIA. The oxygen concentration gradient between the plasmas in the maternal and fetal capillaries of the placenta of the rabbit. Yale J. Biol. Med., 28:197, 1955–56.
32. BARRON, D. H., and G. MESCHIA. A comparative study of the exchange of the respiratory gases across the placenta. Cold Spr. Harb. Symp. quant. Biol., 19:93, 1954.
33. BARTELS, H., W. MOLL, and J. METCALFE. Physiology of gas exchange in the human placenta. Amer. J. Obst. Gynec., 84:1714, 1962.
34. BAUER, D. J. Vagal reflexes appearing in asphyxia in rabbits at different ages. J. Physiol. (Lond.), 95:187, 1939.
35. BEER, R., H. BARTELS, and H. A. RACZKOWSKI. Die Sauerstoffdissoziationskurve des fetalen Blutes und der Gasaustausch in der menschlichen Placenta. Pflügers Arch. ges. Physiol., 260:306, 1955.
36. BERT, P. Leçons sur la physiologie comparée de la respiration. Paris, Baillière, 1870.
37. BERTIN, M. Sur le cours du sang dans le foie du foetus humain. Mém. Acad. Roy. Sci., (Paris), 323, 1753.
38. BICHAT, X. Anatomie générale, appliqueé à la physiologie et à la médecine. Paris, Brosson, Gabon et Cie, 1801.
39. BORN, G. V. R., G. S. DAWES, and J. C. MOTT. The viability of premature lambs. J. Physiol. (Lond.), 130:191, 1955.
40. BORN, G. V. R., G. S. DAWES, and J. C. MOTT. Oxygen lack and autonomic nervous control of the foetal circulation in the lamb. J. Physiol. (Lond.), 134:149, 1956.
41. BORN, G. V. R., G. S. DAWES, J. C. MOTT, and B. R. RENNICK. The relief of central cyanosis caused by pulmonary arteriovenous shunts by construction of an artificial ductus arteriosus. J. Physiol. (Lond.), 130:167, 1955.
42. BORN, G. V. R., G. S. DAWES, J. C. MOTT, and B. R. RENNICK. The constriction of the ductus arteriosus caused by oxygen and by asphyxia in newborn lambs. J. Physiol. (Lond.), 132:304, 1956.

43. BORN, G. V. R., G. S. DAWES, J. C. MOTT, and J. G. WIDDICOMBE. Changes in the heart and lungs at birth. Cold Spr. Harb. Symp. quant. Biol., 19:102, 1954.
44. BORST, H. G., M. McGREGOR, J. L. WHITTENBERGER, and E. BERGLUND. Influence of pulmonary arterial and left atrial pressures on pulmonary vascular resistance. Circulation Res., 4:393, 1956.
45. BOYD, J. D. The nerve supply of the mammalian ductus arteriosus. J. Anat. (Lond.), 75:457, 1941.
46. BOYLE, R. New pneumatical experiments about respiration. Phil. Trans. Roy. Soc., 5:2011, 1670.
47. BRÜCK, K. Temperature regulation in the newborn infant. Biol. Neonat., 3:65, 1961.
48. BURNARD, E. D. A murmur from the ductus arteriosus in the newborn baby. Brit. med. J., I:806, 1958.
49. CARLILL, S. D., H. N. DUKE, and M. JONES. Some observations on pulmonary haemodynamics in the cat. J. Physiol. (Lond.), 136:112, 1957.
50. CHRISTIE, A. Normal closing time of the foramen ovale and ductus arteriosus. Amer. J. Dis. Child., 40:323, 1930.
51. CLARK, G. A. The development of blood-pressure reflexes. J. Physiol. (Lond.), 83:229, 1934.
52. CLEMETSON, C. A. B., and J. CHURCHMAN. Oxygen and carbon dioxide content of umbilical artery and vein blood in toxaemic and normal pregnancy. J. Obstet. Gynaec. Brit. Emp., 60:335, 1953.
53. COHNSTEIN, J., and N. ZUNTZ. Untersuchungen über das Blut, den Kreislauf und die Athmung beim Säugethier-Fötus. Pflügers Arch. ges. Physiol., 34:173, 1884.
54. COHNSTEIN, J., and N. ZUNTZ. Weitere Untersuchungen zur Physiologie des Säugethier-Fötus. Pflügers Arch. ges. Physiol., 42:342, 1888.
55. COMLINE, R. S., and M. SILVER. The release of adrenaline and noradrenaline from the adrenal glands of the foetal sheep. J. Physiol. (Lond.), 156:424, 1961.
56. CONDORELLI, M., A. DAGIANTI, C. POLOSA, and G. GIULIANO. Sulla persistenza di un fisiologico corto circuito attraverso il foramine ovale nei primi giorni della vita extrauterina. Atti Soc. ital. Cardiol. XIX Congresso, 2:165, 1957.
57. COOPER, K. E., and A. D. M. GREENFIELD. A method for measuring the blood flow in the umbilical vessels. J. Physiol. (Lond.), 108:167, 1949.
58. COOPER, K. E., A. D. M. GREENFIELD, and A. ST. G. HUGGETT. The umbilical blood flow in the foetal sheep. J. Physiol. (Lond.), 108:160, 1949.

SPECIAL CIRCULATIONS

59. CROSS, K. W., G. S. DAWES, and J. C. MOTT. Anoxia, oxygen consumption and cardiac output in new-born lambs and adult sheep. J. Physiol. (Lond.), 146:316, 1959.
60. CROSS, K. W., and J. L. MALCOLM. Evidence of carotid body and sinus activity in new-born and foetal animals. J. Physiol. (Lond.), 118:10P, 1952.
61. DALY, I. DE B., and M. DE B. DALY. The effects of stimulation of the carotid body chemoreceptors on pulmonary vascular resistance in the dog. J. Physiol. (Lond.), 137:436, 1957.
62. DANESINO, V. L., S. R. M. REYNOLDS, and I. H. REHMAN. Comparative histological structure of the human ductus arteriosus according to topography, age, and degree of constriction. Anat. Rec., 121:801, 1955.
63. DAWES, G. S. Changes in O_2 supply within the foetal lamb. J. Physiol. (Lond.), 159:44P, 1961.
64. DAWES, G. S. The umbilical circulation. Amer. J. Obstet. Gynec., 84:1634, 1962.
65. DAWES, G. S., J. J. HANDLER, and J. C. MOTT. Some cardiovascular responses in foetal, new-born and adult rabbits. J. Physiol. (Lond.), 139:123, 1957.
66. DAWES, G. S., H. N. JACOBSON, J. C. MOTT, and H. J. SHELLEY. Some observations on foetal and new-born rhesus monkeys. J. Physiol. (Lond.), 152:271, 1960.
67. DAWES, G. S., and J. C. MOTT. Reflex respiratory activity in the newborn rabbit. J. Physiol. (Lond.), 145:85, 1959.
68. DAWES, G. S., and J. C. MOTT. The increase in oxygen consumption of the lamb after birth. J. Physiol. (Lond.), 146:295, 1959.
69. DAWES, G. S., and J. C. MOTT. The vascular tone of the foetal lung. J. Physiol. (Lond.), 164:465, 1962.
70. DAWES, G. S., J. C. MOTT, and B. R. RENNICK. Some effects of adrenaline, noradrenaline and acetylcholine on the foetal circulation in the lamb. J. Physiol. (Lond.), 134:139, 1956.
71. DAWES, G. S., J. C. MOTT, and H. SHELLEY. The importance of cardiac glycogen for the maintenance of life in foetal lambs and newborn animals during anoxia. J. Physiol. (Lond.), 146:516, 1959.
72. DAWES, G. S., J. C. MOTT, H. J. SHELLEY, and A. STAFFORD. The prolongation of survival in asphyxiated immature foetal lambs. J. Physiol. (Lond.), in press, 1963.
73. DAWES, G. S., J. C. MOTT, and J. G. WIDDICOMBE. The foetal circulation in the lamb. J. Physiol. (Lond.), 126:563, 1954.
74. DAWES, G. S., J. C. MOTT, and J. G. WIDDICOMBE. The cardiac murmur from the patent ductus arteriosus in newborn lambs. J. Physiol. (Lond.), 128:344, 1955.

75. DAWES, G. S., J. C. MOTT, and J. G. WIDDICOMBE. The patency of the ductus arteriosus in newborn lambs and its physiological consequences. J. Physiol. (Lond.), 128:361, 1955.
76. DAWES, G. S., J. C. MOTT, and J. G. WIDDICOMBE. Closure of the foramen ovale in newborn lambs. J. Physiol. (Lond.), 128:384, 1955.
77. DAWES, G. S., J. C. MOTT, J. G. WIDDICOMBE, and D. G. WYATT. Changes in the lungs of the newborn lamb. J. Physiol. (Lond.), 121:141, 1953.
78. DEMARSH, Q. B., H. L. ALT, W. F. WINDLE, and D. S. HILLIS. The effect of depriving the infant of its placental blood on the blood picture during the first week of life. J. Amer. med. Ass., 116:2568, 1941.
79. DICKSON, A. D. The ductus venosus of the pig. J. Anat. (Lond.), 90:143, 1956.
80. DONATELLI, L. La funzionalita del seno-carotideo nel feto. Arch. int. Pharmacodyn., 64:93, 1940.
81. DOWNING, S. E. Baroreceptor reflexes in new-born rabbits. J. Physiol. (Lond.), 150:201, 1960.
82. DRAKE, J. Anthropologia Nova, or, a New System of Anatomy. The Appendix. London, W. and J. Innys, 1728.
83. DUKE, H. N. Pulmonary vasomotor responses of isolated perfused cat lungs to anoxia and hypercapnia. Quart J. exp. Physiol., 36:75, 1951.
84. DUKE, H. N. The site of action of anoxia on the pulmonary blood vessels of the cat. J. Physiol. (Lond.), 125:373, 1954.
85. EASTMAN, N. J. Foetal blood studies. I. The oxygen relationships of umbilical cord blood at birth. Johns Hopk. Hosp. Bull., 47:221, 1930.
86. ELDRIDGE, F. L., H. N. HULTGREN, and M. E. WIGMORE. The physiologic closure of the ductus arteriosus in the newborn infant. J. clin. Invest., 34:987, 1955.
87. ELLIOTT, R. H., F. G. HALL, and A. ST. G. HUGGETT. The blood volume and oxygen capacity of the foetal blood in the goat. J. Physiol. (Lond.), 82:160, 1934.
88. EMERY, J. L. The distribution of haemopoietic foci in the infantile human liver. J. Anat. (Lond.), 90:293, 1956.
89. EVERETT, N. B. Early postnatal changes in pulmonary blood volume of the guinea pig. Amer. J. Physiol., 169:34, 1952.
90. EVERETT, N. B., and B. S. SIMMONS. The magnitude of increase in the pulmonary blood volume of the post-natal guinea pig. Anat. Rec., 119:429, 1954.
91. FABRICIUS, H. The Embryological Treatises. Tr. by H. B. Adelmann. Ithaca, N.Y., Cornell University Press, 1942.
92. FAZEKAS, J. F., F. A. D. ALEXANDER, and H. E. HIMWICH. Tolerance of the newborn to anoxia. Amer. J. Physiol., 134:281, 1941.

SPECIAL CIRCULATIONS

93. FELDMAN, W. M. The Principles of Ante-natal and Post-natal Child Physiology Pure and Applied. London, Longmans, Green, 1920.
94. FRANKLIN, K. J. A survey of the growth of knowledge about certain parts of the foetal cardio-vascular apparatus, and about the foetal circulation, in man and some other mammals. Part I: Galen to Harvey. Ann. Sci., 5:57, 1941.
95. FRANKLIN, K. J. Joseph Barcroft 1872–1947. Oxford, Blackwell Scientific Publications, 1953.
96. FRANKLIN, K. J., E. C. AMOROSO, A. E. BARCLAY, and M. M. L. PRICHARD. The valve of the foramen ovale and its relation to pulmonary vein entries. Vet. J., 98:29, 1942.
97. FROMBERG, C. Studien über dem Ductus arteriosus. Arb. path. Anat. Bakt., 9:198, 1914.
98. GAIRDNER, D., J. MARKS, J. D. ROSCOE, and O. R. BRETTALL. The fluid shift from the vascular compartment immediately after birth. Arch. Dis. Childh., 33:489, 1958.
99. GELINEO, S. Développement ontogénétique de la thermorégulation chez le chien. Bull. Acad. Serbe Sci., 18:97, 1957.
100. GÉRARD, G. Le canal artériel. J. Anat. (Paris), 36:1, 1900.
101. GÉRARD, G. De l'oblitération du canal artériel, les théories et les faits. J. Anat. (Paris), 36:323, 1900.
102. GIBSON, G. A. Diseases of the Heart and Aorta, pp. 61, 303, 310–312. Edinburgh, Pentland, 1898.
103. GLASS, H. G., F. F. SNYDER, and E. WEBSTER. The rate of decline in resistance to anoxia of rabbits, dogs and guinea pigs from the onset of viability to adult life. Amer. J. Physiol., 140:609, 1944.
104. GOLLWITZER-MEIER, K. Anoxämie und Kreislauf. Pflügers Arch. ges. Physiol., 220:434, 1928.
105. GRÄPER, L. Die anatomischen Veränderungen kurz nach der Geburt. III. Ductus Botalli, Z. Anat. Entw. Gesch., 61:312, 1921.
106. GROSSER, O. Vergleichende Anatomie und Entwicklungsgeschichte der Eihaute und der Placenta mit besonderer Berücksichtigung des Menschen. Vienna, Wilhelm Braumüller, 1909.
107. GRUENWALD, P. Degenerative changes in the right half of the liver resulting from intra-uterine anoxia. Amer. J. clin. Path., 19:801, 1949.
108. GRUENWALD, P. The pathology of perinatal distress. Arch. Path. (Chicago), 60:150, 1955.
109. GUNTHER, M. The transfer of blood between baby and placenta in the minutes after birth. Lancet I:1277, 1957.
110. HALLER, A. v. Elementa physiologiae corporis humani. Lugduni Batavor, 1757.
111. HAMILTON, W. F., R. A. WOODBURY, and E. B. WOODS. The

relation between systemic and pulmonary blood pressures in the fetus. Amer. J. Physiol., 119:206, 1937.

112. HANDLER, J. J. The foetal circulation and its changes at birth in some small laboratory animals. J. Physiol. (Lond.), 133:202, 1956.

113. HARRISON, T. R., and A. BLALOCK. The regulation of circulation. VI. The effects of severe anoxemia of short duration on the cardiac output of morphinized dogs and trained unnarcotized dogs. Amer. J. Physiol., 80:169, 1927.

114. HARVEY, W. Exercitatio anatomica de motu cordis et sanguinis in animalibus. Francofurti, Fitzeri, 1628.

115. HASELHORST, G., and A. ALLMELING. Die Gewichtszunahme von Neugeborenen infolge postnataler Transfusion. Z. Geburtsh. Gynäk., 98:103, 1930.

116. HASELHORST, G., and K. STROMBERGER. Über den Gasgehalt des Nabelschnurblutes vor und nach der Geburt des Kindes und über den Gasaustausch in der Plazenta. Z. Geburtsh. Gynäk., 100:48, 1931.

117. HAYEK, H. V. Der funktionelle Bau der Nabelarterien und des Ductus Botalli. Z. Anat. Entw. Gesch., 105:15, 1935.

118. HEINRICI, G. Die Zählebigkeit des Herzens Neugeborener. Z. Biol., 26:190, 1890.

119. HILL, J. R. The oxygen consumption of new-born and adult mammals. Its dependence on the oxygen tension in the inspired air and on the environmental temperature. J. Physiol. (Lond.), 149:346, 1959.

120. HOLMES, R. L. Some features of the ductus arteriosus. J. Anat. (Lond.), 92:304, 1958.

121. HOUSTON, C. S., and R. L. RILEY. Respiratory and circulatory changes during acclimatization to high altitude. Amer. J. Physiol., 149:565, 1947.

122. HUGGETT, A. ST. G. Foetal blood-gas tensions and gas transfusion through the placenta of the goat. J. Physiol. (Lond.), 62:373, 1927.

123. INGIULLA, W. Ricerche sperimentali sulla funzione vasomotoria del feto. Atti Soc. ital. Ostet. Ginec., 36:224, 1940.

124. JAGER, B. V., and O. J. WOLLENMAN, JR. An anatomical study of the closure of the ductus arteriosus. Amer. J. Path., 18:595, 1942.

125. JAMES, L. S. In Adaptation to Extrauterine Life, Report of the Thirty-first Ross Conference on Pediatric Research. Columbus, Ross Laboratories, 1959.

126. JAMES, L. S., and R. D. ROWE. The pattern of response of pulmonary and systemic arterial pressures in newborn and older infants to short periods of hypoxia. J. Pediat., 51:5, 1957.

127. JAMES, L. S., I. M. WEISBROT, C. E. PRINCE, D. A. HOLADAY, and V. APGAR. The acid-base status of human infants in relation to birth asphyxia and the onset of respiration. J. Pediat., 52:379, 1958.

SPECIAL
CIRCULATIONS

128. JOST, A. Expériences de décapitation de l'embryon de lapin. C.R. Acad. Sci. (Paris), 225:322, 1947.
129. JOST, A. Hormonal factors in the development of the fetus. Cold Spr. Harb. Symp. quant. Biol., 19:167, 1954.
130. KABAT, H. The greater resistance of very young animals to arrest of the brain circulation. Amer. J. Physiol., 130:588, 1940.
131. KAISER, I. H., and J. N. CUMMINGS. Hydrogen ion and hemoglobin concentration, carbon dioxide and oxygen content of blood of the pregnant ewe and fetal lamb. J. appl. Physiol., 10:484, 1957.
132. KEEN, E. N. The postnatal development of the human cardiac ventricles. J. Anat. (Lond.), 89:484, 1955.
133. KELLOGG, H. B. Time of onset of vagal function in the heart of mammals. Proc. Soc. exp. Biol. (N.Y.), 24:839, 1927.
134. KELLOGG, H. B. The course of the blood flow through the fetal mammalian heart. Amer. J. Anat., 42:443, 1928.
135. KELLOGG, H. B. Studies on the fetal circulation of mammals. Amer. J. Physiol., 91:637, 1930.
136. KENNEDY, J. A., and S. L. CLARK. Observations on the ductus arteriosus of the guinea pig in relation to its method of closure. Anat. Rec., 79:349, 1941.
137. KENNEDY, J. A., and S. L. CLARK. Observations on the physiological reactions of the ductus arteriosus. Amer. J. Physiol., 136:140, 1942.
138. KILIAN, H. F. Ueber den Kreislauf des Blutes im Kinde, welches noch nicht geathmet hat. Karlsruhe, Chr. Fr. Müller, 1826.
139. KIRSTEIN, F. Der Verschluss des Ductus arteriosus (Botalli). Arch. Gynäk., 90:303, 1910.
140. KLAGES, C. Anatomische Untersuchungen des Gefässverlaufs der Leber neugeborener Schafe und geburtsreifer Rinder. Morph. Jb., 68:301, 1931.
141. LANGER, C. Zur Anatomie der fötalen Kreislaufsorgane. Z. Ges. Aertze Wien,. 13:328, 1857.
142. LEECH, C. B. Congenital heart disease. Clinical analysis of seventy-five cases from the Johns Hopkins Hospital. J. Pediat., 7:802, 1935.
143. LIND, J., and C. WEGELIUS. Human fetal circulation: changes in the cardiovascular system at birth and disturbances in the post-natal closure of the foramen ovale and ductus arteriosus. Cold Spr. Harb. Symp. quant. Biol., 19:109, 1954.
144. LINZENMEIER, G. Der Verschluss des Ductus arteriosus Botalli nach der Geburt des Kindes. Z. Geburtsh. Gynäk., 76:217, 1914.
145. LOWER, R. Tractatus de Corde. Item de motu et colore sanguinis et chyli in eum transitu. Londini, Jacobi Allestry, 1669.
146. MACKLIN, C. C. Evidences of increase in the capacity of the pulmo-

nary arteries and veins of dogs, cats and rabbits during inflation of the freshly excised lung. Rev. canad. Biol., 5:199, 1946.

147. McIntyre, D. G., and H. E. Ederstrom. Metabolic factors in the development of homeothermy in dogs. Amer. J. Physiol., 194:293, 1958.

148. Melka, J. Beitrag zur Kenntnis der Morphologie und Obliteration des Ductus arteriosus Botalli. Anat. Anz., 61:348, 1926.

149. Meyer, E. Phénomènes d'inhibition cardio-vasculaire chez le nouveau-né. Arch. Physiol. norm. path., ser. V, 5:475, 1893.

150. Mitchell, S. C. The ductus arteriosus in the neonatal period. J. Pediat., 51:12, 1957.

151. Mount, L. E. The metabolic rate of the new-born pig in relation to environmental temperature and age. J. Physiol. (Lond.), 147:333, 1959.

152. Mulherin, W. A., and J. Krafka, Jr. Intravascular clotting in abandoned fetal channels in the newborn. J. Pediat., 9:318, 1936.

153. Nisell, O. Pulmonary reactions to anoxia and carbon dioxide with regard to their possible significance for new-born infants. In Symposium on Anoxia of the New-born Infant, p. 135. Oxford, Blackwell Scientific Publications, 1953.

154. Opdyke, D. F., J. Duomarco, W. H. Dillon, H. Schreiber, R. C. Little, and R. D. Seely. Study of simultaneous right and left atrial pressure pulses under normal and experimentally altered conditions. Amer. J. Physiol., 154:258, 1948.

155. Patten, B. M. The changes in circulation following birth. Amer. Heart J., 6:192, 1930.

156. Patten, B. M. The closure of the foramen ovale. Amer. J. Anat., 48:19, 1931.

157. Patten, B. M., and K. Toulmin. Certain measurements of the foetal heart and their significance. Anat. Rec., 45:235, 1930.

158. Pohlman, A. G. The fetal circulation through the heart. A review of the more important theories, together with a preliminary report on personal findings. Johns Hopk. Hosp. Bull., 18:409, 1907.

159. Pohlman, A. G. The course of the blood through the heart of the fetal mammal, with a note on the reptilian and amphibian circulations. Anat. Rec., 3:75, 1909.

160. Prec, K. J., and D. E. Cassels. Dye dilution curves and cardiac output in newborn infants. Circulation, 11:789, 1955.

161. Prystowsky, H. Fetal blood studies. VII. The oxygen pressure gradient between the maternal and fetal bloods of the human in normal and abnormal pregnancy. Johns Hopk. Hosp. Bull., 101:48, 1957.

162. von Rauchfuss, C. Ueber Thrombose des Ductus arteriosus Botalli. Virchows Arch. path. Anat., 17:376, 1859.

SPECIAL CIRCULATIONS

163. RECORD, R. G., and T. MCKEOWN. Observations relating to the aetiology of patent ductus arteriosus. Brit. Heart J., 15:376, 1953.
164. RECORD, R. G., and T. MCKEOWN. The effect of reduced atmospheric pressure on closure of the ductus arteriosus in the guinea pig. Clin. Sci., 14:225, 1955.
165. REISS, M., and F. HAUROWITZ. Über das Verhalten junger und alter Tiere bei Erstickung. Klin. Wschr., 8:743, 1929.
166. REYNOLDS, S. R. M. Arterial and venous pressures in umbilical cord of the sheep and nature of venous return from the placenta. Amer. J. Physiol., 166:25, 1951.
167. REYNOLDS, S. R. M. The fetal and neonatal pulmonary vasculature in the guinea pig in relation to hemodynamic changes at birth. Amer. J. Anat., 98:97, 1956.
168. RIBEMONT, A. Recherches sur la tension du sang dans les vaisseaux du foetus et du nouveau-né à propos du moment ou l'on doit lier le cordon ombilical. Arch. tocol., 6:577, 1879.
169. ROEDER, H. Die Histogenese des arteriellen Ganges. Ein Beitrag zur Entwicklungsmechanik der Fötalwege. Arch. Kinderheilk., 33:147, 1902.
170. ROOTH, G., and S. SJÖSTEDT. Oxygen saturation in the umbilical cord. Acta obstet. gynec. scand., 34:442, 1955.
171. ROSSDALE, P. D., and L. W. MAHAFFEY. Parturition in the thoroughbred mare with particular reference to blood deprivation in the newborn. Vet. Rec., 70:142, 1958.
172. ROWE, R. D., and L. S. JAMES. The normal pulmonary arterial pressure during the first year of life. J. Pediat., 51:1, 1957.
173. SABATIER, R. B. Mémoire sur les organes de la circulation du sang du foetus. Mém. Acad. roy. Sci. (Paris), 198, 1778.
174. SABATIER, R. B. Mémoire sur les changements qui arrivent aux organes de la circulation du foetus, lorsqu'il a commencé à respirer. Mém. Inst. nat. (Paris), 3:337, 1802.
175. SCAMMON, R. E., and E. H. MORRIS. On the time of the post-natal obliteration of the fetal blood-passages (foramen ovale, ductus arteriosus, ductus venosus). Anat. Rec., 15:165, 1918.
176. SCHAEFFER, J. P. The behaviour of elastic tissue in the post-fetal occlusion and obliteration of the ductus arteriosus (Botalli) in *Sus scrofa*. J. exp. Med., 19:129, 1914.
177. SCHANZ, F. Ueber den mechanischen Verschluss des Ductus arteriosus. Pflügers Arch. ges. Physiol., 44:239, 1889.
178. SCHARFE, H. Der Ductus Botalli. Beiträge zur Physiologie und Pathologie des Verschlusses. Beitr. Geburtsh. Gynäk., 3:368, 1900.
179. SCHULTZE, B. S. Der Scheintod Neugeborener. Jena, Mauke, 1871.

180. SHELLEY, H. S. Glycogen reserves and their changes at birth. Brit. med. Bull., 17:137, 1961.
181. SINHA, T. P. Increase in pulmonary blood volume during early postnatal life. Anat. Rec., 106:599, 1950.
182. SMITH, C. A. The effect of obstetrical anesthesia upon the oxygenation of maternal and fetal blood with particular reference to cyclopropane. Surg. Gynec. Obstet., 69:584, 1939.
183. SMITH, C. A. The Physiology of the Newborn Infant. 2nd ed. Springfield, Ill., Thomas, 1951.
184. SOLTMANN, O. Ueber das Hemmungsnervensystem der Neugebornen. Jb. Kinderheilk, 11:101, 1887.
185. STAFFORD, A., and J. A. C. WEATHERALL. The survival of young rats in nitrogen. J. Physiol. (Lond.), 153:457, 1960.
186. STAHLMAN, M. T., R. E. MERRIL, and V. S. LEQUIRE. Cardiovascular adjustments in normal newborn lambs. Amer. J. Dis. Child., 104:360, 1962.
187. STIENON, L. Sur la fermeture du canal de Botallo. Arch. Biol. (Paris), 97:801, 1912.
188. STRASSMAN, P. Anatomische und physiologische Untersuchungen über den Blutkreislauf beim Neugebornen. Arch. Gynäk., 45:393, 1894.
189. SWANN, H. G., J. J. CHRISTIAN, and C. HAMILTON. The process of anoxic death in newborn pups. Surg. Gynec. Obstet., 99:5, 1954.
190. SWENSSON, Å. Beitrag zur Kenntnis von dem histologischen Bau und dem postembryonalen Verschluss des Ductus arteriosus Botalli. Z. mikr.- anat. Forsch., 46:275, 1939.
191. TAYLOR, P. M. Oxygen consumption in new-born rats. J. Physiol. (Lond.), 154:153, 1960.
192. VAN HARREVELD, A., and F. E. RUSSELL. Postnatal development of a left-right atrial pressure gradient. Amer. J. Physiol., 186:521, 1956.
193. VIRCHOW, R. Die Thrombosen der Neugebornen. In Gesammelte Abhandlungen zur wissenschaftlichen Medicin. Frankfurt, Meidinger, 1856, p. 591.
194. WALKER, J. Foetal anoxia. J. Obstet. Gyneac. Brit. Emp. 61:162, 1954.
195. WALKHOFF, F. Das Gewebe des Ductus arteriosus und die Obliteration desselben. Z. rat. Med., 36:109, 1869.
196. WELLS, H. G. Persistent patency of the ductus arteriosus. Amer. J. med. Sci., 136:381, 1908.
197. WILSON, E. E., W. F. WINDLE, and H. L. ALT. Deprivation of placental blood as a cause of iron deficiency in infants. Amer. J. Dis. Child, 62:320, 1941.
198. WILSON, R. R. Post-mortem observations on contraction of the human ductus arteriosus. Brit. med. J., I:810, 1958.

SPECIAL CIRCULATIONS

199. WINDLE, W. F. Physiology of the Fetus. Philadelphia, Saunders, 1940.
200. WINDLE, W. F., and R. F. BECKER. The course of the blood through the fetal heart. An experimental study in the cat and guinea pig. Anat. Rec., 77:417, 1940.
201. WOLFF, C. F. De foramine ovali, eiusque usu, in dirigendo motu sanguinis. Observationes novae. Novi Commentarii Acad. Sci. Imp. Petropolitanae, 20:357, 1776.
202. WULF, H. Der Gasaustausch in der reifen Plazenta des Menschen. Z. Geburtsh. Gynäk., 158:134, 1962.
203. ZIETZSCHMANN, O. Lehrbuch der Entwicklungsgeschichte der Haustiere. Berlin, Schoetz, 1924.

Notes and Acknowledgments

GENERAL ACKNOWLEDGMENTS

The editors and authors are particularly indebted to the following institutions and persons for help in preparing this book:

THE COLUMBIA UNIVERSITY MEDICAL LIBRARY. Mr. Thomas P. Fleming, Miss Cecile E. Kramer, Miss Eva H. Eckert, Mr. Philip Weimerskirch, Mr. Samuel J. Waddel, as well as many other members of the staff.

THE NEW YORK ACADEMY OF MEDICINE. Miss Gertrude L. Annan and Mrs. Alice Weaver.

LIBRARY OF THE ROYAL COLLEGE OF PHYSICIANS, LONDON. Mr. L. M. Payne.

WELLCOME HISTORICAL MEDICAL LIBRARY, LONDON. Mr. F. N. L. Poynter and Mr. E. Ashworth Underwood.

OXFORD UNIVERSITY PRESS. Mr. John Begg, Miss Caroline Taylor, Miss Leona Capeless, Mr. William C. Halpin, and Mr. Douglas C. Ross.

COLUMBIA UNIVERSITY COLLEGE OF PHYSICIANS AND SURGEONS. Mrs. Mary Lou Dwyer, Mrs. Vivian Thacker, and Miss Marilyn S. Bongiorno.

CHAPTER I

Fig. 2. Miss Gisela M. A. Richter, whose book "Portraiture of the Greeks" is about to be published by the Phaidon Press, has very kindly given this photograph for use in the present volume. She has also provided the following information about this important discovery:

In the excavations near Ostia (in the Isola Sacra) in 1940, the bust of a bearded elderly man was found in a family tomb erected by Markios Demetrios, a distinguished physician ($\dot{\alpha}\rho\chi\acute{\iota}\alpha\tau\rho$ος) of the late first century A.D. Near by were two pedestals, on one of which is an inscription beginning "Life is short" ($\dot{o}$ $\beta\acute{\iota}os$ $\beta\rho\alpha\chi\acute{v}s$). The face of this bust bears a striking resemblance to that on a first century B.C. Roman coin of Cos. On this coin are found also the letters *I Π* (i.e., Hippocrates) and a caduceus. It is thought that this bust, now in the museum at Ostia, is a copy of an earlier Greek original of Hippocrates, and that both coin and bust represent at least what antiquity believed to be his likeness. As further evidence, that the person thus represented was someone known and revered, it has now been discovered that there are four other busts apparently of the same individual, previously "unknown," one in the museum in Naples, one in the Vatican, one in the Uffizi in Florence, and one in Copenhagen. Unfortunately, the right side of the Ostia head is badly damaged, especially the right eye and the right side of the nose; but the fine modelling of the face can still be made out. Cf. G. Becatti, "Il Ritratto di Ippocrate," Rendicotti della Pontificia Accademia Romana di Archeologia, Vol. XXI, 1945-46, pp. 123 ff.

It may be noted that the British Museum bust of "Hippocrates" is now known to be that of someone else, namely, the philosopher Crisippus of Soloi in Cilicia.

Fig. 7. The following translation of the admission register has been provided by Mr. W. F. Bolton and Mr. Brian Morris of the University of Reading:

"*William Harvey, son of Thomas Harvey, yeoman, a Kentishman from the town of Folkston, educated in the Canterbury grammar school, aged sixteen, was admitted as a Minor Pensioner, companion of scholars, on the last day of May, 1594, under the tutelage of Master George Estey, Fellow of the College, who pledged in faith for him. He has paid three shillings and four pence for this, his admission to college.*"

The marks in the right-hand margin of the facsimile are not part of the text. Instead, they represent the sum Harvey paid upon registration at Caius, i.e., three shillings and four pence (iij ^{s}. iiij ^{d}.).

CHAPTER V

For library assistance and guidance, the authors are indebted to Dr. Genevieve Miller, Assistant Professor of Medical History, Western Reserve University; Miss Ada Floyd and Miss Rose Beckman and the staff of the Cleveland Medical Library; the staff of the History of Medicine Division of the National Library of Medicine, Cleveland, Ohio. Help in translating parts of original manuscripts was afforded by John K. Major, Perkins Professor of Physics, Mrs. Marjorie M. Kupersmith, Instructor in Romance Languages, and Dr. Dieter Koch-Weser, Associate Professor of Medicine, all of Western Reserve University, Cleveland, Ohio; additional help was provided by Miss Edith O. Ray and Miss Laura Althoff of Cleveland, Ohio.

CHAPTER VII

Fig. 26. Sensory receptors in the adventitia of the internal carotid artery at the point of its origin in a mouse of two months. Accompanying this illustration from De Castro (49), is the following footnote (translated):

"It is curious that it is precisely in the mouse that we discovered nearly four years ago the endings at the origin of the internal carotid and that, on account of their arrangement and appearance, we guessed that it had to be concerned with a depressor system, the receptors of which were lodged in this origin. But we have delayed for more than two years the publication of that work. We did not know then the very interesting physiological studies of H. E. Hering which are in perfect accord with our anatomical studies."

CHAPTER X

Fig. 6. Etruscan liver model in bronze. The inscriptions are in early Latin script and difficult to make out. Names of the terrestrial gods and gods of nature may be seen along the bottom margin of the diagram in (B), ranging from Tluscu through Selva, Fufluns to Tecum on the right. Next in counterclockwise distribution may be seen the names of the great celestial deities and to the left above those of Fate and the infernal regions. Presumably alterations in the normal configuration of the liver within the areas marked out by these names indicate changes which would fall under the auspices of the god assigned.

Fig. 10. Translation of the legends describing Galen's concept of the splanchnic circulation. The description appears in the *Tabulae Sex* of Vesalius and the translation is by Charles Singer.[161]

"The Liver, factory of the blood. By the vena porta, *which the Greeks call* stelechiaia *and the Arabs* varidhascoer, *it takes chyle from stomach and intestines and purges away the melancholic fluid into the spleen."*

- A. Cavity or sinus of the liver.
- B. Vena porta, the manus jecoris.
- C. Branches to the gallbladder.
- D. To the pancreas and ecphysis or duodenum.
- E. To the right upper curvature of the stomach.
- F. To the right lower curvature of the stomach.
- G. The great bifurcation of the porta.
- H. This branch is distributed and widely spread out through the lower membrane of the omentum and the pancreas.
- I. Goes to the lower membrane of the omentum in its right part.
- K. Passes via the lesser curvature of the stomach, finally surrounding the os stomachi with numerous branchlets.
- L. Passes to the lower membrane of the omentum in its middle part, first dividing into two, then into many small.
- M. Is divided extensively and passes straight to the hilum of the spleen. By this vessel the impure blood is transmitted to the spleen.
- N. On each side goes firstly to the left gibbosity of the stomach and secondly passes somewhat obscurely to the os stomachi.

O. *Goes to the left side of the fundus of the stomach and the upper membrane of the omentum. I believe that by it no small part of the excretion of the spleen is sent into the stomach.*

P. *Sends forth numerous branches between the membranes of the mesentery. I am not certain whether the* haemorrhoidals *arise from this or from the* vena cava, *because from both veins branches go to that part, and though those from the* porta *are greater, it does not appear that the melancholic blood is purged by the* porta.

The wealth of detail evident in Vesalius' drawing is not apparent in the Galenic descriptions and may be attributed in part at least to an accretion of knowledge during the centuries that passed following Galen's original description of the splanchnic bed.

Figs. 22, 23: Full legends to illustrations from Kiernan.[102].

Fig. 22. Represents the interlobular ducts entering the lobules, and forming the lobular biliary plexuses. a. Two lobules. b,b,b. Interlobular ducts. c,c,c. The interlobular cellular tissue. d,d. The external portions of the lobular biliary plexuses injected. e,e. The intralobular branches of the hepatic vein. f,f. The uninjected central portions of the lobules. No such view of the ducts as that represented in this figure can be obtained in the liver. The interlobular ducts are, in the figure, seen anastomosing with each other: I have never seen these anastomoses, but I have seen the anastomoses of the ducts in the left lateral ligament, and, from the results of experiments related in this paper, I believe the interlobular ducts anastomose. I have never injected the lobular biliary plexuses to the extent represented in the figure.

Fig. 23. Representing the interlobular branches of the portal vein, the lobular venous plexuses, and the intralobular branches of the hepatic veins of these lobules. a,a,a The interlobular veins contained in the spaces. b,b,b. The interlobular veins which occupy the fissures, and which, with the veins in the spaces form venous circles around the lobules. This is the appearance which the venous circles present when examined with a common magnifying glass; they are, however, formed by numerous, and not by single, branches as represented in the figure. c,c,c. The lobular venous plexuses, the branches of which, communicating with each other by intermediate vessels, terminate in the intralobular veins. The circular and ovoid spaces, seen between the branches of the plexuses, are occupied by portions of the biliary plexuses, constituting the acini of Malpighi. d,d,d. The intralobular branches of the hepatic veins, in which the vessels of the plexuses terminate.

List of Illustrations and Sources

CHAPTER I, pages 3 to 70

1. Cities of the ancient world.
2. The "Hippocrates of Ostia." (For further details see pages 817-18.)
3. Galen of Pergamon. (From Galen's *Therapeutica*, Venice, 1500. In the Wellcome Collection of Incunabula. Courtesy of F. N. L. Poynter.)
4. Pulmonary circulation. A page from the manuscript of Ibn Nafis. (From a photographic reproduction in the Columbia University Medical Library. The original manuscript is in the Prussian State Library, Berlin (Mf. 912). For full Arabic text see M. Meyerhof, "Ibn an-Nafis und seine Theorie des Lungenkreislaufs," *Quell. u. Stud. Gesch. der Naturwiss. u. der. Med.* 4: 37, 1933; see also E. E. Bittar, *Ibn Nafis*, Thesis, Yale, 1955.)
5. Title page of *Christianismi Restitutio* of Michael Servetus (Courtesy of the Bibliothèque Nationale, Paris.)
6. Monument where Servetus was burned at the stake. (Photograph by Dr. D. D. Reid.)
7. Admission Register of William Harvey. (Courtesy of Wellcome Historical Medical Museum, London. For translation see page 818.)
8. Robert Boyle. (From *The Philosophical Works of the Honourable Robert Boyle*, London, 1738. Courtesy of Mr. Sidney Edelstein.)
9. Richard Lower. (Courtesy of the Columbia University Medical Library.)
10. Joseph Priestley. (Courtesy of Mr. Sidney Edelstein. Photograph by the American Numismatic Society, New York.)
11. Lavoisier and Madame Lavoisier. (From the portrait by David. Courtesy of the Rockefeller Institute Library, New York.)
12. Lavoisier in his laboratory. (Courtesy of the Archives de l'Académie des Sciences de Paris.)
13. Auguste Chauveau. (Courtesy of the Archives de l'Académie des Sciences de Paris.)
14. Étienne Jules Marey. (Courtesy of the Archives de l'Académie des Sciences de Paris.)

15. Charles Émile François-Franck. (Courtesy of the Archives de l'Académie des Sciences de Paris.)
16. Christian Bohr and his associates. (Courtesy of the late Professor Niels Bohr.)
17. Joseph Barcroft, Lawrence J. Henderson, and F. Gowland Hopkins. (Courtesy of Dr. D. B. Dill.)

Chapter II, pages 71 to 126

1. William Harvey. (Courtesy of the National Portrait Gallery, London, with the permission of Dr. M. Prinzmetal.)
2. William Harvey's notes for his Lumleian Lecture. (Courtesy of the British Museum, London.)
3. Agricola's representation of a water pump. (From Agricola, *De re metallica*. Dover Publications, 1950. With permission.)
4. Stephen Hales. (From the portrait by Thomas Hudson).
5. A table from Stephen Hales's *Haemastaticks*.
6. Jean Léonard Marie Poiseuille (Courtesy of Mr. G. Nicole-Genty.)
7. Carl Friedrich Wilhelm Ludwig. (Courtesy of the Columbia University Medical Library.)
8. Ludwig's kymograph.
9. Adolf Fick. (Courtesy of Professor O. Wyss.)
10. Nathan Zuntz. (From K. E. Rothschuh. *Geschichte der Physiologie*. Berlin, Springer-Verlag, 1953. With permission.)
11. Data from Harvard Fatigue Laboratory. (From L. J. Henderson. *Blood, a Study in General Physiology*. Yale University Press, 1928. With permission.)
12. George Neil Stewart. (Courtesy of Dr. J. M. Rogoff.)
13. Dye dilution curve. (From W. F. Hamilton. *Circulation*, 1953. With permission.)
14. Otto Frank. (Courtesy of Frau Otto Frank.)
15. Pressure curves in the frog heart. (From O. Frank. *Z. Biol.* 1895.)
16. E. H. Starling at work. (From R. Colp, Jr. "Ernest Starling," *Scientific American*, 1951. With permission.)
17. Effect of increased arterial blood pressure on volume changes in the heart. (From S. W. Patterson, H. Piper, and E. H. Starling. *J. Physiol.* (Lond.), 1914. With permission.)

Chapter III, pages 127 to 198

1. Schematic representation of a flexible chain molecule.
2. Shortening and work performance by a spring.
3. Work obtainable from a stretched spring.

4. Length-tension diagram of the spring.
5. Length-tension diagram of skeletal muscle.
6. Length-tension diagram of cardiac muscle.
7. Work obtainable from active muscle.
8. The tipping lever of A. Fick. (From A. Fick. *Mechanische Arbeit und Wärmeentwicklung bei der Muskelthätigkeit*. Leipzig, Brockhaus, 1882.)
9. Relation between various mechanical properties of muscle. (Sections B and C are reproduced from A. V. Hill. *Proc. Roy. Soc.* B, 1939. With permission.)
10. Relation between pressure and volume of the intact heart. (From O. Frank. *Z. Biol.*, 1899.)
11. Effects of arterial resistance and venous return on the volume of the heart. (From E. H. Starling. *The Linacre Lecture on the Law of the Heart*. London, Longmans, Green, 1918.)
12. Fick's work adder. (From S. W. Patterson, H. Piper, and E. H. Starling. *J. Physiol.* (Lond.), 1914. With permission.)
13. Archibald Vivian Hill. (Courtesy of the Columbia University Medical Library.)
14. Performance of work upon a flywheel by a falling weight.
15. The concept of the active state.
16. Effect of stretching a muscle various amounts at the same moment shortly after a maximal shock. (From A. V. Hill. *Proc. Roy. Soc.* B, 1949. With permission.)
17. Records of tension/time curves of frog's sartorius at 0°C. (From J. M. Ritchie. *J. Physiol.* (Lond.), 1954. With permission.)
18. The staircase effect. (From H. P. Bowditch. *Ber. math.-phys. sächs. Ges. Wiss.*, 1871.)
19. Major reactions involved in glycolysis and in reversal of glycolysis.
20. Albert Szent-Györgyi.
21. Actomyosin micell in solution.
22. Electron microscopic appearance of striated muscle. (Courtesy of Professor H. E. Huxley.)

CHAPTER IV, pages 199 to 264

1. A page from the Ebers papyrus. (From *The Papyrus Ebers*. Translated by C. P. Bryan. London, G. Bles, 1930. With permission.)
2. The heart and coronary vessels by Leonardo da Vinci. (From *Quaderni d'Anatomia*, published by O. C. L. Vangensten, A. Fonahn, and H. Hopstock. Christiania, 1911-1916, Vol. II, Folio 4 Recto. With permission.)
3. Andreas Vesalius. (Drawing by Kalkar. From the *Fabrica* of A. Vesalius, 1543.)

4. The coronary vessels, as drawn in the "Six Tables" of Vesalius and Kalkar. (From A. Vesalius. *Tabulae Sex*. Venice, 1538. In *Andreae Vesalii Bruxellensis Icones Anatomicae*. New York Academy of Medicine and the University of Munich, 1934. With permission.)
5. Raymond de Vieussens. (From his *Traité nouveau de la structure et des causes du mouvement naturel du coeur*. Toulouse, 1715.)
6. The heart as drawn by Vieussens. (From his *Traité nouveau* .... Toulouse, 1715.)
7. John Hunter. (Portrait attributed to Thomas Gainsborough. From original portrait in Royal College of Surgeons, England. Courtesy of the Columbia University Medical Library.)
8. William Heberden. (From the mezzotint by James Ward after Sir William Beechey. Courtesy of the Wellcome Historical Medical Library.)
9. Allan Burns. (Courtesy of the Library, University of Glasgow.)
10. Rudolf Ludwig Karl Virchow. (Courtesy of the Columbia University Medical Library).
11. Julius Friedrich Cohnheim. (Courtesy of the Columbia University Medical Library.)
12. Respiration apparatus of Pettenkofer and Voit. (From Robert A. Tigerstedt. *A Textbook of Human Physiology*. Translated by J. R. Murlin. Appleton, 1906. With permission.)
13. Carl von Voit. (Courtesy of the New York Academy of Medicine.)
14. Time course of blood flow through the coronary system in the dog. (Courtesy of Dr. D. E. Gregg and Dr. L. C. Fisher.)
15. The coronary arteries, as demonstrated by injection. (From H. L. Blumgart, P. M. Zoll, A. S. Freedberg, and D. R. Gilligan. *Circulation*, 1950. With permission.)
16. James B. Herrick. (Courtesy of the Columbia University Medical Library.)
17. Fatty acid metabolism of the heart. (From R. J. Bing. Harvey Lect., 1954-55. With permission.)
18. Effects of ventricular fibrillation on cardiac metabolism. (From R. J. Bing. Harvey Lect., 1954-55. With permission.)

Chapter V, pages 265 to 351

1. Gilbert's method of magnetization. (From W. Gilbert. *On the Magnet, Magnetic Bodies also on the Great Magnet, the Earth*. London, Cheswick, 1900. With permission.)
2. Gilbert's versorium. (From W. Gilbert. *On the Magnet* .... London, Cheswick, 1900. With permission.)
3. The torpedo fish. A. From J. Walsh. *Phil. Trans.*, 1773-75. B. From J.

Hunter. *Phil. Trans.*, 1773. (Courtesy of the Columbia University Medical Library.)

4. Galvani's friction machine. (From L. Galvani. *De viribus electricitatis in motu musculari commentarius.* Burndy Library, 1954. With permission.)
5. Experiments by Galvani to show animal electricity. (From L. Galvani. *De viribus electricitatis . . . .* Burndy Library, 1954. With permission.)
6. Alessandro Graf Volta and a voltaic pile. (*Left:* Courtesy of the Columbia University Medical Library. *Right:* Courtesy of the Wellcome Historical Medical Museum, London.)
7. Emil Du Bois-Reymond. (Courtesy of the Columbia University Medical Library.)
8. The rheotome of Burdon-Sanderson and Page. (From J. Burdon-Sanderson and F. J. M. Page. *J. Physiol.* (Lond.), 1879-80.)
9. The mercury capillary electrometer of Lippmann. (From G. Lippmann. *Ann. Chim. (Phys.)*, 1875.)
10. Augustus Waller and friend. (Courtesy of Dr. Howard B. Burchell.)
11. First electrometer record of the human heart. (From A. D. Waller. *Phil. Trans.* B, 1889.)
12. Willem Einthoven and his co-workers. (Courtesy of Dr. Howard B. Burchell.)
13. Einthoven's string galvanometer, Leyden model. (Courtesy of *Ciba Symposia*. With permission.)
14. Evolution of the electrocardiogram from the electrometer. (From W. Einthoven. *Pflügers Arch. ges. Physiol.*, 1903. With permission.)
15. Distribution of potentials produced by the human heart, according to Waller. (From A. D. Waller. *Phil. Trans.* B, 1889.)
16. Axial reference system of Waller. (From A. D. Waller. *The Electrical Action of the Human Heart,* University of London Press, 1922. With permission.)
17. Schema of Waller to show current axis and equator. (From A. D. Waller. *The Electrical Action of the Human Heart,* University of London Press, 1922. With permission.)
18. The equilateral triangle of Einthoven. (From W. Einthoven, G. Fahr, and A. de Waart. *Pflügers Arch. ges. Physiol.*, 1913. With permission.)
19. Frank N. Wilson. (Courtesy of Mrs. Frank N. Wilson.)
20. Diagram of the equilateral triangle that stimulated Burger's interest. (From *Electrocardiografía general, . . . Con un apéndice: Directrices para la valoración de un electrocardiograma por el dr. Elsbeth Koch-Momm.* Traducido por el dr. J. B. Iraeta. Madrid, Espasa-Calpe, s.a., 1942.)
21. Phantom of Burger and van Milaan. (From H. C. Burger and J. B. van Milaan. *Brit. Heart J.*, 1947. With permission.)
22. Triangles of Burger and van Milaan. (From H. C. Burger and J. B. van Milaan. *Brit. Heart J.*, 1947. With permission.)

23. Thomas Lewis. (Courtesy of Dr. Howard B. Burchell.)
24. Lewis's diagram of the excitation process of the human ventricle. (From T. Lewis. *Phil. Trans.* B, 1915. With permission.)
25. Effects of injury during rest and activity.
26. The monocardiogram of Mann. (From H. Mann. *Amer. Heart J.*, 1938. With permission.)
27. First vectorcardiograms recorded with cathode ray oscilloscope. (From R. Sulzer. *Arch. int. Physiol.*, 1936. With permission.)
28. Reversal of polarization following injury of heart muscle. (From J. A. E. Eyster, W. J. Meek, H. Goldberg, and W. E. Gilson. *Amer. J. Physiol.*, 1938. With permission.)
29. Bernstein's membrane theory. (From J. Bernstein. *Pflügers Arch. ges. Physiol.*, 1910. With permission.)
30. First demonstration of overshoot during action potential. (From A. L. Hodgkin and A. F. Huxley. *Nature*, 1933.)
31. Use of microelectrode for recording action potentials of cardiac muscle. (From S. Weidmann. *Ann. N.Y. Acad. Sci.*, 1957. With permission.)
32. Schematic representation of a cardiac membrane action potential. (From P. F. Cranefield and B. F. Hoffman. *Physiol. Rev.*, 1958. With permission.)
33. Potassium efflux during action potential. (From W. S. Wilde. *Ann. N.Y. Acad. Sci.*, 1957. With permission.)

CHAPTER VI, pages 355 to 406

1. Drawings by Malpighi. (From J. Young. *Proc. Roy. Soc. Med.*, 1929. With permission.)
2. Antony van Leeuwenhoek. (Courtesy of the New York Academy of Medicine.)
3. Sketch by Leeuwenhoek of the blood vessels in the tail of the eel. (From A. v. Leeuwenhoek. *Sevende Vervolg der Brieven*. Delft, Holland, 1702. 112th letter, dedicated to Antoni Heinsius, dated 20 Sept. 1698, facing page 57.)
4. Drawing by Leeuwenhoek to show capillary connections. (From A. van Leeuwenhoek. *Arcana Naturae Detecta*. Lugduni Batavorum, Apud Joh: Arnold: Langerak, 1722.)
5. Marshall Hall. (Courtesy of the New York Academy of Medicine.)
6. Marshall Hall's drawing of capillaries in the tail of the stickleback. (From M. Hall. *A Critical and Experimental Essay on the Circulation of the Blood; Especially as Observed in the Minute and Capillary Vessels of the "Batrachia" and of Fishes*. London, 1831.)
7. Johannes Müller. (Courtesy of the Columbia University Medical Library.)

8. August Krogh. (Courtesy of Dr. Bodil Schmidt-Nielsen.)
9. Marie Krogh. (Courtesy of Dr. Bodil Schmidt-Nielsen.)
10. Capillaries of muscle after perfusion with carbon. (From A. Krogh. *J. Physiol.* (Lond.), 1919. With permission.)
11. Krogh's illustration of capillary alternation. (From A. Krogh. *Isis*, 1950. With permission.)
12. Pulmonary circulation in the frog from film by Krogh.
13. Constriction of arteriocapillary sphincter from film by Fulton and Lutz. (From a film strip by G. P. Fulton and B. R. Lutz. With permission.)
14. The minute vessels of the mesoappendix of the rat according to Chambers and Zweifach. (From R. Chambers and B. W. Zweifach. *Amer. J. Anat.*, 1944. With permission.)
15. Micropipette in mesenteric capillary of the frog. (From E. M. Landis. *Amer. J. Physiol.*, 1926. With permission.)
16. Ernest H. Starling and Mrs. Starling. (Courtesy of Professor L. Bayliss.)
17. Blood pressure versus oncotic pressure in four species. (From E. M. Landis. *Physiol. Rev.*, 1934. With permission.)
18. Filtration, absorption, and capillary blood pressure in single capillaries of frog's mesentery. (From E. M. Landis. *Physiol. Rev.*, 1934. With permission.)
19. Filtration, absorption, and capillary blood pressures in perfused hind limb of the cat. (From J. R. Pappenheimer and A. Soto-Rivera. *Amer. J. Physiol.*, 1948. With permission.)
20. Passage of molecules through the capillary wall. (From J. R. Pappenheimer. *Physiol. Rev.*, 1953. With permission.)

Chapter VII, pages 407 to 486

1. Jean-Baptiste de Sénac. (From J.-B. de Sénac. *Méquignon l'aîné*, 1783.)
2. Claude Bernard. (From an original daguerreotype. Courtesy of the late Professor John F. Fulton.)
3. Claude Bernard demonstrating an experiment. (Painting by Lhermitte in the Luxembourg Gallery, Paris.)
4. Charles E. Brown-Séquard. (Courtesy of the Hon. H. Peerbaye, Mayor of Port-Louis.)
5. François Magendie (Courtesy of the Columbia University Medical Library.)
6. William Maddock Bayliss. (Courtesy of Professor Leonard E. Bayliss.)
7. The "Brown Dog Case." (Courtesy of Professor Leonard E. Bayliss.)
8. W. H. Gaskell. (From K. J. Franklin. *Joseph Barcroft*. Oxford, Blackwell, 1953. With permission.)

9. J. Newport Langley. (From W. M. Fletcher. "John Newport Langley. In Memoriam," *J. Physiol.* (Lond.), 1926. With permission.)
10. Walter Bradford Cannon. (Courtesy of Professor E. M. Landis.)
11. Otto Loewi.
12. Henry H. Dale. (Courtesy of the Columbia University Medical Library.)
13. Effect of stimulation of hypothalmus on blood pressure. (From J. P. Karplus and A. Kreidl. *Pflügers Arch. ges. Physiol.*, 1909. With permission.)
14. The depressor nerve in the rabbit. (From E. de Cyon and C. Ludwig. *Arb. physiol. Anstalt.* Leipzig, 1867.)
15. A method for crossed circulation. (From C. Heymans and E. Neil. *Reflexogenic Areas of the Cardiovascular System.* London, Churchill, 1958. With permission.)
16. Cross-circulation experiment by Heymans and Ladon. (From C. Heymans and E. Neil. *Reflexogenic Areas* .... London, Churchill, 1958. With permission.)
17. Carotid artery with carotid sinus according to Scarpa. (From L. M. A. Caldoni and F. Caldoni. Joseph Picotti, 1801-3. Courtesy of the New York Academy of Medicine.)
18. Heinrich Ewald Hering. (Courtesy of Professor Fritz Klenk, University of Cologne.)
19. Hering's experiment involving tugging on common carotid artery. (From H. E. Hering. *Die Karotissinusreflexe auf Herz und Gefasse, vom normalphysiologischen, pathologisch-physiologischen und klinischen Standpunkt.* Dresden, Steinkopff, 1927. With permission.)
20. Infiltration of carotid sinuses with norepinephrine. (From C. Heymans and E. Neil. *Reflexogenic Areas* .... London, Churchill, 1958. With permission.)
21. "Impulse traffic" in baroreceptive fibers after application of epinephrine to sinus wall. (From S. Landgren, E. Neil and Y. Zotterman. *Acta physiol. scand.*, 1952. With permission.)
22. The effect of applying norepinephrine to the walls of both empty carotid sinuses. (From C. Heymans and A. L. Delaunois. *Proc. Soc. exp. Biol.* (N.Y.), 1955. With permission.)
23. Resetting of the arterial blood pressure in a dog with chronic renal hypertension. (From G. Matton. *Arch. int. Pharmacodyn.*, 1957. With permission.)
24. Cardiac-accelerator impulses synchronous with the pulse. (From D. W. Bronk. Harvey Lect., 1933-34. With permission.)
25. Schema of self-regulation of blood pressure.
26. Sensory receptors in the adventitia of the internal carotid artery. (From F. De Castro. *Trab. Lab. Invest. biol.* Univ. Madrid, 1928. For excerpt (translation) from accompanying text, see pages 818-19.)

Chapter VIII, pages 487 to 541

1. Stephen Hales and assistant measuring blood pressure in the horse. (From *Medical Times*, 1944. Courtesy of the late Professor John F. Fulton.)
2. Richard Bright. (From T. J. Pettigrew. *Medical Portrait Gallery*. London, Fischer, 1838-40.)
3. Marey's sphygmograph. (From J. Burdon-Sanderson. *Handbook of the Sphygmograph*. London, Hardwicke, 1867.)
4. Frederick Akhbar Mahomed and his sphygmograph. (From A. Batty Shaw. *Guy's Hosp. Rep.*, 1952. With permission.)
5. Samuel S. K. von Basch and his sphygmomanometer. (Portrait courtesy of New York Academy of Medicine. Apparatus from G. W. Pickering. *High Blood Pressure*. London, Churchill, 1955. With permission.)
6. Franz Volhard. (Courtesy of New York Academy of Medicine.)
7. The Goldblatt clamp. (From H. Goldblatt. *Amer. J. clin. Path.*, 1940. With permission.)
8. The production of persistent hypertension by renal ischemia in the dog. From H. Goldblatt, J. Lynch, R. F. Hanzal, and W. W. Summerville. *J. exp. Med.*, 1934. With permission.)
9. Robert Tigerstedt. (From K. E. Rothschuh. *Geschichte der Physiologie*. Berlin, Springer-Verlag, 1953. With permission.)
10. The Läwen-Trendelenburg method. (From B. A. Houssay and A. C. Taquini. *Rev. Soc. argent. Biol.*, 1938. With permission.)
11. Frequency distribution of systolic and diastolic pressures for females. (From M. Hamilton, G. W. Pickering, J. A. F. Roberts, and G. S. C. Sowry. *Clin. Sci.*, 1954. With permission.)
12. Blood pressure scores of relatives and of propositi. (From W. E. Miall and P. D. Oldham. *Clin. Sci.*, 1955. With permission.)
13. Stature of mid-parent and mean heights of their children. (From F. Galton. *Natural Inheritance*. London, Macmillan, 1889.)

Chapter IX, pages 545 to 606

1. Marcello Malpighi. (Painting by C. Cignani. Collection of Professor Putti, Bologna.)
2. William Bowman. (From an original photograph by Lock and Whitfield in the Wellcome Historical Medical Museum.)
3. Plate from Bowman. (From W. Bowman. *Philos. Trans. Roy. Soc.*, 1842.)
4. The nephron of the human kidney according to Bowman. (From W. Bowman. *Philos. Trans. Roy. Soc.*, 1842.)
5. Carl F. Ludwig. (Courtesy of the Columbia University Medical Library.)

6. Rudolph P. H. Heidenhain. (Courtesy of the Columbia University Medical Library.)
7. The afferent blood supply of the frog's kidney. (From A. R. Cushney. *The Secretion of the Urine*. London, Longmans, Green, 1917. With permission.)
8. Arthur Robertson Cushny. (From F. R. Winton. *Modern Views on the Secretion of Urine*. Boston, Little, Brown, 1956. With permission.)
9. Alfred Newton Richards. (From a film strip photographed by Professor Carl F. Schmidt.)
10. Robert Chambers. (From R. Chambers and E. L. Chambers. *Explorations into the Nature of the Living Cell*. Boston, Harvard University Press, 1961. With permission.)
11. Eli Kennerly Marshall, Jr. (Courtesy of Mrs. E. K. Marshall, Jr.)
12. Lophius piscatorius. (From the manuscript of Edward Tyson in the Royal College of Physicians, London. Courtesy of Mr. L. M. Payne, F.L.A.)
13. Aglomerular kidney of toadfish. (From H. W. Smith. *The Kidney*. New York, Oxford University Press, 1951. With permission.)

CHAPTER X, pages 607 to 701

1. Paleolithic painting in the cave at Lascaux. (From G. Daniel. *Lascaux and Carnac*. London, Lutterworth Press, 1955. Courtesy of the Caisse Nationale des Monuments Historiques, Paris. With permission.)
2. Baked clay tablet describing the appearance of the liver of a sacrificial lamb. (From A. Goetze. *Old Babylonian Omen Texts*. New Haven, Yale University Press, 1947. With permission.)
3. Liver models from Mari. (From M. Rutten. *Rev. Assyriologie et Archéologie Orientale*, 1938. With permission.)
4. Baked clay model of a Babylonian liver. (Courtesy of the British Museum (*BU* 89-4-26.238).)
5. Canopic jars of limestone. (Courtesy of the Walters Art Gallery, Baltimore.)
6. Etruscan liver model in bronze. (From G. Körte. *Mitt. dtsch. archeol. Inst. Rom.*, 1905. The original specimens are in the Civico Museo, Piacenza, Italy. With permission.)
7. Haruspicy in the Forum. (Courtesy of the Louvre, Paris.)
8. Saint Ansano of Siena. (From A. Kemp-Welch. *Burlington Mag.*, 1911. With permission.)
9. The circulatory system according to Diogenes of Apollonia. (From E. Krause. *Janus*, 1909. With permission.)
10. The splanchnic circulation according to Galen. (From A. Vesalius. *Tabulae Sex*. Venice, 1538. For translation of legends by C. Singer

in *Monumenta Medica*, Florence, Lier, 1925, see pages 819-20. With permission.)

11. Physiology of sanguification according to Galen. (From Galen. *Oeuvres anatomiques, physiologiques et médicales*. Paris, Baillière, 1854.)
12. The splanchnic and systemic vasculatures according to Galen. (From Galen. *Oeuvres anatomiques* . . . . Paris, Baillière, 1854.)
13. Medieval concept of the splanchnic circulation. (From K. Sudhoff. *Stud. Gesch. Med.*, 1907. With permission.)
14. "Vein man" from Mondino. (From C. Singer. *Monumenta Medica*. Florence, Lier, 1925. With permission.)
15. Circulation according to Leonardo da Vinci. (From Leonardo da Vinci. *Quaderni d'Anatomia*. Christiania, Dybwad, 1911. With permission.)
16. The splanchnic bed according to Vesalius. (From A. Vesalius. *De humani corporis fabrica libri septum*. Basileae, Oporini, 1543.)
17. Epitaph for the deposed liver by Thomas Bartholin. (From T. Bartholin, translation by J. H. Skavlem. *Ann. med. Hist.*, 1921. With permission.)
18. Glisson working in the anatomical theatre. (From F. Glisson, *Anatomia hepatis*, Hagae, 1681.)
19. The hepatic vasculature according to Glisson. (From F. Glisson, *Anatomia hepatis*, Hagae, 1681.)
20. Frederick Ruysch. (From F. Ruysch. *Opera omnia anatomico-medico-chirurgica*. Amstelodami, 1737.)
21. The splanchnic vasculature according to Ruysch. (*Upper:* From F. Ruysch. *Epistola Anatomica, problematica quarta, ad F. Ruyschium auctore J. J. Campdomerco*. Amstelodami, 1737. *Lower:* From F. Ruysch. *Museum Anatomicum Ruyschianum*. Amstelodami, 1691.)
22. The biliary ductule system according to Kiernan. (From F. Kiernan. *Phil. Trans.*, 1833. For complete legend see page 820.)
23. The intralobular distribution of the sinusoids according to Kiernan. (From F. Kiernan. *Phil. Trans.*, 1833. For complete legend see page 820.)
24. Femoral arterial and portal venous pressures in the dog obtained by Bayliss and Starling. (From W. M. Bayliss and E. H. Starling. *J. Physiol.* (Lond.), 1894.)
25. Apparatus used by Angelo Mosso to study the explanted liver. (From A. Mosso. *Ludwig's Arb. physiol. Anst.* Leipzig, 1875.)
26. Femoral and hepatic arterial pressures and liver volume obtained by François-Franck and Hallion. (From C. E. François-Franck and L. Hallion. *Arch. physiol. norm. path.*, 1896.)

Chapter XI, pages 703 to 742

1. Case 6 in the Smith papyrus. (From J. H. Breasted. *The Edwin Smith Surgical Papyrus*. Chicago, University of Chicago Press, 1930. With permission.)

2. Early coins of Alexandria. (Courtesy of the American Numismatic Society, New York.)
3. The Galenic view of the relations of the cranial nerves. (From L. Choulant. *Geschichte und Bibliographie der anatomischen Abbildung.* Leipzig, Weigel, 1852.)
4. The vessels of the neck according to Leonardo da Vinci. (From Leonardo da Vinci. *Manoscritti di Leonardo da Vinci della Reale Biblioteca di Windsor.* Torino, Roux, 1901.)
5. The *rete mirabile* according to Leonardo da Vinci. (From Leonardo da Vinci. *Manoscritti di Leonardo da Vinci* . . . . Torino, Roux, 1901.)
6. Galen's description of the *rete mirabile*. (From A. Vesalius. *De humanis corporis fabrica, liber VII.* In *Vesalius on the Human Brain*, translated by C. Singer, London, Oxford University Press, 1952. With permission.)
7. The vessels of the brain, from the *Fabrica*. (From A. Vesalius. *De humanis corporis* . . . . In *Vesalius on the Human Brain*, translated by C. Singer. London, Oxford University Press, 1952. With permission.)
8. Thomas Willis. (Courtesy of the Columbia University Medical Library.)
9. The Circle of Willis and the cranial nerves. (From T. Willis. *Cerebri anatome nervorumque descriptio et usus.* Geneva, 1676.)
10. Alexander Monro. (From an engraving by James Heath after Raeburn. Impression in the Wellcome Historical Medical Museum.)
11. Charles S. Sherrington. (Courtesy of the Columbia University Medical Library.)
12. The intracranial volume as a measure of cerebral circulation. (From C. S. Roy and C. S. Sherrington. *J. Physiol.* (Lond.), 1890.)
13. Effects of asphyxia on intracranial volume and systemic blood pressure. (From C. S. Roy and C. S. Sherrington. *J. Physiol.* (Lond.), 1890.)
14. Hill's method of studying the cerebral circulation of the dog. (From L. Hill. *The Physiology and Pathology of the Cerebral Circulation.* London, Churchill, 1896.)
15. Cerebral blood flow in man by nitrous oxide technique. (From S. S. Kety. *Methods in Medical Research*, 1948. With permission.)
16. First study using nitrous oxide method in man. (From S. S. Kety and C. F. Schmidt. *Amer. J. Physiol.*, 1945. With permission.)
17. Autoradiogram for the measurement of local cerebral blood flow. "Local blood flow in neural tissue," in *New Research Techniques in Neuroanatomy.* (From L. Sokoloff, Thomas, 1957. With permission.)

CHAPTER XII, pages 743 to 816

1. The fetal circulation.
2. The principal changes in the circulation at birth. (From G. V. R. Born, G. S. Dawes, J. C. Mott, and J. G. Widdicombe. Cold Spr. Harb. Symp., 1954. With permission.)

3. Raphael Bienvenu Sabatier. (Courtesy of the Columbia University Medical Library.)

4. The entry of the great veins into the heart. (*Left:* From R. B. Sabatier. *Mém. Acad. Roy. Sci.* (Paris), 1778. *Right:* From A. G. Pohlman. *Johns Hopk. Hosp. Bull.*, 1907.)

5. Human fetal heart according to Wolff. (From C. F. Wolff. *Novi Commentarii Acad. Sci. Imp. Petropolitanae*, 1776.)

6. Early illustrations of the foramen ovale. (*Left:* From H. Fabricius. *The Embryological Treatises.* Translated by H. B. Adelmann, Ithaca, N.Y., Cornell University Press, 1942. With permission. *Top right:* From R. Lower. *Tractatus de corde.* London, 1669. *Bottom right:* From J. Drake. *Anthropologia Nova, or, a New System of Anatomy*, Appendix, London, 1728.)

7. Cineradiography in fetus illustrating flow through the foramen ovale. (From A. E. Barclay, K. J. Franklin, and M. M. L. Prichard. *The Foetal Circulation and Cardiovascular System, and the Changes That They Undergo at Birth.* Oxford, Blackwell Scientific Publications, 1944. With permission.)

8. The circulation in the fetal lamb. (From G. V. R. Born, G. S. Dawes, J. C. Mott, and J. G. Widdicombe. Cold. Spr. Harb. Symp., 1954. With permission.)

9. The circulation in the mature fetal lamb. (From G. S. Dawes, J. C. Mott, and J. G. Widdicombe. *J. Physiol.* (Lond.), 1954. With permission.)

10. Joseph Barcroft. (From K. J. Franklin. *Joseph Barcroft.* Oxford, Blackwell Scientific Publications, 1953. With permission.)

11. The first breaths in the mature fetal lamb. (From G. V. R. Born, G. S. Dawes, J. C. Mott, and B. R. Rennick. *J. Physiol.* (Lond.), 1956. With permission.)

12. Underventilation after tying the umbilical cord in a mature fetal lamb. (From G. V. R. Born, G. S. Dawes, J. C. Mott, and B. R. Rennick. *J. Physiol.* (Lond.), 1956. With permission.)

13. Pulmonary vascular changes on expanding the lungs of a mature fetal lamb. (From G. S. Dawes, J. C. Mott, J. G. Widdicombe, and D. G. Wyatt. *J. Physiol.* (Lond.), 1953. With permission.)

14. Closure of the foramen ovale in a mature fetal lamb. (From G. S. Dawes, J. C. Mott, and J. G. Widdicombe. *J. Physiol.* (Lond.), 1955. With permission.)

15. Fetal blood channels according to Fabricius. (From H. Fabricius. De formato foetu. Venice. Franciscum Bolzettam, 1600.

16. Elastic fibers in the large vessels of a human fetus. (Courtesy of Dr. M. M. L. Prichard.)

17. Constriction of the ductus arteriosus when the arterial O_2 saturation is

raised. (From G. V. R. Born, G. S. Dawes, J. C. Mott and B. R. Rennick. *J. Physiol.* (Lond.), 1956. With permission.)

18. Phonocardiogram of an unanesthetized newborn lamb. (From G. V. R. Born, G. S. Dawes, J. C. Mott, and J. G. Widdicombe. Cold Spr. Harb. Symp., 1954. With permission.)

19. Flow through the ductus arteriosus in the newborn lamb. (From G. S. Dawes, J. C. Mott, and J. G. Widdicombe. *J. Physiol.* (Lond.), 1955. With permission.)

20. The venous supply to the fetal liver. (From M. Bertin. *Mém. Acad. Roy. Sci.* (Paris), 1753.)

21. Cineradiograph of an umbilical vein injection into a lamb fetus. (From A. E. Barclay, K. J. Franklin, and M. M. L. Prichard. *The Foetal Circulation*.... Oxford, Blackwell Scientific Publications, 1944. With permission.)

22. First published record, by Cohnstein and Zuntz, showing umbilical arterial and venous pressures. (From J. Cohnstein and N. Zuntz. *Pflügers Arch. ges. Physiol.*, 1884.)

23. Ductus venosus viewed from the umbilical vein in the bovine fetus. (From A. E. Barclay, K. J. Franklin, and M. M. L. Prichard. *The Foetal Circulation* .... Oxford, Blackwell Scientific Publications, 1944. With permission.)

24. The distribution of blood between the fetus and the placenta in sheep. (From J. Barcroft. *Researches on Prenatal Life*. Oxford, Blackwell Scientific Publications, 1946. With permission.)

25. The carbohydrate content of the ventricles of young rats and the mean survival time in nitrogen. (From G. S. Dawes, J. C. Mott, and H. Shelley. *J. Physiol.* (Lond.), 1959. With permission.)

26. Nathan Zuntz. (Courtesy of the Columbia University Medical Library).

Name Index

Abbott, B. C. 143
Abderhalden, Emil 592
Abel, John Jacob 574, 582, 592
Abel, S. 767, 795
Abercrombie, John A. 717
Abernethy, John 240, 684
Abramson, D. I. 297, 520
Ackermann, T. 718, 731
Adams, Forrest H. 786
Addison, Thomas 492
Ader, Clément 292, 336
Aeby, C. T. A. 368
Agricola, Georgius 74, 75, 205
Albertus Magnus 18
Alcmeon of Croton 4, 624, 637, 643, 703, 707, 730
Alexander of Macedon (the Great) 8, 624, 705
Alexander of Tralles 624
Alexander, F. A. D. 799
Alexander, F. G. 734, 735
Alexander, J. 315
Alexander, R. S. 469
Allbutt, Thomas Clifford 502, 504
Alpagos, Andreas 17
Alpagos, Paulus 17
Altschule, M. D. 507, 508
Alzamora, V. 779
Ampère, André Marie 281
Anaxagoras of Clazomenae 624, 635, 640
Anaximander of Miletos 623, 635
Anaximenes of Miletos 4, 623, 635
Anderson, H. K. 433
Anrep, G. V. 456–458
Ansano, Saint 619, 621
Aranzi, Giulio Cesare 745, 778, 787

Aretaeus of Cappadocia 645
Aristotle 8, 77, 202, 203, 207, 360, 548, 624, 628, 629, 632–640, 642, 643, 648, 663, 703–705
Arrhenius, Svante 568
Asclepiades 645
Aselli, Gaspare 389, 658
Asher, L. 393
Ashman, R. 319
Asklepios 12
Atkinson, D. E. 133
Aub, Joseph 727
Audige, J. 598
Auerbach, Leopold 368
Austrian, C. H. 520
Avicenna (Ibn Sinā) 15–18, 203, 207

B

Bacon, Roger 545
Bacq, Z. M. 435, 468
Badoud, E. 53
Baer, R. 687
Baglivi, Giorgio 555, 677
Bainton, R. H. 22, 24
Bancroft, Edward 271
Banks, Joseph 279
Barclay, Alfred E. 674, 753, 754, 767, 768, 772, 789, 792, 795
Barcroft, Joseph 58–61, 689, 735, 751, 753, 758, 760, 761, 765, 768, 772, 779, 781–783, 792, 796
Barker, Lewellys Franklin 315, 325
Barker, P. S. 315
Barlow, Lazarus 394
Barnwell, John B. 590

[835]

Barron, Donald H. 753, 796
Bartels, C. 494
Bartholin, Thomas 390, 658, 659
Basch, Samuel S. K. von 498, 502, 503, 678, 687
Bauer, D. J. 797
Bauer, W. 682, 687
Bayliss, Leonard 590
Bayliss, William Maddock 291, 409, 417–419, 423, 425, 427, 433, 458, 575, 678, 679, 687
Beale, L. S. 674
Belitzer, V. A. 174
Bell, E. T. 512
Bellini, Lorenzo 549–551, 554, 556
Bendall, J. R. 185
Bennet, Abraham 271
Berengario da Carpi, Giacomo 205, 707
Berglund, E. 770
Bergman, P. G. 513–515
Bergmann, Ernst von 94
Bergmann, G. von 506
Berman, M. 171
Bernard, Claude 51, 52, 409–413, 415, 416, 509, 562, 564, 569, 577, 580, 677, 685–687, 731, 733
Bernouilli, Daniel 84, 678
Bernstein, Julius 285, 298, 328, 329
Berres, Joseph B. 565
Bert, Paul 411, 412, 733, 799
Bertin, M. 788
Berzelius, Jöns Jacob 685
Beyne, J. 55
Bezold, Albert von 230, 232, 454
Beutner, A. 49
Bichat, Marie-François-Xavier 367, 672, 673, 677, 684, 766, 767, 789
Bidder, Friedrich Wilhelm 685
Bieter, Raymond Nicholas 599
Billroth, Theodor 105
Binet, Leon 55
Bingel, A. 514
Biot, J. B. 271
Bittar, E. 16, 23
Black, James 377
Black, Joseph 39, 40
Blalock, Alfred 514

Blasius, W. 110
Blix, Magnus 110, 113
Blumgart, H. L. 239
Bochdalek, Victor 240
Bøe, J. 528
Bohr, Christian 56, 57, 60, 90, 92, 236, 379
Boniface VI (Pope) 19
Bordley, James (III) 590
Borelli, Giovanni Alfonso 28, 29, 80, 488, 547, 549, 554, 664, 687, 688
Borst, H. G. 770
Botallo, Leonardo 776
Bott, Phyllis A. 590
Bouckaert, J. J. 458, 470, 510, 724, 732
Bowditch, Henry Pickering 90, 127, 162–164, 327
Bowman, William 556–561, 564–567, 573, 577, 600
Boyle, Robert 29–33, 37–39, 73, 79, 82, 269, 799
Brachet, I. L. 731
Bradford, J. R. 54, 55
Bradley, R. C. 590
Brady, A. J. 165
Brahe, Tycho 215
Bramwell, J. C. 91
Braun-Menéndez, E. 516, 518
Brecher, G. A. 154
Bréguet, L. 85
Bright, Richard 492, 493, 496, 497, 501
Brissaud, E. 674
Brodie, Benjamin Collins 685
Broen, J. 217
Bronk, D. W. 468
Brouha, L. 468
Brown, E. D. 459
Brown, J. G. 387, 448
Brown-Séquard, Charles-Édouard 53, 409, 412–414, 418, 686
Bruisson, C. 681
Brüke, Ernst Wilhelm von 235, 564
Budin, Pierre 794
Bumpus, F. M. 517
Bunsen, Robert W. 87
Burch, G. E. 152
Burchell, H. B. 314

Burdon-Sanderson, John 284–286, 289, 319, 418, 494, 495, 499
Burger, H. C. 305–307, 336
Burian, Richard 598
Burnard, Eric D. 786, 787
Burns, Allan 218, 222, 223, 225
Burns, John 222
Burrows, G. 718
Burton, A. C. 151, 152, 426
Burton-Opitz, Russell 679, 687
Byrom, F. B. 508, 519

C

Caesalpinus, Andreas 25, 214
Caldani, Leopoldo 273, 274
Calvin, John 20, 25
Cannon, Walter Bradford 431, 432, 435, 687
Canton, John 271
Carlill, S. D. 770
Carlisle, Anthony 280
Cartier, Jacques 205
Carrier, E. B. 388
Cassels, D. E. 785
Catherine of Russia 223
Cavazzani, E. 681, 687
Cavendish, Henry 39, 271
Cayla, Ch. 565
Cellini, Benvenuto 205
Celsus 645
Cesi, Frederigo (Prince) 545
Chambers, Robert 384, 385, 388, 401, 588, 589
Chapman, C. B. 111
Charles I of England 71
Charles V (Emperor) 19, 205, 212, 213
Chaucer, Geoffrey 204, 625
Chauveau, Auguste 48–50, 91, 97, 448, 678
Chelius, Max Joseph von 681
Child, C. G. 507
Chinard, F. P. 402
Chirac, Pierre 215
Chittenden, Russell Henry 582
Chorobski, Jerzy 732
Christiansen, J. 61
Christopherson, A. R. 331

Chrzonszczewsky, N. 570, 674
Cicero, Marcius Tullius 619
Clark, G. A. 797, 798
Clark, S. L. 779
Clausius, Rudolph Julius Emmanuel 94
Cobb, S. 718, 724, 731, 732, 735
Cohn, F. 319
Cohnheim, Julius 52, 230–232, 239, 378, 448, 585
Cohnstein, J. 750, 765, 791, 793, 794, 802
Colbert, Jean-Baptiste 80
Cole, K. S. 328
Colladon, Germain 20
Columbus, Christopher 205
Columbus, Realdus 23–26, 76, 77, 213, 712
Comline, R. S. 798
Comroe, J. H., Jr. 473
Concato, L. 458, 470
Condorelli, M. 772, 774
Constantine of Africa 18, 203
Cooper, Astley 458
Cooper, Keith E. 758
Copernicus, Nicholas 72, 77, 205, 215
Cori, Carl Ferdinand 132, 171, 179
Cori, Gerty T. 132, 171
Cori, Osvaldo 133
Corso, F. 733
Cortez, Hernando 207
Corvisart, Jean-Nicolas 225
Cosimo, Duke (of Pisa) 213
Cotton, T. F. 378
Coulomb, Charles Augustin 271
Cournand, André 104, 108, 727
Cowper, William 676
Craib, W. H. 303, 313
Crane, Marian M. 595
Crowe, Samuel 593
Cserna, S. 734
Ctesibios of Alexandria 85, 665
Cullen, William 676
Cummings, J. N. 761
Cuneus, Gabriel 269
Curtis, H. J. 328
Curtius, Matthaeus 207, 209
Cushny, Arthur Robertson 573–582, 586, 591, 594, 596

Cyon, Elias von (Elie de) 89, 90, 453, 454, 468

D

Dagianti, A. 772
Dale, Henry Hallett 370, 378, 419, 433–436, 575, 682, 687
Daly, Ivan de Burgh 456, 457, 770
Daly, Michael de Burgh 770
Daniel, P. M. 674
d'Arsonval, Jacques Arsène 52
Darwin, Erasmus 794
Dastre, A. 416
Davis, David Melvin 593
Davy, Humphry 280
Dawes, Geoffrey S. 451, 473
Dawson, W. R. 201
Dean, Henry Percy 54, 55, 718
de Haan, J. 595
della Porta, Giovanni 79
Dell'Oro, E. 518
Democritos of Abdera 624, 635, 640, 704, 707
Denis, Willy 598
Derow, H. A. 507, 508
Descartes, René 214, 215, 217, 713
Deuticke, H. J. 171
de Vries, Hugo 568
de Waart, A. 302, 323
Deysach, L. J. 674
Diocles of Caryostos 8
Diogenes of Apollonia 4, 626–628, 649, 704, 707
di Paolo, Giovanni 488
Disse, J. 674
Dittmar, Carl 90
Dogiel, Jan 90, 679
Dollond, John 362, 672
Donaldson, Frank, Jr. 152
Donders, Frans Cornelius 319, 718, 723, 731
Donker, H. J. L. 169
Donnan, Frederick George 61, 399, 400
Dontas, A. S. 469
Dorough, M. E. 518
Douglas, Claude G. 61

Doyère, Louis 556
Drake, J. 752
Draper, M. H. 331, 334
Drebbel, Cornelius 30
Dreser, Hermann 110, 568
Drinker, Cecil K. 400, 584
Drury, D. R. 518
Du Bois-Reymond, Emil 87, 277, 282–284, 287, 327, 328, 336, 365, 564
Dudley, H. W. 435
Du Fay, Charles 269
Duhamel, J. M. C. 85
Duke, Helen N. 770
Dumke, P. R. 723, 724
Durrer, D. 312
Duverney, Joseph-Guichard 675

E

Ebbecke, U. 370, 378
Eberth, Carl J. 368
Eck, Nikolai Vladimirovich 685
Eckhard, Carl 416
Edelstein, L 210
Edsall, J. T. 181, 182
Edwards, John Graham 598
Einthoven, Willem 188, 290–296, 298–300, 302–309, 323, 336, 455
Eldridge, F. L. 784
Elias, H. 675
Elizabeth I 71
Ellinger, P. 674
Elliott, D. F. 517
Elliott, T. R. 433–435
Ellis, Arthur 494
Embden, Gustav 132, 171
Empedocles of Acragas 4, 29, 624, 636, 638, 642, 704
Engelhardt, E. 435
Engelhardt, W. A. 174, 182
Engelmann, Theodor Wilhelm 285, 296, 327, 329
Eppinger, Hans 315, 316
Erasistratos of Iulis 9, 10, 12, 74, 202, 203, 624, 629, 633–636, 640, 643–645, 655, 661, 707
Erasmus, Desiderius 205

Erichsen, John E. 228
Erlanger, Joseph 110, 318
Euler, H. von 132
Euler, Ulf S. von 55
Euripides 266
Evans, C. L. 246
Everett, N. B. 795
Ewald, Carl Anton 496
Eyster, J. A. E. 297, 327, 455

F

Fabricius ab Aquapendente, Hieronymus 73, 74, 76, 78, 213, 743, 752, 776, 777
Fahr, George 57, 302, 323
Fahr, Theodor 502, 504, 507
Faivre, J. 497
Falkenheim, H. 718
Fallopius, Gabriel 213, 214
Fano, G. 90
Fantoni, J. 676
Faraday, Michael 280
Farrington, B. 643
Fasciolo, J. C. 515, 516
Fazekas, J. F. 799
Fenn, Wallace O. 156, 159
Ferdinand II, Grand Duke of Tuscany 547
Fernel, Jean 20, 24, 207
Ferrein, Antoine 669–671
Ferris, E. B., Jr. 726
Fick, Adolph 53, 87, 93–97, 110, 112, 113, 146, 154, 391, 678
Fick, Ludwig 87
Fierst, S. M. 521
Findley, T., Jr. 590
Finesinger, Jacob E. 732
Flack, Martin 297
Flasher, J. 518
Fleisch, A. 373, 474
Fleischl, E. 90
Fleming, D. 13, 25
Flexner, Louis B. 796
Flint, Austin, Sr. 685
Flourens, M.-J.-P. 681
Fog, M. 425

Folin, Otto 598
Fontana, Felice 273
Forbes, H. S. 718, 724, 731
Forssmann, Werner 103
Foster, Michael 59, 429, 430, 555
Fothergill, John 218, 222
Fourier, Jean B. J. 94
Fracastorius 127
Francis I 205
François-Frank, Charles-Émile 53–55, 681, 686, 687
Frank, E. 506
Frank, Otto 90, 99, 110–113, 150–152
Franklin, Benjamin 39, 270, 271, 273, 276, 278
Franklin, Kenneth J. 34, 753, 754, 768, 771, 772, 788, 789, 792, 795
Frederiq, P. 678
Freedberg, A. S. 239
Friedman, B. 514
Fuchs, Leonhard 20
Führer, H. 52
Fulton, G. P. 384
Fulton, John F. 38
Funcke, Otto 56

G

Gad, Johannes 680
Galeazzi, Domenico Maria Gusmano 274
Galen of Pergamon 7, 10–18, 20, 22–27, 74, 76, 202–205, 207, 209, 210, 212, 244, 549, 601, 622, 624, 625, 629–642, 644–648, 651, 657, 706, 707, 709–711, 771, 774, 776
Galilei, Galileo 72, 74, 76, 77, 79, 215, 488, 545, 546, 655, 665, 666
Galton, Francis 529
Galvani, Luigi 273–278, 281, 282, 284, 326
Gama, Vasco da 205
Gammon, G. D. 510
Gärtner, G. 723
Gaskell, P. 426
Gaskell, Walter Holbrook 90, 296, 335, 429, 430, 433, 448, 575
Gasser, H. S. 159

Gauer, O. H. 472
Gayda, T. 734
Geddes, L. A. 85
George IV 499
Geraghty, John Timothy 594
Gérard, G. 776
Gerard, Ralph Waldo 331, 333, 735
Gerard of Cremona 18
Gerhardt, Carl 94
Gernandt, B. 469
Gibbs, E. L. 726
Gibbs, F. A. 729
Gibbs, Josiah W. 399, 400
Gibson, G. A. 782
Gilbert, William 267–269, 280
Gilligan, D. R. 239
Giuliano, G. 772
Glisson, Francis 632, 658–665, 675, 683
Gmelin, Leopold 685
Goldblatt, H. 507, 510–513, 516
Goll, F. 566, 569
Goltz, Friedrich Leopold 415
Goodale, W, T. 256
Gordon, D. B. 518
Gorlin, R. 248
Graefe, Albrecht von 505
Grafflin, Allan Lyle 598
Grant, R. T. 510, 520
Gray, Stephen 269
Green, D. E. 244
Green, J. H. 467
Greenfield, A. David M. 758
Gregg, Donald E. 237
Grehant, N. 97
Grew, Nehemiah 547
Grollman, A. 102, 103, 105
Gross, L. 239
Grotte, G. 402
Gudbjarnason, S. 257
Guericke, Otto von 30, 269
Guinand, Pierre Louis 672
Guinther, Johann (of Andernach) 20, 207
Guitel, F. 598
Gull, William 495–497, 500, 501
Gunther, Mavis 794
Gürber, A. 61

H

Haas, E. 516
Hackel, D. B. 256
Hagemann, O, 97, 98
Hajdu, S. 127, 164
Haldane, John Scott 58–61, 575
Hales, Stephen 38, 39, 81–85, 91, 215, 373–377, 386, 489–491, 676, 678
Hale-White, W. 496
Hall, Chester Moor 672
Hall, Marshall 37, 218, 228, 362–365, 375, 377, 386, 389
Haller, Albrecht von 50, 51, 240, 366, 367, 377, 669, 676, 677, 684, 788
Hallion, L. 681, 686, 687
Halloran, R. D. 726
Hamilton, M. 527, 529
Hamilton, William F. 105, 108, 767
Handley, C. A. 734
Hanson, J. 185
Hanzal, R. F. 511, 512
Harden, A. 171, 173
Harris, A. S. 311
Harrison, Tinsley R. 514
Hartwich, A. 515
Harvey, William 12, 14, 24–28, 48, 71–80, 83, 90, 127, 213–215, 269, 355–357, 361, 373, 386, 403, 488, 545, 547, 548, 555, 556, 622, 647, 648, 651, 655–657, 659, 661–666, 675, 678, 690, 707, 712–714, 716, 745, 748, 766, 771, 775, 776, 788
Hasselbalch, K. A. 57
Hawksbee, Francis 270
Hayman, Joseph M., Jr. 549, 590
Heberden, William 218, 220–222, 225
Hecht, H. H. 331
Héger, P. 51, 52, 90
Heidenhain, Rudolph P. H. 392, 393 399, 570–573, 577, 578, 581, 585, 586, 594
Heintz, W. 685
Heller, H. 514
Helmer, O. M. 516
Helmholtz, Hermann L. F. von 87, 129, 225, 227, 285, 301, 303, 307, 336, 365, 564, 577, 733

Henderson, Lawrence J. 58, 60–62
Henderson, Yandell 99, 120, 154, 415
Hendrix, James Paisley 590, 735
Henle, Jacob 365, 409, 565, 673, 677
Henley, William 271
Henriques, V. 106, 236
Henry VIII 205
Henry, J. P. 471
Heracleitos of Ephesus 624, 635, 637
Hering, Ewald 92, 458, 459
Hering, Heinrich Ewald 459, 461–464, 510
Hèrisson, J. 497
Hermann, M. 566, 569, 587
Herodotus 617
Herophylos of Chalcedon 9, 10, 12, 202, 624, 629, 705–707
Herrick, James B. 223, 227, 242, 243
Herter, Christian A. 582
Heseler, Baldesar 209, 212
Hess, W. R. 447, 474
Hessel, G. 515
Heymans, Corneille 455, 458, 464, 465, 468, 470, 472, 510, 724
Highmore, Nathaniel 549
Hill, Archibald Vivian 91, 92, 147, 149, 155–160, 162, 164, 177, 189
Hill, Leonard 720–723, 731, 734
Himwich, H. E. 799
Hippocrates of Cos 5, 201, 203, 207, 210, 625, 635, 704
Hirsch, H. L. 726
Hirschfelder, A. D. 315
Hirt, A. 674
Hirt, Ludwig 454
His, Wilhelm, Jr. 297
Hoang-ti (Emperor) 266
Hodgkin, A. L. 328, 331, 336
Hodgkin, Thomas 492
Hodgson, Joseph 225
Hoff, H. E. 85
Hofmeister, Franz 60, 433
Holbein, Hans 205
Hollmann, H. E. 325
Hollmann, W. 325
Homer 266
Hooke, Robert 29, 30, 32, 35, 37, 38, 82, 85, 547

Hooker, D. R. 110, 455
Hopkins, Frederick Gowland 59, 575
Hoppe-Seyler, Felix 56, 568, 578, 685
Hou, C. L. 734
Houssay, B. A. 515
Houston, C. S. 762
Howell, William Henry 152
Howland, John 584
Huchard, Henri 502
Hudson, C. L. 590
Hüfner, G. von 90
Huggett, Arthur St. George Joseph McCarthy 750, 751, 759, 802
Hultgren, H. N. 784
Humboldt, Alexander von 277
Hunt, Reid 435
Hunter, John 218–220 222, 271, 273, 367, 458
Huot, A. 598
Hürthle, Karl 678
Huschke, Emil H. 556, 565
Huxley, A. F. 328, 331, 336
Huxley, H. E. 185
Huxley, Thomas Henry 601
Hyrtl, Josef 674

I

Ibn Nafis 15–17, 23
Ibn Sīnā (Avicenna) 15–18, 203, 207

J

Jackson, Hughlings 494
Jacobs, Merkel H. 388
Jaffé, Max 685
James I 71
James, L. Stanley 785
Janeway, Theodor Caldwell 504
Jenner, William 218, 221
Jensen, P. 724
Johnson, George 494–497
Johnson, J. A. 104
Johnston, F. D. 325
Jones, Muriel 771
Jores, L. 496
Jost, Alfred 797, 798

[841]

Joule, James Prescot 129
Jourdan, F. 732
Julian The Apostate 15

K

Kahn, J. R. 516, 522
Kahn, R. H. 378, 457
Kaiser, I. H. 761
Kalckar, H. M. 133, 174
Katchalsky, A. 136
Katz, B. 331, 336
Katz, Louis N. 152, 245
Kaufmann, M. 448
Kaufmann, P. 459
Keen, E. N. 775
Keilin, D. 170
Keith, Arthur 297
Kellie, George 717
Kellogg, H. B. 751
Kelvin, Lord (William Thomson) 292, 306, 336
Kemp, Tage 527
Kennedy, J. A. 779
Kepler, Johannes 77, 215
Kiernan, Francis 670–672, 684
Kilian, Hermann Friedrich 747, 748, 750, 751, 754, 766, 789
Kinsman, J. M. 105
Kirchoff, Gustav Robert 287
Kirsch, M. 241
Kisch, B. 459
Kissin, M. 510, 514
Kleinerman, J. 256
Kleist, Ewald von 269
Klug, F. 235
Kluyver, A. J. 169–171
Knisely, M. H. 674, 680
Knoll, Philipp 459, 718
Knoop, Franz 171
Koch, E. 464, 510
Koch, Robert 227
Kohlrausch, Friedrich Wilhelm Georg 94
Kölliker, Albert von 93, 283, 284, 319, 409, 673
Kolls, Alfred Conrad 594, 596
Korányi, A. v. 568

Korotkoff, N. S. 498
Korteweg, D. J. 91
Köster, G. 455
Kovalcík, Vladimir 781
Kraft, G. 171
Kramer, K. 772
Krause, C. 367
Krause, Karl Friedrich Theodor K. 565
Krayer, O. 152
Krebs, H. A. 171
Kries, Johannes Adolph von 90, 387
Krogh, August 57, 58, 60, 102, 369–372, 379–383, 386–388, 402, 491, 586, 680, 689
Krogh, Marie 58, 379
Kronecker, Hugo K. 245
Kühne, Willy 287
Kupffer, C. von 674

L

Ladon, A. 455
Laënnec, René-T.-H. 225, 229
Laffont, Marc 417
Lagrange, Joseph Louis 43
Lalesque, Fernand 54
Lamfrom, H. 516
Landis, Eugene M. 515
Langendorff, O. 236, 237
Langer, C. 778
Langer, L. J. 240
Langley, John Newport 429, 430
Laplace, Pierre Simon, Marquis de 46, 168, 226, 271
Lardy, H. A. 178
Lavoisier, Antoine Laurent 29, 37, 38, 41–48, 56, 168, 225, 242, 733
Lavoisier, Madame (Marie Anne Pierette Paulze) 43
Lawrence, William 733
Leake, C. 77
Leboucq, G. 6, 7
van Leeuwenhoek, Antony 79, 358–361, 367, 371–373, 386, 547, 548
Leloir, L. F. 516
Lennox, W. G. 726
Lentz, K. I. 516

Lenz, E. 284
Leonardo da Vinci 71, 205, 651–653, 708, 709
Le Quire, V. S. 772
Leucippos of Miletos 624, 635
Leupold of Leipzig 85
Levin, A. 146
Lewis, B. M. 729
Lewis, G. N. 131
Lewis, Thomas 290, 299, 303, 308–312, 314–316, 318, 323, 336, 370, 378, 387, 449
Lewis, Warren Harmon 598
Leyden, Ernst von 232, 233
Lichtheim, Ludwig 51, 52
Liebig, Justus von 56, 242
Liebreich, Richard 505
Liljestrand, Göran 55, 58, 102, 118, 469
Limbeck, R. von 61
Lind, James 772, 784, 786
Lindhard, J. 58, 102
Ling, G. 331, 333
Linzenmeier, G. 778
Lipmann, F. 133, 171, 173
Lippmann, Gabriel 287, 288, 336
Lister, J. L. 377
Litten, Moritz 52
Littré, Émile 6
Ljubimowa, M. N. 182
Locke, F. S. 245
Loeb, Jacques 564
Loewi, Otto 433–435
Loewy, A. 99
Lombard, J. S. 733
Longcope, Warfield 494
Longet, François-Achille 416
Lower, Richard 29, 32–38, 80, 82, 216, 217, 407, 408, 752, 766
Lucas, Keith 575
Lucretius 266
Ludwig, Carl Friedrich Wilhelm von 48, 49, 56, 85, 87–90, 92, 93, 162, 233, 390–393, 398, 399, 418, 429, 453, 454, 468, 562–570, 572, 573, 575, 577–581, 585, 587, 590, 591, 600, 678, 679, 681, 686, 688
Lumière, Auguste 50

Luther, Martin 205
Lutz, B. R. 384
Lynch, J. 511, 512
Lysolm, E. 118

M

McClurkin, T. 796
McCubbin, J. W. 467
McDowell, Muriel C. 590
McGregor, M. 770
McKeown, Thomas 779
McLean, Franklin C. 62
McMichael, J. 508
McWilliam, J. A. 296
MacGillavry, T. H. 674
MacKenzie, D. W., Jr. 674
Mackenzie, James 299, 309
MacLeod, A. G. 315
Magendie, François 51, 391, 393, 413, 414, 416, 677, 685, 733
Magnus, Gustav 48, 56
Magnus, Rudolph 90
Mahomed, Frederick Akhbar 497, 499, 500–502, 509, 523
Mall, Franklin Paine 674, 680, 687
Malpighi, Marcello 28, 79, 80, 356, 357, 360, 366, 367, 403, 546–557, 568, 665, 666, 669, 670, 674, 683, 688
Manca, G. 681, 687
Mangold, R. 736
Mann, H. 323–325
Marchand, R. 285
Marcus Aurelius 12
Marey, Étienne-Jules 48–50, 92, 97, 110, 289, 497–499, 678, 681
Markoff, I. 102
Markwalder, J. 113, 236
Marsh, B. B. 185
Marsh, B. S. 158
Marsh, W. H. 516
Marshall, Eli Kennerly, Jr. 591–596, 598, 600
Martius, C. 171
Mascagni, Paolo 366
Mason, M. F. 514, 779
Matteucci, Carlo 282, 283

Matton, G. 467
Mautner, H. 682
Mayer, Julius R. 56
Mayer, Robert 129, 227
Mayow, John 37, 38, 716
Mayrs, Edward Brice Cooper 595, 596
Meek, W. J. 297, 327
Meerson, F. Z. 252
Meissner, George 319
Melka, J. 778
Mendel, Gregor 227
Merril, R. E. 772
Meschia, Giacoma 796
Metcalfe, Thomas 429, 433
Meyer, F. 236
Meyer, Hans H. 433, 575
Meyer, K. H. 134
Meyer, Lothar 56, 90
Meyerhof, Otto 132, 146, 171
Meyerhoff, Max 23
Miall, W. E. 529, 530
Michelangelo 205
Mies, H. 510
Millikan, G. A. 772
Milovanovich, J. B. 326
Moens, A. J. 91
Mondino de'Luzzi 204, 205, 651, 707
Montanus (Monte, G. B. da) 209
Montgomery, Hugh 515, 590
Moore, B. 681
Moore, J. W. 105
Morat, J. P. 416
Morawitz, P. 236, 237
Morgagni, Giovanni Battista 214, 218, 273, 676
Morin, Arthur Jules 284
Moritz, A. R. 512
Mosso, Angelo 564, 681, 682, 725, 733, 734
Müller, Fritz 102
Müller, Heinrich 283, 284, 319
Müller, Johannes 282, 365–367, 377, 556, 562, 565, 577, 670, 673
Muñoz, J. M. 516
Monro, Alexander II 716, 717
Muralt, A. L. von 181
Myerson, Abraham 726

N

Nachmanson, D. 171
Nägeli, Carl Wilhelm von 168
Nasse, Christian Fredrich 415
Nastuk, W. L. 331
Naunyn, Bernard Gustav Julius 433, 718
Neckam, Alexander 267
Needham, D. M. 182
Needham, J. 182
Newell-Martin, H. 235
Newton, Isaac 82, 215, 226, 672, 678, 690
Nicholls, F. 754, 756
Nicholson, William 280
Nisell, O. 770
Nobili, Leopoldo 281, 282
Noll, D. 182
Noll, Friedrich W. 390
Nollet, Jean-Antoine (Abbé) 270
Nothnagel, Hermann 718, 731
Nussbaum, Moritz 572, 573
Nylin, G. 118, 729
Nymann, Gregor of Wittenberg 713

O

Ochoa, S. 174
Oersted, Hans Christian 281
Ohm, Georg Simon 271
Oldham, P. D. 529, 530
Oldt, M. R. 512
Oliver, George 418, 419, 687
Oliver, Jean 590
Olson, R. E. 256
Ons-en-Bray 85
Opdyke, D. F. 775
Oppenheimer, B. S. 316
Oppenheimer, Robert A. 63
Oribasios of Pergamon 15, 624
Osler, William 495
Ostwald, Wilhelm 181
Overton, Ernst 331

P

Pagano, G. 458, 459
Page, Charles Grafton 284

Page, F. J. M. 285, 286, 319
Page, Irvine H. 467, 516, 517
Paintal, A. S. 454
Pal, J. 687
Pamm, Peter Ludwig 230, 232
Pappenheimer, John R. 398, 400–402
Paracelsus, Aureolus 32
Paré, Ambröise 213
Parkinson, John 316, 317
Parnas, J. K. 132, 171
Parry, Caleb Hillier 218, 220, 221, 223, 225
Pasteur, Louis 169, 227, 242
Patten, B. M. 767, 774, 776
Patterson, S. W. 113, 116, 151, 154
Patterson, T. S. 37, 38
Pattison, Granville Sharp 223
Paul of Aegina 624
Pavy, Frederick William 686
Pearson, R. S. B. 520
Peart, W. S. 517, 522
Pecquet, Jean 658
Penfield, Wilder 732, 735
Perera, George A. 508
Pericles 266
Peter the Great 667
Pétrequin, Joseph-P.-E. 675
Pettenkofer, Max von 233, 242
Pfeffer, Wilhelm Friedrich Philipp 394, 568
Pflüger, Eduard F. W. 56, 90, 97
Philalaus of Croton 624, 636, 637
Philip II 213
Philip of Macedon 8
Philistion of Locroi 6, 7, 624, 634
Pick, E. P. 682
Piegu, Alexandre 681
Pierce, J. A. 590
Piper, H. 113, 116, 154
Pizarro, Francisco 207
Plant, Oscar H. 584–586, 590
Plato 7, 85, 266, 610, 624, 634, 636, 637, 639, 640, 643, 648
Platt, Robert 527
Plesch, J. 99
Poggendorff, J. C. 281
Pohlman, A. G. 747, 748, 750, 751

Poiseuille, Jean Léonard Marie 51, 84, 86, 87, 90, 386, 387, 390, 409, 491, 497, 677, 678, 680, 690
Poisson, Siméon Denis 271
Polosa, C. 772
Polybus of Cos 635
Portzehl, H. 184
Potter, V. R. 178
Pouillet, C. S. M. 86, 87, 284
Poulsson, L. T. 682, 687
Pourfour du Petit, Francois 408
Pourtales, Guy de 180
Pratt, Frederick H. 240
Praxagoras of Cos 8, 9
Prec, K. J. 785
Prendergast, J. 14
Prichard, Marjorie M. L. 754, 768, 781, 789, 792, 795
Priestley, Joseph 29, 37, 39–41, 44, 56, 81, 271
Prince, A. L. 99, 120
Prinzmetal, Myron 514, 520
Ptolemy I Soter 9, 705
Purkinje, Johannes Evangelista 297
Pythagoras of Samos 624, 703

Q

Quain, Richard 228
Quincke, Heinrich 94
Quinquand, C. E. 97

R

Rabelais, François 205
Rabinovitz, M. 178
Ramsey, R. W. 144
Randall, J. H., Jr. 226
Randall, M. 131
Ranvier, Louis-Antoine 164
Rashkind, W. J. 469
Rauchfuss, C. 776
Réaumur, René A. F. de 270
Rebatel, F. 235
Recklinghausen, H. von 368, 498, 510
Record, Reginald Graham 779
Regnault, H. V. 233
Rehberg, P. B. 388

[845]

Rein, H. 118, 470, 734
Reiset, J. 233
Révécz, G. 735
Reynolds, S. R. M. 241, 770
Richard I (the Lion-Hearted) 267
Richards, Alfred Newton 370, 378, 582–588, 590, 591, 596, 600
Richards, Dickinson W. 682, 687, 727
Richmann, Georg Wilhelm 273
Riley, Richard L. 762
Rindfleisch, Eduard von 93
Ringer, Sidney 576
Riolan, Jean 76, 79, 214, 714
Ritchie, A. D. 136
Ritchie, J. M. 161
Riva-Rocci, Scipione 498
Roberts, J. A. F. 527, 528
Robison, John 271
Rokitansky, Carl 229
Röntgen, Wilhelm K. 94, 96, 228
Rosenblueth, A. 431
Rosenheim, Otto 245
Rössler, R. 687
Rothberger, C. J. 299, 315, 316
Rothschild, M. A. 310, 311, 315, 316
Rothschild, P. 510
Rouget, Charles 378
Rous, P. 400
Rowe, Richard D. 786
Rowntree, Leonard G. 593, 594
Roy, Charles Scott 387, 448, 585, 678, 681, 718, 720–724, 731, 732, 735
Rubner, Max 90, 92, 113, 233, 234
Rudbeck, Olaf 658
Ruffer, Marc A. 201
Rufus of Ephesus 645
Rumford, Count (Benjamin Thompson) 129
Runnström, J. 174
Rushmer, R. F. 117, 118
Russell, F. E. 774, 775
Ruysch, Frederik 555, 667–670

S

Sabatier, Raphael Bienvenu 746–748, 750, 751, 754, 756

Sabourin, C. 674
Sakai, S. 459
Salathé, A. 718
Salvenmoser, (Ludwig's assistant) 564
Sanctorius 664
Santorini, Giovanni Domenico 676
Saunders, J. B. de M. 209
Savjoloff, V. V. 323
Saxton, Joseph 284
Schäfer, Edward A. (Sharpey-Schafer) 97, 399, 419, 514, 681, 687
Schaltheiss-Rechberg, A. von 232
Schanz, F. 776
Scheele, Carl Wilhelm 37, 44
Schellong, F. 325
Scher, A. M. 314
Schiff, Moritz 415, 416, 686, 733
Schleiden, Matthias Jacob 673
Schmid, J. 687
Schmidt, Carl Frederic 586–588, 685, 723–725, 727, 732, 734, 735
Schmiedeberg, Oswald 433
Schneider, D. 468
Schneider, J. W. 134
Schrötter, H. von 99
Schultén, Maximus Widekind von 718
Schultze, Bernhard Sigismund 765
Schumlansky, Alexander 556
Schwann, Theodor 365, 673
Schwarz, H. 517
Schweigger, Johannes S. C. 281
Schwyzer, R. 517
Sedgwick, William Thompson 235
Segall, H. N. 456
Seguin, Armand 46
Sénac, Jean-Baptiste de 215, 217, 408
Seneca, Lucius Annaeus 199
Seneviratne, R. D. 674
Sérégé, H. 680
Serota, H. M. 735
Servetus, Michael 18–25, 72, 77
Setschenow, Ivan Michailowitsch 90
Severini, L. 448
Sewall, Henry 454, 455
Sherrington, Charles Scott 459, 575, 718–723, 731, 732, 735
Shumway, N. P. 516, 522

Siciliano, L. 459
Siekevitz, P. 178
Silver, M. 798
Singer, Charles 210
Sinha, T. P. 795
Simmons, B. S. 795
Sjöstrand, F. S. 185
Skeggs, L., Jr. 516, 522
Slade, J. G. 378
Slegel, Paul Marquart 27, 78
Smith, Clement 795
Smith, Lorrain 58
Søbye, P. 527
Sodi-Pallares, D. 312, 314
Soemerring, Samuel T. von 365
Sokoloff, L. 735, 736
Sollman, Torald 459
Solomon (King) 266
Soranus of Ephesus 645
Soskin, Samuel 724
Soulé E. 680
Sowry, G. S. C. 527
Spallanzani, Lazaro 90, 367, 415, 681
Spalteholz, Werner 239
Sparkman, D. 515
Spehl, E. 51, 52
Spigelius (van den Spiegel, Adrian) 662
Staehelin, R. 506
Stahl, George Ernst 38, 41, 47
Stahlman, Mildred T. 772
Stannius, Hermann 296
Starling, Ernest Henry 52, 113–117, 127, 151, 152, 154, 155, 157, 236, 291, 376, 393, 394, 397–399, 418, 419, 433, 456–458, 568, 575, 576, 585, 590, 678, 679, 687
Starr, Isaac 110
Steinach, Eugen 378
Steiner, D. W. 454, 455
Stelling, Carl 409
Stelluti, Francesco 545
Steno (Stensen, N.) 683
Stevinus, Simon 678
Stewart, George Neil 105, 106
Stienon, L. 776
Stirling, William 105, 562
Stoerk, O. 316

Strassmann, P. 778
Strato (or Stratōn of Lampsacos) 643, 644
Straub, F. B. 152
Strecker, Adolf 685
Street, S. F. 144
Stricker, Salomon 378, 416
Stukeley, William 81
Sue, P. 274
Sulzer, R. 325
Summerville, W. W. 511, 512
Sutton, H. G. 495–497, 500, 501
Swammerdam, Jan 360, 547
Sylvius, Franciscus 664
Sylvius, François de la Boe 713
Sylvius, Jacobus (Jacques Dubois) 20, 207, 213
Szent-Györgyi, Albert 127, 164, 170, 182–185

T

Taggart, John 518
Takeuchi, T. 592
Talbott, J. H. 735
Tammann, G. 569, 579
Tannenberg, J. 384
Tanzi, Eugenio 733
Taquini, A. C. 515
Tarquinius Superbus 617
Tatawi, Muhyi Ad-Din At- 16
Taveau, René de M. 435
Tawara, S. 297
Temkin, Owsei 23
Thales of Miletos 266, 623, 635
Thebesius, Adam Christian 217, 218, 240
Theophrastos of Erosos 643
Thiry, Ludwig 468
Thorel, C. 297
Thornton, J. B. 3
Tiedemann, Friedrich 685
Tigerstedt, Robert A. 244, 513–515, 680
Titian 205, 210
Torrens, D. S. 758
Torricelli, Evangelista 678
Toulmin, K. 767
Traube, Ludwig 496, 497, 502, 568
Trotter, Wilfred 530

Tschermak, J. N. 455, 458, 461
Tsibakova, E. T. 174
Tubby, Alfred H. 393

U

Ustimovitsch, C. 566, 570

V

Valverde, Juan 25
Van Harreveld, A. 774, 775
van Helmont, Jean Baptiste 30, 664
van Kalkar, Jan Stefan 208, 210, 212
van Leersum, Evert Cornelis 510
van Milaan, J. B. 306, 307
van Musschenbroek, Pieter 269, 270
Van Slyke, Donald D. 62, 583
van't Hoff, Jacobus Henricus 568
Ventris, Michael 623
Verney, E. B. 456, 457
Verworn, Max 564, 577
Vesalius, Andreas 20, 23, 71, 205, 207–214, 218, 549, 651, 654, 655, 706, 708, 710–712, 787
Vickers, James Leonard 594, 595
Vierordt, Karl 92, 96, 497, 499
Vieussens, Raymond de 214–218, 240
Virchow, Rudolph Ludwig 229, 365, 778
Visscher, M. B. 104, 155
Vogt, Karl 564
Voit, Carl von 110, 111, 233, 234, 242, 248
Volhard, Franz 502, 504–507, 519
Volkmann, Alfred Wilhelm 96
Volta, Alessandro 276–281
Vulpian, E.-F.-A. 686

W

Wagner, J. 723
Wagner, Rudolph W. 565
Wainewright, J. 669
Wakim, K. G. 674
Walker, Arthur M. 590
Walkhoff, F. 776

Wallace, George Barclay 575, 584
Waller, Augustus Desiré 288–291, 295, 296, 299–302, 308, 323, 336
Waller, Augustus Volney 289, 409, 414, 415, 686
Walsh, John 271–273
Warburg, Otto 132, 169
Warren, James W. 492
Wasserman, E. 111
Watson, William 270
Wearn, Joseph Treloar 241, 588, 589, 596
Weber, Ernst Heinrich 91, 409, 565, 673
Weber, Eduard Friedrich 91, 144
Weber, H. H. 182, 184
Webfer, Johann Jacob 666
Webster, T. B. L. 623
Wegelius, Carl 772, 784
Weidmann, S. 331, 334
Weigert, Carl 232
Weitz, Wilhelm 525, 527
Wellman, H. 178
Wenckebach, Karl Friedrich 299
Wertheim, M. G. 85
Westfall, B. B. 590
Whalen, W. J. 165
Wharton, Thomas 659, 661
Wheatstone, Charles 85, 86
White, Harvey Lester 590
White, Paul D. 316, 317
Whitehead, A. N. 79
Whittenberger, J. L. 770
Whytt, Robert 372
Wiegand, W. B. 134
Wieland, H. 169, 170
Wiggers, Carl J. 49, 152, 188, 231, 239, 242, 254
Wigmore, M. E. 784
Wilde, W. S. 334
Wilkie, D. R. 134, 142, 143, 147, 159
Wilks, Samuel 494
William IV 499
Williams, H. B. 323
Willis, Thomas 32–34, 80, 548, 664, 713–715
Wilson, C. 507, 508, 519, 520
Wilson, Frank N. 303, 304, 307, 310, 313, 315, 316, 319, 325, 336

Windle, William F. 765, 767, 782, 783, 795
Winterberg, H. 299
Winterstein, L. 245
Wisenbaugh, P. E. 522
Wislicenus, Johannes 94, 95
Wislocki, George 593
Wöhlisch, E. 134, 135
Wolff, Caspar Friedrich 747–751, 754
Wolff, H. G. 718, 724
Wolff, L. 316, 317
Wolton, William 22
Woodbury, L. A. 331
Woodbury, R. A. 767
Woods, E. B. 767
Woods, K. R. 516
Woods, R. H. 151
Woodworth, R. S. 162
Wooldridge, Leonard Charles 90
Wren, Christopher 79, 85, 715
Wu, H. 62
Wyman, J. 146

Y

Young, James 28
Young, J. Z. 329
Young, Thomas 96, 489, 678
Young, W. J. 171, 173

Z

Zahn, A. 236, 237
Zayats, T. L. 252
Ziegler, Ernst 232, 233
Zilboorg, G. 210
Zoll, P. M. 239
Zotterman, Y. 469
Zuntz, Nathan 61, 97, 98, 102, 750, 765, 791, 793, 794, 802
Zweifach, B. W. 384, 385, 401

Subject Index

A

Acetylcholine, 433–5, 438, 451
Actin, 184, 186
Action potentials (*see* Transmembrane potentials)
    first studies, 280–85, 326, 327
    of cardiac muscle, 327, 287–91, 331–3
    of pacemaker tissues, 334, 335
    of skeletal muscle and nerve, 282, 326, 328–31
    of squid axon, 328–31, 333
Active state of muscle, 159–65
Actomyosin, 182–5, 252
Aglomerular fish, 596–600
Air
    basic element, 635–7, 643
    physical properties, 30, 32, 38, 39
Alexandria, Museum of, 8, 9, 10, 624, 629, 705
Alexandria, two famous physicians, 9, 11, 202, 203
"All-or-none principle," 164
Alveolar-capillary gas exchange, 56–62
Amber, 265
Angina pectoris, 199, 218–25
Aortic (depressor) nerve, 453–8
Aristotelian corpus, 18, 201, 202
Arteriocapillary sphincters, 384
Athens (*see* School)
Autonomic nervous system, 429–31, 441–7
Avicenna's Canon, Commentary on, 16, 17
Angiotensin (Angiotonin), 516–19, 522
Arterial hypertension (*see* Hypertension)
Ascites (according to Galen), 644

Anatomia hepatis, 659
Asphyxia, in newborn, 762, 763, 765, 766, 781, 787, 797–802

B

Baroreceptor reflexes
    effect of drugs on, 464–6
    effect on blood flow through organs, 470
    effect on veins, 469
    from aortic arch, 453–8
    from arteries, 471
    from carotid sinus, 458–71
    from heart, 471, 472
    from pulmonary circulation, 471
    in fetus, 798
Bernstein's membrane theory, 328, 329
Bile, ideas about, 634, 635, 640, 645, 661, 663, 683–5
Birth
    blood volume, 793–5
    cardiac output, 795, 796
    pulmonary circulation, 766–71
    respiratory changes, 764
    systemic circulation, 763, 765, 766
Blood
    concepts about motion, 4, 11–13, 18, 21, 22, 25, 643
    formation from food (*see* Sanguification)
    function in gas exchange, 41, 60
    identification of, 4
    nature of, 10
    transfusion of, 37
    transport of, 8, 10
Blood flow, velocity of, 83, 90–92

Blood gases, 90, 97–9
Blood pressure
    measurement of, 678
        pulmonary arterial, first measurements, 49
        systemic arterial, first measurement, 489, 490, hypertension (see Hypertension), in giraffe, 492, measurement in man, 497–504, regulation of, 470, 489, 491
Blood vessels
    ideas about contents, 5, 8, 9, 24, 548, 637, 644, 707
    identification of, 4
Bohr effect, 57
Bowman's capsule, original description, 557, 558
Bradykinin, 451
Brain (see also Cerebral)
    ideas about function, 8, 11, 703–12, 733
    nerves of (see Cranial nerves)
    vascular anatomy, 704, 705, 707–14
Bright's disease, 492–502, 504–9, 522–4
British clinicians, 218–25, 228
"Brown Dog Case," 418

C

"Caloric," 46, 47
Calorimetry, 177, 226, 233
Capillaries
    alternation, 380–82
    blood flow, 39, 372, 373, 376, 377, 379–83
    blood pressure, 386–99
    contractility, 375, 377–86
    definition of, 361, 365, 377
    density, 382
    discovery of, 28, 29, 355–61, 548
    exchange, 366, 376, 389–403, 439, 441, 492, 566, 567
    filtration, 390
    functional anatomy, 361–72
    in tissue respiration, 379–83
    microscopy, 356–60, 377, 586–8
    of kidney (see Glomerulus)
    of liver, 633, 661, 665, 673, 674, 677
    of lungs, 28, 29, 39, 357, 358, 383, 547, 548
    of muscle, 381
    of tail, 359, 364
    pores, 366, 390, 402
    quantitative histology, 361–72
    resistance to blood flow, 375, 387
    vasomotor activity (see Capillaries, contractility)
    wall, as membrane, 399–403
Capsule of liver (Glisson's), 675, 676
Carbon dioxide
    discovery of, 39, 40, 226
    early observations, 45–7
    transport in blood, 59, 61
Cardiac (see also Heart)
Cardiac catheterization, 92, 103–5
Cardiac output (see also Pulmonary blood flow)
    acetylene method, 102, 103, 105
    ballistocardiography, 110
    empiric methods, 109, 110
    Fick principle, 95–7
    Fick method, direct, 97–9, 102–5, 107–9
    Fick method, indirect, 99–102, 105
    in newborn, 795, 796
    indicator-dilution method, 96, 102, 103, 105–10
    measurement in horse, 83
    nitrous oxide method, 98, 102
    regulation, rest and exercise, 119
Cardiac size, 116–18
Cardiovascular reflexes, 453–75
Cardiovascular system (see also Circulation)
    before Galen, 8, 11
    according to Galen, 12, 212, 214
    according to Harvey, 25, 26, 27
Carotid sinus (baroreceptor) reflex, 458–71
    anatomy of, 460, 461
    discovery of, 459–64
    effect of drugs, 464–6
    efferent pathways, 468–70

initiation of, 464–6
in chronic hypertension, 467
Catechol amines, 418, 419, 433–5, 438
Central terminal of Wilson, 304, 305
Cerebral blood flow
    determinants of, 719, 722–5, 730–32
    direct measurements in animals, 723–5, 727, 732, 734, in clinical disorders, 730–31, in normal man, 725–30
    direct observations of, 718, 723
    effect of drugs, 730
    first experiments, 716–23
    Hill's method, 721–23, 726
    indirect methods, 718–23
    "Monro-Kellie Doctrine," 718, 720, 721
    neurogenic control, 731, 732
    nitrous oxide method, 726–9
    reflex regulation, 459, 470, 471
    regional, 729, 735, 736
Cerebral blood volume, 717
Cerebral cortex, in vasomotor control, 442–7
Cerebral metabolism
    and mental function, 734–7
    in animals, 734, 735
    in clinical disorders, 735
    in normal man, 734–7
Cerebri Anatome, 32, 713
Chemical (neurohumoral) transmitters (*see* Nerve impulse)
Chemical vasodilators, 447–53
Chemoreceptor reflexes, 472–4, 798
Choroid plexus, 707
Christianismi Restitutio, 19–21, 77
Cineradiography in fetus, 753, 767, 772, 784, 789, 790, 792
"Circle of Willis," 713, 715
Circulation, arterial contraction in, 676, 678
Circulation
    ideas before Galen, 627, 633, 634, 651
    according to Galen, 12, 212, 214, 633, 634, 646, 647
    according to Harvey, 25–7, 71, 77, 548, 551, 634, 655–7, 659, 663–5

Circulation, coronary (*see* Coronary)
Circulation, in fetus (*see* Fetal circulation)
Circulation time, 92, 105, 106, 108, 109
Cnidus (*see* School)
"Coction," 639
Conservation of energy, 227, 233
Cos (*see* School)
Coronary blood flow
    determinants, 237–8, 247
    effect of drugs, 248
    experimental physiology and pathology, 228–35
    measurement of, 235–7, 246, 247
    phasic nature, 237, 238
Coronary circulation
    16th and 17th century ideas, 212, 214, 217
    18th century ideas, 218–25
    19th century ideas, 228
    "irrigation coefficient," 236
Coronary heart disease, 218–25, 228, 232, 233, 242
Coronary sinus catheterization, 236, 237, 246
Coronary vessels
    collaterals, 239
    injection studies, 239
    Thebesian veins, 216, 218, 240–42
Cranial nerves, 703, 706, 713, 715, 732
"Crasis," 639
Crossed circulation, 455–7
Currents of rest and injury (*see* Action potentials)

D

De corde, 33–7, 407
De humanis corporis fabrica, 205, 210–13, 655, 710–12
De magnete, 268
De motu cordis, 25–8, 72, 74, 76–9, 127, 356, 488, 656–8, 712–14
De profundis, 658
De sedibus et causis morborum, 218
De viribus electricitatis, 277
Depressor nerve (*see* Aortic nerve)
Diffusion, 391, 392

[853]

Dilution methods (*see* Cardiac output)
Dipole, 306, 308
Dissection
    before Vesalius, 4, 203
    Vesalius, 209–11
    human, 651, 660
Dissociation curves (*see* Bohr effect, Haldane effect)
    of fetal blood, 751
Divination, 610–23, 639, 648
Donnan equilibrium, 61
Ductus arteriosus
    anatomy and function, 77, 745, 747, 759, 774, 776, 777, 780, 781
    blood flow after birth, 781–6
    closure, 776, 778, 779
    in neonatal circulation, 786, 787
    murmur of patency, 782–5
Ductus venosus, 787–93
"Dynamis," 639, 640, 645

E

Ebers papyrus (*see* Papyrus Ebers)
Eck fistula, 685
Einthoven's triangle, 303–5
Electricity
    animal, 271–3, 276–8
    first observations and experiments, 265–7, 269, 270
    frictional, 269, 275, 278
    Galvanic, 276–8
Electrocardiogram, first, 289, 290
Electrochemistry, 278
Electromagnetism, 280, 281
Electrometer, capillary, 287–91, 295, 296
Elements, four, 4, 635–8, 643, 664
"Eminently respirable air" (*see* Oxygen)
Epidemiology of essential hypertension, 525–31
Epinephrine, 433–5
    action on carotid sinus, 465, 466
    paradox, 585–7
Epitome, 212
Essential hypertension (*see* Hypertension)
Excitation of heart
    activation of atria, 312, 313
    activation of ventricles, 313, 314
    activation of ventricular septum, 311, 314, 315
    activation, wave of, 308–11, 315, 318
    after injury, 321
    after intraventricular block, 315, 316
    "arborization block," 316
    recovery process, 318–20
Excitation of muscle, 159–65
Eustachian valve, 747, 748

F

Fabrica (*see* De humanis corporis fabrica)
Fenn effect, 155, 156, 159
Fetal circulation
    cineradiography, 753, 767, 777, 784, 789, 790, 792
    early concepts, 77, 743–59
    nervous control, 797–9
    physiological studies, 750, 753–9
Fetal environment, 759–63
Fick principle
    for pulmonary blood flow (*see* Cardiac output)
    for cerebral blood flow, 726, 727
Fick's tipping lever, 146
Fick's work adder, 154
Filtration rate (glomerular), 600, 601
Fire, 637, 639, 643
First Principle, 4
"Fixed air" (*see* Carbon dioxide)
Force-velocity relation
    of flywheel, 157, 158
    of skeletal muscle, 149, 158, 159, 164
Foramen ovale
    anatomy and function, 77, 745, 747–53, 755, 758, 771, 777
    closure of, 771–4
Frank-Starling law (*see* Starling's law of the heart)

G

Galvanometer
    early models, 280–5
    Einthoven's, 292–6
    string, 291–6, 298, 299

"Gas sylvestre," 30
Genetics of arterial hypertension, 525–31
Glisson's capsule, 661, 675, 676
Glomerulus, renal
    arrangement of capillaries, 566, 567
    blood flow by direct visualization, 587
    blood pressure in, 585
    direct examination, 586–8
    filtration rate, 600–601
    first accurate description, 557, 559, 567
    identification of, 555, 556
    micropuncture, 588–92
    original description, 551–4
Goosefish (*Lophius piscatorius*) (see Aglomerular fish)
Glycolysis, in fetus, 799, 800

H

H-substance, 449
Haemastatics, 83, 84, 489, 490
Haldane effect, 61
Haruspicy, 611–23, 639, 648
Heart
    action potentials, 287
    anatomy and function, ancient concepts, 6–8, 10, 13, 199, 201–3, 214, Descartes' "ferment," 217, Lower's ideas, 37, 80, 81, 117–19, Medieval concepts, 204, 205
    as engine (or pump), 128, 134, 138, 664, 677
    beat, myogenic origin of, 429
    conduction system, 296–8
    efficiency of, 245, 247, 256
    electrical field, 299–305
    excitation of (see Excitation of heart)
    failure, contractile proteins in, 252–3, dilated heart in, 155, metabolic basis of, 253, 255
    force of (Borelli), 489
    innate heat of, 637, 640, 657
    metabolism, 247–50
    muscle (see also Myocardial), mechanical properties, 147–54, work and metabolism, 155, 157
    rate, regulation of, 117, 118
    reflex regulation, 117–19
    seat of soul, 636
    size, 116–18
    transplantation, 257, 258
    vector, 299–305
Heart-lung preparation, 245, 246
Hemoglobin, 56, 57
Hepatic (see also Liver)
    capillaries (see Capillaries of liver)
    nerves, 662, 663
    sphincters, 682
Hippocratic documents (corpus), 4–7, 202, 634, 704, 733
Histamine, 434, 449, 451
Humors, 634–40, 659, 664, 704
Hydrogen, discovery of, 39
Hyperemia, reactive, 448–53
Hyperpiesis, 504
Hypertensin (see Angiotensin)
Hypertension
    systemic arterial, benign versus malignant, 504–8
    Bright's disease and, 492–7
    classification of, 504–8
    early observations, 488
    experimental, 507–19
    genetic and environmental factors, 525–31
    in animals, 509–12
    in man, 492
    malignant, 504–8, 512
    mechanisms in man, 520–24
    natural history, 508, 509
    neurogenic, 510
    organ blood flow in, 520, 521, 523
    pheochromocytoma, 522–4
    primary versus secondary, 499–502, 504–6, 508, 509
    renal (see Renal hypertension)
Hypothalamus, in vasomotor control, 442–7

I

Indicator-dilution principle
    for cerebral blood flow, 728, 729

for pulmonary blood flow (see Cardiac output)
Interventricular septum (see Ventricular septum)
Ionia (see School)
Innate heat of heart, 637, 640, 657
Intrinsic deflection, 311, 312

K

Kidney
    comparative anatomy, 550, 557–9, 566
    function (see Urine formation)
    injection studies, 555, 556, 566
    nerves, 570, 594
Kymograph, invention of, 85–7, 89

L

Laplace's law, 151, 152, 155
Lascaux, Cavern of, 608, 609
Lead field and vector, 306–8
Length-tension diagrams
    of heart muscle, 143, 147
    of skeletal muscle, 142–6, 149
    of spring, 139–42
Leyden jar, 270, 273
Liver (see also Hepatic)
    anatomy of, 629, 651, 655, 659, 665, 666, 670–75
    fetal circulation of, 787–93
    histology of, 671, 672
    vessels of, 661–3 (see also Splanchnic vascular structures)
Lodestone, 266
Lophius piscatorius (goosefish), 597 (see also Aglomerular fish)
Lumleian lecture (Harvey), 73
Lungs
    ancient ideas about function, 6, 9, 29, 202
    before Lower, 27–9
    in aeration of blood, 29, 30, 33
    in arterialization of blood (Lower), 33, 34
Lymph and lymphatics, 389–92, 658, 659

M

Magnetic needle, 267
Malpighian corpuscle, 551–4 (see also Glomerulus)
Manometers, 86, 87
Mechanical work
    efficiency of, 145, 155
    maximal, 145
    of contractile tissues, 137–9
    of heart muscle, 139
    of skeletal muscle, 138, 139, 144, 145
    of spring, 139–41
Mental function and cerebral blood flow, 734–7
Metabolism
    ancient ideas, 202
    as combustion, 168, 169, 226
    cellular, 168–80
    during muscular contraction, 177–80
    energy transformations, 168, 169, 226
    of heart, 242–58
    of homotransplanted heart, 257, 258
    of tissues, 233, 234, 242–4
Micropuncture, 588–91
"Minute vessels," 378
"Monocardiogram," 323–5
Monro-Kellie doctrine, 717, 718
Muscle, cardiac (see Myocardial)
    "linear" mechanical properties, 143, 147
Muscle, skeletal
    energetics of contraction, 155, 156
    excitation and active state, 159–65
    "linear" mechanical properties, 138–49, 151
    mechanical efficiency, 156
    mechanical model, 159
    molecular model, 186, 187
    relaxation factor, 185
    versus heart muscle, 188
    work, metabolism and energy, 155–7
Muscular activity
    cardiovascular adjustments, 442, 443, 446, 447
    vasodilator substances, 448–53

Myocardial contraction
    economy, 137
    energetics, 130–38
    mechanical efficiency, 134, 136, 147
    mechanochemical coupling, 129, 135, 136
    physical concepts, 129
    staircase effect ("Treppe"), 127, 162–4
    topochemical coupling, 129, 135
    "Weber's paradox," 144
Myocardial metabolism
    in cardiac disorders, 251–5
    of homotransplanted heart, 257, 258
Myocardial oxygen consumption, 247
Myogenic automaticity, 423–7, 453
Myosin
    of failing heart, 252, 253
    of skeletal muscle, 181–6

N

Neck, vessels of, 704, 708
Neonatal circulation
    blood volume, 793–5
    cardiac output, 795, 796
    ductus arteriosus, 781–6
    general features, 786, 787, 793–6
    neurohumoral regulation, 797–9
    pulmonary blood volume, 795
Nerve impulse, chemical transmission of, 425, 428, 433–8
Nerve plexuses in vessel walls, 424, 428, 452, 453
Nerves, ancient ideas, 11
"Nitre," 30
Nitrogen, 39, 41, 46
Nitrous oxide
    for cardiac output, 98, 102
    for coronary blood flow, 246, 247
Norepinephrine
    as neurohumoral transmitter, 437
    on carotid sinus, 464–7

O

Opsanus Tau (toadfish), 599, (see also Aglomerular fish)

Osmotic pressure
    of intestinal contents, 575
    of plasma, 568, 569
    of proteins, 393–7, 492, 568, 569
    of urine, 568, 569
Oxygen consumption during hypoxia, 761, 762, 796
Oxygen, discovery of, 37, 39, 44–7, 226
Oxygen secretion in lungs, 57–9

P

Padua (*see* School)
Papyrus
    Ebers, 200, 201, 626, 703
    Smith, 8, 199, 201, 626, 703
    Westcar, 201
Pergamon (*see* School)
Permeability, capillary (*see* Capillary wall)
Phlogiston, 41, 44, 47
Pinocytosis, 403
Pneuma, 4, 10, 12, 14, 636, 644, 657, 664, 704
Poiseuille's law, 86, 678
Pores
    in capillary wall, 400–403
    in ventricular septum (*see* Ventricular septal pores)
Portal vein (*see also* Splanchnic vascular structures) concepts from Aristotle to Galen, 628–32
    in fetus, 787–91
Pre-excitation syndrome, 316–18
Presclerosis, 502
Proteins, osmotic pressure of, 393–7, 492
Pulmonary arterial pressure, first measurements, 49
Pulmonary blood flow
    distribution of, 52
    effect of respiration, 50–52
Pulmonary blood volume, 52
Pulmonary capillaries
    discovery of, 28, 29
    rate of blood flow, 39
Pulmonary circulation
    discovery of, 15–17, 21–5
    heart-lung preparation, 52

ideas about function, 9, 13, 14, 25, 33, 34
perfusion of, by Harvey, 78
regulation of, 52-4
Pulse, 644
Pulse wave, 90, 91
Pumps, history of, 74, 75

R

Reactive hyperemia (*see* Hyperemia, reactive)
Reciprocity theorem, 307
Recording devices (clocks), 85, 86
Red blood cells, 360
Relaxation factor, 185
Renal hypertension
experimental, 511, 512
in man, 520-24
mechanisms of, 512-19
Renin, 513-19
Respiration
alveolar-capillary, 56-62
as combustion, 43, 46, 47, 168, 169, 226
for cooling, 637
site of, 47, 48, 56, 226
Respiratory gases, in blood, 56
Rete mirabile, 705-11, 723
Rheotome, 284-6
Royal Society, 79, 81, 82

S

Salerno (*see* School)
Sanguification, 637-42, 644, 646, 655, 663, 683
Sarcomere, structure of, 186, 187
Scalene triangle, 306, 307
School
of Alexandria, 8-11
of Athens, 8
of Cnidus, 10, 634
of Cos, 8, 201
of Ionia, 3, 4
of Padua, 23-5, 73, 209, 213
of Pergamon, 11
of Salerno, 203

Scientific Societies, 79
Six Tables, 211, 212, 631, 655
Smith Papyrus (*see* Papyrus)
Solid conductors, 299-303
Sphygmograph, 497-500
Sphygmomanometer, 502, 503
Spirit
animal, 11, 12, 707, 713, 714, 716
natural, 636, 707
vital, 11, 14, 21, 22, 205, 707
"*Spiritus Aeris Nitrosus*," 30, 32, 38, 716
Splanchnic circulation
according to Galen, 631
according to Leonardo, 652, 653
according to Ruysch, 668
according to Vesalius, 652, 653
medieval concepts, 631
Splanchnic vascular bed
blood flow, 651, 679
dynamics, 642-7, 678-89
function, 637-47
innervation, 662, 663, 679, 681, 686, 689
integrations, 683-9
physiology, 675-89
structure, 625-34, 650-53, 665-75
Spleen, function of, 639-41
Squid axon, 328-31, 333
Staircase effect ("Treppe"), 127, 162-4
Starling's law
of capillary exchange, 376, 393-9, 492, 568
of the heart, 110-20, 152-4
Statical Essays, 39, 82-4
Stroke volume
first measurements, 78, 83
regulation of, 110-20
Sympathin E and I, 435-7

T

T-wave, 285, 287, 318-20, 322
Tabulae sex (*see* Six Tables)
Terrestrial lightning, 267
Thebesian veins, 216, 218, 240-42
Tone, vascular (*see* Vascular tone)
Torpedo fish, 265, 271, 272, 280

Transmembrane potentials (*see also* Action potentials)
   Bernstein's theory, 328, 329
   during injury, 326, 327
   ionic hypothesis, 331
   of cardiac muscle, 331–3
   of squid axon, 328–31, 333
   recording of, 328–35

U

U-wave, 320
Umbilical vessels, hemodynamics, 758, 787–93
Urea, distribution in body, 593, 595
Uric acid, renal excretion, 595, 596
Urine formation
   filtration-reabsorption theory, Ludwig, 562, 565–70, Richards, 582, 588–91
   ideas before Malpighi, 549, 550
   Malpighi's concept, 553–4
   "Modern view" of Cushny, 573–82
   secretory theory, Bowman, 560–2, Heidenhain, 570–73, Marshall, 591, 594–600

V

"Vagusdruckversuch," 458, 461
Vascular smooth muscle, 409, 420, 423–7
Vascular segments
   capacitance vessels, 422, 440, 441
   functional classification, 420–22
   resistance vessels, 421, 422, 438, 439
   sphincters, 421, 439
Vascular tone
   assessment, 422
   basal, 422, 423
   determinants, 422–7
   first concepts, 407, 408
   myogenic versus extrinsic factors, 423–7
   nerve plexuses in walls, 424, 428, 452, 453
   nervous influences, 422, 423, 428
   neurohumoral substances, 418, 419, 423, 425
Vasodilator nerves, 416, 417, 428, 438, 447–9
Vasodilator substances, 448–53
Vasomotor centers
   discovery of, 415, 417
   effect on vasomotor fibers, 441, 442
   influence of higher centers, 442–5, 447
   reciprocal interaction (Bayliss), 417, 418, 427, 438
   spinal, 441, 442
Vasomotor control
   first insights, 409–20
Vasomotor nerves (*see also* Vasomotor centers)
   discharge rate, 431–3, 437, 438
   discovery of, 408
   functional organization, 427, 428
   in vascular tone, 408–15
   to capacitance vessels, 440, 441
   to resistance vessels, 438, 439
   to sphincters, 439
Vasomotor reflexes, 453–75
Vectorcardiogram, 322–6
Vegetable Statics, 82
Veins, baroreceptor control, 469
Venous valves, 73
Ventricular septal pores, 13, 16, 21–5, 76, 212, 214
Ventricular septum
   activation, 311, 314, 315
   block, 315, 316
"Virtuosi," 666
Vitalism, 564, 569, 573, 574, 577–9, 581, 582, 709, 716, 733
Voltaic pile, 279, 280

W

"Wallerian degeneration," 414, 415
Westcar papyrus (*see* Papyrus)
Wolff-Parkinson-White syndrome, 316–18
Work (*see* Mechanical work)